AF571161

Informatik aktuell

Reihe herausgegeben von

Gesellschaft für Informatik e.V. (GI), Berlin, Deutschland

Ziel der Reihe ist die möglichst schnelle und weite Verbreitung neuer Forschungs- und Entwicklungsergebnisse, zusammenfassender Übersichtsberichte über den Stand eines Gebietes und von Materialien und Texten zur Weiterbildung. In erster Linie werden Tagungsberichte von Fachtagungen der Gesellschaft für Informatik veröffentlicht, die regelmäßig, oft in Zusammenarbeit mit anderen wissenschaftlichen Gesellschaften, von den Fachausschüssen der Gesellschaft für Informatik veranstaltet werden. Die Auswahl der Vorträge erfolgt im allgemeinen durch international zusammengesetzte Programmkomitees.

Heinz Handels · Katharina Breininger ·
Thomas M. Deserno · Andreas Maier ·
Klaus H. Maier-Hein · Christoph Palm ·
Thomas Tolxdorff
(Hrsg.)

Bildverarbeitung für die Medizin 2026

Proceedings, German Conference on Medical Image Computing, Lübeck March 15–17, 2026

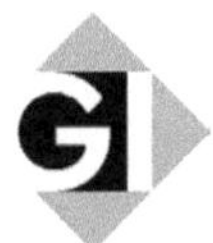

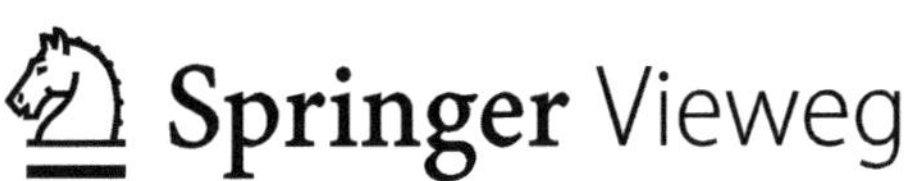

Hrsg.
Heinz Handels
Institut für Medizinische Informatik
Universität zu Lübeck
Lübeck, Deutschland

Thomas M. Deserno
Peter L. Reichertz Institut für Medizinische Informatik
Technische Universität Braunschweig und Medizinische Hochschule Hannover
Braunschweig, Deutschland

Klaus H. Maier-Hein
Medical Image Computing E230
Deutsches Krebsforschungszentrum (DKFZ)
Heidelberg, Deutschland

Thomas Tolxdorff
Institut für Medizinische Informatik
Charité - Universitätsmedizin Berlin
Berlin, Deutschland

Katharina Breininger
Center for Artificial Intelligence and Data Science (CAIDAS)
Universität Würzburg
Würzburg, Deutschland

Andreas Maier
Lehrstuhl für Mustererkennung
Friedrich-Alexander-Universität Erlangen-Nürnberg
Erlangen, Deutschland

Christoph Palm
Fakultät für Informatik und Mathematik
Ostbayerische Technische Hochschule Regensburg
Regensburg, Deutschland

ISSN 1431-472X ISSN 2628-8958 (electronic)
Informatik aktuell
ISBN 978-3-658-51099-2 ISBN 978-3-658-51100-5 (eBook)
https://doi.org/10.1007/978-3-658-51100-5

Die Deutsche Nationalbibliothek verzeichnet diese Publikation in der Deutschen Nationalbibliografie; detaillierte bibliografische Daten sind im Internet über https://portal.dnb.de abrufbar.

Dieses Werk wurde gefördert durch Universitätsklinikum Augsburg AöR. This research was partially funded by the German Childhood Cancer Foundation under grant number A 2024/05 / DKS 2025.01, the Intramural Research Funding “Precision Medicine for pHGG” of the Faculty of Medicine, University of Augsburg, the Bavarian Center for Cancer Research as part of the Lighthouse “Local Therapies”, as well as by the Bavarian Ministry of Economic Affairs, Regional Development and Energy (StMWi) under grant number DIK-2310-0004// DIK0556/02. This research was partially funded by the Intramural Research Funding “MultiPro” of the Faculty of Medicine, University of Augsburg, the Bavarian Center for Cancer Research as part of the Lighthouse “Local Therapies,” as well as by the Bavarian Ministry of Economic Affairs, Regional Development and Energy (StMWi) under Grant Number DIK-2310-0004// DIK0556/02, as well as the Bavarian Ministry of Economic Affairs, Regional Development and Energy (StMWi) Grant Number: LSM-2403-0017

© Der/die Herausgeber bzw. der/die Autor(en), exklusiv lizenziert an Springer Fachmedien Wiesbaden GmbH, ein Teil von Springer Nature 2026

Die Kapitel „Label, Refine, Repeat: Extending nnInteractive with Dataset Traversal and nnU-Net Proposals“, „AI-based Automated Framework for Quantitative PET/CT Image Analysis“ und „Anatomy-informed 3D Reconstruction of Tracked Ultrasound Sweeps: A Proof of Concept“ werden unter der Creative Commons Namensnennung 4.0 International Lizenz (http://creativecommons.org/licenses/by/4.0/deed.de) veröffentlicht. Weitere Details zur Lizenz entnehmen Sie bitte der Lizenzinformation im Kapitel.

Das Werk einschließlich aller seiner Teile ist urheberrechtlich geschützt. Jede Verwertung, die nicht ausdrücklich vom Urheberrechtsgesetz zugelassen ist, bedarf der vorherigen Zustimmung des Verlags. Das gilt insbesondere für Vervielfältigungen, Bearbeitungen, Übersetzungen, Mikroverfilmungen und die Einspeicherung und Verarbeitung in elektronischen Systemen.
Die Wiedergabe von allgemein beschreibenden Bezeichnungen, Marken, Unternehmensnamen etc. in diesem Werk bedeutet nicht, dass diese frei durch jede Person benutzt werden dürfen. Die Berechtigung zur Benutzung unterliegt, auch ohne gesonderten Hinweis hierzu, den Regeln des Markenrechts. Die Rechte des/der jeweiligen Zeicheninhaber*in sind zu beachten.
Der Verlag, die Autor*innen und die Herausgeber*innen gehen davon aus, dass die Angaben und Informationen in diesem Werk zum Zeitpunkt der Veröffentlichung vollständig und korrekt sind. Weder der Verlag noch die Autor*innen oder die Herausgeber*innen übernehmen, ausdrücklich oder implizit, Gewähr für den Inhalt des Werkes, etwaige Fehler oder Äußerungen. Der Verlag bleibt im Hinblick auf geografische Zuordnungen und Gebietsbezeichnungen in veröffentlichten Karten und Institutionsadressen neutral.

Planung/Lektorat: Petra Steinmueller
Springer Vieweg ist ein Imprint der eingetragenen Gesellschaft Springer Fachmedien Wiesbaden GmbH und ist ein Teil von Springer Nature.
Die Anschrift der Gesellschaft ist: Abraham-Lincoln-Str. 46, 65189 Wiesbaden, Germany

Wenn Sie dieses Produkt entsorgen, geben Sie das Papier bitte zum Recycling.

Bildverarbeitung für die Medizin 2026

Veranstalter

Institut für Medizinische Informatik, Universität zu Lübeck und
Deutsches Forschungszentrum für Künstliche Intelligenz (DFKI), Lübeck

Unterstützende Fachgesellschaften

CURAC	Computer- und Roboterassistierte Chirurgie
DAGM	Deutsche Arbeitsgemeinschaft für Mustererkennung
DGBMT	Fachgruppe Medizinische Informatik der Deutschen Gesellschaft für Biomedizinische Technik im Verband Deutscher Elektrotechniker
GI	Gesellschaft für Informatik – Fachbereich Informatik in den Lebenswissenschaften
GMDS	Gesellschaft für Medizinische Informatik, Biometrie und Epidemiologie
IEEE	Joint Chapter Engineering in Medicine and Biology, German Section

Tagungsvorsitz

Prof. Dr. Heinz Handels
Institut für Medizinische Informatik, Universität zu Lübeck
Deutsches Forschungszentrum für Künstliche Intelligenz, Lübeck

Tagungssekretariat

Susanne Petersen
Institut für Medizinische Informatik, Universität zu Lübeck

Anschrift:	Ratzeburger Allee 160, D-23562 Lübeck
Telefon:	+49 451 3101 5601
E-Mail:	`orga-2026@bvm-conf.org`
Web:	`https://bvm-conf.org`

Lokale BVM-Organisation

Heinz Handels, Mattias Heinrich, Jan Ehrhardt, Marja Fleitmann, Susanne Petersen, Jan-Hinrich Wrage, u. a.

Verteilte BVM-Organisation

Begutachtung	Heinz Handels und Jan-Hinrich Wrage – Institut für Medizinische Informatik, Universität zu Lübeck
Mailingliste	Klaus Maier-Hein – Medical Image Computing, Deutsches Krebsforschungszentrum (DKFZ) Heidelberg
Special Issue	Andreas Maier – Lehrstuhl für Mustererkennung, Friedrich-Alexander Universität Erlangen-Nürnberg
Tagungsband	Thomas M. Deserno und Paulo Haas – Peter L. Reichertz Institut für Medizinische Informatik, TU Braunschweig
Web & News	Christoph Palm und Sümeyye Yildiran – Regensburg Medical Image Computing (ReMIC), OTH Regensburg

BVM-Komitee

Prof. Dr. Katharina Breininger, Center for Artificial Intelligence and Data Science (CAIDAS), Universität Würzburg

Prof. Dr. Thomas M. Deserno, Peter L. Reichertz Institut für Medizinische Informatik der TU Braunschweig und der Medizinischen Hochschule Hannover

Prof. Dr. Heinz Handels, Institut für Medizinische Informatik, Universität zu Lübeck und DFKI Lübeck

Prof. Dr. Andreas Maier, Lehrstuhl für Mustererkennung, Friedrich-Alexander-Universität Erlangen-Nürnberg

Prof. Dr. Klaus Maier-Hein, Medical Image Computing, Deutsches Krebsforschungszentrum Heidelberg

Prof. Dr. Christoph Palm, Regensburg Medical Image Computing (ReMIC), OTH Regensburg

Prof. Dr. Thomas Tolxdorff, Institut für Medizinische Informatik, Charité-Universitätsmedizin Berlin

Programmkomitee

Marc Aubreville, Hochschule Flensburg
Katharina Breininger, Universität Würzburg
Thomas Deserno, TU Braunschweig
Jan Ehrhardt, Universität zu Lübeck
Sandy Engelhardt, Universitätsklinik Heidelberg
Floris Ernst, Universität zu Lübeck
Nils Forkert, University of Calgary, Canada

Michael Götz, Universitätsklinikum Ulm
Horst Hahn, Fraunhofer MEVIS, Bremen
Heinz Handels, Universität zu Lübeck
Tobias Heimann, Siemens Healthineers, Erlangen
Mattias Heinrich, Universität zu Lübeck
Anja Hennemuth, Charité-Universitätsmedizin Berlin
Alexander Horsch, The Arctic University of Norway, Tromsø, Norwegen
Dagmar Kainmüller, MDC Berlin
Bernhard Kainz, FAU Erlangen-Nürnberg
Timo Kepp, DFKI Lübeck
Ron Kikinis, Harvard Medical School, Boston, USA
Andreas Kist, FAU Erlangen-Nürnberg
Roman Klöckner, UKSH Campus Lübeck
Dagmar Krefting, Universität Göttingen
Jan Lellmann, Universität zu Lübeck
Andreas Maier, FAU Erlangen-Nürnberg
Klaus Maier-Hein, DKFZ Heidelberg
Lena Maier-Hein, DKFZ Heidelberg
Thomas Martinetz, Universität zu Lübeck
André Mastmeyer, Jade Hochschule, Wilhelmshaven
Dorit Merhof, Universität Regensburg
Jan Modersitzki, Fraunhofer MEVIS, Lübeck
Nassir Navab, TU München
Christoph Palm, OTH Regensburg
Bernhard Preim, Universität Magdeburg
Annika Reinke, DKFZ Heidelberg
Karl Rohr, Universität Heidelberg
Daniel Rückert, TU München
Sylvia Saalfeld, UKSH Campus Kiel
Dennis Säring, FH Wedel
Julia Schnabel, Helmholtz München & TU München
Ingrid Scholl, FH Aachen
Stefanie Speidel, HZDR/NCT Dresden
Nicolai Spicher, Technical University of Denmark
Thomas Tolxdorff, Charité-Universitätsmedizin Berlin
Klaus Tönnies, OvG Universität Magdeburg
Hristina Uzunova, Universitätsmedizin Greifswald
Gudrun Wagenknecht, Forschungszentrum Jülich
René Werner, UKE Hamburg
Thomas Wittenberg, Fraunhofer IIS, Erlangen
Ivo Wolf, Hochschule Mannheim

Sponsoren und Unterstützer der BVM 2026

Wir freuen uns sehr über die langjährige kontinuierliche Unterstützung mancher Firmen sowie auch über das neue Engagement anderer. Die BVM wäre ohne diese finanzielle Unterstützung nicht durchführbar.

Platin-Sponsor

- **Siemens Healthineers AG**, Siemensstr. 3, 91301 Forchheim
  `https://www.siemens-healthineers.com/`

Gold-Sponsor

- **Nexus Chili GmbH**, Friedrich-Ebert-Str. 2, 69221 Dossenheim
  `https://nexus-chili.com/`

Silber-Sponsoren

- **Heidelberg Engineering GmbH**, Max-Jarecki-Str. 8, 69115 Heidelberg
  `https://www.heidelbergengineering.com/`
- **ImFusion GmbH**, Agnes-Pockels-Bogen 1, 80992 München
  `https://imfusion.com/`

Sponsor

- **MiE - medical imaging electronics GmbH**, Hauptstr. 112, 23845 Seth
  `https://mie-scintron.com/`

Microsoft CMT

Das Microsoft Conference Management Toolkit (CMT) wurde für die Durchführung des Peer-Review-Prozesses für diese Konferenz genutzt. Dieser Dienst wurde von Microsoft kostenlos zur Verfügung gestellt, wobei Microsoft alle Kosten übernahm, einschließlich der Kosten für Azure-Cloud-Dienste sowie für Softwareentwicklung und Support.

Preisträgerinnen und Preisträger der BVM 2025 in Regensburg

BVM Award 2025 für die beste Abschlussarbeit im Bereich der Medizinischen Bildverarbeitung

Dr. Azade Farshad
(Computer Aided Medical Procedures, TUM School of Computation, Information and Technology, Technische Universität München)
Learning to Learn Neural Representations with Limited Data and Supervision
Doktorarbeit

BVM-Preise 2025 für die besten wissenschaftlichen Arbeiten

1. **Wiebke Heyer**
   (Institut für Medizinische Informatik, Universität zu Lübeck)
   Heyer W, Weihsbach C, Otte C, Lichtenstein J, Lippross S, Heinrich MP, Hansen L
   Autocalibration for 3D Ultrasound Reconstruction in Infant Hip Dysplasia Screening
2. **Maximilian Weiherer**
   (FAU Erlangen-Nürnberg und OTH Regensburg)
   Weiherer M, Riedheim von A, Brébant V, Egger B, Palm C
   iRBSM: A Deep Implicit 3D Breast Shape Model
3. **Timo Kepp**
   (DFKI Lübeck)
   Kepp K, Andresen J, Falta F, Handels H
   Bridging Gaps in Retinal Imaging

Pitt-Meinzer-Vortragspreis 2025

Jasmin Arjomandi
(Department Artificial Intelligence in Biomedical Engineering, FAU Erlangen-Nürnberg)
Arjomandi J, Neubig L, Kist AM
LLM-driven Baselines for Medical Image Segmentation

BVM-Posterpreis 2025

Joshua Niemeijer
(DLR Braunschweig, Institut für Medizinische Informatik, Universität zu Lübeck)
Niemeijer J, Ehrhardt J, Uzunova H, Handels H
TSynD Targeted Synthetic Data Generation for Enhanced Medical Image Classification: Leveraging Epistemic Uncertainty to Improve Model Performance

Vorwort

Die German Conference on Medical Image Computing (Bildverarbeitung für die Medizin, BVM) wird in diesem Jahr vom Institut für Medizinische Informatik an der Universität zu Lübeck gemeinsam mit dem Deutschen Forschungszentrum für Künstliche Intelligenz (DFKI) Lübeck ausgerichtet. Nach der erfolgreichen Durchführung der BVM 2001, 2011 und 2019 ist dies nun das vierte Mal, dass diese zentrale Tagung zu neuen Entwicklungen in der Medizinischen Bildverarbeitung in Deutschland in der traditionsreichen Hansestadt Lübeck unter Leitung von Prof. Dr. Heinz Handels stattfindet.

Die Bedeutung des Themas Bildverarbeitung für die Medizin hat über die Jahre deutlich zugenommen. Die Bildverarbeitung ist in verschiedenen medizinischen Bereichen wie der Diagnoseunterstützung, der Operationsplanung, der Strahlentherapie und der computergestützten Chirurgie von zentraler Bedeutung. Sie hält aber auch zunehmend Einzug in die Bereiche der Prävention und Rehabilitation. Diese Entwicklungen haben maßgeblich dazu beigetragen, dass sich die Medizinische Bildverarbeitung an der Schnittstelle zwischen Informatik und Medizin als eine Schlüsseltechnologie zur Digitalisierung des Gesundheitswesens etabliert hat.

Hierbei spielen die Methoden des Deep Learning eine zentrale Rolle, die schon seit Jahren die auf der BVM vorgestellten Arbeiten thematisch dominieren und an deren Weiterentwicklung die BVM-Community intensiv mitgearbeitet hat. An der Universität zu Lübeck bildet der Bereich für Künstliche Intelligenz in der Medizin einen zentralen Forschungsfokus, der in den letzten Jahren systematisch ausgebaut wurde. Vor diesem Hintergrund ist es für uns eine besondere Freude, dass die BVM 2026 erstmalig gemeinsam vom Institut für Medizinische Informatik und dem DFKI Lübeck ausgerichtet wird.

Zentraler Aspekt der BVM ist neben der Diskussion aktueller Forschungsergebnisse aus der vielfältigen BVM-Community die Förderung des wissenschaftlichen Nachwuchses. Die Tagung bietet vor allem Promovierenden, aber auch Studierenden mit hervorragenden Abschlussarbeiten, eine Plattform, um ihre Ergebnisse zu präsentieren, dabei in den fachlichen Diskurs mit der Community zu treten und Netzwerke mit anderen Forschenden zu knüpfen.

Die hohe Attraktivität der BVM 2026 spiegelt sich auch darin wider, dass im Vergleich zum letzten Jahr 50 % mehr Einreichungen eingegangen sind. Es wurden 86 Originalarbeiten und 55 Abstracts eingereicht. Über ein anonymisiertes Review-Verfahren mit jeweils drei Reviews wurden aus 141 Beitragseinreichungen 24 Vorträge, 68 Posterbeiträge und 6 Softwaredemonstrationen angenommen. Die besten Arbeiten werden auch in diesem Jahr wieder mit Preisen ausgezeichnet.

Inhaltlich können wir uns auf ein attraktives und hochklassiges Programm freuen. Neben 98 begutachteten Präsentationen als Vortrag, Poster oder Softwaredemonstration werden interessante Tutorials und inspirierende eingeladene Vorträge das Programm bereichern.

Tutorial Kaapana Demo: HandsOn
Prof. Dr. Klaus Maier-Hein und sein Team, DKFZ, Heidelberg

Kaapana ist eine Open-Source-Plattform für die medizinische Bildverarbeitung, die sich an Kliniker, Datenwissenschaftler und Entwickler richtet. Sie ermöglicht groß angelegte Machine-Learning-Forschung auf Basis realer Daten, indem sie modernste KI-Tools in Kliniken und Forschungszentren einführt. Das Tutorial beginnt mit einem Überblick über die Kaapana-Plattform und ihre Funktionen. Anschließend wird eine praktische Demo mit Kaapana-Instanzen durchgeführt. Es wird ein vollständiger End-to-End-Analyse-Workflow der Plattform vorgestellt, wobei der Schwerpunkt auf der Erstellung und Kuratierung von Datensätzen, der Verarbeitung medizinischer Bilder, der Verwendung von Machine-Learning-Modellen in der Plattform und der Erforschung von Möglichkeiten zur Erweiterung der Plattform in verschiedenen Anwendungsfällen liegt.

Tutorial Foundation Models for Few-shot Medical Image Analysis
Dr. Johannes Lotz und sein Team, MeVis Lübeck

Foundation Models verändern die medizinische Bildgebungsforschung rasant, indem sie robuste, übertragbare Merkmalsräume bereitstellen, die den Annotationsaufwand reduzieren und gleichzeitig eine schnelle Modellentwicklung für klinisch relevante Aufgaben ermöglichen. Dieses Tutorial verwendet das Foundation Model Medical Multitask Modeling als Beispiel und zeigt, wie vorab trainierte Backbones für (i) Few-Shot-Klassifizierung, (ii) Few-Shot-Segmentierung und (iii) Multiple-Instance-Learning (MIL) auf 2D-, 3D- und Gigapixel-Pathologiedaten angepasst werden können.

Weiterhin finden auf BVM 2026 inspirierende Keynote-Vorträge zu aktuellen Themen der Medizinischen Bildverarbeitung und KI statt, für die wir uns herzlich bei unseren Gastredner*innen bedanken.

Responsible Use of Responsible AI
Prof. Dr. Aasa Feragen
DTU Compute, Technical University of Denmark, Denmark

Verantwortungsbewusste KI-Tools wie algorithmische Fairness, erklärbare KI oder Unsicherheitsquantifizierung werden oft sowohl gefördert als auch gefordert, um eine stärker ethisch geprägte KI zu ermöglichen. In diesem Vortrag werden einige der potenziellen Fallstricke diskutiert, die mit der Verwendung verantwortungsbewusster KI-Tools verbunden sind: Algorithmische Fairness-Tools können Verzerrungen hervorrufen, erklärbare KI-Tools können zu Fehlinterpretationen führen und Tools zur Quantifizierung von Unsicherheiten können zu übermäßigem Vertrauen in falsche Vorhersagen führen. Im Anschluss werden aktuelle Best Practices und offene technische Probleme diskutiert.

Fairness and Bias Mitigation in Medical Image Analysis AI
Prof. Dr. Nils Forkert
Departments of Radiology, Clinical Neurosciences and Electrical and Software Engineering, University of Calgary, Canada

Künstliche Intelligenz (KI) ist bereits zu einem unverzichtbaren Werkzeug geworden, um die riesigen Mengen an medizinischen Daten in greifbare Vorteile umzuwandeln. In diesem Vortrag werden neueste Arbeiten vorgestellt, die darauf abzielen, Verzerrungen in medizinischen Bilddaten und ML-Modellen zu identifizieren und zu verstehen. Es wird ein neuartiger Rahmen für die Simulation synthetischer Daten vorgestellt, der eine kontrollierte, systematische Bewertung ermöglicht, wie sich bestimmte Bildverzerrungen auf die Modellleistung auswirken und wie Risikominderungsstrategien die Unterschiede zwischen Untergruppen verringern können. Auf dieser Grundlage wird gezeigt, wie neuronale Faltungsnetze verschiedene Arten von Verzerrungen über ihre Schichten hinweg kodieren und wie diese Kodierungen zum Shortcut-Lernen beitragen. Darüber hinaus wird erläutert, wie fortschrittliche KI-Methoden eingesetzt werden können, um die zugrunde liegenden Mechanismen unfairen Modellverhaltens aufzudecken. Der Vortrag unterstreicht die Bedeutung kontrollierter Experimente, Erklärbarkeit und soziotechnischen Bewusstseins bei der Entwicklung von KI-Systemen, die nicht nur genau, sondern auch fair und vertrauenswürdig in der klinischen Praxis sind.

Towards AI Excellence: Focus on European Innovation and Regulation
Prof. Dr. Antonio Krüger
CEO des Deutschen Forschungszentrums für Künstliche Intelligenz (DFKI), Saarbrücken

In diesem Vortrag werden die Chancen der Künstlichen Intelligenz mit Schwerpunkt auf Deutschland und Europa skizziert. Er beleuchtet Forschungsansätze und aktuelle Trends in der KI-Landschaft. Außerdem werden wichtige politische Initiativen wie die nationale Hightech-Agenda und Vorschläge zum Ausbau von KI-Rechenzentren diskutiert, um Forschung und praktische Anwendung voranzutreiben. Abschließend wird der Rechtsrahmen des EU-KI-Gesetzes und dessen Auswirkungen auf Innovation, Sicherheit und soziales Vertrauen analysiert. Der Vortrag betont die Bedeutung gezielter politischer Maßnahmen, einer leistungsfähigen Infrastruktur und wissenschaftlicher Exzellenz für die Förderung der KI in Europa.

A Living Lens of Spontaneous Slow Oscillations: Illuminating Dark Brain Energy
Prof. Dr. Xi-Nian Zuo
McGovern Institute for Brain Research at Beijing Normal University, Bejing, China

In den letzten zehn Jahren haben fMRT-Studien frequenzabhängige Eigenschaften der spontanen langsamen Oszillationen (SSOs) im Gehirn aufgedeckt, von denen angenommen wird, dass sie die Grundlage für die „dunkle Energie“ im Gehirn bilden. Die Entschlüsselung der „dunklen Energie” des Gehirns – seiner SSOs und kortikalen Wanderwellen – treibt die Grundlagenforschung in den Neurowissenschaften voran und legt den Grundstein für neue KI-Paradigmen. Indem man versteht, wie das Gehirn Oszillationen selbst organisiert, um eine flexible, energieeffiziente Informationsverarbeitung zu erreichen, können diese Prinzipien in Algorithmen und Hardware mit verbesserter Robustheit und Energieeffizienz umgesetzt werden. Mit seinem Team hat Prof. Zuo Studien zu Multi-Band-Frequenzen von SSOs der letzten 15 Jahre untersucht und ein Modell vorgeschlagen, um die hierarchische Organisation von Multi-Band-SSOs durch die Integration ihrer Funktionen zu verdeutlichen. Neuere Arbeiten im Bereich der neuromorphen KI untersuchen wellenbasierte Dynamiken für die Echtzeit-Sensorverarbeitung sowie wann und warum oszillatorische Berechnungen herkömmliche Architekturen übertreffen. Sie erweitern gleichzeitig das Modell der „dunklen Energie des Gehirns" zu einem falsifizierbaren, skalenübergreifenden Framework für Gehirnfunktionen und vom Gehirn inspiriertes Computing.

Weitere Informationen zur BVM 2026 finden sich auf der Webseite der Konferenz unter:

`https://www.bvm-conf.org`

Abschließend möchten wir allen, die zum Gelingen der BVM 2026 beigetragen haben, unseren herzlichen Dank für ihr Engagement aussprechen: den Verfasserinnen und Verfassern der wissenschaftlichen Beiträge, den eingeladenen Gastredner*innen, den Lehrenden der Tutorials, den Industrievertretenden, dem Programmkomitee, den unterstützenden Fachgesellschaften, den Mitgliedern des dezentralen und des lokalen BVM-Organisationsteams sowie allen Mitarbeitenden des DFKI Labors Lübeck und des Instituts für Medizinische Informatik der Universität zu Lübeck.

Wir wünschen allen Teilnehmenden der BVM 2026 inspirierende Vorträge und Diskussionen, interessante neue Kontakte sowie vielfältige neue Eindrücke aus der Welt der Medizinischen Bildverarbeitung.

Januar 2026

Heinz Handels (Lübeck)
Katharina Breininger (Würzburg)
Thomas M. Deserno (Braunschweig)
Andreas Maier (Erlangen)
Klaus Maier-Hein (Heidelberg)
Christoph Palm (Regensburg)
Thomas Tolxdorff (Berlin)

Inhaltsverzeichnis

Die fortlaufende Nummer am linken Seitenrand entspricht den Beitragsnummern, wie sie im endgültigen Programm des Workshops zu finden sind. Dabei steht V für Vortrag, P für Poster, und S für Softwaredemonstration.

Session 1: Classification and Detection

V1 *Sofija Engelson, Jan Ehrhardt, Yannic Elser, Malte M. Sieren, Julia Andresen, Stefanie Schierholz, Tobias Keck, Daniel Drömann, Jörg Barkhausen, Heinz Handels*
Interpretable Mediastinal Lymph Node Station Classification and N-staging on CT and PET/CT Images 1

V2 *Adarsh Bhandary Panambur, Tri-Thien Nguyen, Siming Bayer, Andreas Maier*
Breast MRI Evaluation with Weakly-informed Slice-level Explanation: BE-WISE 10

V3 *Jonas Ammeling, Jonathan Ganz, Frauke Wilm, Katharina Breininger, Marc Aubreville*
Abstract: Investigation of Class Separability within Object Detection Models in Histopathology 18

Session 2: Image Acquisition and Reconstruction

V4 *Bipin Yadav, Adarsh Raghunath, Franziska Weber, Andreas Maier*
Self-supervised Dual-domain Swin Transformer for Sparse-view CT Reconstruction: DuDoSwin 19

V5 *Temke Kohlbrandt, Kai Geissler, Stefan Heldmann*
How Predictable is the Human Body? Predicting Organ Bounding Boxes With a Statistical Atlas Based on Four Keypoints . . . 26

V6 *Ziad Al-Haj Hemidi, Eytan Kats, Mattias P. Heinrich*
Abstract: PrIINeR: Towards Prior-informed Implicit Neural Representations for Accelerated MRI . . . 33

V7 *Yipeng Sun, Linda-Sophie Schneider, Siyuan Mei, Chengze Ye, Mingxuan Gu, Fabian Wagner, Siming Bayer, Andreas Maier*
Interpretable Framework for Zero-shot 4D Low-dose CT Denoising: Filter2Noise-4D . . . 34

Session 3: Foundation Models

V8 *David Lurz, Luisa Neubig, Markus Kopp, Andreas Kist*
Foundation Models in Medical Image Segmentation: How Foundational Are Foundation Models Really? . . . 40

V9 *Jan Tagscherer, Sarah de Boer, Lena Philipp, Fennie van der Graaf, Dré Peeters, Joeran Bosma, Lars Leijten, Bogdan Obreja, Ewoud Smit, Alessa Hering*
Modular Pipeline for Rapidly Evaluating Foundation Models in Medical Imaging: EvalBlocks . . . 48

V10 *Maeen Alikarrar, Christopher Syben, Joshua Scheuplein, Christian Hümmer, Ludwig Ritschl, Steffen Kappler, Andreas Maier*
Parameter-efficient Finetuning of Foundational Models for Text-guided X-ray Image Segmentation . . . 55

V11 *Marc S. Seibel, Nele S. Brügge, Timo Kepp, Bennet Kahrs, Jan Ehrhardt, Heinz Handels*
Revealing Eye-dentity: Foundation Models Enable Reidentification from Retinal OCT . . . 63

Session 4: Segmentation

V12 *Selina Baumgart, Nikolas Deubner, Andreas M. Kist*
Quantifying Anatomical Bias in Coronary Segmentation: Why Your Model Prefers the LCA More Than the RCA 70

V13 *Dominik Hirsch, Jan Ehrhardt, Heinz Handels*
Exploring Cross-dataset Transferability in Lung Nodule Segmentation via Weak Supervision and Synthetic Anomalies 76

V14 *Maximilian Rokuss, Yannick Kirchhoff, Seval Akbal, Balint Kovacs, Saikat Roy, Constantin Ulrich, Tassilo Wald, Lukas T. Rotkopf, Heinz-Peter Schlemmer, Klaus Maier-Hein*
Abstract: LesionLocator: Zero-shot Universal Tumor Segmentation and Tracking in 3D Whole-body Imaging 83

Session 5: Vision-Language Models

V15 *Md Badhon Miah, Lukas Buess, Andreas Maier*
Vision-language Models for Structured Report Generation in Radiology: Towards Consistent and Reliable Chest X-ray Reporting 84

V16 *Daniel Wolf, Heiko Hillenhagen, Billurvan Taskin, Alex Bäuerle, Meinrad Beer, Michael Götz, Timo Ropinski*
Abstract: Your other Left! Vision-language Models Fail to Understand Relative Positions in Medical Images 90

V17 *Luc Builtjes, Joeran Bosma, Mathias Prokop, Bram van Ginneken, Alessa Hering*
Abstract: Leveraging Open-source Language Models for Clinical Information Extraction: A Study in Resource-constrained Healthcare Settings 92

Session 6: Image Registration and Deformations

V18 *Julia Andresen, Bennet Kahrs, Heinz Handels, Timo Kepp*
Pathology-aware Implicit Neural Registration for Change Analysis in Retinal OCT Data: FRINR 93

V19 *Michael Schwimmbeck, Christopher Auer, Thomas Wittenberg, Stefanie Remmele*
Forecasting Organ Deformations in Navigated Liver Surgery using Exponential Smoothing 100

V20 *Johannes Bostelmann, Jan Lellmann*
Abstract: Liemorph: Transformer-based Image Registration using Flows on Lie Groups 106

Session 7: Unsupervised and Self-supervised Learning

V21 *Yuan Bi, Lucie Huang, Ricarda Clarenbach, Reza Ghotbi, Angelos Karlas, Nassir Navab, Zhongliang Jiang*
Abstract: Synomaly Noise and Multi-stage Diffusion: A Novel Approach for Unsupervised Anomaly Detection in Medical Images 108

V22 *Constantin Ulrich, Tassilo Wald, Jonathan Suprijadi, Sebastian Ziegler, Michal Nohel, Robin Peretzke, Gregor Köhler, Klaus Maier-Hein*
Abstract: An OpenMind for 3D Medical Vision Self-supervised Learning 109

V23 *Maja Schlereth, Moritz Schillinger, Katharina Breininger*
Abstract: Faster, Self-supervised Super-resolution for Anisotropic Multi-view MRI using a Sparse Loss 110

Poster Session 1

P1 *Franziska Weber, Thomas Gorges, Adarsh Raghunath, Andreas Maier*
Anomaly Detection in Thoracic CT: A Public Benchmark Based on CT-RATE 111

P2 *Robin Peretzke, Marlin Hanstein, Maximilian Fischer, Lars Wessel, Obada Alhalabi, Sebastian Regnery, Andreas Kudak, Maximilian Deng, Tanja Eichkorn, Philipp Hoegen-Saßmannshausen, Fabian Allmendinger, Jan-Hendrik Bolten, Philipp Schröter, Christine Jungk, Jürgen Debus, Peter Neher, Laila König, Klaus Maier-Hein*
Multimodal Classification of Radiation-induced Contrast Enhancement and Tumor Recurrence using Deep Learning 118

P3 *Alexia Rizoudis, Santiago Cepeda, Frank Kramer, Dominik Müller*
Comparative Analysis of Machine Learning Models for 3-month Survival Prediction in Aneurysmal Subarachnoid Hemorrhage 124

P4 *Leonard Klausmann, Tobias Rueckert, David Rauber, Raphaela Maerkl, Suemeyye R. Yildiran, Max Gutbrod, Christoph Palm*
Abstract: DIY Challenge Blueprint: From Organization to Technical Implementation in Biomedical Image Analysis 131

P5 *Luisa Gallée, Catharina S. Lisson, Christoph G. Lisson, Daniela Drees, Felix Weig, Daniel Vogele, Meinrad Beer, Michael Götz*
Abstract: Minimum Data, Maximum Impact: 20 Annotated Samples for Explainable Lung Nodule Classification 132

P6 *Dishantkumar Sutariya, Eike Petersen*
Impact of Preprocessing Methods on Racial Encoding and Model Robustness in CXR Diagnosis 133

S1 *Sonja Adomeit, Lukas Förner, Elisabeth Scheurer, Jan Bäßler, Elina Gastreich de Llanes, Jonas Böhringer, Ralph A. Bundschuh, Constantin Lapa, Kartikay Tehlan, Thomas Wendler*
AI-based Automated Framework for Quantitative PET/CT Image Analysis 139

P7 *Lina Felsner, Sevgi G. Kafali, Hannah Eichhorn, Agnes A. J. Leth, Aidas Batvinskas, André Datchev, Fabian Klemm, Jan Aulich, Puntika Leepagorn, Ruben Klinger, Daniel Rueckert, Julia A. Schnabel*
Master Class on Reproducibility: A Student Hackathon on Advanced MRI Reconstruction Methods 146

P8 *Julius Werner, Veronica Ferrero, Francesco Pennazio, Elisa Fiorina, Jona Kasprzak, Jorge Roser, Magdalena Rafecas*
Abstract: Adding the Temporal Dimension in Image Reconstruction for Proton Therapy Verification 154

P9 *Laura Hellwege, Johann C. Engster, Moritz Schaar, Thorsten M. Buzug, Maik Stille*
Reversible Image Augmentations for Unsupervised Deep Learning in Computed Tomography 156

P10 *Zeineb Azouzi, Linda Vorberg, Rainer Schneider, Andreas Maier, Fabian Wagner*
Automatic Patient Positioning Control and Correction on MRI Localizer Images 162

P11 *Xuesong Li, Nassir Navab, Zhongliang Jiang*
Abstract: Speckle2Self: Self-supervised Ultrasound Speckle Reduction Without Clean Data 169

P12 *Jennifer Ochmann, Johanna P. Müller, Franciskus X. Erick, Bernhard Kainz*
Distil or Cluster? Data-efficient Learning for Ultrasound in Practice 170

P13 *Anna-Lisa Allgaier, Katrin Volk, Anja Zillner, Luise Robra, Jonas Bornmann, Andreas Leiniger, Rainer Brucher, Alfred M. Franz*
Scanliner with Integrated Fiducial Markers for 3D-reconstruction of Residual Limbs using Ultrasound Imaging 177

P14 *Alexander Furtner, Zoe Reinke, Thomas Wendler*
Anatomy-informed 3D Reconstruction of Tracked Ultrasound Sweeps: A Proof of Concept 185

P15 *Emely Rosbach, Jonas Ammeling, Christof A. Bertram, Andreas Riener, Marc Aubreville*
Abstract: When Two Wrongs Don't Make a Right: Examining Confirmation Bias and the Role of Time Pressure During Human-AI Collaboration in Computational Pathology 193

P16 *Maximilian Fischer, Peter Neher, Peter Schüffler, Sebastian Ziegler, Shuhan Xiao, Robin Peretzke, David Clunie, Constantin Ulrich, Michael Baumgartner, Alexander Muckenhuber, Silvia Dias Almeida, Michael Götz, Jens Kleesiek, Marco Nolden, Rickmer Braren, Klaus Maier-Hein*
Abstract: Unlocking the Potential of Digital Pathology: Novel Baselines for Compression 194

P17 *Ding Xin, Verena Wally, Chrstina Guttmann-Gruber, Bernadette Liemberger, Johann Bauer, Andreas Uhl*
Towards a Visual Distinction of Benign and Tumorous Wound Surface in Epidermolysis Bullosa 195

S2 *Sweta Banerjee, Timo Gosch, Sara Hester, Viktoria Weiss, Thomas Conrad, Taryn A. Donovan, Nils Porsche, Jonas Ammeling, Christoph Stroblberger, Robert Klopfleisch, Christopher Kaltenecker, Christof A. Bertram, Katharina Breininger, Marc Aubreville*
Enabling Fast and Mobile Histopathology Image Annotation through Swipeable Interfaces: SWAN 203

P18 *Joshua Scheuplein, Björn Kreher, Andreas Maier*
Prediction of Patient and Mobile C-arm Orientation in Orthopedic Trauma Procedures 210

P19 *Joshua Scheuplein, Maximilian Rohleder, Andreas Maier, Björn Kreher*
Abstract: DINO Adapted to X-ray (DAX): Foundation Models for Intraoperative X-ray Imaging 217

P20 *Serouj Khajarian, Michael Schwimmbeck, Konstantin Holzapfel, Johannes Schmidt, Christopher Auer, Stefanie Remmele, Oliver Amft*
Abstract: Automated Multimodel Segmentation and Tracking for AR-guided Open Liver Surgery using Scene-aware Self-prompting 218

P21 *Janine Rothert, Judith L. Salz, Joy Rakshit, Viola Ehses, Florentine Huettl, Tobias Huber, Hauke Lang, Georg Rose, Sylvia Saalfeld, Georg Hille*
Perfusion-aware Surgical Planning: Simulating the Effects on Planned Hepatic Resection Zones using Graph-based Vessel Modeling 219

S3 *Mohamed Tababi, Timo Baumgärtner, Charissa Morales, Jan Komposch, Johannes Roßkopf, Till Malzacher, Michael Braun, Bernd Schmitz, Alfred M. Franz*
Software Prototyping in Java: Examples on Automatic Annotation and AI-based Instrument Tracking for Stroke Treatment 226

Poster Session 2

P22 *Georgii Kolokolnikov, Marie-Lena Schmalhofer, Lennart Well, Inka Ristow, René Werner*
Deep Radiomics with DINOV3 for MRI-based Differentiation of Peripheral Nerve Sheath Tumors in Neurofibromatosis Type 1 233

P23 *Christopher J. Hansen, Paula Kloehn, Anna-Louisa Kollster, Toni Gehrmann, Jonas Conrad, Christian Graetz, Christof Dörfer, Claus-C. Glüer, Jan-Bernd Hövener, Coenraad Mouton*
Is DINOv3 Ready for Caries Detection on Panoramic Dental X-ray Images? 239

P24 *Caroline v. Dresky, Claus von der Burchard, Monty Santarossa, Julia Andresen, Marc S. Seibel, Timo Kepp, Johann Roider, Heinz Handels*
Visual Acuity Assessment from Uni- and Multimodal Retinal Image Data using the Foundation Model MIRAGE 245

P25 *Luisa Neubig, Deirde Larsen, Takeshi Ikuma, Melda Kunduk, Andreas M. Kist*
Characterization of Foundation Models for Longitudinal Similarity Measurement in Medical Video Data 252

S4 *David Lurz, Luisa Neubig, Andreas Kist*
Adaptive Automatic Prompt Generation Assistant for Segmentation Foundation Models 259

P26 *Stefan M. Fischer, Lina Felsner, Richard Osuala, Johannes Kiechle, Daniel M. Lang, Jan C. Peeken, Julia A. Schnabel*
Abstract: Progressive Growing of Patch Size: Curriculum Learning for Accelerated and Improved Medical Image Segmentation 267

P27 *Balint Kovacs, Goran Stanic, Fabian Weykamp, Florian Ebert, Dimitrios Bounias, Bouchra Tawk, Martin Niklas, Jakob Liermann, Oliver Jäkel, Klaus H. Maier-Hein, Ralf Floca, Kristina Giske*
Abstract: Cross-Modality Supervised Prostate Segmentation on CBCT for Adaptive Radiotherapy 269

P28 *Anqi Wang, Florian Putz, Yixing Huang, Andreas Maier*
Comparative Study of Deep Learning Models for Brain Metastases Autosegmentation 270

P29 *Kai Geissler, Markus Wenzel, Susanne Diekmann, Robert Grimm, Heinrich von Busch, Torbjörn Vik, Hans Meine*
Applying Active Learning to Nipple Segmentation in Breast MRI 277

P30 *Jacopo Bracci, Alexander Katzmann, Leonhard Rist, Linda Vorberg, Michael Sühling, Andreas Maier*
Hybrid Vessel Wall Segmentation for Assisted Annotation in CT Angiography 285

P31 *Michal Nohel, Katerina Krejci, Constantin Ulrich, Maximilian Rokuss, Yannick Kirchhoff, Jiri Chmelik, Stefan Reguli, Jan Hrubovcak, Lubomir Martinek, Lukas Knybel*
Automatic Deep Learning-Based Segmentation of Abdominal Vessels in CT Scans 292

P32 *Hartmut Häntze, Myrthe Buser, Alessa Hering, Lisa C. Adams, Keno K. Bressem*
Abstract: Sex-based Bias Inherent in the Dice Similarity Coefficient: A Model Independent Analysis for Multiple Anatomical Structures 298

P33 *Georg Wimmer, Christof Kauba, Christian Puttinger, Pamina Schlager, Roland Zauner, Carolin Gemeier, Tobias Welponer, Christine Prodinger, Anja Diem, Katharina Ude-Schoder, Martin Laimer, Johann W. Bauer, Andreas Uhl*
Medical Image Annotations for AI-based Wound Segmentation: The Rocky Road to High-quality Training Data 299

P34 *Nico Schmutzenhofer, Lukas Förner, Sina Wendrich, Kartikay Tehlan, Thomas Wendler*
Label, Refine, Repeat: Extending nnInteractive with Dataset Traversal and nnU-Net Proposals 307

S5 *Nilesh P. Rijhwani, Titus J. Brinker, Neher Peter, Nolden Marco, Klaus Maier-Hein, Christoph Wies, Maximilian Fischer*
Bridging Radiology and Pathology: A DICOM-based Framework for Multimodal Mapping and Integrated Visualization 315

S6 *Maja Schlereth, Filippo Fagni, Moritz Schillinger, Katharina Breininger*
Flexible Multiplanar Viewer with Easy Adaptability for Expert Studies, Questionnaires, and Investigational Imaging Biomarker Assessment 321

P35 *Chengze Ye, Linda-Sophie Schneider, Yipeng Sun, Siyuan Mei, Siming Bayer, Paula A. Pérez-Toro, Andreas Maier*
Differentiable Approximate Truncation Robust CBCT Reconstruction via Known Operator Learning 328

P36 *Chengze Ye, Linda-Sophie Schneider, Yipeng Sun, Mareike Thies, Siyuan Mei, Andreas Maier*
Abstract: DRACO: Differentiable Reconstruction for Arbitrary CBCT Orbits 334

P37 *Sonja Wichelmann, Florian Weiler, Thomas Friedrich, Joerg Barkhausen, Roman Kloeckner, Franz Wegner, Malte M. Sieren*
Abstract: Bake Your Phantom: Low-cost Recipes for Dough-based, Tissue-mimicking CT Phantoms 335

P38 *Shadi Khamseh, Florian Wolz, Joshua Scheuplein, Thorsten Ergler, Andreas Maier*
AI-based Dual-domain Framework for Gridline Suppression in Digital Radiography 337

P39 *Manuel Laufer, Julius Haas, Dominik Mairhöfer, Malte Sieren, Hauke Gerdes, Fabio Leal dos Reis, Arpad Bischof, Thomas Käster, Erhardt Barth, Jörg Barkhausen, Thomas Martinetz*
Evaluation of Time-of-flight Camera Positioning for AI-based Patient Pose Assessment in Radiography 345

P40 *Kartikay Tehlan, Thomas Wendler*
Abstract: Physiological Neural Representations in Dynamic Imaging 353

P41 *Sorel T. Djoumsi, Laura Lemberger-Viehmann, Tatyana Ivanovska, Christian Bergler, Thiha Aung, Silke Härteis*
Einsatz Künstlicher Intelligenz zur Zellsegmentierung und Klassifikation in histologischen Bildern von Pankreaskarzinomen 354

P42 *Max Gutbrod, David Rauber, Christoph Palm*
Improving Generalization in Mitotic Cell Detection via Domain Transformations 362

P43 *Thomas Eixelberger, Philipp Maisch, Christian Bolenz, Thomas Wittenberg*
Computer-assisted Detection of Lesions in Cystoscopy: Continuous Improvement by Data Extension and Model Selection 368

P44 *Nils Porsche, Flurin Müller-Diesing, Sweta Banerjee, Miguel Goncalves, Marc Aubreville,*
Filtering Scheme for Confocal Laser Endomicroscopy (CLE)-video Sequences for Self-supervised Learning 375

Poster Session 3

P45 *Luc Builtjes, Alessa Hering*
Tracking Cancer Through Text: Longitudinal Extraction from Radiology Reports using Open-source Large Language Models . . . 381

P46 *Jiajun Wang, Yipeng Sun, Siming Bayer, Andreas Maier*
Explainable Radiologist-aligned VLM for CT Image Quality Assessment . . . 387

P47 *Marc Aubreville, Taryn A. Donovan, Christof A. Bertram*
Exploring General-purpose Autonomous Multimodal Agents for Pathology Report Generation . . . 393

P48 *Siyuan Mei, Fuxin Fan, Mareike Thies, Mingxuan Gu, Fabian Wagner, Oliver Aust, Ina Erceg, Zeynab Mirzaei, Georgiana Neag, Yipeng Sun, Yixing Huang, Andreas Maier*
Abstract: BigReg: An Efficient Registration Pipeline for High-resolution X-ray and Light-sheet Fluorescence Microscopy . . . 400

P49 *Lukas Förner, Thomas Wendler*
Abstract: Bone-guided Semi-supervised Registration . . . 401

P50 *Ole Gildemeister, Johannes Bostelmann, Pia Schulz, Andra Oltmann, Phillip Rostalski, Jan Modersitzki, Jan Lellmann*
Abstract: Time-continuous Sliding Motion Image Registration using Stationary Velocity Fields for Respiratory Motion Interpolation . . . 402

P51 *Marten J. Finck, Sina P. Lücke, Niklas C. Koser, Yu Sun, Jan-B. Hövener, Wojtek Palubicki, Sören Pirk*
Resource-efficient Fine-tuning of Stable Diffusion for Synthetic Hand Radiograph Generation . . . 403

P52 *Jen Dusseljee, Sarah de Boer, Alessa Hering*
Kidney Cancer Detection Using 3D-based Latent Diffusion Models . . . 411

P53 *Joshua Niemeijer, Jan Ehrhardt, Heinz Handels, Hristina Uzunova*
Abstract: Uncertainty-aware ControlNet Bridging Domain Gaps with Synthetic Image Generation 419

P54 *Marvin Seyfarth, Salman U. H. Dar, Sandy Engelhardt*
Rethinking Diversity Metrics in Medical Imaging with Wasserstein Distance 420

P55 *Yaqiong Ni, Adarsh Bhandary Panambur, Chang Liu, Tri-Thien Nguyen, Siming Bayer, Huang Juan, Sun Jiayu, Lv Su, Andreas Maier*
Opportunistic Breast Cancer Risk Stratification From Low-dose Chest CT Using Multiple Instance Learning 427

P56 *Katharina Eckstein, Constantin Ulrich, Michael Baumgartner, Jessica Kächele, Dimitrios Bounias, Tassilo Wald, Ralf Floca, Klaus H. Maier-Hein*
Abstract: The Missing Piece: A Case for Pre-training in 3D Medical Object Detection 435

P57 *Marco Pawłowski, Dennis Säring, Jochen Herrmann, Eilin Jopp-van Well, Heinz Handels*
Comparison of Modern Transformer Architectures and CNN-based Models for MRI-based Age Estimation of the Knee 436

P58 *Ole H. Martensen, Tobias Strauß, Majid Ramedani, Martin Dyrba*
Comparison of Post-hoc Calibration Methods for Neural Network Likelihood Scores 443

P59 *Daiqi Liu, Tomás Arias-Vergara, Jana Hutter, Andreas Maier, Paula A. Pérez-Toro*
Abstract: Audio-vision Contrastive Learning for Phonological Class Recognition 450

P60 *Cassandra Krause, Mattias P. Heinrich, Ron Keuth*
Fracture Morphology Classification: Local Multiclass Modeling for Multilabel Complexity 451

P61 *Xinghao Wang, Marco Maass, Yuanheng Zhang, Chen Li, Xinyu Huang, Hongzan Sun, Marcin Grzegorzek*
Deep Learning Framework for Brain Age Prediction Integrating Gray Matter Structure and White Matter Microstructure: MN-FNet 458

P62 *Jessica Kächele, Markus Wennmann, Arvin von Salomon, Peter Neher, Heinz-Peter Schlemmer, Klaus Maier-Hein*
Abstract: Automated Detection of Focal Bone Marrow Lesions from MRI: A Multi-center Feasibility Study in Patients with Monoclonal Plasma Cell Disorders 464

P63 *Lena Philipp, Maarten de Rooij, John Hermans, Matthieu Rutten, Horst Hahn, Bram van Ginneken, Alessa Hering*
Abstract: Annotation-efficient 3D Body Composition Segmentation 465

P64 *Tassilo Wald, Benjamin Hamm, Julius Holzschuh, Rami El Shafie, Andreas Kudak, Balint Kovacs, Irada Pflüger, Bastian von Nettelbladt, Constantin Ulrich, Michael A. Baumgartner, Philipp Vollmuth, Jürgen Debus, Klaus H. Maier-Hein, Thomas Welzel*
Abstract: Enhancing Deep Learning Methods for Brain Metastasis Detection Through Cross-technique Annotations on SPACE MRI 466

P65 *Mattias P. Heinrich*
Abstract: BinaryFormer: Differentiable 1-bit Self-attention for Long-range Transformers in Medical Segmentation and 3D Diffusion Models 467

P66 *Sina Walluscheck, Vanja S. Cangalovic, Tanja Lossau, Stefan Heldmann, Jan H. Moltz*
Neural Instance Optimization for Lesion Segmentation in Follow-up CT 468

P67 *Lukas Mechs, Stefan B. Ploner, Yunchan Hwang, Muhammad U. Jamil, Nadia K. Waheed, James G. Fujimoto, Andreas Maier*
Automated Segmentation and Biomarker Analysis in OCT Images using a Transformer-based Framework 475

P68 *Rianne Weber, Niels Rocholl, Max de Grauw, Mathias Prokop, Ewoud Smit, Alessa Hering*
Data-driven Model Adaptation Enhances Lesion Segmentation: ULS+ 482

Interpretable Mediastinal Lymph Node Station Classification and N-staging on CT and PET/CT Images

Sofija Engelson [1,2], Jan Ehrhardt [1,2], Yannic Elser [3], Malte M. Sieren [3,4], Julia Andresen [1], Stefanie Schierholz [5], Tobias Keck [5,6], Daniel Drömann [7], Jörg Barkhausen [3], Heinz Handels [1,2]

[1]Institute of Medical Informatics, University of Luebeck
[2]AIMedI, German Research Center for Artificial Intelligence
[3]Dept. of Radiology & Nuclear Medicine, Univ. Medical Center Schleswig-Holstein (UKSH)
[4]Dept. of Interventional Radiology, UKSH
[5]Dept. of Surgery, UKSH
[6]Fraunhofer Research Institution for Individualized and Cell-Based Medical Engineering
[7]Dept. of Pulmonology, UKSH
sofija.engelson@uni-luebeck.de

Abstract. We present an interpretable approach for automated lymph node station (LNS) classification and N-staging on PET/CT and CT only by extending two established segmentation algorithms with probabilistic atlas-based LNS mapping. Our results show that a probabilistic approach for LNS mapping improves the detection accuracy by over 40 percentage points. The proposed method yields an accuracy of 0.74 for LNS classification and 0.68 for N-staging on PET/CT, representing a significant improvement toward human-level performance compared with the baseline approach. A performance drop for CT only evaluation indicates the PET scan adds valuable information to lymph node assessment, which is in alignment with according literature.

1 Introduction

In the commonly used TNM classification, the N-stage indicates the extent of metastatic spread to regional lymph nodes. The four N-stages provide an ordinal measure of lung cancer progression, increasing with the distance of malignant lymph nodes from the primary tumor. Rule-based N-staging according to Amin et al. [1] requires classification of lymph nodes into malignant and benign, as well as mapping of individual mediastinal lymph nodes to lymph node stations (LNS) according to Mountain and Dresler [2]. Differentiation between malignant and benign lymph nodes can be achieved by various methods. Histopathological examination after surgical resection or biopsy remains the diagnostic gold standard, whereas non-invasive imaging methods such as PET/CT are widely used beforehand. PET/CT combines metabolic and morphological information, but is costly and not always available. For diagnosis on CT only, lymph nodes with a short-axis diameter greater than 10 mm

© Der/die Autor(en), exklusiv lizenziert an
Springer Fachmedien Wiesbaden GmbH, ein Teil von Springer Nature 2026
H. Handels et al. (Hrsg.), *Bildverarbeitung für die Medizin 2026*,
Informatik aktuell, https://doi.org/10.1007/978-3-658-51100-5_1

are considered pathological [3]. However, both PET/CT and CT assessments are prone to false positives due to inflammatory or sarcoid-like reactions.

Manual N-staging remains a labor-intensive and error-prone process. Thus, AI-based approaches for subtasks of N-staging offer promising potential for improving N-staging accuracy and efficiency. Approaches for automatic lymph node classification on CT and PET/CT often use radiomics features from manual segmentations or annotated regions of interest. Iuga et al. [4] carry out N-staging as a proof-of-concept study based on automated LNS mapping on CT using a deep-learning framework. Previous work from our working group consisted of training a CNN-based approach from sampled patches for LNS classification and N-staging [5]. However, learning-based approaches are difficult to verify and interpret. Cao et al. [6] and Hofman et al. [7] propose LNS mapping based on atlas-based registration and lymph node segmentation masks. Yet, both methods use the centroid of the lymph node to map it to a LNS, and rely on the lymph node size as the defining criterion for malignancy.

We propose to extend two segmentation algorithms developed as part of MICCAI challenges by adding probabilistic atlas-based LNS mapping as a basis for rule-based N-staging. Our methodological contributions are 1.) improved atlas-based LNS mapping through a probabilistic approach to account for the ambiguity in LNS delineation, and 2.) a fully-automated pipeline for verifiable N-staging. Interpretability is achieved through visualization of malignant LNS, enabling traceability of the N-stage determination. Furthermore, we assess the performance of our method based on different input modalities (PET/CT and CT only) and use histology as the ground-truth reference standard.

2 Methods and materials

We differentiate two scenarios – *A* evaluation on PET/CT and *B* evaluation on CT only. The proposed workflow consists of three steps: 1.) segmentation of malignant regions, 2.) mapping of malignant regions to LNS, and 3.) rule-based N-staging. An overview of the proposed workflow can be reviewed in Fig. 2.

2.1 Segmentation of malignant regions

In the first step of scenario *A*, we predicted segmentation masks of lesions with high tracer uptake, including the primary tumor and the metastases with the algorithm that won the autoPET Challenge in 2022 [8]. For the evaluation on CT images only in scenario *B*, segmentation masks of enlarged lymph nodes were produced (LNQ Challenge 2024) [9].

2.2 Probabilistic mapping of malignant regions to LNS

The second step aims to map the areas segmented in step 1 to the corresponding station in order to identify pathological LNS. The boundaries between LNS are anatomically ambiguous and difficult to define due to substantial anatomical variability. Consequently, interobserver variability is high [10], and traditional multi-atlas fusion strategies, such as majority voting, often yield unreliable results. To address this, we employ a probabilistic approach, in which lymph node assignment to stations is defined by a continuous weight map reflecting the fuzziness of the boundary definitions. More concretely, five atlases with annotated LNS masks [11] were registered to our data using rigid, affine, and deformable registration based on the segmentation masks of the TotalSegmentator algorithm [12]. Details on the registration approach can be reviewed in our previous works [5, 9]. Then, a weight map $W^l = (w^l_{ijk})$ at pixel index (i, j, k) was calculated for each LNS $l \in L$ based on the atlas-based probabilities and geometrical properties, i.e., $W^l = B^l \odot D^l$ where $\odot$ denotes element-wise multiplication.

Given the binary segmentation mask $M^{a,l} = (m^{a,l}_{ijk})$ of LNS l from the registered atlases $a \in \{1, ..., A\}$, the probabilistic map $B^l = (b^l_{ijk})$ is computed by

$$b^l_{ijk} = \begin{cases} \frac{\sum_{a=1}^{A} m^{a,l}_{ijk}}{A} & \frac{\sum_{a=1}^{A} m^{a,l}_{ijk}}{A} > \frac{1}{A} \\ 0 & \text{otherwise} \end{cases} \quad (1)$$

As geometric properties, we use the normalized Euclidean distances (e^l_{ijk}) from the centroid of the non-zero probability region for LNS l, i.e., $D^l = (1 - e^l_{ijk})$. The process of weight map generation is presented in Fig. 1. Further, we identified a LNS l as pathological, if the maximum probability $p = \max_{ijk} s_{ijk} \odot w^l_{ijk}$, that a malignant region in segmentation mask $S = (s_{ijk}) \in \{0, 1\}$ generated in step 1 of our pipeline lies within the LNS, exceeds a threshold value t. Threshold t is a hyperparameter, which was tuned via grid search over $\{0, 0.1, 0.25, 0.5, 0.75, 0.9\}$. The optimal threshold was selected by maximizing balanced accuracy for LNS classification as well as accuracy for N-staging. We assume that one connected-component of segmentation mask S can cover multiple stations.

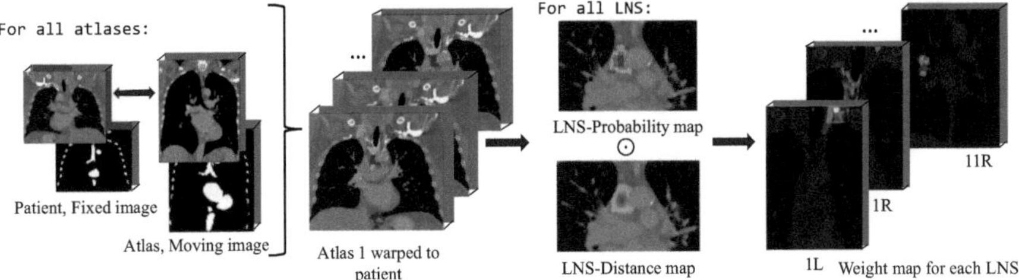

Fig. 1. Generation process for LNS weight map. From the segmentation masks of L LNS obtained via multi-atlas segmentation with A atlases, we compute a weight map for each LNS that encodes both probabilistic and geometric properties.

2.3 Rule-based n-staging

Given the primary tumor side, LNS were grouped into LNS groups and the N-staging rules [1] were applied for the last step of the pipeline.

2.4 Experiments

To assess the improvement of LNS mapping using the proposed probabilistic LNS mapping approach, we compared the detection accuracies per LNS of the standard and the probabilistic LNS mapping approach using a publicly available dataset, for which enlarged lymph nodes and stations are annotated on pixel-level [13, 14]. For each segmented lymph node, the corresponding LNS was assigned either by the station whose centroid lies within it or by the station with the highest weight map probability. In an extension of this experiment, we aim to assess how segmentation errors propagate into mapping errors. For this, we extend the original setup by replacing the ground truth [13, 14] with predicted segmentation masks from the algorithm of scenario *B* and transferring the ground-truth station number to the predicted lymph node mask before the evaluation of atlas-based LNS mapping. In order to transfer the station number as a ground-truth reference to each connected

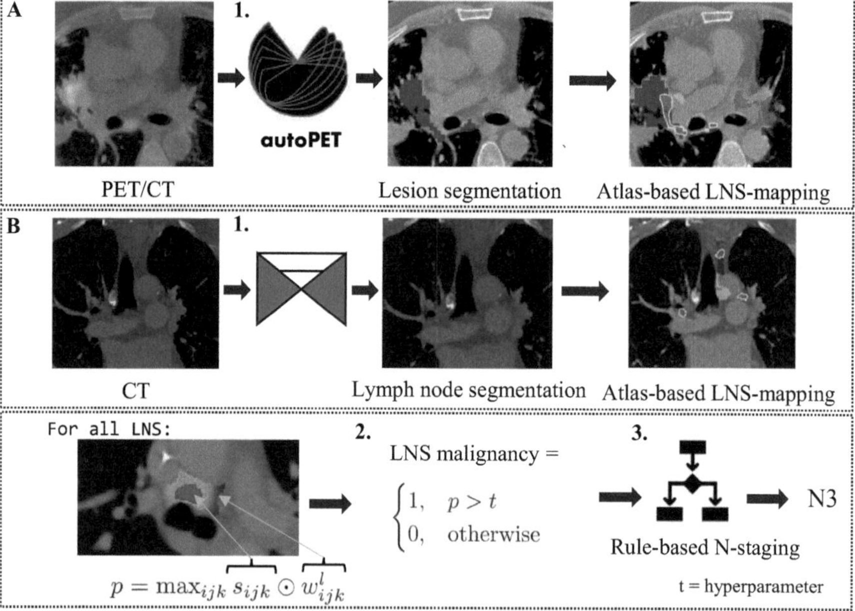

Fig. 2. Overview of proposed methods. We generate PET-lesion (scenario *A*) or lymph node segmentations (scenario *B*) and label an LNS l as pathological, if the maximum value of the according weight map within the lymph node/lesion mask exceeds a threshold t. Rule-based N-staging follows.

component in the predicted mask, we counted overlapping voxels to the ground-truth mask per station number and assigned the station with the highest pixel count to the lymph node. Since the lymph node segmentation algorithm was trained on the same dataset [13, 14] as used for experiment evaluation, only unseen test cases were included in this follow-up experiment.

For LNS classification and N-staging performance assessment, we used an in-house dataset consisting of 353 patients and the publicly available Radiogenomics dataset [15]. LNS classification can be understood as a combination of lymph node classification and LNS mapping, where classification accuracy quantifies the ability to distinguish malignant from benign LNS. As the Radiogenomics dataset does not provide labels on LNS-level, only the in-house dataset was used for the evaluation of LNS classification. The datasets were split into five stratified folds based on N-stage and pathological LNS count, with patient-level separation across training and test sets. In addition to the proposed algorithms, a thresholding approach serves as a comparison method. In clinical practice, a lymph node station is considered pathological when the maximum standardized uptake value $SUV_{\max}$ within a manually defined volume exceeds a threshold o. To reproduce this baseline, we computed $SUV_{\max}$ for LNS segmentations from multi-atlas registration with majority-vote fusion and selected the optimal threshold via grid search over $\{3, 3.5, 4, 4.5, 5, 5.5, 6\}$.

3 Results

The left plot of Fig. 3 shows the correctly and incorrectly mapped LNS through matching the centroid of the lymph node mask with the LNS masks from multi-atlas segmentation fused through majority voting. In Fig. 3 on the right, the LNS were assigned to the lymph nodes using the proposed method. The average detection accuracy over all lymph nodes can be improved from 0.31 to 0.73 using the proposed probabilistic approach. When predicted, instead of ground-truth, lymph node segmentation masks are used for this experiment, the average LNS mapping detection accuracy across all predicted lymph nodes is 0.72.

The five-fold cross-validated results of the comparison of different approaches for LNS classification and N-staging based on PET/CT or CT only can be reviewed in Tab. 1. To provide further context, we additionally report medical experts' performance by correlating information extracted from radiology reports with the histopathological ground truth.

Among PET/CT-based methods, the proposed algorithm achieves higher balanced accuracy for LNS classification and higher accuracy for N-staging. The examination of confusion matrices shows that the thresholding approach is heavily oversensitive, while the proposed algorithm shows a more balanced distribution of false negatives and positives. A performance assessment on LNS-level shows few positive cases in station 1R and 1L, however, the balanced accuracy is comparable across the remaining stations and shows no correlation to the LNS that are more difficult to map according to the LNS mapping analysis presented above. Nevertheless, none of the algorithmic results surpass human performance. When comparing the performance for the two input modalities, we observe a severe performance drop

Algorithm	ImgMod	Acc.	Bal. Acc.	Sens.	Spec.
		LNS Classification			
Ours (t = 0.9)	CT	0.92 ± 0.00	0.58 ± 0.02	0.21 ± 0.05	0.95 ± 0.00
Thresholding (o = 4)	PET/CT	0.84 ± 0.01	0.72 ± 0.02	**0.58** ± 0.03	0.85 ± 0.01
Ours (t = 0.25)	PET/CT	**0.91** ± 0.00	**0.74** ± 0.02	0.55 ± 0.04	**0.92** ± 0.00
Doctors	PET/CT	0.95	0.80	0.63	0.97
		N-staging			
		0.48 ± 0.02		0.34 ± 0.09	0.78 ± 0.02
		0.56 ± 0.03		**0.56** ± 0.02	0.83 ± 0.01
		0.68 ± 0.02		0.55 ± 0.08	**0.86** ± 0.01
		0.70		0.71	0.89

Tab. 1. Results for lymph-node assessment in predicting the histologically confirmed N-stage. Best algorithmic performance is shown in bold. Physician performance was available only for the in-house dataset. For PET/CT evaluation, the proposed method differs significantly from thresholding for both LNS classification (McNemar's test) and N-staging (permutation test) with a p-value < 0.05. ImgMod = image modality.

for CT only evaluation, especially the sensitivity on LNS-level and N-staging. As shown in Fig. 4, primarily involve incorrect delineation of lymph nodes, particularly confusion with adjacent fat tissue, neighboring lymph nodes, or the primary tumor (failure case 4a to 4c). In addition, discrepancies between image-based assessment and histopathological findings occur in some cases (failure case 4d).

4 Discussion

In this work, we present an interpretable approach for LNS classification and N-staging using different imaging modalities and evaluate its performance in regard to the true malignancy status confirmed by histopathological examination. Our comparison shows that the proposed approach for PET/CT has better performance for

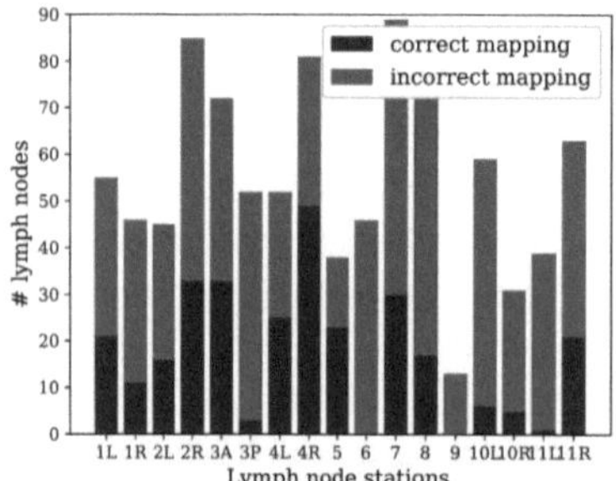

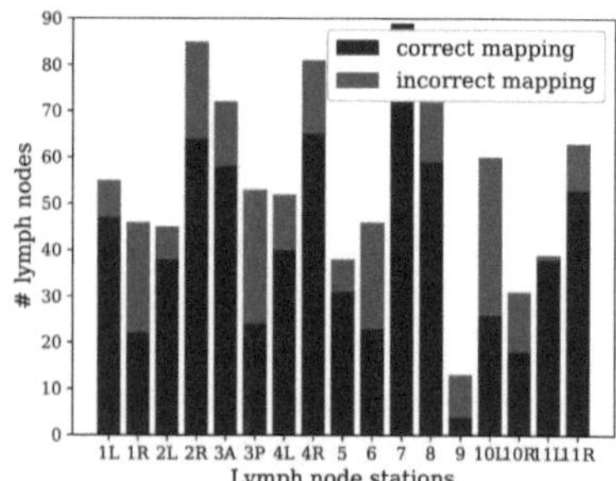

Fig. 3. Assessment of atlas-based LNS mapping per LNS for multi-atlas segmentation (left) and the proposed probabilistic approach (right).

N-staging than thresholding of $SUV_{\max}$ based on LNS segmentation masks from multi-atlas registration fused through majority voting. Errors in LNS classification directly affect and propagate into the N-staging accuracy, because one wrongly predicted LNS can lead to a change from N0 to N3 or the other way around. The algorithmic performance on PET/CT is higher than for CT only. Our experiments show that segmentation errors have only a marginal influence on the LNS mapping performance. However, the differentiation between healthy and pathological lymph nodes is hampered due to errors in delineation of segmented lymph nodes from surrounding fat tissue, collocated lymph nodes, and the primary tumor. The inability to accurately identify individual instances has been identified as the main limitation in previous work for mediastinal lymph node segmentation [14]. Furthermore, we hypothesize that errors in LNS classification can also be led back to the task definition of the segmentation algorithm in scenario *B*. The algorithm is trained to segment enlarged lymph nodes, but lymph node size alone may not be a reliable criterion for lymph node malignancy [16, 17]. The observed performance drop for CT only in comparison to PET assessment is in alignment with according literature [18] and suggests that the PET scan does provide important information about the true malignancy status of lymph nodes. The gap to human performance indicates that there are still other factors that are indicative of the malignancy status that are not sufficiently captured by the algorithms. Possible factors considered by physicians include proximity to the primary tumor, lymphatic drainage pathways, and combined imaging features, i.e., PET lesion segmentation masks were annotated based on tracer uptake, ignoring CT morphology [19]. However, the proposed N-staging pipeline serves as a valuable decision-support tool for radiologists for evaluation on PET/CT and CT only, as all sub steps are verifiable through the visualization of malignant LNS.

Acknowledgement. This work was supported by grants of the collaborative research project "AI ecosystem in health care" within the subproject titled "Health system-

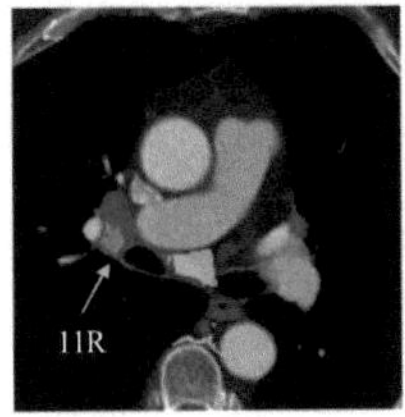

(**a**) Delineation from surrounding fat tissue fails.

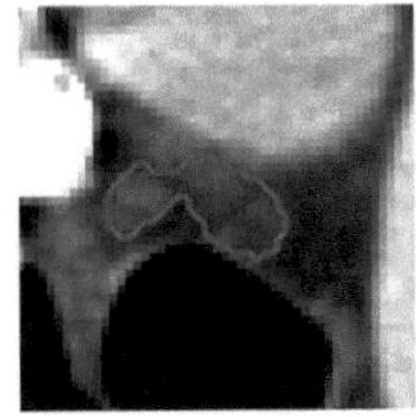

(**b**) Delineation of collocated lymph nodes fails.

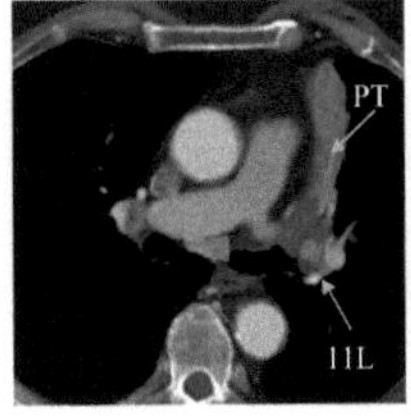

(**c**) Primary tumor invades adjacent lymph nodes.

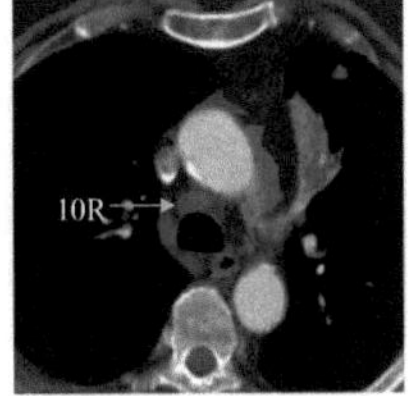

(**d**) Image (N1) and histology (N0) assessment do not align.

Fig. 4. Failure cases for scenario *B*. The lymph node segmentation outline is colored in red. LNS segmentation masks from multi-atlas registration fused via majority voting are overlayed over the CT image (soft tissue window: −200, 400 Hounsfield units). LNS segmentation masks are omitted in Fig. 4b for better border visibility of lymph nodes. PT = primary tumor.

based analysis of disease patterns using lung diseases as an example" financed by the federate state Schleswig-Holstein, Germany.

References

1. Amin MB, Greene FL, Edge SB, Compton CC, Gershenwald JE, Brookland RK et al. The eighth edition AJCC cancer staging manual: continuing to build a bridge from a population-based to a more "personalized" approach to cancer staging. CA Cancer J Clin. 2017;67(2):93–9.
2. Mountain CF, Dresler CM. Regional lymph node classification for lung cancer staging. Chest. 1997;111(6):1718–23.
3. Eisenhauer E, Therasse P, J. B, Schwartz L, Sargent D, Ford R et al. New response evaluation criteria in solid tumours: revised RECIST guideline (version 1.1). Eur J Cancer. 2009;45(2):228–47.
4. Iuga AI, Lossau T, Caldeira LL, Rinneburger M, Lennartz S, Große Hokamp N et al. Automated mapping and N-staging of thoracic lymph nodes in contrast-enhanced CT scans of the chest using a fully convolutional neural network. Eur J Radiol. 2021;139:109718.
5. Engelson S, Elser Y, Sieren MM, Ehrhardt J, Andresen J, Schierholz S et al. Deep learning-based mediastinal lymph node assessment on PET/CT images without pixel-level annotations. J Med Imaging. 2025. In submission.
6. Cao Y, Feng J, Wang C, Yang F, Wang X, Xu J et al. LNAS: a clinically applicable deep-learning system for mediastinal enlarged lymph nodes segmentation and station mapping without regard to the pathogenesis using unenhanced CT images. Radiol Med. 2024;129(2):229–38.
7. Hoffman J, Liu J, Turkbey E, Kim L, Summers RM. Automatic identification of IASLC-defined mediastinal lymph node stations on CT scans using multi-atlas organ segmentation. Proc SPIE MI. 2015:94141R.
8. Ye J, Wang H, Huang Z, Deng Z, Su Y, Tu C et al. Exploring vanilla U-net for lesion segmentation from whole-body FDG-PET/CT scans. arXiv: 2210.07490. 2022.
9. Engelson S, Ehrhardt J, Kepp T, Niemeijer J, Schierholz S, Berkel L et al. Comparison of anatomical priors for learning-based neural network guidance for mediastinal lymph node segmentation. Proc SPIE MI. 2024:1292719.
10. Kepka L, Bujko K, Garmol D, Palucki J, Zolciak-Siwinska A, Guzel-Szczepiorkowska Z et al. Delineation variation of lymph node stations for treatment planning in lung cancer radiotherapy. Radiother Oncol. 2007;85(3):450–5.
11. Lynch R, Pitson G, Ball D, Claude L, Sarrut D. Computed tomographic atlas for the new international lymph node map for lung cancer: a radiation oncologist perspective. Pract Radiat Oncol. 2013;3(1):54–66.
12. Wasserthal J, Breit HC, Meyer MT, Pradella M, Hinck D, Sauter AW et al. Totalsegmentator: robust segmentation of 104 anatomic structures in CT images. Radiol Artif Intell. 2023;5(5):e230024.
13. Roth HR, Lu L, Seff A, Cherry KM, Hoffman J, Wang S et al. A new 2.5D representation for lymph node detection using random sets of deep convolutional neural network observations. Proc MICCAI. 2014:520–7.
14. Bouget D, Pedersen A, Vanel J, Leira HO, Langø T. Mediastinal lymph nodes segmentation using 3D convolutional neural network ensembles and anatomical priors guiding. Comput Methods Biomech Biomed Engin. 2022;11:44–58.

15. Bakr S, Gevaert O, Echegaray S, Ayers K, Zhou M, Shafiq M et al. A radiogenomic dataset of non-small cell lung cancer. Sci Data. 2018;5:180202.
16. Arita T, Matsumoto T, Kuramitsu T, Kawamura M, Matsunaga N, Sugi K et al. Is it possible to differentiate malignant mediastinal nodes from benign nodes by size? reevaluation by CT, transesophageal echocardiography, and nodal specimen. Chest. 1996;110(4):1004–8.
17. Prenzel KL, Mönig SP, Sinning JM, Baldus SE, Brochhagen HG, Schneider PM et al. Lymph node size and metastatic infiltration in non-small cell lung cancer. Chest. 2003;123(2):463–7.
18. Wu Y, Li P, Zhang H, Shi Y, Wu H, Zhang J et al. Diagnostic value of fluorine 18 fluorodeoxyglucose positron emission tomography/computed tomography for the detection of metastases in non-small-cell lung cancer patients. Int J Cancer. 2013;132(2):E37–E47.
19. Gatidis S, Hepp T, Früh M, La Fougère C, Nikolaou K, Pfannenberg C et al. A whole-body FDG-PET/CT dataset with manually annotated tumor lesions. Sci Data. 2022;9(1):601.

Breast MRI Evaluation with Weakly-informed Slice-level Explanation

BE-WISE

Adarsh Bhandary Panambur [1†], Tri-Thien Nguyen [1,2†], Siming Bayer [1,3], Andreas Maier [1]

[1]Pattern Recognition Lab, Friedrich-Alexander-University Erlangen-Nuremberg, Erlangen, Germany
[2]Radiological Institute, University Clinic Erlangen, Erlangen, Germany
[3]Siemens Healthineers, Erlangen, Germany
adarsh.bhandary.panambur@fau.de

Abstract. Breast MRI provides superior soft-tissue contrast and lesion conspicuity compared to mammography but its large-scale deployment is hampered by the need for fine-grained annotations. We propose BE-WISE, a transformer-based framework for interpretable breast MRI classification that jointly learns breast-level diagnosis and slice-level lesion localization from minimal radiologist input. The approach integrates a Swin transformer backbone into an attention-based multiple-instance learning scheme and optimizes a unified Gaussian-based objective that couples global and local supervision. On the multicenter ODELIA Breast MRI dataset, BE-WISE with focal loss attains a test AUC of 0.8683 and an Odelia score of 0.7098, improving over the medical slice transformer baseline by more than 7% in AUC and 14% in odelia score. Slice-wise prediction profiles align with expert-indicated lesion slices, supporting the interpretability of the model. These findings indicate that weak, slice-level expert guidance can substantially enhance diagnostic performance and enable human-in-the-loop AI for breast MRI.

1 Introduction

Breast cancer is the most common malignancy in women, affecting roughly one in twenty globally, with an estimated 2.3 million new cases and 670,000 deaths each year [1, 2]. Mammography is currently regarded as the standard imaging modality for population-based breast cancer screening. However, its sensitivity decreases significantly in women with dense breast tissue, where lesions may be masked by fibroglandular structures. In such cases, breast magnetic resonance imaging (MRI) serves as an alternative or supplementary modality due to its superior soft-tissue contrast and ability to detect occult lesions. Although breast MRI improves diagnostic

†These authors contributed equally to this work.

© Der/die Autor(en), exklusiv lizenziert an
Springer Fachmedien Wiesbaden GmbH, ein Teil von Springer Nature 2026
H. Handels et al. (Hrsg.), *Bildverarbeitung für die Medizin 2026*,
Informatik aktuell, https://doi.org/10.1007/978-3-658-51100-5_2

accuracy in dense breast populations, it remains more expensive and time-consuming compared to mammography and is therefore used predominantly for diagnostic purposes rather than for screening [3]. Over the past decade, artificial intelligence (AI) and deep learning (DL) techniques have shown considerable promise in advancing breast cancer detection and diagnosis using breast MRI [4]. Nevertheless, developing robust DL models for this task remains difficult due to the need for precise lesion- or voxel-level annotations across three-dimensional MRI volumes. The complexity of volumetric acquisition and inter-sequence variability further hinders large-scale, high-quality dataset curation necessary for reliable model training and validation.

Recent studies, such as the medical slice transformer [5], highlight the efficacy of pretrained 2D feature extractors for case-level breast MRI classification. Hirsch et al. [6] showed that large, well-annotated datasets enable strong diagnostic performance even with simple architectures, while Oviedo et al. [7] proposed an explainable anomaly detection framework that identifies malignancies without lesion-level labels. However, most existing methods still overlook the complementary diagnostic information within dynamic contrast-enhanced MRI sequences. The combination of pre-contrast, post-contrast, and subtraction images captures essential morphological and temporal enhancement patterns, with early enhancement serving as a key malignancy biomarker [8]. However, temporal variability across institutions due to differences in protocols, contrast timing, and acquisition parameters [9] limits model generalization in multicenter settings. Furthermore, most existing methods rely solely on image-level analysis, neglecting auxiliary clinical or radiological cues and failing to leverage complementary diagnostic information from dynamic contrast-enhanced MRI.

In this work, we address dynamic contrast-enhanced (DCE) T1-weighted breast MRI using pre-contrast, earliest post-contrast, and subtraction volumes, guided by a single radiologist-marked slice per exam as minimal supervision. The proposed BEWISE framework couples a Swin transformer with attention-based multiple-instance learning and a unified Gaussian objective to jointly learn breast-level diagnosis and slice-level lesion localization, improving robustness across heterogeneous MRI protocols. Our contributions are: (i) a multi-sequence, Swin-transformer-based pipeline that achieves accurate and interpretable breast MRI classification from sparse expert input; (ii) a unified Gaussian-based supervision objective that links global and slice-level signals for joint optimization; and (iii) evidence that adding even one lesion-indicative slice markedly boosts diagnostic performance, enabling a practical human-in-the-loop refinement workflow.

2 Materials and methods

2.1 Dataset description and preprocessing pipeline

We use the ODELIA Breast MRI Challenge 2025 dataset [10], consisting of 500 dynamic contrast-enhanced breast MRI cases from multiple European institutions. Each breast was labeled as normal, benign, or malignant, yielding 1,000 breasts split into 814 training, 102 validation, and 104 test samples via stratified sampling to maintain class and institutional balance. The dataset composition is approximately 67% normal, 13% benign, and 20% malignant. A board-certified radiologist with over five years of experience additionally provided rapid annotations for benign and malignant cases, identifying a representative slice suspected to contain the lesion, based on ODELIA reference labels. The BreastDivider model [11] was used to automatically segment and crop left and right breast regions from whole-body MRI volumes. Given the clinical importance of early enhancement for lesion assessment and the variability in contrast timing across institutions, three sequences were used for model training: pre-contrast, early post-contrast, and subtraction. Subtraction volumes were generated by subtracting pre-contrast images from the latest available post-contrast phase, thereby incorporating delayed enhancement and washout information into the input representation. Each breast volume was resampled to 32 axial slices at 224×224 resolution. For each slice, pre-contrast, late post-contrast, and subtraction images were stacked as three-channel inputs, with subtraction computed after geometric alignment of sequences. Image intensities were min-max normalized per channel and per sample to reduce scanner- and subject-level variability.

2.2 Method

Figure 1 shows the proposed Swin-based framework for weakly supervised breast MRI analysis. The pre-contrast, late post-contrast, and subtraction sequences are stacked to form an input tensor of size $(B, 32, 3, 224, 224)$. Each slice is processed by a shared Swin-tiny transformer [12], generating contextual embeddings of dimension $(B, 32, 768)$. The model comprises two key modules: (1) slice-level lesion predictor, which performs weak localization of lesion-containing slices using

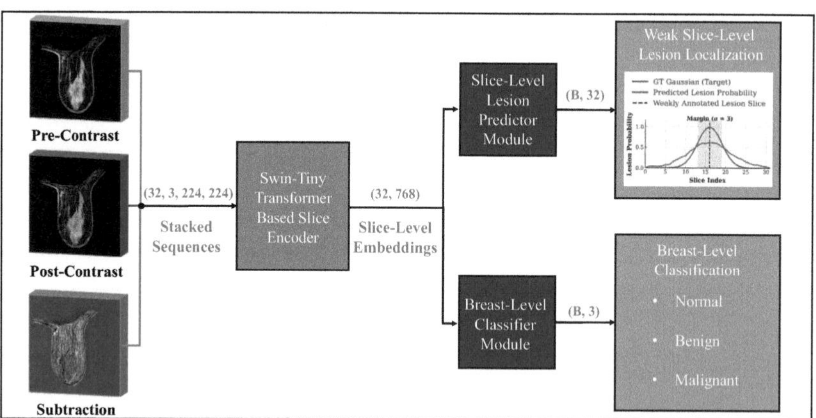

Fig. 1. Overview of the proposed framework. Pre-, post-, and subtraction MRI sequences are stacked and encoded using a shared Swin-tiny transformer to produce slice-level embeddings. The slice-level lesion predictor estimates weak lesion probabilities per slice, while the breast-level classifier aggregates embeddings for global diagnosis.

Tab. 1. Classification performance on the test dataset.

Model	Test AUC	Odelia score
Med-Slice Transformer (CE)[5]	0.7968 (0.019)	0.5695 (0.026)
Breast-Level Classifier Module only (CE)	0.8147 (0.007)	0.5899 (0.025)
Breast-Level Classifier Module (Focal)	0.8447 (0.002)	0.6629 (0.010)
BE-WISE (CE)	0.8580 (0.002)	0.6810 (0.04)
BE-WISE (Focal)	**0.8683 (0.014)**	**0.7098 (0.02)**

radiologist-provided reference annotations, and (2) breast-level classifier, which aggregates slice embeddings to predict the overall diagnostic category (normal, benign, or malignant). Together, these components enable joint slice-level lesion localization and breast-level classification in a unified method.

2.2.1 Slice-level lesion predictor module. The slice-level lesion predictor (SLP) operates on the encoded slice embeddings to estimate the probability of each slice containing a lesion. Each slice feature vector is processed through a lightweight multilayer perceptron consisting of Layer Normalization, a linear projection, GELU activation, dropout, and a final linear layer followed by a sigmoid activation, producing slice-wise probabilities of shape $(B, 32)$ for each breast volume. For benign and malignant cases, weak supervision is derived from radiologist-provided lesion slice indices. To model spatial uncertainty along the axial dimension, a Gaussian target distribution is generated as

$$t_i = \exp\left(-\frac{(i - s_0)^2}{2\sigma^2}\right), \quad i \in [1, S] \tag{1}$$

where t_i denotes the target value for the i-th slice, s_0 is the annotated lesion slice index, S is the total number of slices per breast, and σ is the Gaussian margin controlling the spread of the supervision. The distribution is normalized such that $\max_i t_i = 1$. For normal cases, all target values are set to zero. The slice-level localization loss is computed using binary cross-entropy between predicted probabilities and Gaussian targets. This formulation enables weak slice-level lesion localization while maintaining stability against uncertain or coarse annotations.

2.2.2 Breast-level classifier module. The breast-level classifier aggregates slice embeddings using an attention-based pooling mechanism inspired by the attention-based multiple instance learning (ABMIL) framework [13]. Two learnable linear projections generate attention scores that are normalized through a softmax operation, assigning higher weights to diagnostically relevant slices while suppressing non-informative regions. The weighted aggregation of slice embeddings yields a compact breast-level representation, which is subsequently normalized, regularized with dropout, and passed through a linear classifier to produce three-class logits corresponding to normal, benign, and malignant categories.

2.2.3 Loss function. The network is trained with a joint objective combining breast-level classification and slice-level localization losses

$$\mathcal{L}_{\text{total}} = \alpha\, \mathcal{L}_{\text{global}} + (1 - \alpha)\, \mathcal{L}_{\text{slice}} \tag{2}$$

where $\mathcal{L}_{\text{global}}$ can be either a cross-entropy loss or focal loss for breast-level diagnosis, and $\mathcal{L}_{\text{slice}}$ is the binary cross-entropy (CE) loss between predicted slice probabilities and Gaussian targets centered at the annotated lesion slice. The margin parameter σ controls the spread of the Gaussian, balancing precise and broader lesion localization. The loss is designed with the intuition that lesions manifest across varying local regions in consecutive slices. The weighting factor α governs the trade-off between global classification and slice-level supervision. By jointly optimizing these losses, the model effectively integrates localized lesion cues with global contextual information, potentially enhancing diagnostic robustness and interpretability.

3 Results and discussion

All experiments were repeated with multiple random seeds with mean and standard deviation reported for assessing the stability. Performance was assessed using the area under the ROC curve (AUC) micro and the odelia score. While AUC reflects overall discrimination, it overlooks clinically relevant thresholds. Therefore, sensitivity at 90 % specificity and specificity at 90 % sensitivity were additionally computed, and averaged together with AUC to form the odelia score [10]. For focal loss-based experiments, we explore various gamma values and report the best test results (γ=0.5 in our case) based on the validation performance. Tab 1 shows the classification performance on the test dataset and subsequently discuss the absolute gains of our proposed approach. Relative to the medical slice transformer (MST) baseline [5], replacing it with our breast-level classifier already yields a clear improvement, increasing test AUC by about 1.8% and odelia score by about 2%. This confirms that a dedicated breast-level aggregation tailored to our dataset is more effective than the generic slice-to-patient sequence modeling of MST. Furthermore,

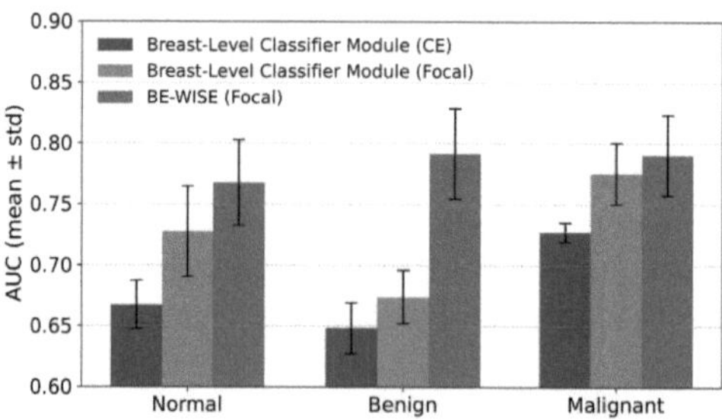

Fig. 2. Per-class AUC performance on the test set for: the breast-level classifier module with cross-entropy (CE), breast-level classifier module with focal, and BE-WISE with focal loss.

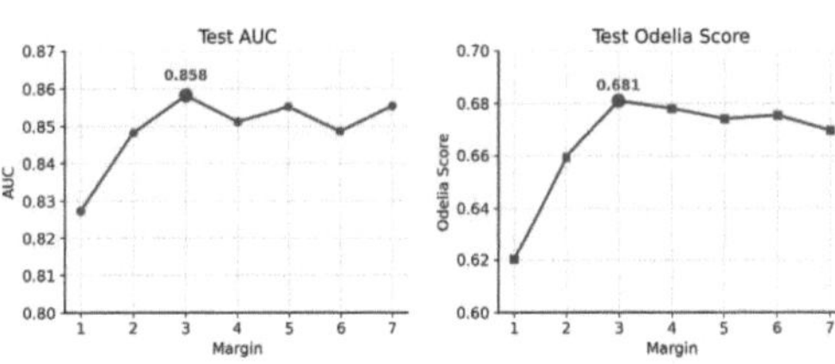

Fig. 3. Effect of margin parameter (σ) on test performance while using cross entropy loss. Performance peaks at σ=3, where moderate smoothing enhances robustness, while larger margins lead to over-smoothing and reduced precision.

given the pronounced class imbalance in our cohort, applying focal loss instead of cross-entropy to the same breast-level classifier leads to a further AUC increase of about 3% and a substantially larger odelia score gain of about 7%, indicating that down-weighting easy negatives improves calibration of clinically relevant positives. On top of this, integrating the slice-level guidance module and jointly learning with both breast-level and slice-aware signals (our BE-WISE architecture) improves over the focal-loss breast-level classifier by more than 1% in AUC and 2% in odelia score, showing that even weak lesion-location supervision provides complementary information to global labels. Finally, using focal loss also within BE-WISE yields an additional improvement of about 1 percentage point in AUC and about 3% in odelia, and these gains were confirmed to be statistically significant ($p < 0.001$ for AUC; $p < 0.01$ for odelia), demonstrating that focal re-weighting and slice-level supervision provides strong classification support to the network.

Figure 2 shows the per-class AUC performance comparing the breast-level classifier module trained with cross-entropy, the breast-level classifier module trained with focal loss, and the proposed BE-WISE framework with focal loss. BE-WISE improves discrimination across all classes despite pronounced class imbalance. For normal cases, which are critical in screening and lack lesion-centered cues, BE-WISE achieves higher AUC, indicating that the model reliably recognizes the absence of suspicious findings. Notably, the most pronounced improvement is observed for benign cases, where BE-WISE substantially outperforms breast-level baselines, while malignant cases also show consistent gains, demonstrating improved recognition of lesion-related patterns that are insufficiently captured by classification-only models. Figure 3 shows the sensitivity of BE-WISE to the margin parameter σ, which controls the spread of Gaussian supervision during slice-level training. Both AUC and odelia score peak at σ=3, indicating that moderate smoothing improves robustness, while larger values cause over-smoothing and reduced localization precision.

Figure 4 shows slice-wise prediction distributions for correctly and incorrectly classified cases, illustrating BE-WISE's interpretability. Each plot presents lesion probabilities across 32 slices with the radiologist-annotated slice indicated by a Gaussian prior. Correct cases show aligned peaks, reflecting accurate localization under weak supervision, while misclassified ones exhibit flatter or shifted activations from subtle enhancements or artifacts. Normal cases maintain uniformly low responses, demonstrating that BE-WISE achieves strong diagnostic accuracy with inherent spatial interpretability and implicit lesion localization without voxel-level labels.

The use of a single annotated slice provides only approximate lesion guidance, and a detailed analysis of annotation variability, lesion extent, or lesion-size-dependent performance is beyond the scope of this work. In a clinical reporting setting, BE-WISE is intended to function as an assistive cue rather than an automated decision system. By highlighting slices most relevant to the breast-level prediction through slice-level probability profiles, the model enables radiologists to quickly verify, correct, or disregard its suggestions during routine interpretation. When available, such minimal expert feedback can be incorporated as weak supervision in subsequent training cycles, enabling a lightweight human-in-the-loop refinement process without requiring voxel-level annotations. The proposed BE-WISE model establishes a robust and interpretable baseline for weakly supervised breast MRI analysis. Using minimal slice-level annotations, it improves diagnostic accuracy while preserving spatial interpretability, supporting scalable AI-assisted breast cancer screening. Future work will extend the framework to semi-supervised and active learning settings with expert-in-the-loop refinement. We aim to extend this work by making the margin parameter learnable, enabling adaptive Gaussian supervision that dynamically adjusts to lesion characteristics rather than relying on

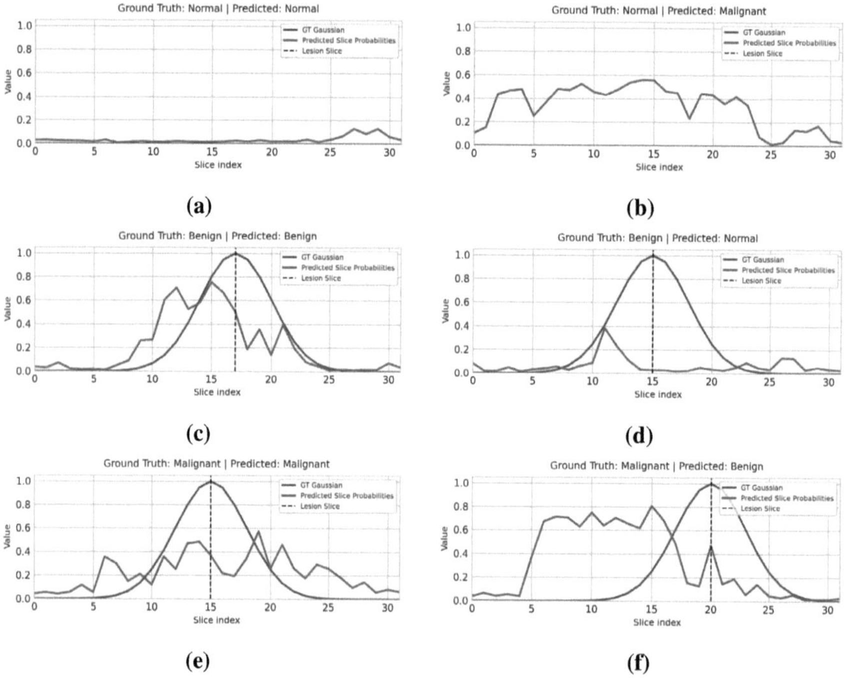

Fig. 4. Illustrative slice-level prediction profiles for breast MRI cases. The left column shows correctly classified cases and the right column shows misclassified cases. Predicted slice-level probabilities (red) are shown alongside the Gaussian lesion prior (green); the dashed line indicates the radiologist-annotated lesion slice, which is absent for normal cases.

manually tuned hyperparameters. In addition, radiologist-led evaluations will be incorporated to quantitatively assess localization reliability and validate the clinical applicability of the proposed framework.

Acknowledgement. The authors thank the creators and organizers of the ODELIA Breast MRI dataset [10]. The authors gratefully acknowledge the scientific support and HPC resources provided by the Erlangen national high performance computing center (NHR@FAU) of the Friedrich-Alexander-Universität Erlangen-Nürnberg (FAU). The hardware is funded by the german research foundation (DFG).

References

1. Sung H, Ferlay J, Siegel RL, Laversanne M, Soerjomataram I, Jemal A et al. Global cancer statistics 2020: GLOBOCAN estimates of incidence and mortality worldwide for 36 cancers in 185 countries. CA Cancer J Clin. 2021;71(3):209–49.
2. Kim J, Harper A, McCormack V, Sung H, Houssami N, Morgan E et al. Global patterns and trends in breast cancer incidence and mortality across 185 countries. Nat Med. 2025;31(4):1154–62.
3. Wekking D, Porcu M, De Silva P, Saba L, Scartozzi M, Solinas C. Breast MRI: clinical indications, recommendations, and future applications in breast cancer diagnosis. Curr Oncol Rep. 2023;25(4):257–67.
4. Lo Gullo R, Brunekreef J, Marcus E, Han LK, Eskreis-Winkler S, Thakur SB et al. AI applications to breast MRI: today and tomorrow. J Magn Reson Imaging. 2024;60(6):2290–308.
5. Müller-Franzes G, Khader F, Siepmann R, Han T, Kather JN, Nebelung S et al. Medical slice transformer for improved diagnosis and explainability on 3D medical images with DINOv2. Sci Rep. 2025;15(1):23979.
6. Hirsch L, Sutton EJ, Huang Y, Kayis B, Hughes M, Martinez D et al. High-performance open-source AI for breast cancer detection and localization in MRI. Radiol Artif Intell. 2025;7(5):e240550.
7. Oviedo F, Kazerouni AS, Liznerski P, Xu Y, Hirano M, Vandermeulen RA et al. Cancer detection in breast MRI screening via explainable AI anomaly detection. Radiology. 2025;316(1):e241629.
8. Macura KJ, Ouwerkerk R, Jacobs MA, Bluemke DA. Patterns of enhancement on breast MR images: interpretation and imaging pitfalls. RadioGraphics. 2006;26(6):1719–34.
9. Mann RM, Cho N, Moy L. Breast MRI: state of the art. Radiology. 2019;292(3):520–36.
10. Escudero Sánchez L, Müller-Franzes G, Saldanha O, Payne N, Abdullah K bin, Zhang T et al. ODELIA breast MRI challenge 2025. Zenodo, 2025.
11. Rokuss M, Hamm B, Kirchhoff Y, Maier-Hein K. Divide and conquer: A large-scale dataset and model for left–right breast MRI segmentation. arXiv preprint: 2507.13830. 2025.
12. Liu Z, Lin Y, Cao Y, Hu H, Wei Y, Zhang Z et al. Swin transformer: hierarchical vision transformer using shifted windows. Proc IEEE/CVF ICCV. 2021:10012–22.
13. Ilse M, Tomczak J, Welling M. Attention-based deep multiple instance learning. Proc ICML. 2018:2127–36.

Abstract: Investigation of Class Separability within Object Detection Models in Histopathology

Jonas Ammeling [1], Jonathan Ganz [2], Frauke Wilm [2], Katharina Breininger [3], Marc Aubreville [4]

[1]Technische Hochschule Ingolstadt, Ingolstadt, Germany
[2]MIRA vision Microscopy GmbH, Göppingen, Germany
[3]Center for AI and Data Science, Julius-Maximilians-Universität Würzburg, Würzburg, Germany
[4]Flensburg University of Applied Sciences, Flensburg, Germany
jonas.ammeling@thi.de

Object detection is central to histopathological image analysis, yet standard metrics (e.g. AP, F1-score) reveal little about where and why models fail, especially under domain shifts across scanners, tissues, or laboratories. In this study [1], we propose a quantitative, non-invasive framework to assess and class separability directly in the latent spaces of dense, fully convolutional object detectors with local correspondences. By aggregating object-level activations into size-invariant descriptors and computing separability per layer, our method reveals how discrimination emerges, propagates, or collapses within backbone, feature pyramid network (FPN), and detection heads. We adapt two metrics: an adapted generalized discrimination value (aGDV), contrasting inter- vs. intra-class distances, and a hellinger distance-based discrimination value (HDV), quantifying distribution overlap via the Bhattacharyya coefficient with variance-based channel selection and adaptive binning. On three real world datasets covering mitotic figure detection and multi-class cell detection, separability is modest in early backbone layers, increases through deeper backbone and FPN, and peaks in detection heads aligned with the relevant object scale. Layer-wise HDV further differentiates domains with good generalization from those with severe domain shift and reflects class-specific confusion in multi-class settings. The framework provides actionable guidance for architecture and training decisions, indicating where discrimination is gained or lost, the impact of multi-domain training, stain augmentation, or self-supervised learning.

References

1. Ammeling J, Ganz J, Wilm F, Breininger K, Aubreville M. Investigation of class separability within object detection models in histopathology. IEEE Trans Med Imaging. 2025;44:3162–74.

© Der/die Autor(en), exklusiv lizenziert an
Springer Fachmedien Wiesbaden GmbH, ein Teil von Springer Nature 2026
H. Handels et al. (Hrsg.), *Bildverarbeitung für die Medizin 2026*,
Informatik aktuell, https://doi.org/10.1007/978-3-658-51100-5_3

Self-supervised Dual-domain Swin Transformer for Sparse-view CT Reconstruction

DuDoSwin

Bipin Yadav, Adarsh Raghunath, Franziska Weber, Andreas Maier

Pattern Recognition Lab, Friedrich-Alexander-Universität Erlangen-Nürnberg (FAU), Germany
bipin.yadav@fau.de

Abstract. Sparse-view computed tomography (CT) reconstruction suffers from streak artifacts and loss of fine detail after filtered back-projection (FBP). To alleviate these issues, we propose a self-supervised dual-domain swin transformer (DuDoSwin) that performs sinogram angular super-resolution and image-domain refinement, connected via a differentiable FBP bridge for end-to-end optimization. On the AAPM Low-Dose CT dataset, DuDoSwin achieves superior reconstruction quality and perceptual fidelity compared to existing learning-based and interpolation-based methods, improving quantitative (PSNR/SSIM/LPIPS) metrics under severe angular undersampling (4×, 8×, 16×). By jointly modeling projection and image domains, the proposed dual-domain design restores sharp anatomical structures and enhances perceptual quality, contributing to higher-quality low-dose CT reconstruction. The implementation is available at `https://github.com/bipin-y-lab/DuDoSwin`.

1 Introduction

Computed tomography (CT) remains a cornerstone of diagnostic imaging, yet the ionizing radiation involved poses inherent risks, creating a persistent trade-off between image quality and patient safety. Reducing radiation dose by lowering tube current or performing angular undersampling degrades photon statistics and introduces artifacts in filtered back-projection (FBP) reconstructions, ultimately compromising diagnostic fidelity.

Traditional analytic methods such as frequency-consistency-based sinogram completion [1] and modified FBP algorithms for sparse-view acquisition [2] offered early insights into mitigating information loss under limited-angle constraints. More recently, differentiable physics-driven reconstruction frameworks, e.g., DRACO [3], have enabled end-to-end gradient propagation through the imaging pipeline, supporting arbitrary geometries and improving adaptability across diverse acquisition trajectories. Meanwhile, the prompted contextual transformer (ProCT) [4] was introduced for incomplete-view CT reconstruction, addressing both sparse-view and

© Der/die Autor(en), exklusiv lizenziert an
Springer Fachmedien Wiesbaden GmbH, ein Teil von Springer Nature 2026
H. Handels et al. (Hrsg.), *Bildverarbeitung für die Medizin 2026*,
Informatik aktuell, https://doi.org/10.1007/978-3-658-51100-5_4

limited-angle settings. The method incorporates a projection-view aware prompting mechanism to inform the network of specific acquisition patterns, and an artifact-aware contextual module that learns from paired image contexts to recognize and correct diverse unseen artifact structures. In our work, we adopt ProCT (image-domain) as a strong baseline.

In addition, learning-based strategies have sought to bridge the dose-quality gap by coupling data-driven priors with physical models. Dual-domain architectures such as DuDo-Trans [5] demonstrate that jointly learning in projection and image domains improves information consistency, while Self-supervised dual-domain denoising schemes reduce reliance on paired supervision [6]. Complementary Generative (cycle-consistent) approaches have also been explored for unsupervised super-resolution in X-ray imaging modalities [7].

We present a self-supervised Dual-Domain Swin Transformer architecture for sparse-view CT reconstruction. The proposed model operates in two stages: (i) Refinement of low-resolution (LR) sinogram by a Swin module followed by angular super-resolution (SR) using a residual upsampler with a bicubic skip connection, which is then reconstructed via differentiable FBP, and (ii) Reconstructed image refinement using a Swin module.

Our working hypothesis is that explicitly restoring missing angular information in the projection domain, followed by image-domain refinement, reduces view-aliasing streaks and improves reconstruction quality under severe angular undersampling.

1.1 Contributions

- We propose a dual-domain pipeline (sinogram angular super-resolution $\longrightarrow$ differentiable FBP $\longrightarrow$ image refinement) that supports end-to-end training while remaining parameter-efficient, using 1.36–1.80 M trainable parameters depending on the upsampling factor (ProCT baseline: 6.5 M in our setup).
- We evaluate on the AAPM Low-Dose CT dataset and achieve quantitative improvements: 45.64 dB PSNR / 0.981 SSIM / 0.011 LPIPS at 4×, 44.11 dB / 0.975 / 0.020 at 8×, and 42.02 dB / 0.963 / 0.035 at 16× (Tab. 1).

2 Materials and methods

2.1 DuDoSwin model

Fig. 1 illustrates the complete processing pipeline of DuDoSwin. Let $X_{\mathrm{LR}} \in \mathbb{R}^{1 \times H_\theta/s \times W_d}$ denote a sparse-view sinogram with H_θ/s angular views and W_d detector elements. An initial convolutional head and Swin-based feature extraction module with window size ω generate intermediate feature representations [8]. These features are processed by a Residual SinoUpsampler that employs PixelShuffle along the angular dimension combined with a bicubic skip connection, producing the super-resolved sinogram $\hat{X}_{\mathrm{SR}}$. A scan-specific differentiable FBP operator reconstructs the initial image Y_0, which is subsequently refined by a Swin module to produce the final output $\hat{Y}$. A global 1×1 residual connection preserves low-frequency image content throughout the refinement stage.

The Swin module (Fig. 2) implements windowed self-attention with bilateral-style guidance for edge-aware refinement. This design allows the network to sharpen anatomical structures while controlling noise amplification, particularly important in regions where FBP reconstruction introduces artifacts.

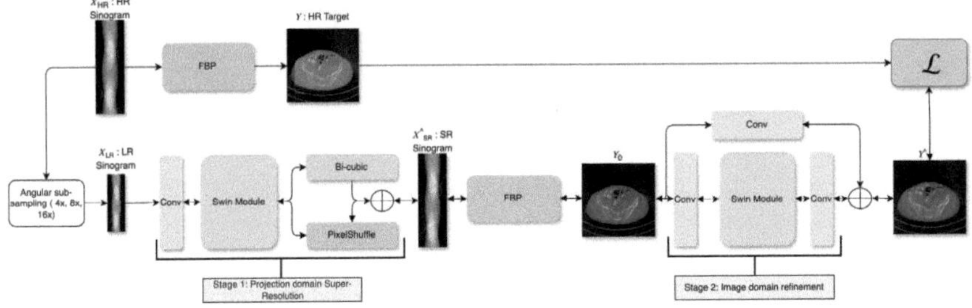

Fig. 1. Overview of the proposed DuDoSwin pipeline for sparse-view CT reconstruction. In Stage 1 (Projection domain), the low-view sinogram is processed by a Swin-based feature extractor and upsampled angularly using PixelShuffle with a bicubic skip connection to recover missing projection views. A differentiable FBP layer then reconstructs an initial image Y_0. In Stage 2 (Image domain), a Swin module further enhances anatomical details and suppresses streak artifacts, producing the final reconstruction $\hat{Y}$.

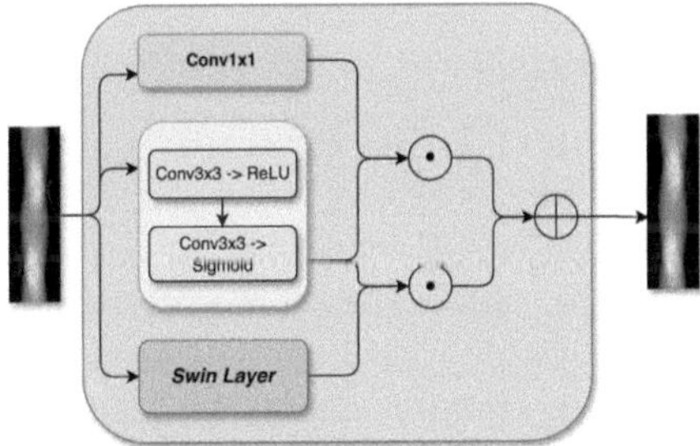

Fig. 2. Illustration of the proposed Swin Module, which integrates convolutional local filtering with transformer-based global reasoning. The Conv1×1 block (top-left) represents a lightweight convolutional branch $S(x)$ that preserves local spatial detail. The guidance branch (center) consists of two 3×3 convolutions with ReLU and Sigmoid activations, producing a learnable gating map $g(x)$ that adaptively balances local and global features. The Swin layer (bottom-left) corresponds to $F_{\text{swin}}(x)$, implemented using a BasicLayer-a hierarchical Swin Transformer block comprising window-based multi-head self-attention with cyclic shift and MLP sublayers operating on flattened feature tokens. The outputs of the convolutional and Swin branches are fused through adaptive gated blending, where $g(x)$ modulates the contribution of each path using element-wise multiplications ($\odot$). The final output is computed as: $y = g(x) \odot F_{\text{swin}}(x) + (1 - g(x)) \odot S(x)$, yielding a convex combination of transformer-derived global context and convolution-based local structure.

2.2 Losses and metrics

We minimize a HU-aware weighted sum of L_1 and MSE on reconstructions $\hat{Y}$ and targets Y in Hounsfield units (HU), respectively. The total training loss is

$$\mathcal{L} = \alpha \frac{\|\hat{Y} - Y\|_1}{100} + \beta \frac{\|\hat{Y} - Y\|_2^2}{10000} \tag{1}$$

with α=1.0 and β=0.1.

L_1 and L_2-type reconstruction losses are widely used in CT restoration, with complementary behavior (detail preservation vs. penalizing large errors), recent LDCT work discusses these tradeoffs [9], and some modern approaches explicitly combine L_1 and L_2 terms [10].

We normalize the training loss by scaling HU error terms with fixed constants to improve numerical stability (preventing overflow in mixed-precision squared-error computations and reducing excessive gradient clipping). All reported metrics (PSNR/SSIM/LPIPS) are computed on raw HU with a fixed dynamic range of 4000 HU (window $[-1000, 3000]$), making PSNR a monotonic transform of HU-MSE: $\text{MSE}_{\text{HU}} = 4000^2/10^{\text{PSNR}/10}$ and $\text{RMSE}_{\text{HU}} = 4000/10^{\text{PSNR}/20}$. For reference, our DuDoSwin PSNR values correspond to RMSE of approximately 20.9 HU (4×), 24.9 HU (8×), and 31.7 HU (16×) under this fixed range. LPIPS is computed after clipping to $[-1000, 3000]$ and mapping to $[-1, 1]$.

We selected (α, β) via a small validation sweep (PSNR at 16×): $(1.0, 0.1)$ achieved 40.69 dB vs. 40.33 dB $(1.0, 0.01)$, 40.25 dB $(1.0, 0.05)$, and 39.29 dB $(0.5, 0.1)$.

2.3 Dataset and training details

We use the AAPM Low-Dose CT dataset (AAPM Low-Dose CT Grand Challenge, `http://www.aapm.org/GrandChallenge/LowDoseCT/`), which provides clinical abdominal CT scans together with fan-beam projection geometry metadata (projection angles, DSO, DDO, detector pitch d_u). We perform a patient-wise split with 7 training patients (1173 slices) and 3 held-out patients (511 slices); one held-out patient (139 slices) is used for validation/model selection. Due to limited data, we report slice-wise statistics aggregated over all held-out patients. Sparse-view sinograms are synthesized by uniform angular subsampling with $s \in \{4, 8, 16\}$ while preserving detector sampling. Projections are standardized to a consistent orientation and detector alignment, converted to single precision, and reconstructed into HU targets using a fan-beam FBP implementation with a Hann filter and spatial resolution of 256×256 pixels.

DuDoSwin is implemented in PyTorch and trained for 10 epochs on an NVIDIA Quadro RTX 8000 using mixed precision (avg. per-epoch time ~45 min). ProCT is used as our primary baseline and is trained for 50 epochs on the same split (avg. per-epoch time ~6 min). Results are reported as mean ± standard deviation over all evaluated test slices (Tab. 1); we report slice-wise variability rather than multi-seed averaging due to compute constraints. Trainable parameters for DuDoSwin scale with the upsampling factor: 1.36 M (4×), 1.51 M (8×), 1.80 M (16×).

Tab. 1. Quantitative results (mean ± std over test slices) for angular super-resolution at 4×, 8×, and 16×.

Scale	Method	PSNR ↑ [dB]	SSIM ↑	LPIPS ↓	Time [ms] ↓
4×	Ours (DuDoSwin)	**45.64 ± 1.47**	**0.981 ± 0.006**	**0.011 ± 0.003**	**396.81 ± 1.01**
4×	ProCT	45.50 ± 0.80	0.979 ± 0.003	0.026 ± 0.010	107.10 ± 7.91
4×	FBP	40.65 ± 1.08	0.958 ± 0.013	0.029 ± 0.013	6.67 ± 1.28
4×	Bilinear	40.10 ± 0.93	0.963 ± 0.010	0.017 ± 0.008	7.03 ± 1.31
4×	Bicubic	39.70 ± 0.91	0.958 ± 0.011	0.023 ± 0.010	7.07 ± 1.30
8×	Ours (DuDoSwin)	**44.11 ± 1.29**	**0.975 ± 0.007**	**0.020 ± 0.006**	**268.92 ± 0.95**
8×	ProCT	42.88 ± 1.00	0.970 ± 0.005	0.037 ± 0.013	102.94 ± 7.71
8×	FBP	37.45 ± 1.10	0.894 ± 0.024	0.089 ± 0.027	6.00 ± 0.79
8×	Bilinear	37.28 ± 1.02	0.936 ± 0.014	0.036 ± 0.014	6.64 ± 0.80
8×	Bicubic	36.83 ± 1.00	0.928 ± 0.016	0.041 ± 0.016	6.64 ± 0.81
16×	Ours (DuDoSwin)	**42.02 ± 1.18**	**0.963 ± 0.009**	**0.035 ± 0.010**	**451.89 ± 2.93**
16×	ProCT	39.65 ± 1.35	0.950 ± 0.010	0.051 ± 0.015	105.32 ± 14.04
16×	Bilinear	33.99 ± 1.07	0.880 ± 0.020	0.090 ± 0.023	7.84 ± 1.07
16×	Bicubic	33.61 ± 1.06	0.869 ± 0.022	0.090 ± 0.026	7.84 ± 1.10
16×	FBP	33.14 ± 0.95	0.753 ± 0.035	0.212 ± 0.031	7.12 ± 1.11

3 Results

Tab. 1 and Fig. 3 summarize quantitative and qualitative results across 4×, 8×, and 16×. At 4×, interpolation and FBP baselines exhibit streaking and loss of angular detail, while ProCT tends to be smoother (slight over-regularization). DuDoSwin achieves the best overall fidelity (PSNR/SSIM) and the strongest perceptual score (LPIPS), consistently across sparsity levels. Runtime shows DuDoSwin is slower than ProCT and classical baselines, motivating acceleration strategies discussed below.

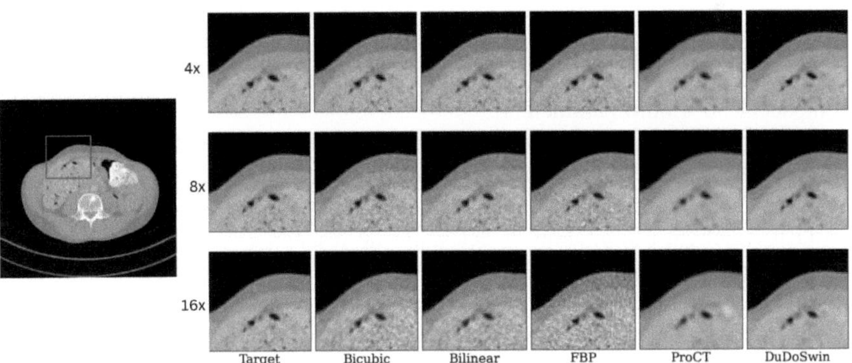

Fig. 3. Qualitative comparison at 4×, 8×, and 16× angular sparsity. These results are shown for a test patient slice and all methods are visualized using identical windowing.

Tab. 2. Ablation at 8× (3 epochs per variant): component-wise performance on the AAPM evaluation data split (511 slices; includes the validation patient). All trainable variants are trained from scratch using the same patient-wise split, loss, and optimizer/scheduler configuration. The checkpoint with the lowest validation loss is evaluated. Values are mean ± std PSNR over slices. Given the limited training budget, results indicate component trends rather than fully converged rankings.

Model Variant	Description	Params	PSNR ↑ [dB]
Full Model (Baseline)	Complete architecture with all components enabled	1.51M	42.01 ± 1.04
No Global Residual	Remove the global residual skip from the FBP reconstruction Y_0 to the final output	1.51M	42.57 ± 1.16
Simplified Upsampler	Remove the bicubic residual skip connection in the angular upsampler	1.47M	42.50 ± 1.14
Bicubic Upsampler	Replace the sinogram angular upsampler with fixed bicubic interpolation (projection domain)	1.17M	42.52 ± 1.17
No Image Swin	Bypass Swin Module in image domain with identity	0.74M	41.79 ± 1.11
No Sinogram Swin	Bypass Swin Module in sinogram domain with identity	1.10M	41.46 ± 0.98
No Swin Processing	Disable both sinogram and image Swin Modules	0.33M	39.49 ± 0.82
Baseline Interpolation	Non-learnable baseline: bicubic + FBP only (no training)	0.00M	36.96 ± 1.08

4 Discussion

Our results (Tab. 1; Fig. 3) support the working hypothesis that dual-domain learning (restoring missing angular information in the projection domain, followed by image-domain refinement) yields reconstructions that are perceptually sharper and structurally more consistent under severe sparse-view sampling. Across all undersampling factors, DuDoSwin provides stronger perceptual fidelity (LPIPS) and higher quantitative scores than ProCT and interpolation-based reconstructions, while remaining compact (1.36–1.80M parameters).

However, the sinogram angular upsampler can occasionally introduce faint streak artifacts along previously missing angular lines. A temporary mitigation was achieved by integrating a bicubic-upsampled residual into the network output. These artifacts highlight a limitation of deterministic reshaping operations in modeling view-correlated dependencies. Future research will explore learned anisotropic upsampling or implicit angular interpolation modules that jointly model spatial and angular correlations to infer missing projections more accurately.

Additionally, DuDoSwin is slower than ProCT (Tab. 1), motivating future acceleration through reduced model depth (fewer Swin blocks) and deployment-oriented optimizations (e.g., compilation and kernel fusion via torch.compile or ONNX/TensorRT).

Beyond this, future work will also focus on coupling the dual-domain Swin architecture with deep unrolling principles. Integrating DuDoSwin into an unrolled optimization framework would allow each projection-image iteration to emulate a physics-informed reconstruction step, combining the interpretability of iterative methods with the representational power of transformers. Such a "DuDoSwin-Unrolled" variant could further enforce data fidelity at every stage, reducing reliance on explicit supervision.

References

1. Pohlmann M, Berger M, Maier A, Hornegger J, Fahrig R. Estimation of missing fan-beam projections using frequency consistency conditions. Proc CT Meeting. 2014:203–7.
2. Wu M, Maier A, Yang Q, Fahrig R. A novel filtered backprojection-based algorithm for sparse-view CT image reconstruction. Proc Fully3D. 2015:202–5.
3. Ye C, Schneider LS, Sun Y, Thies M, Mei S, Maier A. DRACO: differentiable reconstruction for arbitrary CBCT orbits. arXiv: 2410.14900. 2024.
4. Ma C, Li Z, He J, Zhang J, Zhang Y, Shan H. Prompted contextual transformer for incomplete-view CT reconstruction. arXiv: 2312.07846. 2024.
5. Wang C, Shang K, Zhang H, Li Q, Hui Y, Zhou SK. DuDoTrans: dual-domain transformer provides more attention for sinogram restoration in sparse-view CT reconstruction. arXiv: 2111.10790. 2021.
6. Wagner F, Thies M, Pfaff L, Aust O, Pechmann S, Weidner D et al. On the benefit of dual-domain denoising in a self-supervised low-dose CT setting. Proc IEEE ISBI. 2023:1–5.
7. Raghunath A et al. Unsupervised super resolution in X-ray microscopy using a cycle-consistent generative model. Proc BVM. 2023:105–10.
8. Liu Z, Lin Y, Cao Y, Hu H, Wei Y, Zhang Z et al. Swin transformer: hierarchical vision transformer using shifted windows. arXiv: 2103.14030. 2021.
9. Li Q, Li S, Li R, Wu W, Dong Y, Zhao J et al. Low-dose computed tomography image reconstruction via a multistage convolutional neural network with autoencoder perceptual loss network. Quant Imaging Med Surg. 2022;12(3):1929–57.
10. Fang T, Hu J, He X, Yang J. MAN: latent diffusion enhanced multistage anti-noise network for efficient and high-quality low-dose CT image denoising. arXiv: 2509.23603. 2025.

How Predictable is the Human Body?

Predicting Organ Bounding Boxes With a Statistical Atlas Based on Four Keypoints

Temke Kohlbrandt [1], Kai Geissler [2], Stefan Heldmann [1]

[1]Fraunhofer MEVIS Lübeck
[2]Fraunhofer MEVIS Bremen
temke.kohlbrandt@mevis.fraunhofer.de

Abstract. Optimizing patient positioning during CT and MRI examinations is crucial to enhance imaging efficiency and reduce radiation exposure. This study explores the accuracy of bounding box prediction for internal body structures gained from statistical atlases based on four key points in comparison to a regression model. Therefore, we utilized a dataset including 10 828 whole-body MR volumes and extracted corresponding segmentation masks. We evaluated how effectively these boxes encompass the target structures, considering also the size. Our method yields results comparable to the regression model. However, it offers the advantage of rapid adaptability to diverse research questions, making it more flexible for various analytical scenarios.

1 Introduction

The initial step in any CT and MRI examination is to position the patient and the table to ensure that the target area is centered within the scanner's field of view. This process can consume a considerable portion of the overall procedure time and often necessitates additional navigation scans to confirm the patient's placement. Thus, optimizing table positioning can enhance the efficiency of imaging workflows in clinical settings and has the potential to reduce radiation dose by omitting navigation scans. Recent methods involve utilizing sensors and camera systems within the examination room to determine the patient's position. This information, combined with anatomical models of patients, can be used to derive the optimal table position for the scanner before an MRI or CT examination. In this context, several techniques based on depth imaging with time-of-flight sensors have been proposed. Gange et al. [1] focus on identifying key points on the body surface and selecting the scan range based on these identified anatomical markers. In addition, they compute a body contour from the depth image and compute the vertical geometric center of the patient for the required table elevation.

Henrich [2] (LOOC) utilizes point clouds extracted from depth images to predict internal body structures, while Geißler [3] and Kats [4] solely rely on depth images achieving a mean Average Symmetric Surface Distance under 10 mm for the structure

© Der/die Autor(en), exklusiv lizenziert an
Springer Fachmedien Wiesbaden GmbH, ein Teil von Springer Nature 2026
H. Handels et al. (Hrsg.), *Bildverarbeitung für die Medizin 2026*,
Informatik aktuell, https://doi.org/10.1007/978-3-658-51100-5_5

segmentations. In contrast to complex deep learning-based methods, we investigate whether a sufficient estimate of organ position can be achieved using four key points in combination with a statistical atlas based on a training cohort. Our focus is to predict axis-aligned bounding boxes relevant for table positioning, and we compare our statistical atlas approach with a linear regression model. Our study aims to evaluate not only how well each structure is covered by its prediction, but also the size of the predicted bounding box and thus the resulting radiation exposure in the CT context.

2 Materials and methods

2.1 Data

We use images from the MR imaging study within the german national cohort study (NAKO, 2014-2019) [5], which includes 10 828 whole-body MR volumes from volunteers in a breath-hold examination (VIBE). The volumes have an image size of 320×260 for axial slices with an isotropic resolution of 1.4 mm and consist of four table positions with a total of 316 slices and a slice thickness of 3 mm. The data was divided into a training and test group with 8 956 and 1 054 subjects, respectively. Since we extract our key points from segmentation, we employ the pretrained, publicly available segmentation model VIBESegmentator [6] to generate segmentation masks for the MRI volumes. It was trained on the NAKO dataset and covers all major bones, organs, and vessels from thigh to neck. As it only provides a joint vertebra label for all the vertebrae, the individual vertebrae were segmented using TotalSegmentator MRI [7]. For simplicity, we limit our evaluation to a grouped selection of 13 organs covering all different types of large and small structures.

2.2 Methods

2.2.1 Extraction of keypoints. For our method, we extract keypoints for each shoulder and hip joint, which are commonly extracted in pose estimation, as in the COCO dataset [8], by defining the center of the humerus and femur bone heads. Therefore, we calculate a Euclidean distance transformation of the segmentation masks for the scapula and hip, set a threshold of 20 mm, and intersect them with the masks for the humerus and femur. We then estimate the four bone head centers by calculating the center of gravity of these intersected masks. Finally, we perform an orthogonal projection of the detected points along the anterior-posterior axis onto the anterior body surface. The extracted keypoints are used in place of pose estimation keypoints for initial experiments.

2.2.2 Keypoint-based registration. We select one case as reference and calculate affine transformations that map all other cases to its coordinates based on four key points. Since the keypoints are often located almost in the same coronal plane, estimating a full 3D affine transformation is numerically unstable. Therefore, we only consider 2D affine transformations for the superior-inferior and medial-lateral axes, with additional translations along the anterior-posterior axis, to align keypoints centers in the AP direction.

2.2.3 Prediction of organ bounds. For our statistical atlas, we extract the bounding boxes for each organ for all training cases and determine the percentiles for the six sides. We then use these as bounds for the prediction of organ positions for all test cases.

That is, for each of our $N = 8956$ samples in our training set, we have segmentations $\mathcal{S}_j^\omega$ $(j = 1, \ldots, N)$ of all organs $\omega \in \Omega = \{$"liver", "heart", "kidney", …$\}$ For simplicity, let ω be an arbitrary but fixed organ, and let

$$\mathcal{B}_j^\omega = [x_j^{\min}, x_j^{\max}] \times [y_j^{\min}, y_j^{\max}] \times [z_j^{\min}, z_j^{\max}]$$

be the bounding box of that organ for the j-th sample $\mathcal{S}_j^\omega$, where

$$x_j^{\min} = \min\{x : (x, y, z) \in \mathcal{S}_j^\omega\}$$
$$x_j^{\max} = \max\{x : (x, y, z) \in \mathcal{S}_j^\omega\}$$

and analogously for the y and z directions.

On this basis, we calculate empirical upper and lower percentiles $x_{(p)}^{\min}, x_{(p)}^{\max}, \ldots,$ such that a percentage p of samples lie above and below these values, i.e.

$$\#\{j : x_j^{\min} \geq x_{(p)}^{\min}\} \geq N \cdot p \quad \text{and} \quad \#\{j : x_j^{\max} \leq x_{(p)}^{\max}\} \geq N \cdot p$$

and analogously for the remaining directions.

Finally, we define a box from the p-th percentile bounds for the structure ω as

$$\mathcal{B}_p^\omega := [x_{(p)}^{\min}, x_{(p)}^{\max}] \times [y_{(p)}^{\min}, y_{(p)}^{\max}] \times [z_{(p)}^{\min}, z_{(p)}^{\max}]$$

Note that all percentile bounds are spatially independent of each other and that the definition of our (one-sided) percentile box does *not* imply

$$\#\{j : \mathcal{S}_j^\omega \subseteq \mathcal{B}_p^\omega\} \geq N \cdot p$$

In extreme cases, especially for small p, it may occur that $x_{(p)}^{\max} \leq x_{(p)}^{\min}$, or analogously in the y and z directions. In such cases, we discard the predicted box. In the following, we refer to $\mathcal{B}_p^\omega$ as the predicted bounds box at confidence level p.

2.3 Evaluation

Let $\mathcal{S}_k^\omega$ $(k = 1, \ldots, M)$ be the segmentation mask of structure $\omega \in \Omega$ for one of our $M = 1054$ samples in our test set, with $\mathcal{B}_k^\omega$ the corresponding bounding box, and let $\mathcal{B}_p^\omega$ be the predicted bounds box at confidence level p.

We want to assess how well the predicted box covers the whole segmentation. Therefore, we compute the F_1 score, also known as the Dice coefficient, and define

$$\text{overlap score} := \mathrm{F}_1\left(\mathcal{S}_k^\omega, \mathcal{S}_k^\omega \cap \mathcal{B}_p^\omega\right) \tag{1}$$

Although we want $\mathcal{B}_p^\omega$ to cover the entire structure or most of it, it should still be compact and have a similar size to $\mathcal{B}_k^\omega$. To this end, we define the following measure

$$\text{box volume ratio} := \ln\left(\frac{|\mathcal{B}_p^\omega|}{|\mathcal{B}_k^\omega|}\right)^2 \tag{2}$$

Note that this measure is zero when the volumes are equal, and it is symmetric in the sense that using $|\mathcal{B}_k^\omega|/|\mathcal{B}_p^\omega|$ instead of $|\mathcal{B}_p^\omega|/|\mathcal{B}_k^\omega|$ yields the same value.

As mentioned above, due to the construction of our percentile bounds box, we cannot infer that the bounding box is contained with certain probability. However, to evaluate the correlation between the bounds box and the probability that at least $x\%$ of the organs are contained for a specific confidence level p, we define the

$$x\% \text{ containment probability} := \#\left\{k : \frac{|\mathcal{S}_k^\omega \cap \mathcal{B}_p^\omega|}{|\mathcal{S}_k^\omega|} \geq x\right\}/M \tag{3}$$

For comparison, we trained a linear (ridge) regression model using the keypoints as input. It uses 12 input variables (4 points × 3 spatial dimensions as flattened input vector) and predicts the bounding box for each structure. We used the Ridge model of `scikit-learn 1.6.1` and the L_2 regularization with a weight of 1 for numerical stability.

3 Results

We compute our metrics for $M = 1054$ samples and 13 organs. Figure 1a shows the overlap score and the box volume ratio for the different predicted bounds boxes based on confidence levels p and different structures. In addition, the mean value over all structures is shown as a black line, as well as the mean value over all structures for the baseline regression model. Since the latter is not dependent on the different confidence levels, it is plotted as a gray dashed horizontal line.

The plot shows that the bounds boxes based on a confidence level of 57% or greater have a better overlap score on average over all structures compared to the regression model (0.9405). Furthermore, we analyzed the performance of each structure individually. For the hips, our predicted boxes outperform the regression box regarding the overlap score starting from the confidence level of 0.18. Conversely, the predicted bounds boxes perform worse for the vertebrae T5 and the stomach, as the overlap score for the latter exceeds that of the regression boxes from the confidence level 0.82 onwards. In particular, the bounds boxes for vertebra T5 with $p < 10$ were excluded, as they exhibited a negative extent in at least one of the three dimensions. In comparison, the box volume ratios are lower than the regression model (0.1237) only for the predicted bounds boxes with a confidence level between 41 and 60%.

In Fig. 1b, the containment probabilities for thresholds of 100%, 95% and 90% are displayed as a function of the confidence levels p and the various structures.

While the curve for 100% shows an exponential relationship for both all structures and the individual structures, the curve for the lower threshold of 95% approaches a diagonal, indicating a linear relationship between p and the 95% containment probability. However, for smaller threshold, the percentage of structures contained within the box varies considerably across individual structures. For the hip, scapula, and lung lobes, 95% of the structures are more frequently contained within the predicted box at lower confidence levels p compared to the stomach, kidneys, and clavicula. While the hip already contains more structures than the regression model at a confidence level of 0.29, the kidney only achieves this at a confidence level of around 0.81. The plots also show the difficulty for the regression model to predict bounding boxes that encompass the entire structure. Only 1.95% of the samples

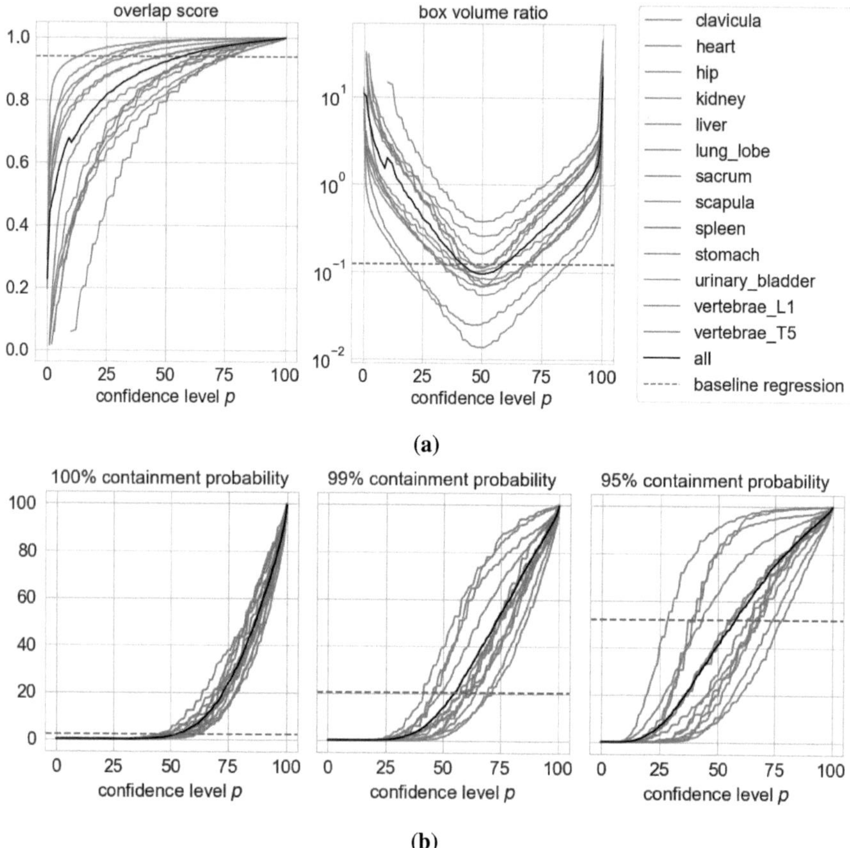

Fig. 1. (a) Left: overlap score, right: box volume ratio per structure. (b) Containment probabilities for three different thresholds. The black line indicates the mean performance across all structures depending on the confidence levels p, while the gray dashed line represents the mean performance for the results of the baseline regression model.

across all structures have the structure entirely within the box. In 20.41% of the samples, 99% of the structure is contained within the box, while 52.06% of the samples have 95% of the structure inside the bounding box. Our boxes achieve better results across all containment probabilities for confidence levels above 54%.

4 Discussion

Our evaluation shows that our method consistently outperforms the baseline regression approach across all metrics for confidence levels between 54% and 57%. Furthermore, the results indicate that our method performs well for larger and less deformable anatomical structures like hips and also the lung lobes, which shows an above-average outcome. However, challenges arise when dealing with smaller structures as well as with variable structures, such as the clavicula, vertebrae, and stomach. Since the box boundaries depend on the voxel size, they have a particular effect on predicting smaller structures. One important observation is the difficulty in predicting boxes that fully encompass the entire structure, a limitation present in both the regression model and our proposed method. An advantage of our method is the ability to select a confidence level p, giving users the flexibility to prioritize either a smaller bounding box – reducing radiation exposure – or a larger box that maximizes organ containment. In contrast, our baseline approach is limited to generating bounding boxes of similar sizes, offering less adaptability to specific clinical needs. It is important to note that, even with our method, a high overlap score results in an increased box volume ratio, but the flexibility could enhance clinical diagnostics by prioritizing safety or the accurate coverage of anatomical structures, depending on the clinical question. Since we observe a negative correlation for small structures far away from the keypoints, we conclude that our four peripheral keypoints may be a limitation of our method. Thus, including keypoints located in the body center is of high interest for future work, as is a more detailed analysis of the individual structures. Additionally, the applicability of statistical atlases for a wider range of structures and different datasets should be explored to enhance the robustness and generalizability of the model.

Acknowledgement. This work was supported within the Fraunhofer and DFG transfer programme.

References

1. Gang Y, Chen X, Li H, Wang H, Li J, Guo Y et al. A comparison between manual and artificial intelligence–based automatic positioning in CT imaging for COVID-19 patients. Eur Radiol. 2021;31(8):6049–58.
2. Henrich P, Mathis-Ullrich F. LOOC: localizing organs using occupancy networks and body surface depth images. IEEE Access. 2025.
3. Geißler K, Mensing D, Kohlbrandt T, Hirsch JG, Heldmann S. Predicting anatomical structures from 2D depth images of patients. Proc SPIE MI IP. 2025;13406:407–11.

4. Kats E, Geißler K, Hirsch JG, Heldman S, Heinrich MP. Internal organ localization using depth images: a framework for automated MRI patient positioning. Proc BVM. 2025:324–9.
5. Bamberg F, Kauczor HU, Weckbach S, Schlett CL, Forsting M, Ladd SC et al. Whole-body MR imaging in the German national cohort: rationale, design, and technical background. Radiology. 2015;277(1):206–20.
6. Graf R, Platzek P, Riedel EO, Ramschütz C, Starck S, Möller HK et al. VIBESegmentator: full body MRI segmentation for the NAKO and UK biobank. Eur Radiol. 2025:1–15.
7. D'Antonoli TA, Berger LK, Indrakanti AK, Vishwanathan N, Weiss J, Jung M et al. TotalSegmentator MRI: robust sequence-independent segmentation of multiple anatomic structures in MRI. Radiology. 2025;314(2):e241613.
8. Jin S, Xu L, Xu J, Wang C, Liu W, Qian C et al. Whole-body human pose estimation in the wild. Proc CV ECCV. 2020:196–214.

Abstract: PrIINeR

Towards Prior-informed Implicit Neural Representations for Accelerated MRI

Ziad Al-Haj Hemidi [†], Eytan Kats [†], Mattias P. Heinrich

Institut für Medizinische Informatik, Universität zu Lübeck
z.alhajhemidi@uni-luebeck.de

Magnetic resonance imaging (MRI) provides excellent diagnostic detail but suffers from long scan times. Accelerated imaging through undersampling reduces acquisition but introduces aliasing, while parallel imaging and compressed sensing degrade quality at higher acceleration. Deep learning methods trained on large datasets suppress artifacts effectively, yet often over-smooth or hallucinate features. Implicit neural representations (INRs), which optimize continuous image functions per-instance, preserve fine details but remain under-constrained, leaving residual artifacts.

We propose PrIINeR (prior-informed implicit neural representation) [1], a framework that unites population-trained priors with INR optimization. PrIINeR employs a hash-grid encoded implicit network jointly optimized with coil sensitivity maps and guided by a dual data consistency objective, enforcing fidelity to both undersampled k-space and prior-informed reconstructions. Total variation regularization further suppresses aliasing while maintaining sharp edges.

On the NYU fastMRI [2] knee dataset (4–10× undersampling), PrIINeR consistently improves reconstruction quality over both INR-only methods and population-trained priors of varying complexity. Gains in SSIM and PSNR are statistically significant ($p < 0.05$) across nearly all settings, while qualitative results confirm better artifact suppression and preservation of anatomical detail.

By combining global priors with instance-specific fidelity, PrIINeR offers a robust, flexible approach to accelerated MRI. Code is publicly available at: `https://github.com/multimodallearning/PrIINeR`.

References

1. Al-Haj Hemidi Z, Kats E, Heinrich MP. PrIINeR: towards prior-informed implicit neural representations for accelerated MRI. Proc BMVC. 2025.
2. Zbontar J, Knoll F, Sriram A, Murrell T, Huang Z, Muckley MJ et al. fastMRI: an open dataset and benchmarks for accelerated MRI. arXiv preprint: 1811.08839. 2018.

[†] These authors contributed equally to this work.

© Der/die Autor(en), exklusiv lizenziert an
Springer Fachmedien Wiesbaden GmbH, ein Teil von Springer Nature 2026
H. Handels et al. (Hrsg.), *Bildverarbeitung für die Medizin 2026*,
Informatik aktuell, https://doi.org/10.1007/978-3-658-51100-5_6

Interpretable Framework for Zero-shot 4D Low-dose CT Denoising

Filter2Noise-4D

Yipeng Sun [1], Linda-Sophie Schneider [1], Siyuan Mei [1], Chengze Ye [1], Mingxuan Gu [1], Fabian Wagner [2], Siming Bayer [1], Andreas Maier [1]

[1]Friedrich-Alexander-Universität Erlangen-Nürnberg, Erlangen
[2]Siemens Healthineers AG, Forchheim
yipeng.sun@fau.de

Abstract. Four-dimensional CT (4D-CT) tracks tumor motion throughout the breathing cycle for radiation therapy planning, but dose reduction per phase introduces spatio-temporal noise compromising tumor delineation. Existing learning-based denoising methods are either clinically impractical (requiring paired data) or lack interpretability (black-box networks). We present Filter2Noise-4D (F2N-4D), a zero-shot interpretable framework employing content-adaptive bilateral filtering that exploits spatio-temporal information from neighboring slices. Self-supervised training uses interpolation of neighboring slices to construct training pairs. With only 1.8k parameters, F2N-4D achieves competitive performance while maintaining transparency.

1 Introduction

In radiation therapy, managing respiratory motion is essential for treating thoracic and abdominal tumors. Four-dimensional computed tomography (4D-CT) has become the clinical standard for tracking tumor motion throughout the breathing cycle. This temporal data is essential for delineating the Internal target volume (ITV), which encompasses the complete trajectory of tumor movement, ensuring the prescribed radiation dose covers the tumor while minimizing exposure to surrounding healthy tissues [1].

However, acquiring data for each respiratory phase necessitates limiting the radiation dose per 3D volume to adhere to the ALARA (as low as reasonably achievable) principle. This dose reduction in 4D low-dose CT (4D-LDCT) introduces spatio-temporal noise that is correlated both spatially within each volume and temporally across breathing phases. This noise obscures tumor boundaries and introduces artifacts, compromising delineation accuracy and potentially impacting treatment efficacy and patient safety [2, 3].

Existing denoising paradigms are ill-suited for this challenge. Supervised deep learning methods [4] are clinically impractical, as their requirement for large datasets

© Der/die Autor(en), exklusiv lizenziert an
Springer Fachmedien Wiesbaden GmbH, ein Teil von Springer Nature 2026
H. Handels et al. (Hrsg.), *Bildverarbeitung für die Medizin 2026*,
Informatik aktuell, https://doi.org/10.1007/978-3-658-51100-5_7

of registered noisy and clean image pairs cannot be ethically met. Self-supervised and zero-shot methods have emerged as alternatives, but universally rely on deep, black-box architectures like U-Nets. This opacity impedes clinical adoption, as radiologists and physicists cannot verify the model's decision-making process, raising concerns about potential alterations or hallucination of diagnostic information [5].

This work introduces Filter2Noise-4D (F2N-4D), a framework addressing the dual challenges of performance and clinical trust in 4D-LDCT denoising. To our knowledge, this is the first zero-shot, interpretable denoising method for 4D-CT. Building on the Filter2Noise approach [6], we replace black-box function approximators with learnable, content-aware bilateral filters. By building the denoising process around a known mathematical operator whose parameters can be visualized, F2N-4D provides a verifiable, clinician-controllable, and parameter-efficient (1.8k parameters) solution for enhancing 4D-LDCT in clinical practice.

2 Methods

2.1 Attention-guided bilateral filters (AGBF)

The foundation of F2N-4D is an interpretable, mathematically defined denoising operator, which replaces the conventional black-box network. We process a 4D-

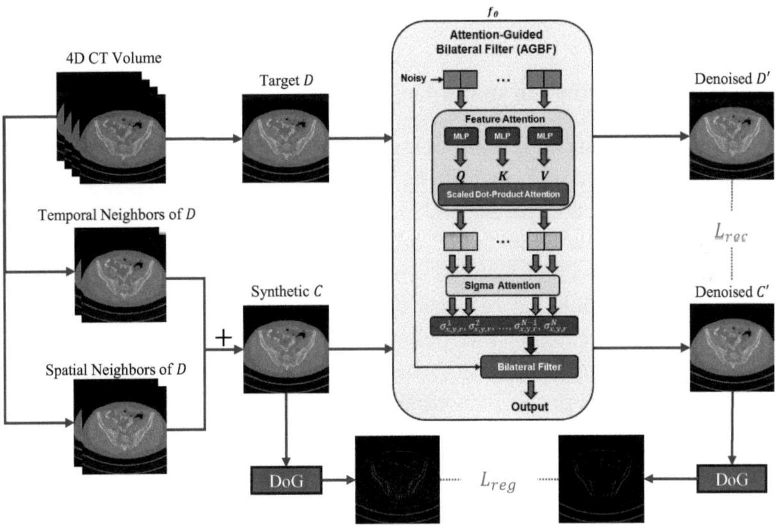

Fig. 1. Overview of the F2N-4D self-supervised training pipeline. (1) From a single noisy 4D-CT volume, a target slice $\boldsymbol{D}$ is selected, along with its adjacent spatial and temporal neighbors. (2) The neighbors are warped and combined via spatio-temporal morphing to create a synthetic input slice $\boldsymbol{C}$. (3) The pair $(\boldsymbol{C}, \boldsymbol{D})$ is used for training. The core reconstruction loss ($\mathcal{L}_{\text{rec}}$) enforces consistency between the denoised versions of the two slices, $f_\theta(\boldsymbol{C})$ and $f_\theta(\boldsymbol{D})$. An edge-preserving regularizer ($\mathcal{L}_{\text{reg}}$) maintains structural fidelity by comparing edge maps.

LDCT volume, $\boldsymbol{Y} \in \mathbb{R}^{T\times D\times H\times W}$, in a slice-wise manner. For each 2D slice, we apply a single AGBF layer, denoted by the function f_θ. The key principle is that a lightweight attention network, $\mathcal{A}_\theta$, does not predict the denoised image directly. Instead, it predicts the spatially varying parameters $(\sigma_r, \sigma_x, \sigma_y)$ that govern the behavior of the bilateral filter for each local patch.

The denoised value of a pixel at coordinate $\boldsymbol{p} = (y, x)$ is a weighted average of its neighbors in the neighborhood $\mathcal{N}$

$$f_\theta(\boldsymbol{y})_{\boldsymbol{p}} = \frac{1}{W_{\boldsymbol{p}}} \sum_{\boldsymbol{q}\in\mathcal{N}_{\boldsymbol{p}}} \boldsymbol{y}_{\boldsymbol{q}} \cdot w_s(\boldsymbol{p}, \boldsymbol{q}; \sigma_x, \sigma_y) \cdot w_r(\boldsymbol{y}_{\boldsymbol{p}}, \boldsymbol{y}_{\boldsymbol{q}}; \sigma_r) \tag{1}$$

where $W_{\boldsymbol{p}}$ is the normalization factor. The spatial kernel w_s and range kernel w_r are defined by the locally predicted standard deviations

$$w_s(\boldsymbol{p}, \boldsymbol{q}; \sigma_x, \sigma_y) = \exp\left(-\frac{(p_y - q_y)^2}{2\sigma_y^2} - \frac{(p_x - q_x)^2}{2\sigma_x^2}\right) \tag{2}$$

$$w_r(\boldsymbol{y}_{\boldsymbol{p}}, \boldsymbol{y}_{\boldsymbol{q}}; \sigma_r) = \exp\left(-\frac{\|\boldsymbol{y}_{\boldsymbol{p}} - \boldsymbol{y}_{\boldsymbol{q}}\|^2}{2\sigma_r^2}\right) \tag{3}$$

This design makes the denoising process transparent. The learned parameter maps can be visualized, providing a direct and verifiable insight into how the model adapts its smoothing strategy across different anatomical regions.

2.2 Zero-shot training via spatio-temporal morphing

To train the AGBF on a single noisy 4D scan, we introduce a self-supervised strategy that generates synthetic training pairs by leveraging the spatio-temporal redundancy of the data. For a given target slice $\boldsymbol{D} \triangleq \boldsymbol{Y}_{z,t}$ at spatio-temporal coordinates (z, t), we construct a synthetic input slice $\boldsymbol{C}$ through a two-stage process.

First, we create two intermediate synthetic slices. A temporal intermediate, $\boldsymbol{Y}'_t$, is generated by interpolating between the adjacent temporal neighbors. A spatial intermediate, $\boldsymbol{Y}'_z$, is created by interpolating between the adjacent spatial neighbors. Second, these two intermediate slices are themselves interpolated to create the final synthetic input $\boldsymbol{C}$. This process is formally defined as

$$\boldsymbol{Y}'_t \triangleq \frac{1}{2}\left(\boldsymbol{Y}_{z,t-1} + \boldsymbol{Y}_{z,t+1}\right) \qquad \text{(Temporal Intermediate)} \tag{4}$$

$$\boldsymbol{Y}'_z \triangleq \frac{1}{2}\left(\boldsymbol{Y}_{z-1,t} + \boldsymbol{Y}_{z+1,t}\right) \qquad \text{(Spatial Intermediate)} \tag{5}$$

$$\boldsymbol{C} \triangleq \frac{1}{2}\boldsymbol{Y}'_t + \frac{1}{2}\boldsymbol{Y}'_z \qquad \text{(Final Synthetic Input)} \tag{6}$$

The resulting pair $(\boldsymbol{C}, \boldsymbol{D})$ is used for training. While both slices represent the same underlying anatomy, the synthetic slice $\boldsymbol{C}$ contains a different realization of noise due to the averaging of four different neighbor slices. By training the AGBF to produce consistent results from these two different inputs, it learns to be robust to noise and preserve the common anatomical signal, ensuring spatio-temporal coherence in the final denoised volume.

A key advantage of our framework is its training efficiency. The self-supervised training does not require the entire 4D volume. Instead, it is performed on a representative subset of the interior slices where valid neighbors exist for spatio-temporal morphing. Once the attention network $\mathcal{A}_\theta$ is trained on this subset, it has learned a general, content-aware function that maps local image patches to optimal filter parameters. This learned function is then applied in a single inference pass to denoise the entire 4D volume, including the boundary slices and any interior slices not used for training. This approach is effective because the model learns relationships between anatomical structures and noise characteristics, which generalize across the entire scan, eliminating the need to train on every slice.

2.3 Self-supervised loss function

The AGBF network is trained end-to-end by minimizing a composite loss function that balances noise reduction with the preservation of structural details, as depicted in Fig. 1. The total loss for each training pair $(\boldsymbol{C}_i, \boldsymbol{D}_i)$ is

$$\mathcal{L}_{\text{total}} = \mathcal{L}_{\text{rec}} + \lambda \mathcal{L}_{\text{reg}} \tag{7}$$

where λ is a hyperparameter that controls the trade-off.

The reconstruction loss, $\mathcal{L}_{\text{rec}}$, is based on the principle of self-supervised consistency. Since both the synthetic input $\boldsymbol{C}_i$ and the target slice $\boldsymbol{D}_i$ are different noisy observations of the same underlying anatomy, their denoised versions should be identical. This constraint forces the network to learn a mapping that is invariant to the specific noise realization

$$\mathcal{L}_{\text{rec}} = \|f_\theta(\boldsymbol{C}_i) - f_\theta(\boldsymbol{D}_i)\|_1 \tag{8}$$

To prevent the blurring of anatomical structures, the regularization loss, $\mathcal{L}_{\text{reg}}$, penalizes inconsistencies in edge information. It compares the absolute edge maps of the denoised output and the target, where edges are detected by a Difference-of-Gaussians (DoG) operator

$$\mathcal{L}_{\text{reg}} = \Big\| |\text{DoG}(\boldsymbol{D}_i)| - |\text{DoG}(f_\theta(\boldsymbol{C}_i))| \Big\|_1 \tag{9}$$

The DoG operator is defined as the convolution $(*)$ with two Gaussian kernels, $\mathcal{G}_{s1}$ and $\mathcal{G}_{s2}$, of different standard deviations: $\text{DoG}(\boldsymbol{y}) = (\boldsymbol{y} * \mathcal{G}_{s1}) - (\boldsymbol{y} * \mathcal{G}_{s2})$. This term explicitly guides the model to maintain edge sharpness.

3 Experiments & results

3.1 Experimental setup

Experiments were conducted using the publicly available thoracic 4D-CT dataset from the University of Texas MD Anderson Cancer Center [7]. We simulated 4D-LDCT data by adding signal-dependent Poisson noise directly to the image volumes.

Method	PSNR (dB) ↑	SSIM ↑	RMSE ↓
Noisy Input	35.83	0.9390	0.0155
F2N-4D	**37.31**	**0.9769**	**0.0137**

Tab. 1. Quantitative evaluation of F2N-4D on the simulated 4D-LDCT dataset.

The F2N-4D model was implemented in PyTorch 2.0.1 with Python 3.11 and trained for 100 epochs using the AdamW optimizer with a learning rate of 1×10^{-3} on an NVIDIA A100 GPU.

3.2 Quantitative results

Tab. 1 presents the quantitative evaluation of F2N-4D across the test dataset. All metrics are computed on the entire 4D volume. The model achieves improvements in all metrics compared to the noisy input, demonstrating noise reduction while preserving structural information. The PSNR and SSIM values indicate reconstruction quality, while the RMSE confirms the accuracy of the denoised outputs.

3.3 Qualitative results

Fig. 2 presents qualitative results for six representative cases. The denoised images exhibit visual improvements compared to the noisy inputs, appearing closer to the ground truth. Notably, noises are removed, while anatomical structures are preserved. This demonstrates the framework's capability to learn a denoising function that maintains structural fidelity.

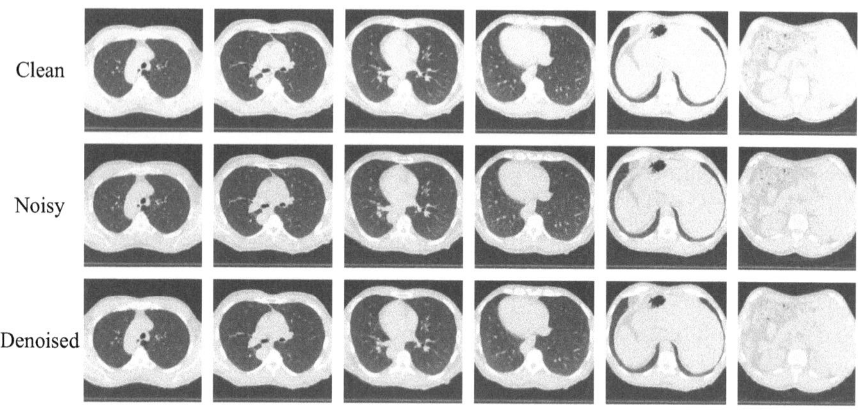

Fig. 2. Qualitative denoising results of F2N-4D on six representative cases from the simulated 4D-LDCT dataset are presented. All images are shown with a window level (WL) of −600 HU and a window width (WW) of 1500 HU.

4 Conclusion

In this work, we introduced Filter2Noise-4D, a framework for interpretable, zero-shot denoising of 4D low-dose CT images. By adapting the principles of the Filter2Noise framework, we developed a system that applies a transparent Attention-Guided Bilateral Filter to each slice of the 4D volume. This operator's behavior is controlled by a lightweight attention network and is trained from a single noisy scan using a self-supervised strategy featuring a spatio-temporal morphing technique. Our results on realistic simulated 4D-CT data show that F2N-4D achieves performance in image fidelity. Crucially, this is achieved by training on only a representative subset of the 4D data, demonstrating that the learned content-aware filter function generalizes to the entire volume. This efficiency, combined with the model's parameter efficiency of only 1.8k parameters (orders of magnitude fewer than conventional deep networks), underscores its practicality. By combining performance with interpretability and user control, F2N-4D provides a trustworthy and clinically viable tool to enhance 4D-LDCT, with potential to improve the accuracy and safety of radiotherapy planning and other imaging applications.

Acknowledgement. This work was supported by the German Federal Ministry of Education and Research (BMBF) under the grant "Verbundprojekt 05D2022 – KI4D4E: Ein KI-basiertes Framework für die Visualisierung und Auswertung der massiven Datenmengen der 4D-Tomographie für Endanwender von Beamlines. Teilprojekt 5." Grant number: 05D23WE1.

References

1. Schwarz A, Schmidt S, Wohlfahrt P, Dickmann J, Maier A. Trainable spatio-temporal bilateral filters: 4D-filtering for 4DCT denoising. Proc MIPMI. 2025;13405:919–23.
2. Chen H, Zhang Y, Zhang W, Liao P, Li K, Zhou J et al. Low-dose CT denoising with convolutional neural network. Proc IEEE ISBI. 2017:143–6.
3. Wagner F, Thies M, Gu M, Huang Y, Pechmann S, Patwari M et al. Ultralow-parameter denoising: trainable bilateral filter layers in computed tomography. Med Phys. 2022;49(8):5107–20.
4. Tian C, Fei L, Zheng W, Xu Y, Zuo W, Lin CW. Deep learning on image denoising: an overview. Neural Netw. 2020;131:251–75.
5. Huang Y, Preuhs A, Lauritsch G, Manhart M, Huang X, Maier A. Data consistent artifact reduction for limited angle tomography with deep learning prior. Proc MLMIR. 2019:101–12.
6. Sun Y, Schneider LS, Gu M, Mei S, Ye C, Wagner F et al. Filter2Noise: interpretable self-supervised single-image denoising for low-dose CT with attention-guided bilateral filtering. arXiv preprint: 2504.13519. 2025.
7. Castillo R, Castillo E, Guerra R, Johnson VE, McPhail T, Garg AK et al. A framework for evaluation of deformable image registration spatial accuracy using large landmark point sets. Phys Med Biol. 2009;54(7):1849.

Foundation Models in Medical Image Segmentation

How Foundational Are Foundation Models Really?

David Lurz[1], Luisa Neubig[1], Markus Kopp[2], Andreas Kist[1]

[1]Department Artificial Intelligence in Biomedical Engineering, Friedrich-Alexander-University Erlangen-Nürnberg
[2]Institute Radiology, University Hospital Erlangen
david.lurz@fau.de

Abstract. Task-constrained deep learning models have shown strong performance for medical image segmentation. Recently, generalist segmentation foundation models have emerged, showing promising results across different scenarios. However, we lack large-scale studies comparing the performance of 2D image, video, and volume segmentation across multiple models and modalities. To unmask how foundational the models truly are, we comprehensively evaluate the segmentation performance of SAM2.1, SAM3, MedSAM2, SAM-Med2D, SAM-Med3D, nnInteractive and VISTA3D on more than 80 medical datasets. MedSAM2 stands out as the most foundational of all models, while SAM-Med3D and VISTA3D excel in 3D CT segmentation scenarios, but require noticeably more computational power and memory. nnInteractive seems to be a promising model, featuring very fast inference time and rather high segmentation performance. Our code and evaluation results are openly available at `https://github.com/DavidL-11/med-seg-fm`.

1 Introduction

Medical image segmentation is a major part of medical image processing. Advances in deep learning have shown deep neural networks to be exceptionally good for image segmentation, but they are commonly task-specific and limited to predicting only the classes on which they were trained; thus, they cannot generalize to unseen anatomical structures. Foundation models (FMs), such as the segment anything model (SAM), have the promise to overcome this limitation by being trained on large amounts of data with zero-shot capabilities, potentially segmenting anything the user requests and adapting to new tasks. This greatly reduces the number of models required, as there would not need to be a model for each object of interest and each imaging modality. In recent years, many foundation models for segmentation have been released, some even tailored for medical usage. Most of these models require some kind of input prompt, e.g. a point, a bounding box or a text label, to indicate which areas to segment.

© Der/die Autor(en), exklusiv lizenziert an
Springer Fachmedien Wiesbaden GmbH, ein Teil von Springer Nature 2026
H. Handels et al. (Hrsg.), *Bildverarbeitung für die Medizin 2026*,
Informatik aktuell, https://doi.org/10.1007/978-3-658-51100-5_8

Previous work has highlighted some of these models and compared them to each other. Dongjie Cheng et al. [1] compared the three prompt modes `auto`, `point`, and `box` of the original SAM. Scientists in [2] evaluated MedSAM against SAM and specialist models, such as a U-Net, while being largely focused on MRI, CT, and endoscopy images. The MedSAM2 paper [3] compared its performance to various SAM2.1 checkpoints. The IMIS-Bench [4] provides a large dataset collection and evaluates SAM(2), SAM-Med2D, MedSAM, and their own IMIS-Net on the dataset, but only contains 2D images and is missing newer models like MedSAM2 or SAM2.1.

While recent studies have compared individual or small subsets of such models, a systematic evaluation encompassing multiple newly released FMs is lacking. Furthermore, existing evaluations are predominantly conducted by the creators of the respective models, potentially limiting the objectivity of the reported results. A large study evaluating many models on a large amount of diverse datasets, including 2D/3D images and videos, is still missing, which would be necessary to truly call them "foundation "models. The impact of prompt type and its susceptibility to human error during prompt creation also needs to be further researched.

2 Materials and methods

The segmentation FMs SAM2.1 [5], SAM3 [6], SAM-Med2D [7], SAM-Med3D [8], MedSAM2 [3], nnInteractive [9] and VISTA3D [10] are chosen for our comparison.

The datasets include an extension of BAGLS (glottis + vocal fold segmentation) [11], brain electron microscopy (mitochondria segmentation) [12], NeoPolyp [13] (Polyp segmentation), Endoscapes [14] (organ and tool segmentation), IMed361-M [4] (>50 datasets of varying modalities and segmentation targets, mainly CT/MRI), MedSegBench [15] (35 datasets of more rare segmentation targets), AMOS22 and FLARE22 (Grand Challenge multi-organ abdomen CT/MRI and CT segmentation), ToothFairy3 [16, 17] (segmentation of 70 classes in CBCT head scans), medical segmentation decathlon [18] (10 different 3D segmentation tasks), and our own VFSS dataset for bolus segmentation in videofluoroscopic swallowing studies. For applicable datasets (FLARE22, AMOS22) and models (SAM2, MedSAM2), CT windowing was performed.

Prompts are generated from the ground truth using one of the following methods:

- *Point (center)*: Prompt at the center of mass, or a random point if the prompt would not be contained in the ground truth.
- *Point (random)*: Point prompt in a random location of the eroded ground truth.
- *Point (rim)*: Point prompt at the edge of the ground truth.
- *Box*: Box prompt with optional padding to simulate human error.

SAM3 uses the same prompts, but differs in the sense that it has a visual mode (like SAM2) and a context segmentation mode (automatically segments other visually similar structures with just one prompt). Our evaluations use its visual mode. The intersection-over-union (IoU) and normalized surface distance (NSD) are chosen as segmentation quality metrics.

3 Results

Using the aforementioned datasets, we evaluated the models on the test splits to unveil their capabilities. With BAGLS and VFSS, we determined the zero-shot capabilities of FMs, as both feature somewhat rare segmentation tasks that are probably not included in the training data of the models. For BAGLS-VF, Fig. 1a highlights that the larger SAM2.1 checkpoints mostly showed noticeable improvement over their smaller counterparts when using point prompts. SAM3's visual point/box prompt performance is roughly the same as SAM2.1 Large. It required the most computation time and more than 3 GB VRAM. MedSAM2$_{\text{latest}}$ displays much better point prompt performance, but slightly worse box prompt performance than all the SAM-models. Fine-tuning the SAM2.1-Tiny checkpoint on 300, 500, and 1000 images has shown a steady increase in segmentation quality (mIoU of 0.71, 0.76, and 0.80), almost reaching the large checkpoint with box prompts. As a downside, its generalizability is completely removed, as a model fine-tuned only on the glottis was only able to segment the glottis and no vocal folds, showing an overall mIoU of 0.27.

Fig. 1b highlights that placing a point in the center of mass or a random location does not significantly impact segmentation quality, only when they are placed near the edge of the structure.

Fig. 2a shows that using more point prompts can drastically improve segmentation performance, but depending on the object size, using too many can also have a negative impact, as the metrics for the small glottis saturate more quickly than for the larger vocal folds. Slightly smaller box prompts with a negative padding showed an improvement over theoretically perfect boxes in Fig. 2b, but also negatively affect performance much faster after a certain threshold. This is because boxes with a −50% padding (= subtract half the box width/height on all sides) already have an area of 0. The metrics for VFSS video segmentation peaked when supplying the model with 10 positive and 3 negative point prompts every 5 frames at an IoU of 0.55 and an NSD of 0.65. The largest negative impact on segmentation quality seems

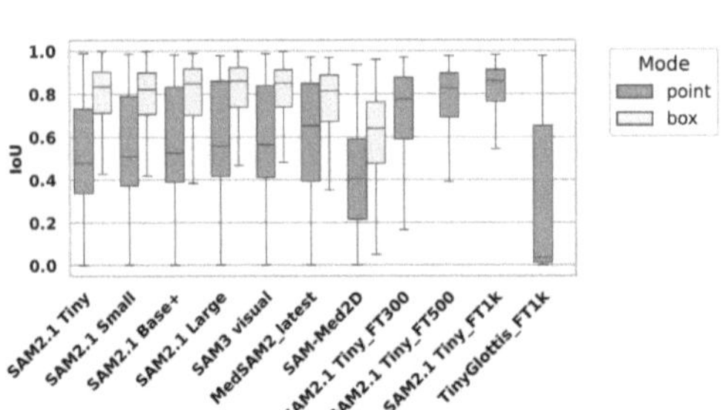

(a) Checkpoint and model comparison vs. fine-tuning (FT) SAM2.1 Tiny on 300, 500 and 1k images.

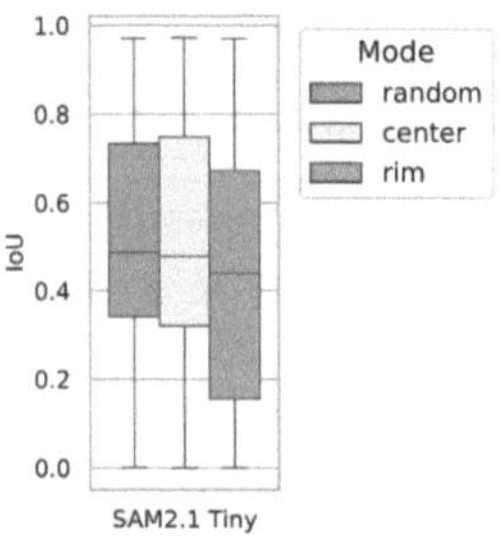

(b) SAM2.1 Tiny point prompt IoU per prompt placement strategy.

Fig. 1. Influence of Model/Checkpoint and Point Placement on mIoU.

to be unclear boundaries, as indicated by the VFSS performance and the difference between the unclear boundaries for endoscapes with box (0.737 IoU) and point (0.465 IoU) prompts, as well as the significantly better results of the brain electron microscopy dataset (0.870 IoU for box, 0.787 IoU for point) with clear boundaries. Also, SAM2.1 ($mIoU_{box}$ = 0.783) and SAM3 ($mIoU_{box}$ = 0.782) performed better than $MedSAM2_{latest}$($mIoU_{box}$ = 0.737) in endoscapes, showing a better adaptability and zero-shot performance, even though endoscopy images should be included in MedSAM2. Since typical task-constrained deep learning models have to perform both localization and segmentation of objects, whereas FMs with given prompts only need to perform segmentation, the FMs performed really good in images where the localization task is hard, like polyp segmentation in NeoPolyp, where FMs could achieve an $mIoU_{box}$ of 0.940 (MedSAM2), 0.914 (SAM2.1 Tiny), 0.917 (SAM3) and 0.823 (SAM-Med2D).

In most medical segmentation tasks, the models performed considerably well, as indicated by the large amount of datasets in IMed361M (Fig. 3a) and MedSegBench (Fig. 3b). SAM3 achieved strong point prompt performance, even without special tuning for medical images, and was more robust to bad prompts, i.e. single points or box prompts with a padding. $MedSAM2_{latest}$ with box prompts achieved an impressive median IoU of more than 0.8 for both collections. By using box prompts, we could also reduce the impact of a rather weak model, meaning that the IoU difference compared to a better model was much smaller than when using point prompts. Box prompts with a 10% padding on each side also outperformed point prompts for all models. SAM3's text prompts with context segmentation resulted in an mIoU of 0.455 with a very large standard deviation of 0.407, meaning it often either segments very good or not at all.

In 3D images, the most difficult structures for FMs were also very small (e.g., pulps), featured unclear boundaries (tumor and edema), or were of complex structure (hepatic vessels). FMs have been found to be well-suited for locating and segmenting areas of unusual tissue, such as a tumor and its surrounding edema, as in MSD

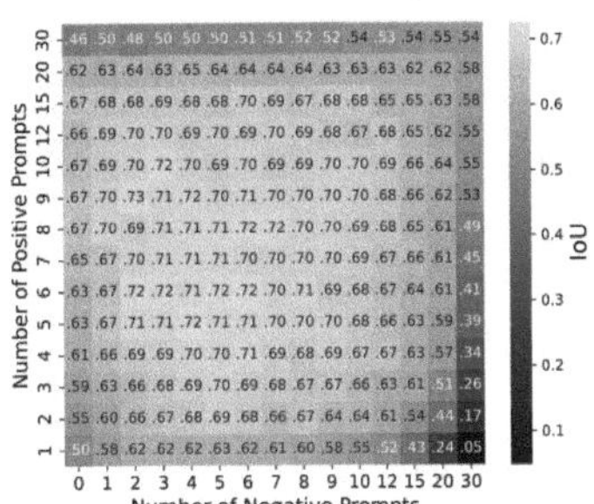

(a) SAM2.1 Tiny mIoU heatmap per point prompt amount.

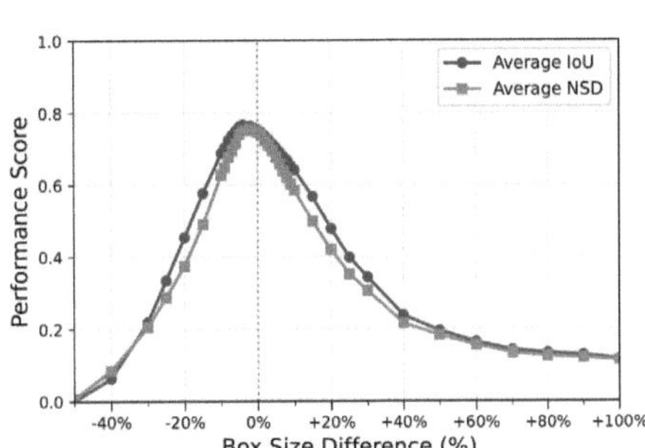

(b) Average box prompt IoU per box padding size.

Fig. 2. Influence of prompt amount and quality on performance for SAM2.1 Tiny.

Glioma. When combining both classes, MedSAM2 achieves an mIoU of almost 0.8. When only trying to segment the tumor alone, the unclear boundaries cause mIoU score to drop to around 0.4.

MedSAM2 requires CT windowing as preprocessing, as shown by the AMOS22 dataset (CT/MRI scans), where MedSAM2 without windowing achieved an mIoU of 0.454 and with windowing 0.648, a more than 40% increase. This allows it to be even with SAM-Med3D and nnInteractive for this dataset. Still, it can't compete with VISTA3D point (mIoU = 0.673) or label (mIoU = 0.750) prompts. CT images displayed a 15% higher mIoU across all models compared to MRI scans. FLARE22 contains easier CT segmentation cases, allowing the models to reach an mIoU of 0.83±0.10 (VISTA3D-label), 0.77±0.18 (VISTA3D-point), 0.75±0.20 (nnInteractive), 0.75±0.21 ($\text{MedSAM2}_{\text{latest}}$), 0.74±0.14 (SAM-Med3D). The hardest objects to segment include the duodenum, pancreas, and the adrenal glands. While VISTA3D achieves outstanding results for known objects using label prompts in CT images, its zero-shot performance is very bad when only using a few prompts, often achieving less than a 0.1 mIoU (e.g., for ToothFairy3, MSD Glioma). MedSAM2 is much better in that regard, but also struggles with three-dimensional small objects, as it achieves an mIoU of only around 0.2 for the ToothFairy3 classes pulp, jawbone, canal, and sinus, whereas the teeth (0.785) and pharynx (0.9) don't pose a problem (Tab. 1). nnInteractive produces much better results for some classes, especially pulp, sinus and jawbone. For jawbone, it also segmented all teeth automatically, which could be removed with more interactive prompts, leading to even higher mIoU scores.

Speed and memory requirements of the models tested can be seen in Tab. 2. Since the speed is highly variable between images, the measurements are relative to SAM2.1-Base+ (100%).

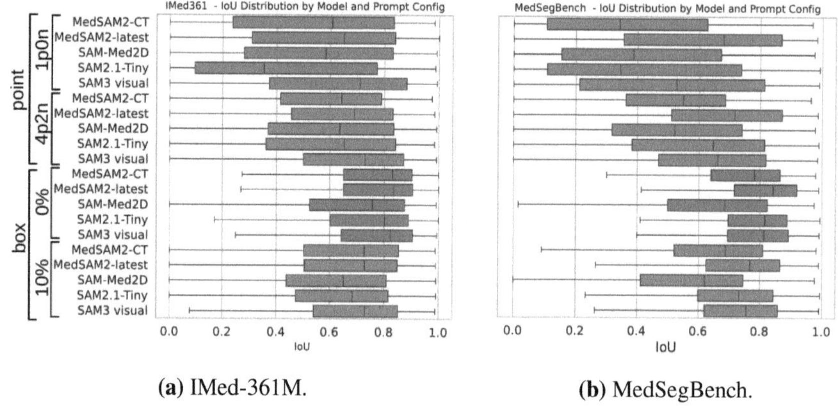

(a) IMed-361M. **(b)** MedSegBench.

Fig. 3. Influence of prompt choice (point, box) and quality (10% box padding) on performance for our models (XpYn = X positive, Y negative point prompts).

Tab. 1. ToothFairy3 evaluation results for MedSAM2 (MS2) and nnInteractive.

Object	MS2_CT		MS2_latest		nnInteractive	
	mIoU↑	mNSD↑	mIoU↑	mNSD↑	mIoU↑	mNSD↑
Pulp	0.131	0.331	0.057	0.187	0.437	0.724
Canal	0.212	0.394	0.274	0.467	0.302	0.526
Sinus	0.677	0.750	0.556	0.729	0.878	0.935
Jawbone	0.188	0.336	0.238	0.443	0.721	0.775
Bridge	0.673	0.816	0.650	0.823	0.576	0.681
Crown	0.610	0.690	0.571	0.655	0.496	0.624
Implant	0.136	0.413	0.137	0.385	0.114	0.330
Pharynx	0.900	0.918	0.882	0.898	0.838	0.863
Tooth	0.785	0.881	0.795	0.881	0.863	0.920

Tab. 2. Summary and comparison of segmentation foundation models.

	Input Type	Prompts	VRAM↓	Time↓
SAM2.1	2D/Video/(3D)	Point/Box/Mask	900 MB	80%-180%
SAM3	2D/Video/(3D)	Point/Box/Mask/Test	>4 GB	200%
MedSAM2	2D/3D/Video	Point/Box	650 MB	50%
SAM-Med2D	2D	Point/Box	2 GB	60%
SAM-Med3D	3D	Point	2 GB	70%
VISTA3D	3D	Point/Label	>3.5 GB	120%-300%
nnInteractive	3D	Point/Box/ Scribble/Lasso	>6 GB	40% (very fast for small objects)

4 Discussion

While the results were mostly very good, it should be noted that these results of the FMs can only be achieved with perfect box prompts, which might not be attainable in real conditions. In addition, datasets where the localization of objects might be the most difficult task, such as polyp segmentation, the results are skewed towards the FMs. Nevertheless, with the acquired results, we can compare how FMs perform against specialized deep neural networks, measured by multiple public results of the same or similar datasets. Scientists in [19] found that humans achieve an average IoU of 0.772 with an intra-rater reliability of 0.77 and an inter-rater reliability of 0.70, calculated by their IoU. Additionally, their U-Net with a ResNet50 and an EfficientNet50 backbone achieved an agreement of 0.788, which led them to classify glottis segmentation with an IoU of larger than 0.7 as "good quality". We could surpass these values on average, even with SAM2.1 Tiny at an mIoU of 0.765 ± 0.165, up to an mIoU of 0.803 with SAM2.1-Large ± 0.149. For VFSS, the performance is lacking, requiring many prompts and only achieving a maximum mIoU of 0.55 with 13 prompts every 5 frames, while other methods on similar datasets were able to achieve an mIoU of around 0.73 without requiring any input [20]. MedSegBench's best baseline network, DenseNet121 (DN121), could be beaten with both SAM2.1-Tiny and MedSAM2$_{\text{latest}}$, achieving an mIoU of 0.717 and 0.714, respectively, compared to DN121's 0.702. Especially, MedSAM2$_{latest}$'s median IoU of 0.808 is improved compared to DN121's 0.738. The datasets the FMs struggled with the most were related to vessel segmentation. For FLARE22, the best models from the official Grand Challenge leaderboard achieved a mean IoU of 0.835 on the validation set, theoretically placing VISTA3D in the top 10 out of 1100 submissions. However, the true ranking of these models can't be determined because these results rely on our own test split. Overall, MedSAM2 seems to be the best all-around multimodal 2D/3D/video medical segmentation foundation model right now, especially in resource-constrained environments. SAM-Med3D and especially VISTA3D work great in 3D CT segmentation when these constraints are not a problem. nnInteractive is the fastest model for 3D segmentation if sufficient VRAM is available, and shows strong performance with a variety of different input prompt types, as well as much better zero-shot accuracy than SAM-Med3D and VISTA3D, leading us to recommend it if only 3D segmentation is necessary. SAM-Med2D was always the worst model and cannot be recommended.

SAM3's new concept of context segmentation, which segments visually similar objects with a single prompt is promising for images with lots of similar objects, but poses the problem of segmenting wrong objects (especially when there's only one correct instance among a visually similar group, e.g. vocal folds look similar to surrounding tissue). Its text-based context segmentation mode works great for simple objects like the Spleen (MSD Spleen 2D: SAM3 with $mIoU_{text} = 0.894$ and $mIoU_{box} = 0.897$) in X-ray, CT and MRI images. Nevertheless, it has a certain ambiguity of prompts, as SAM3 can find and segment the mitochondria in brain electron microscopy fine with the prompt "cells", but segments nothing with a prompt "mitochondria". It also cannot detect some structures like the vocal folds or polyps automatically. Therefore, its visual mode is often superior for uncommon and more complicated medical image segmentation tasks.

Although models frequently yield commendable results, several issues persist. Primarily, the generalization and zero-shot capability of most medical FMs do not quite reach their counterpart for natural images, mostly due to the lack of training data and unclear boundaries. Additionally, segmentation of intricate or small structures, such as pulps, vessels, tumors, or adrenal glands, remains quite limited, especially in multi-dimensional images. Many models that address some of these limitations have already been published, such as Vessel-SAM2, but mostly fall into the task-specific category, as they lose some of their foundational capabilities. Moreover, many such structures are contained within larger regions, like hepatic vessels inside the liver, which complicates prompt placement because models tend to favor segmenting simpler objects. Given that these interactive FMs are heavily dependent on prompt quality and quantity, a significant amount of manual effort by humans is often still necessary. Our work presented here is limited by the fact that we mostly focused on single-prompt segmentation for each object, leaving out iterative prompting strategies like human-in-the-loop or more complex prompts like mask or scribble prompts. We compared seven of the available FMs.

References

1. Cheng D, Qin Z, Jiang Z, Zhang S, Lao Q, Li K. SAM on medical images: a comprehensive study on three prompt modes. arXiv: 2305.00035. 2023.
2. Ma J, He Y, Li F, Han L, You C, Wang B. Segment anything in medical images. Nat Commun. 2024;15(1):654.
3. Ma J, Yang Z, Kim S, Chen B, Baharoon M, Fallahpour A et al. MedSAM2: segment anything in 3D medical images and videos. arXiv: 2504.03600. 2025.
4. Cheng J, Fu B, Ye J, Wang G, Li T, Wang H et al. Interactive medical image segmentation: a benchmark dataset and baseline. arXiv: 2411.12814. 2024.
5. Ravi N, Gabeur V, Hu YT, Hu R, Ryali C, Ma T et al. SAM 2: segment anything in images and videos. arXiv: 2408.00714. 2024.
6. Carion N, Gustafson L, Hu YT, Debnath S, Hu R, Suris D et al. SAM 3: segment anything with concepts. arXiv: 2408.00714. 2025.
7. Cheng J, Ye J, Deng Z, Chen J, Li T, Wang H et al. SAM-Med2D. arXiv: 2308.16184. 2023.
8. Wang H, Guo S, Ye J, Deng Z, Cheng J, et al. SAM-Med3D: towards general-purpose segmentation models for volumetric medical images. arXiv: 2310.15161. 2024.
9. Isensee F, Rokuss M, Krämer L, Dinkelacker S, Ravindran A, Stritzke F et al. nnInteractive: redefining 3D promptable segmentation. arXiv: 2503.08373. 2025.
10. He Y, Guo P, Tang Y, Myronenko A, Nath V, Xu Z et al. VISTA3D: a unified segmentation foundation model for 3D medical imaging. arXiv: 2406.05285. 2024.
11. Gómez P, Kist AM, Schlegel P, Berry DA, Chhetri DK, Dürr S et al. BAGLS: a multihospital benchmark for automatic glottis segmentation. Sci Data. 2020;7(1):186.
12. Lucchi A, Li Y, Fua P. Learning for structured prediction using approximate subgradient descent with working sets. Proc IEEE CVPR. 2013:1987–94.
13. Ngoc Lan P, An NS, Hang DV, Long DV, Trung TQ, Thuy NT et al. NeoUNet : towards accurate colon polyp segmentation and neoplasm detection. Proc ISVC. 2021:15–28.
14. Murali A, Alapatt D, Mascagni P, Vardazaryan A, Garcia A, Okamoto N et al. The endoscapes dataset for surgical scene segmentation, object detection, and critical view of safety assessment. Sci Data. 2025;12(1):331.
15. Kuş Z, Aydin M. MedSegBench: a comprehensive benchmark for medical image segmentation in diverse data modalities. Sci Data. 2024;11(1):1283.
16. Bolelli F, Marchesini K, Nistelrooij N van, et al. Segmenting maxillofacial structures in CBCT volume. Proc IEEE/CVF CVPR. 2025:1–10.
17. Bolelli F, Lumetti L, Vinayahalingam S, et al. Segmenting the inferior alveolar canal in CBCTs volumes: the toothfairy challenge. IEEE Trans Med Imaging. 2024:1–17.
18. Antonelli M, Reinke A, Bakas S, Farahani K, AnnetteKopp-Schneider, Landman BA et al. The medical segmentation decathlon. Nat Commun. 2022;13(1):4128.
19. Kist AM, Razi S, Groh R, Gritsch F, Schützenberger A. Predicting semantic segmentation quality in laryngeal endoscopy images. PLoS One. 2025;20(7):e0314573.
20. Park D, Kim Y, Kang H, Lee J, Choi J, Kim T et al. PECI-Net: bolus segmentation from video fluoroscopic swallowing study images using preprocessing ensemble and cascaded inference. Comput Biol Med. 2024;172:108241.

Modular Pipeline for Rapidly Evaluating Foundation Models in Medical Imaging

EvalBlocks

Jan Tagscherer, Sarah de Boer, Lena Philipp, Fennie van der Graaf, Dré Peeters, Joeran Bosma, Lars Leijten, Bogdan Obreja, Ewoud Smit, Alessa Hering

Diagnostic Image Analysis Group, Radboud University Medical Center, Nijmegen, The Netherlands

jan.tagscherer@radboudumc.nl

Abstract. Developing foundation models in medical imaging requires continuous monitoring of downstream performance. Researchers are burdened with tracking numerous experiments, design choices, and their effects on performance, often relying on ad-hoc, manual workflows that are inherently slow and error-prone. We introduce *EvalBlocks*, a modular, plug-and-play framework for efficient evaluation of foundation models during development. Built on Snakemake, EvalBlocks supports seamless integration of new datasets, foundation models, aggregation methods, and evaluation strategies. All experiments and results are tracked centrally and are reproducible with a single command, while efficient caching and parallel execution enable scalable use on shared compute infrastructure. Demonstrated on five state-of-the-art foundation models and three medical imaging classification tasks, EvalBlocks streamlines model evaluation, enabling researchers to iterate faster and focus on model innovation rather than evaluation logistics. The framework is released as open source software at `https://github.com/DIAGNijmegen/eval-blocks`.

1 Introduction

Foundation models have shown great promise in medical imaging, learning semantically rich embeddings from large-scale pretraining that can then be used for few-shot adaptation to data-scarce tasks. When integrated into downstream pipelines, these pretrained models can substantially accelerate development and improve performance across diverse clinical applications. While this quality is appealing, developing these models involves a multitude of design choices, such as data sampling, architecture selection, and training strategy. This results in an iterative development process during which it is important to continuously estimate a model's downstream performance and gain insights into the impact of training and architecture choices.

The evaluation of foundation models is often performed using bespoke scripts while also managing compute resources and organizing experiments. This unnec-

© Der/die Autor(en), exklusiv lizenziert an
Springer Fachmedien Wiesbaden GmbH, ein Teil von Springer Nature 2026
H. Handels et al. (Hrsg.), *Bildverarbeitung für die Medizin 2026*,
Informatik aktuell, https://doi.org/10.1007/978-3-658-51100-5_9

essary difficulty slows iteration, complicates reproducibility, and shifts focus away from improving models themselves.

The emergence of foundation models has prompted the creation of benchmarks to compare their downstream performance on various medical imaging tasks. Wang et al. [1] define clinically relevant tasks for a systematic comparison, Jin et al. [2] assess fairness across datasets, tasks, and sensitive attributes, and the UNICORN challenge [3] evaluates submitted models on multimodal tasks. While valuable for standardized comparison, these benchmarks focus on comprehensiveness over rapid evaluation during model development.

Similar needs for lightweight evaluation have been addressed in other domains. Hugging Face's LightEval [4] supports the rapid assessment of large language models, and NVIDIA's NeMo Evaluator SDK [5] aims to make LLM evaluation robust, reproducible, and scalable.

In medical imaging, however, a comparable tool for efficient and reproducible model evaluation is lacking. We address this gap with *EvalBlocks*, a modular, extensible, and cluster-ready pipeline based on Snakemake [6] and designed for efficient, reproducible assessment of foundation models in medical imaging. We demonstrate the utility of our pipeline by evaluating five recent foundation models across three malignancy classification tasks.

In summary, our contributions include:

- A modular, extensible, and efficient evaluation framework for foundation models in medical imaging that is available as open source software.
- A demonstration of the pipeline that evaluates five foundation models on three medical imaging classification tasks.

2 Materials and methods

2.1 Architecture overview

Fig. 1 illustrates the pipeline, composed of independent Snakemake rules that define their input-output dependencies and resource requirements. They are automatically executed when their required inputs are available. Rules are grouped into three categories: (1) feature models that transform input patches into embeddings, (2) optional aggregation steps, and (3) evaluation procedures. Intermediate outputs are cached for efficient reuse.

Experiments are recorded declaratively in a configuration file, specifying datasets, models, and evaluation methods. The pipeline can run selected experiments or all configured combinations on demand and supports distributed execution in cluster environments such as Slurm [7], running computational steps in parallel wherever possible.

We demonstrate the framework's utility by implementing a set of blocks that allow for the evaluation of five foundation models across three medical imaging classification tasks. The goal of these experiments is not to advance state-of-the-art performance, but to demonstrate how EvalBlocks accelerates experimental iteration.

2.2 Datasets

We evaluate on three patch-level malignancy classification tasks derived from the AMARA (in-house), PANORAMA [8], and PI-CAI [9] datasets. Each dataset provides training and test splits across five folds. For all datasets, we extract patches of size 224 × 224 × 16 along with malignancy labels. Input data is preprocessed according to the specifications provided by each model's authors. For models that can handle three-dimensional input data, we use the entire patch. For two-dimensional architectures, we input the central slice. Finally, DINOv2 [10] and DINOv3 [11] have been trained on natural images. For these models, we interpret the input slices as grayscale images with values between 0 and 255.

From the AMARA dataset's CT scans, we extract 161 malignant and 502 benign pulmonary nodules from 320 patients with ground-truth labels determined by pathological confirmation.

The PANORAMA dataset [8] yields 675 CT patches of healthy pancreatic tissue and 675 patches with ductal adenocarcinoma.

Finally, we produce 219 MR patches depicting prostate carcinoma and 219 patches with healthy prostate tissue from the public test set of the PI-CAI challenge [9].

2.3 Foundation models

We evaluate five foundation models: CT-FM [12] is the only model that has been trained on three-dimensional CT scans as its only modality, while the remaining medically-focused models process two-dimensional but multi-modal input data. Curia [13] has been created through unsupervised training on a large dataset of medical

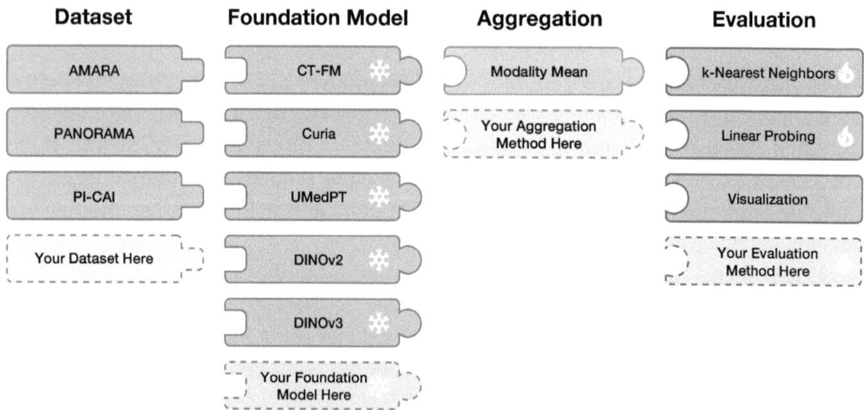

Fig. 1. In our framework, pipeline steps are implemented as self-contained blocks. Foundation models embed input patches, and these feature embeddings can be optionally aggregated and then evaluated. The pipeline blocks can be freely extended and plugged into each other, enabling fast, reproducible, and customizable evaluation during foundation model development.

images. UMedPT [14] is the only model in our evaluation that has been trained in a supervised manner. Finally, we also include DINOv2 [10] and DINOv3 [11], which have been trained on natural images rather than medical imaging data. The public release includes preconfigured blocks for these models, including all necessary preprocessing steps, enabling immediate plug-and-play use.

2.4 Aggregation methods

For demonstration purposes, we aggregate the embeddings of our MRI dataset by computing the element-wise mean of feature vectors across modalities to assess whether combining complementary contrasts improves downstream performance.

Beyond this example, the framework supports defining custom aggregation modules, enabling more complex strategies such as weighted averaging, attention-based fusion, or case-level pooling.

2.5 Evaluation strategies

We implement three interchangeable evaluation strategies that operate on the optionally aggregated feature embeddings.

First, we fit a k-nearest neighbors classifier with $k \in \{10, 20, 100, 200\}$ on the training features and report accuracy and AUC on the test split; results for $k = 20$ are shown in the following. Second, we train a single linear layer using cross entropy loss with a learning rate of $1e-5$ and evaluate its accuracy and AUC. Third, we generate visual analyses by applying linear discriminant analysis, principal component analysis, and t-SNE to the feature embeddings, providing interpretable plots of the learned representations.

3 Results

We evaluated all combinations of foundation models, aggregation methods, and evaluation strategies using the EvalBlocks pipeline. This produced a comprehensive set of metrics and visualizations for each configuration, demonstrating that the pipeline executes and records experiments in an automated and reproducible manner.

Fig. 2 depicts model performance on our two CT datasets, showcasing how EvalBlocks can be used to estimate the difficulty of a downstream task and compare models.

Fig. 3 focuses on our framework's ability to evaluate across modalities and aggregation methods, allowing for fast prototyping of the latter and informed selection of inputs.

Finally, Fig. 4 showcases how the visualization block can enable a more thorough analysis of feature embeddings produced by the foundation models.

During the evaluation of these models, caching avoided recomputing embeddings across experiments. In combination with the framework's parallel execution capabilities, this reduced wall-time substantially.

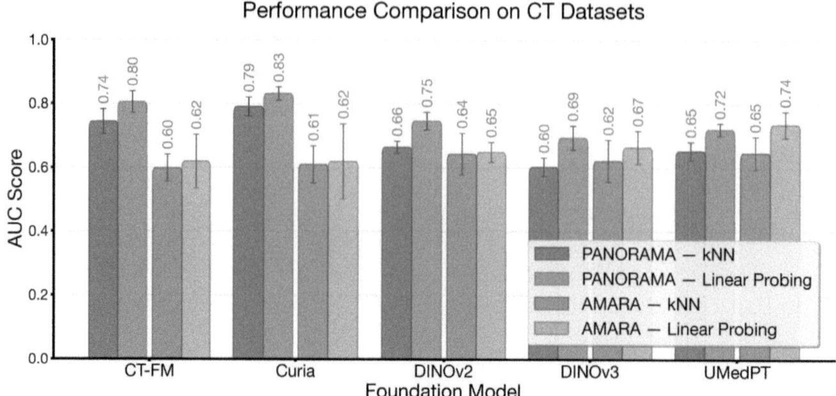

Fig. 2. A visualization of model results on our CT datasets created by running EvalBlocks, with error bars depicting the standard deviation across folds. While CT-FM [12] and Curia [13] perform best on PANORAMA [8], UMedPT [14] is slightly more accurate on AMARA. Our pipeline allows for fast and automated comparison between models and checkpoints.

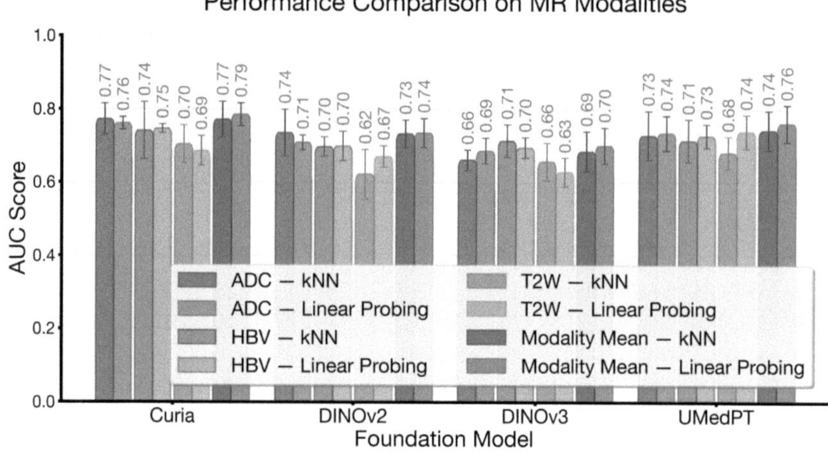

Fig. 3. EvalBlocks also enables evaluation across modalities and aggregation methods, here for the PI-CAI [9] dataset. Error bars denote the standard deviation across folds. Overall, ADC is the most informative modality for malignancy discrimination. The modality mean aggregation emerges as a well-performing strategy for this task. Our framework enables researchers to easily prototype aggregation methods.

4 Discussion

EvalBlocks provides a modular and efficient framework for evaluating foundation models in medical imaging. In this study, we demonstrated its flexibility and utility by evaluating five foundation models across three downstream classification tasks with minimal configuration effort. The modular design facilitates the rapid integration of datasets, models, aggregation strategies, and evaluation methods. The framework's efficient caching and centralized experiment tracking substantially reduces both computational and manual effort. Furthermore, EvalBlocks can run locally, which made the assessment of foundation models on in-house datasets possible.

We note that, as the number of datasets and models grows, the combinatorial space of possible evaluations expands quickly. EvalBlocks mitigates this by lever-

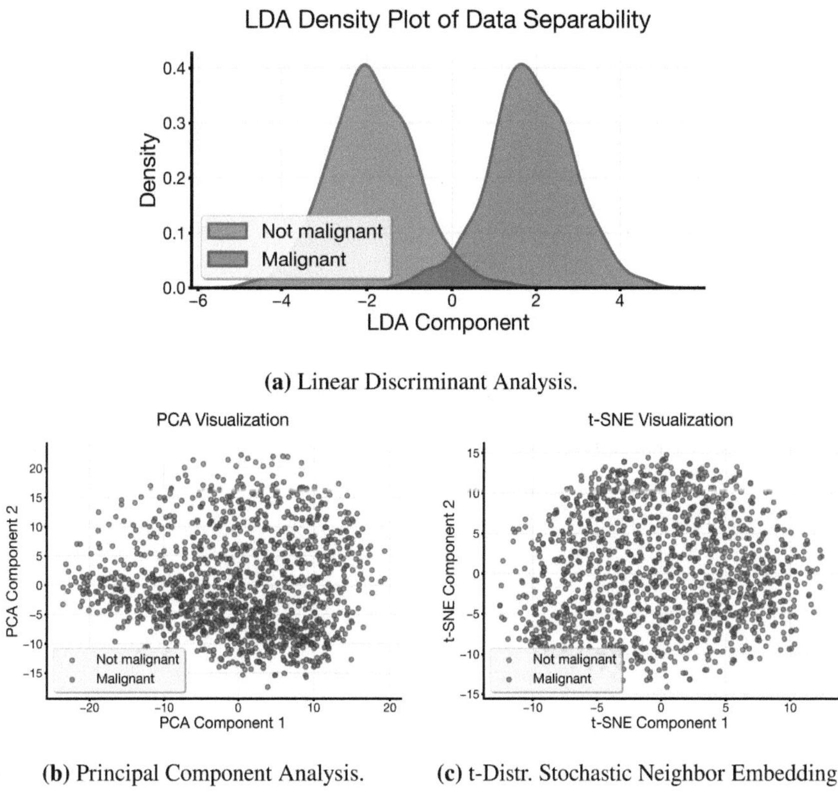

(a) Linear Discriminant Analysis.

(b) Principal Component Analysis.

(c) t-Distr. Stochastic Neighbor Embedding.

Fig. 4. Visualizations of the feature embeddings of Curia [13] on the first fold of the PANORAMA dataset [8]. While PCA and t-SNE yield no clusters, LDA shows two distinct peaks for the two classes. This reveals that the model produces linearly separable feature embeddings for this task in label-dependent directions, but not in directions of maximum variance or local neighborhood structures. EvalBlocks produces these visualizations for all folds, datasets, and models, allowing deeper analysis where necessary.

aging Snakemake's caching and parallelization capabilities and by allowing users to selectively run subsets of experiments.

While existing benchmarks are useful as static leaderboards for foundation models, they are not suited for iterative model development. EvalBlocks fills this gap by enabling reproducible, transparent, and scalable evaluation during model development, thus bridging the gap between large-scale benchmarking and practical experimentation.

Future work will expand EvalBlocks to additional task types such as segmentation and detection. Integrating the framework with existing popular platforms like Hugging Face will allow for better community collaboration. By reducing the burden of evaluation logistics, EvalBlocks allows researchers to focus on improving model architectures, training strategies, and downstream adaptation.

References

1. Wang D, Wang X, Wang L, Li M, Da Q, Liu X et al. A real-world dataset and benchmark for foundation model adaptation in medical image classification. Sci Data. 2023;10(1):574.
2. Jin R, Xu Z, Zhong Y, Yao Q, QI D, Zhou SK et al. FairMedFM: fairness benchmarking for medical imaging foundation models. Proc NeurIPS. 2024;37:111318–57.
3. D'Amato M, Weber R, Lefkes J, van der Graaf F, Stegeman M, Grisi C et al. The UNICORN challenge: public few-shots. Version 7.0. Zenodo, 2025.
4. Habib N, Fourrier C, Kydlíček H, Wolf T, Tunstall L. LightEval: a lightweight framework for LLM evaluation. Version 0.11.0. 2023.
5. NVIDIA-NeMo. NeMo evaluator SDK. URL: `https://github.com/NVIDIA-NeMo/Evaluator/`.
6. Mölder F, Jablonski KP, Letcher B, Hall MB, van Dyken PC, Tomkins-Tinch CH et al. Sustainable data analysis with Snakemake. F1000Res. 2025;10:33.
7. Yoo AB, Jette MA, Grondona M. Slurm: simple Linux utility for resource management. Proc JSSPP. 2003:44–60.
8. Alves N, Schuurmans M, Rutkowski D, Yakar D, Haldorsen I, Liedenbaum M et al. The PANORAMA study protocol: pancreatic cancer diagnosis: radiologists meet AI. Zenodo, 2024.
9. Saha A, Bosma JS, Twilt JJ, van Ginneken B, Bjartell A, Padhani AR et al. Artificial intelligence and radiologists in prostate cancer detection on MRI (PI-CAI): an international, paired, non-inferiority, confirmatory study. Lancet Oncol. 2024;25(7):879–87.
10. Oquab M, Darcet T, Moutakanni T, Vo H, Szafraniec M, Khalidov V et al. DINOv2: learning robust visual features without supervision. arXiv preprint: 2304.07193. 2023.
11. Siméoni O, Vo HV, Seitzer M, Baldassarre F, Oquab M, Jose C et al. DINOv3. arXiv preprint: 2508.10104. 2025.
12. Pai S, Hadzic I, Bontempi D, Bressem K, Kann BH, Fedorov A et al. Vision foundation models for computed tomography. arXiv preprint: 2501.09001. 2025.
13. Dancette C, Khlaut J, Saporta A, Philippe H, Ferreres E, Callard B et al. Curia: a multi-modal foundation model for radiology. arXiv preprint: 2304.07193. 2025.
14. Schäfer R, Nicke T, Höfener H, Lange A, Merhof D, Feuerhake F et al. Overcoming data scarcity in biomedical imaging with a foundational multi-task model. Nat Comput Sci. 2024;4(7):495–509.

Parameter-efficient Finetuning of Foundational Models for Text-guided X-ray Image Segmentation

Maeen Alikarrar [1,2], Christopher Syben [2], Joshua Scheuplein [1,2], Christian Hümmer[2], Ludwig Ritschl[2], Steffen Kappler[2], Andreas Maier [1]

[1]Pattern Recognition Lab, Department of Computer Science, Friedrich-Alexander-Universität Erlangen-Nürnberg, Erlangen, Germany
[2]X-ray Department, Siemens Healthineers AG, Forchheim, Germany
maeen.alikarrar@fau.de

Abstract. Radiographic image segmentation presents unique challenges due to overlapping anatomical structures, projection ambiguity, and the scarcity of high-quality annotations. Recently, segmentation foundation models such as *MedSAM* have emerged as powerful tools for automated medical image analysis. Trained on large-scale and diverse image-mask pairs, MedSAM has achieved broad generalization across a wide range of medical image segmentation tasks. Despite this, its exposure to X-rays was primarily limited to chest radiographs annotated with lung masks, and the model relied on spatial prompts like bounding boxes, which are labor-intensive to draw precisely during inference and prone to ambiguity. To overcome these limitations, we propose a parameter-efficient adaptation of MedSAM designed for X-ray image segmentation. The approach integrates lightweight low-rank adaptation (LoRA) fine-tuning to enable efficient model updating while incorporating text-based conditioning to guide mask prediction. This design facilitates intuitive, non-expert human interaction without requiring precise geometric prompts. Evaluated on internal chest and lower-limb radiographic datasets, the model achieves a mean Dice (mDice) score of 92.42 and a mean intersection-over-union (mIoU) of 86.46 while unfreezing only a small fraction of parameters. These results demonstrate that parameter-efficient, language-conditioned adaptation offers an effective strategy for enhancing segmentation performance in projection-based medical imaging.

1 Introduction

Medical image segmentation is a fundamental task in biomedical image analysis, enabling the delineation of anatomical structures and providing precise shape information for improved diagnosis, treatment planning, and disease monitoring [1, 2]. Although deep learning has significantly advanced segmentation, leading to the creation of sophisticated models, these models typically require extensive datasets with high-quality manual annotations and are often tailored to specific tasks, limiting their generalization across diverse domains [3]. This challenge has sparked interest

© Der/die Autor(en), exklusiv lizenziert an
Springer Fachmedien Wiesbaden GmbH, ein Teil von Springer Nature 2026
H. Handels et al. (Hrsg.), *Bildverarbeitung für die Medizin 2026*,
Informatik aktuell, https://doi.org/10.1007/978-3-658-51100-5_10

in foundational models [4, 5] that promise broad generalization with minimal labeled data. Among these, the segment anything model (SAM) [6] represents a major shift, introducing a prompt-driven segmentation framework capable of generalizing to unseen natural images in zero- or few-shot settings. However, SAM's pretraining on natural image datasets results in a domain gap when applied to medical data, where fine anatomical structures, uncertain and complex object boundaries, and wide-ranging object scales make segmentation inherently challenging [7]. This limitation drove the need for adapting or fine-tuning SAM to bridge the domain gap between medical and natural images [2].

MedSAM [8] extended SAM through large-scale fine-tuning on over 1.5 million medical image-mask pairs spanning modalities such as CT, MRI, ultrasound, and X-ray. While MedSAM demonstrates impressive cross-modality generalization, it remains constrained by its reliance on bounding-box prompting, which requires expert anatomical knowledge to define accurate regions of interest. Moreover, X-ray data are underrepresented in its training corpus. Unlike volumetric modalities such as CT and MRI, which provide spatially resolved anatomical context, X-rays capture 2D projections of complex 3D structures, leading to spatial ambiguity and overlapping anatomies that make accurate segmentation challenging. Most publicly available X-ray datasets consist primarily of chest radiographs – often limited to lung masks – further restricting generalization. As a result, foundation models tailored specifically for X-rays have mainly focused on chest radiography, supported by large public resources such as CheXpert, MIMIC-CXR, and NIH CXR14. Notable examples include *CheXFound* [9], *CXR-CLIP* [10], and *DINO-CXR* [11].

Vision-language foundation models such as CLIP [12] have demonstrated that textual supervision serves as a powerful learning signal, aligning images and language within a shared semantic space. Recent work suggests that natural language provides a richer and more flexible conditioning signal that can complement visual representations and help disambiguate overlapping anatomy [13]. *FluoroSAM* [14], a language-promptable variant of SAM, addresses data scarcity by training from scratch on synthetic X-ray projections derived from CT volumes paired with anatomical text labels. The dataset comprised different human anatomies and viewing angles. However, FluoroSAM's evaluation on real X-rays show limited performance, reporting an average Dice of 0.60 and IoU of 0.47.

In this work, we propose a parameter-efficient framework for adapting MedSAM to real X-ray segmentation using text-based guidance. Our method integrates textual prompts that correspond to anatomical targets and fine-tunes MedSAM through LoRA [15], enabling efficient domain adaptation without full network retraining. By conditioning the model on textual context, we aim to resolve the ambiguity of overlapping structures and localize anatomically relevant regions. We validate our approach on two X-ray datasets – chest and lower-limb radiographs – demonstrating that text-guided LoRA fine-tuning achieves substantial performance gains while maintaining computational efficiency.

2 Materials and methods

2.1 Dataset

We utilize two internally collected radiographic datasets with polygon-based JSON annotations describing anatomical structures. DICOM images were exported based on clinical collaboration and following all required local regulations and the general data protection regulation (GDPR) of the European Union. Additional ethical approval was not required. The first dataset consists of 4,094 chest X-ray images containing four labeled regions: vertebral column, scapula, clavicle, and lungs, including both left-right instances when applicable. The second dataset includes 2,614 lower-limb radiographs with annotations for femur, patella, tibia, and fibula. As illustrated in Figure 1, both datasets exhibit substantial anatomical overlap inherent to projection imaging (e.g., clavicle/lung or patella/femur), making them suitable for evaluating segmentation models under spatial ambiguity and overlap.

A unified preprocessing pipeline is applied to prepare the data for model training. All images are resized to 1024×1024 to satisfy SAM input requirements, followed by percentile-based intensity clipping (0.5–99.5) and normalization to the $[0, 1]$ range. Polygon annotations are rasterized into binary masks and subsequently resized to 256×256 to match the model output resolution. Both datasets were first split independently into 70% training, 10% validation, and 20% test subsets, then the respective splits were merged to form unified training, validation, and test sets.

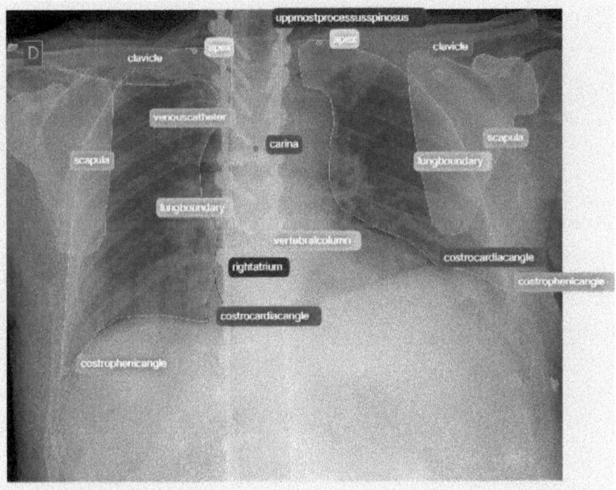

(a) Chest X-ray sample with annotated regions.

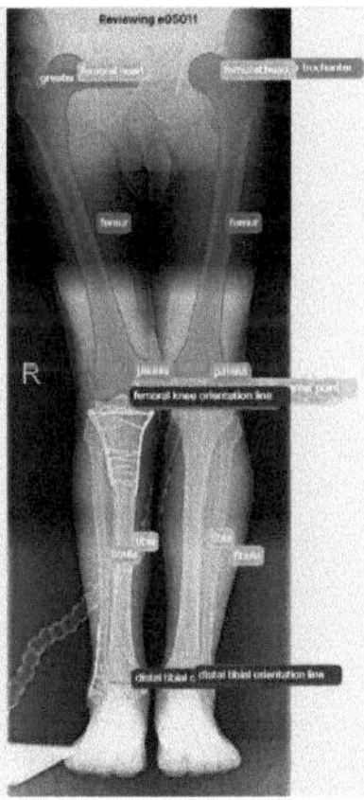

(b) Lower-limb radiograph sample with annotated bones.

Fig. 1. Example samples from our radiographic datasets showing annotated regions. Left: chest X-ray; right: lower-limb radiograph.

2.2 Model architecture

Figure 2 illustrates the proposed framework. The model is initialized with pretrained *MedSAM* weights. Image features are extracted using the ViT-B image encoder, while a CLIP-based text encoder is incorporated to enable text prompting. In the CLIP text encoder, The *[EOS]* (End of Sequence) token marks the end of the input text. Its embedding represents the overall meaning of the entire text prompt and is used as the final text feature in our framework. Both the image and text embeddings, each projected to a 256-dimensional latent space, are jointly processed by the mask decoder to generate the final segmentation output. Our LoRA design, including rank, scaling factor, and initialization strategy, strictly follows the configuration proposed in SAMed [16]. LoRA weights are injected to the query q and value v projections in every transformer block. Therefore, for multiheaded attention, the process becomes

$$\mathrm{Att}(Q, K, V) = \mathrm{Softmax}\left(\frac{QK^\top}{\sqrt{d}}\right)V$$

where

$$Q = W_q U + B_q A_q U, \quad K = W_k U, \quad V = W_v U + B_v A_v U$$

Here, W_q, W_k, and W_v are the frozen pretrained weights from MedSAM, U is the layer input, while A_q, B_q, A_v, and B_v are the trainable LoRA parameters.

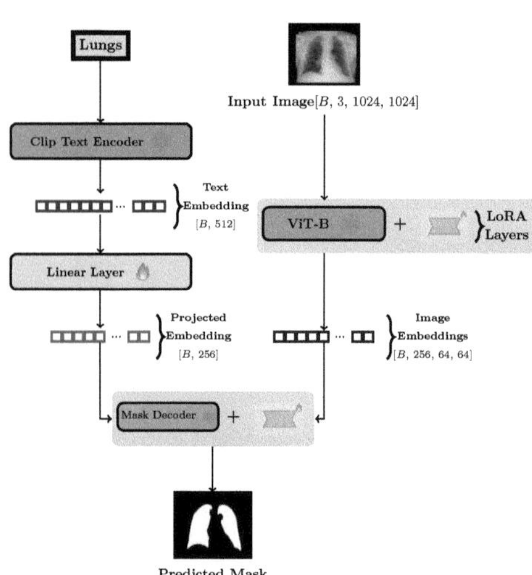

Fig. 2. Overview of the proposed framework. Trainable LoRA layers are injected into the frozen MedSAM ViT-B image encoder and mask decoder. A frozen CLIP text encoder extracts text embeddings, which are projected via a trainable linear layer. The mask decoder then processes the image and text embeddings and outputs the binary segmentation mask.

Unless otherwise stated, all training and optimization settings follow the MedSAM implementation. We adopt the same loss formulation, optimizer, learning rate schedule, and number of training epochs as MedSAM. The batch size is set to 8,

Tab. 1. Segmentation performance comparison (mDice and mIoU) for different fine-tuning strategies applied to MedSAM.

Method	mDice [%]	mIoU [%]
MedSAM (bbox prompting)	59.46	46.63
LoRA on decoder	84.21	74.12
Decoder full fine-tuning	87.84	79.43
LoRA on encoder + LoRA on decoder	92.42	86.46
LoRA on encoder + decoder full fine-tuning	92.19	86.11
Full fine-tuning (encoder + decoder)	93.63	88.55

consistent with MedSAM, except in experiments where the image encoder is fine-tuned, for which a batch size of 4 is used due to increased memory requirements. No additional hyperparameter tuning or architectural modifications are introduced, ensuring that performance gains can be attributed to the incorporation of anatomical text prompting and LoRA-based adaptation rather than differences in training configuration

3 Experiments and results

We first establish a baseline using the original MedSAM model with bounding-box prompting and no fine-tuning. This configuration achieves an mDice of 59.46 and an mIoU of 46.63, reflecting the limited transferability of the pretrained model to our radiographic datasets.

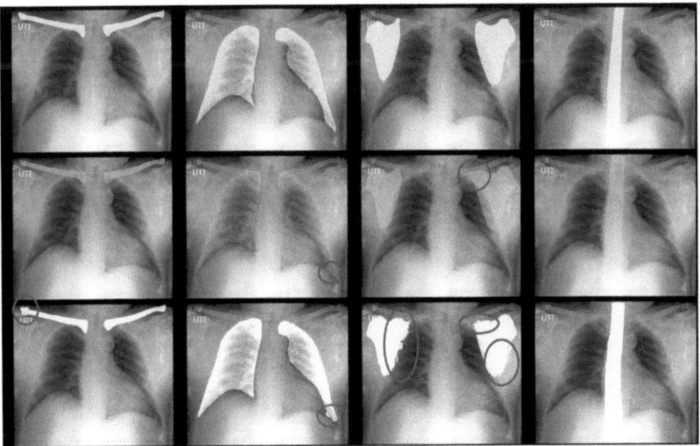

Fig. 3. Comparison of text-prompted segmentation results across chest labels. *Row 1:* Ground truth masks. *Row 2:* Predictions from full fine-tuning (Image encoder + decoder). *Row 3:* Predictions from LoRA fine-tuning (Image encoder + decoder).

We then fine-tune only the decoder while keeping the image encoder frozen, as the decoder is responsible for translating visual and textual features into spatially precise segmentation maps. Two adaptation strategies are explored: traditional full-parameter fine-tuning and LoRA. Conventional fine-tuning yields substantial performance gains (mDice 87.84, mIoU 79.43), whereas LoRA-based tuning reaches 84.21 and 74.12, respectively (Tab. 1). The strong improvement of both methods over the baseline underscores the decoder's pivotal role in domain adaptation, though LoRA alone results in a 3.63% mDice and 5.31% mIoU gap compared to full fine-tuning.

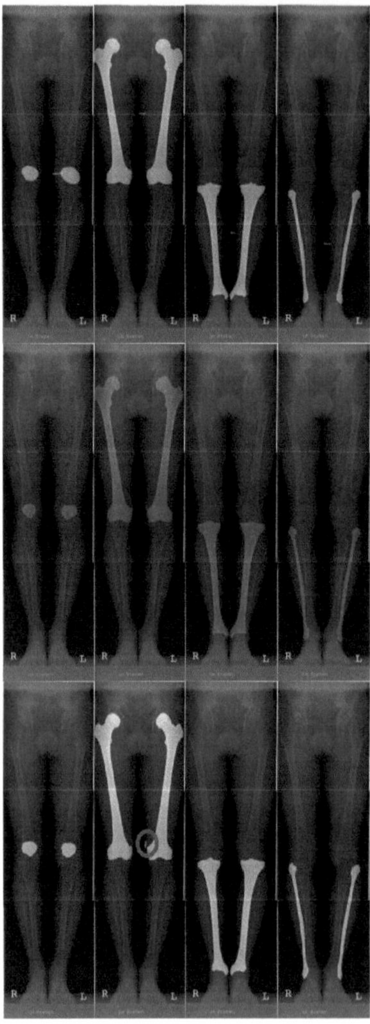

Fig. 4. Comparison of text-prompted segmentation results across legs labels. *Row 1:* Ground truth masks. *Row 2:* Predictions from full fine-tuning (Image encoder + decoder). *Row 3:* Predictions from LoRA fine-tuning (Image encoder + decoder).

To improve text-guided segmentation while maintaining parameter efficiency, we next adapted the encoder – which contains the majority of the model's representational capacity (≈89M parameters) – using LoRA, adding fewer than 150K trainable weights. The decoder, being comparatively lightweight (≈4M parameters), was again the main target for adaptation. We first applied LoRA to both encoder and decoder, achieving strong results (mDice 92.42, mIoU 86.46). To test whether fully optimizing the small decoder could offer additional gains, we also combined encoder LoRA with full decoder fine-tuning; however, the difference (mDice 92.42% vs. 92.19%; mIoU 86.46% vs. 86.11%) proved negligible.

Full fine-tuning of both encoder and decoder achieved the highest overall performance (mDice 93.63, mIoU 88.55), but the modest 1–2% margin over the parameter-efficient LoRA setup suggests diminishing returns relative to the vastly larger number of trainable parameters. Collectively, these findings demonstrate that LoRA applied to both encoder and decoder offers an optimal balance between segmentation accuracy and computational efficiency, making it a practical strategy for adapting large segmentation models to radiographic domains. A qualitative comparison of the segmentation results across both datasets is shown in Figures 3 and 4.

4 Discussion

This work presented a text-guided approach for adapting MedSAM to X-ray segmentation. MedSAM's limited transferability to X-ray images necessitates targeted adaptation. By applying lightweight LoRA updates to the encoder and decoder, we achieved mDice of 92.42 % and mIoU of 86.46 %, with minimal additional parameters. These findings highlight LoRA's efficiency for scalable, text-aware medical segmentation. The current work is limited to fixed anatomical labels, which restricts open-vocabulary segmentation and limits the expressive potential of language conditioning. Future work should explore richer textual descriptions.

Disclaimer. The presented methods in this paper are not commercially available and their future availability cannot be guaranteed.

References

1. Yan Z, Sun W, Zhou R, Yuan Z, Zhang K, Li Y et al. Biomedical SAM 2: segment anything in biomedical images and videos. arXiv: 2406.03286. 2024.
2. Litjens G, Kooi T, Bejnordi BE, Setio AAA, Ciompi F, Ghafoorian M et al. A survey on deep learning in medical image analysis. Med Image Anal. 2017;42:60–88.
3. Fu Y, Lei Y, Wang T, Curran WJ, Liu T, Yang X. A review of deep learning based methods for medical image multi-organ segmentation. Phys Med. 2021;85:107–22.
4. Wang X, Chen G, Qian G, Gao P, Wei XY, Wang Y et al. Large-scale multi-modal pre-trained models: a comprehensive survey. Mach Intell Res. 2023;20(4):447–82.
5. Liang PP, Zadeh A, Morency LP. Foundations and recent trends in multimodal machine learning: principles, challenges, and open questions. arXiv: 2209.03430. 2022.
6. Kirillov A, Mintun E, Ravi N, Mao H, Rolland C, Gustafson L et al. Segment anything. arXiv: 2304.02643. 2023.

7. Huang Y, Yang X, Liu L, Zhou H, Chang A, Zhou X et al. Segment anything model for medical images? Med Image Anal. 2024;92:103061.
8. Ma J, He Y, Wu T et al. Segment anything in medical images. Nat Commun. 2024;15(1):654.
9. Yang Z, Xu X, Zhang J, Wang G, Kalra MK, Yan P. Chest X-ray foundation model with global and local representations integration. IEEE Trans Med Imaging. 2025;44(12):4787–99.
10. You K, Gu J, Ham J, Park B, Kim J, Hong EK et al. CXR-CLIP: toward large scale chest X-ray language-image pre-training. Proc MICCAI. 2023:101–11.
11. Shakouri M, Iranmanesh F, Eftekhari M. DINO-CXR: a self supervised method based on vision transformer for chest X-ray classification. Proc AVC. 2023:320–31.
12. Radford A, Kim JW, Hallacy C, Ramesh A, Goh G, Agarwal S et al. Learning transferable visual models from natural language supervision. arXiv: 2103.00020. 2021.
13. Zhao Z, Zhang Y, Wu C, Zhang X, Zhou X, Zhang Y et al. Large-vocabulary segmentation for medical images with text prompts. NPJ Digit Med. 2025;8(1):566.
14. Killeen BD, Wang LJ, Inigo B, Zhang H, Armand M, Taylor RH et al. FluoroSAM: a language-promptable foundation model for flexible X-ray image segmentation. arXiv: 2403.08059. 2025.
15. Hu EJ, Shen Y, Wallis P, Allen-Zhu Z, Li Y, Wang S et al. LoRA: low-rank adaptation of large language models. Proc ICLR. 2022.
16. Zhang K, Liu D. Customized segment anything model for medical image segmentation. arXiv: 2304.13785. 2023.

Revealing Eye-dentity

Foundation Models Enable Re-identification from Retinal OCT

Marc S. Seibel [1†], Nele S. Brügge [2†], Timo Kepp [2], Bennet Kahrs [1], Jan Ehrhardt [1], Heinz Handels [1,2]

[1]Institute of Medical Informatics, University of Luebeck
[2]German Research Center for Artificial Intelligence, Luebeck
nele.bruegge@dfki.de

Abstract. Foundation models have become central to medical imaging research, yet subject re-identification implications remain unclear. In this work, we study whether optical coherence tomography (OCT)-derived B-scan features extracted using frozen generalist and specialist foundation models allow re-identification of subjects intra- and cross-device. A lightweight binary classifier was trained to predict whether two feature sets originate from the same individual. Results show that specialist models such as RETFound reach 78 % re-identification accuracy (Rank-1) on high-resolution OCT data, while generalist models perform only slightly worse. Performance decreased substantially on the lower-resolution data and was near chance across devices. These findings suggest that general foundation models extract subject-related information, potentially entangled with recording device-related information.

1 Introduction

Optical coherence tomography (OCT) is the gold standard for non-invasive imaging of retinal structures, enabling early detection and monitoring of diseases such as age-related macular degeneration, diabetic retinopathy, and glaucoma [1]. While OCT supports clinical and longitudinal research, its full potential increasingly depends on modern deep learning approaches for image analysis. Such systems could benefit from content-based image retrieval, enabling OCT image databases to be queried for similar image features to support automatic diagnosis [2]. However, the ability of deep learning models to re-identify subjects from anonymized images raises significant privacy concerns [3, 4].

Previous studies have demonstrated that deep learning models can re-identify individuals from chest X-rays [3], CT scans [5], MRI scans [6], and fundus photographs [7], even after metadata removal. These findings indicate that anatomical and biometric features – such as vascular patterns or structural morphology – can serve as unique identifiers. In OCT, retinal layer geometry, choroidal patterns, and

[†]These authors contributed equally to this work.

© Der/die Autor(en), exklusiv lizenziert an
Springer Fachmedien Wiesbaden GmbH, ein Teil von Springer Nature 2026
H. Handels et al. (Hrsg.), *Bildverarbeitung für die Medizin 2026*,
Informatik aktuell, https://doi.org/10.1007/978-3-658-51100-5_11

vessel organization could similarly enable subject recognition, potentially exposing sensitive health information when datasets, feature representation, and models are shared. For color fundus photographs and OCT B-scans, Nebbia et al. [7] demonstrated that features extracted from the frozen, domain-specialized RETFound model are vulnerable to re-identification.

An unresolved question is whether the type of feature extractor affects re-identification risk, and whether re-identification is possible across different OCT devices, e.g. factors that would influence content-based image retrieval systems. General-purpose (generalist) foundation models, such as DINO [8, 9], are pretrained on large natural image corpora and provide broad visual representations. In contrast, domain-specific (specialist) models are pretrained on ophthalmic data and capture anatomical features with greater precision [10]. While specialist models typically outperform generalist ones in diagnostic tasks [10, 11], it remains unclear whether this improved feature sensitivity also increases the risk of encoding subject-specific information.

We address this gap by systematically evaluating re-identification performance using OCT-derived features under two scenarios: 1) intra-device (scans of the same eye from the same device) and 2) cross-device (scans of the same eye across different devices). We hypothesize that generalist models, lacking domain-specific priors, may be less sensitive to biometric details, whereas specialist models, tuned for retinal anatomy, may inadvertently amplify identifiable features.

2 Material and methods

2.1 OCT datasets

We evaluated re-identification performance on a paired in-house OCT dataset acquired from 50 healthy subjects (100 eyes in total) using two different OCT devices. The first device is the *spectralis* OCT, which provided clinical grade images. For each subject, two imaging sessions were available: a low-resolution (LR) and a high-resolution (HR) scan. These sessions capture the same anatomical region and serve as matched pairs. The self-examination low-cost full-field optical coherence tomography (SELFF-OCT) has been developed for self-monitoring of neovascular age-related macular degeneration at home [12]. For each eye, up to 45 recordings are contained in the dataset. Since SELFF-OCT volumes exhibit more artifacts and higher noise levels compared to spectralis SD-OCT, recordings where the retina was not clearly visible were automatically removed as described in Seibel et al. [13].

2.2 Feature extraction

We use various pretrained frozen foundation models for feature extraction to obtain slice-level representations from OCT volumes. The SimCLR family [14] (*ResNet-18, ResNet-50, ResNet-101*) represents contrastive learning approaches trained on large-scale natural image datasets. *DINOv2* and *DINOv3* [8, 9] extend self-distillation with vision transformers (ViT) and ConvNeXT architectures, capturing rich hierarchical features. We use the base and large ViT and ConvNeXT variants of the model. *RETFound-DINOv2* [10] serves as a domain-specialized model, pretrained on ophthalmic data to enhance the sensitivity to retinal structures.

To ensure consistent processing across both devices, SELFF-OCT and spectralis HR scans were resampled to match spectralis LR scans. From each 3D volume, 30 central B-scans with a distance of 25 μm were selected to capture the foveal region. Slices were resized to 224×224 pixel resolution, normalized according to the model's pretrained statistics, and cropped to span the same field of view.

2.3 Re-identification

We formulated eye re-identification as a binary classification task on pairs of OCT volumes. An overview of our re-identification training and inference process is given in Fig. 1. For each configuration, we generated 50,000 training pairs by sampling features from the training set: for the same-device scenario with Spectralis, pairs compared high- (HR) and low-resolution (LR) scans, while for SELFF-OCT, pairs compared scans from different sessions. Positive pairs contained slices from the same eye but always from a different volume of a given eye. In the cross-device scenario (Spectralis vs. SELFF-OCT), pairs were constructed using one sample from each device. All models were trained with subject-disjoint splits (70 % train,

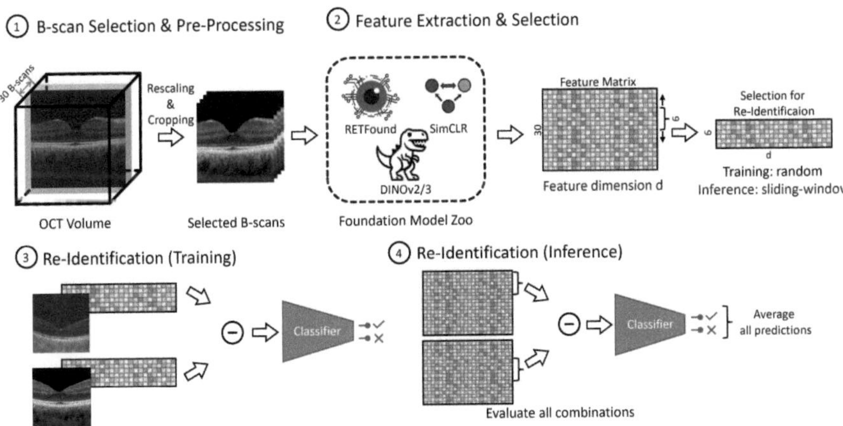

Fig. 1. Overview of the re-identification training and inference process based on OCT images and foundation model features. 1) B-scan selection: We extract 30 central slices per volume, which are then rescaled and cropped to a standardized field of view. 2) These slices are passed through frozen foundation models to obtain per-slice feature embeddings. Six slices are sampled and combined via subtraction to form input representations. 3) A shallow binary classifier is trained on the difference between two such representations to predict whether they originate from the same eye. 4) During inference, slice combinations are generated in a sliding-window manner, and the resulting similarity scores are aggregated to compute re-identification metrics.

10 % validation, 20 % test) to ensure generalization to unseen subjects. In the training phase, six consecutive features $f_i^{(1)} \in \mathbb{R}^d$ from one volume were combined with six consecutive features $f_i^{(2)} \in \mathbb{R}^d$ from a second volume by calculating the difference $\Delta_i = f_i^{(2)} - f_i^{(1)}$. Six such difference vectors $\{\Delta_i, \Delta_{i+1}, \ldots, \Delta_{i+5}\}$ were concatenated and used as input to the classification head.

The evaluation on the test set used slice-level and eye-level retrieval-based protocols. Since we combine six consecutive slices at a time, we get 25 non-overlapping difference vectors per eye-level comparison. For the SELFF-OCT images, we paired the slices of only two different volumes per eye to limit the number of possible combinations (up to 45 volumes per eye). For the retrieval-based metrics, for each query volume from a held-out eye, we computed the similarity scores against a gallery containing one positive match and multiple negative samples. We averaged the predicted similarity values for all slices per eye and matched the eye in the gallery with the highest average similarity to the query eye.

As a model for the feature-based approaches, we trained a shallow 1D convolutional classification head to predict whether two B-scan volumes belong to the same eye. The network operates on the spatial dimension of slice-level feature embeddings using convolutions with a kernel size of 3. A final sigmoid layer produces the similarity score, optimized using binary cross-entropy loss and Adam optimization with a learning rate of 0.001, and early stopping based on the validation loss of a small held-out validation set.

To get an upper bound on the re-identification performance, we also evaluated re-identification based on OCT B-scan images, the processing of which requires more complex models. For this, we employed a ConvNeXt Tiny model pretrained on ImageNet. Input pairs were concatenated along the channel dimension, creating a 3-channel input: slice from volume 1, slice from volume 2, zero channel. This input was normalized using ImageNet statistics, and processed through the backbone with global max pooling. A two-layer classification head (256 hidden units, 50 % dropout) predicted the pair label. The model was trained using AdamW optimization with a learning rate of $5 \cdot 10^{-5}$, batch size 64 and early stopping to prevent overfitting. For image-level models, data augmentation included random rotations (±15°), random gamma intensity shifts, and randomly adding Gaussian noise during training.

3 Results

We evaluated re-identification performance using frozen generalist and specialist foundation models across intra-device (Spectralis, SELFF-OCT) and cross-device settings over five random seeds. Eye-level (averaged predictions) retrieval results are reported as mean Rank-1, Rank-3, and mean average precision (mAP). For assessing the classification performance of a single slice-level feature pair, we report the balanced accuracy. The results are summarized in Tab. 1.

Re-identification was successful when both query and gallery scans originated from the same device. For Spectralis SD-OCT, re-identification performance reached Rank-1 = 0.78 ± 0.10 and mAP = 0.87 ± 0.06 using the RETFound-DINOv2

Tab. 1. Re-identification metrics for intra-device (Spectralis, SELFF-OCT) and inter-device settings between the two devices (Cross Device). We use retrieval metrics (rank 1 and rank 3 accuracy and mAP) and balanced accuracy (BA). All values are reported in %. The best results across all feature extraction methods are highlighted in bold.

Data	Spectralis				SELFF-OCT				Cross Device			
	mAP	BA	R-1	R-3	mAP	BA	R-1	R-3	mAP	BA	R-1	R-3
B-Scan	95	92	93	97	83	88	73	91	65	74	43	80
SimCLR (ResNet-101)	85	85	75	95	53	78	35	63	**23**	**63**	**7**	**25**
Dinov2 (ViT 87M)	85	**87**	75	93	**65**	**82**	**48**	**81**	17	48	5	15
Dinov2 (ViT 0.3B)	84	85	73	93	57	79	39	73	16	48	5	13
Dinov3 (ConvNext 0.2B)	57	77	40	71	52	75	35	63	17	55	5	15
Dinov3 (ViT 0.3B)	82	84	73	89	56	80	39	65	14	47	4	13
RETFound	**87**	86	**78**	**96**	53	78	33	67	19	50	6	17

model, closely followed by DINOv2-base (Rank-1 = 0.75) and SimCLR-ResNet101 (Rank-1 = 0.75). At higher retrieval ranks, performance exceeded Rank-3 = 0.96 and Rank-5 = 0.97, indicating that the correct eye is almost always among the top few candidates. Balanced accuracy values were consistently high across models, reaching values up to 0.87 for DINOv2-base, confirming reliable binary classification between same- and different-eye pairs.

For the SELFF-OCT data, re-identification performance was lower but remained above random: based on DINOv2-base, Rank-1 accuracy was 0.48 ± 0.06 and mAP = 0.65 ± 0.05, while other models ranged between 0.33 and 0.43 Rank-1 accuracy. Despite lower single-rank accuracy, higher-rank retrieval of Rank-3 = 0.81 and Rank-5 = 0.87 showed that correct matches were often retrieved within the top five candidates. Balanced accuracy for DINOv2-base reached a balanced accuracy of 0.82, indicating that even with noisier, lower-resolution scans, the classification model maintained its performance. The high mAP values across both datasets suggest that feature-based similarity remains stable over multiple queries. When matching SELFF-OCT queries to Spectralis galleries (and vice versa), performance dropped sharply across all models. Rank-1 values ranged from 0.04 to 0.07, and mAP values were below 0.23, indicating near-chance retrieval performance.

4 Discussion

The results showed that for our OCT datasets, frozen foundation models retain sufficient information for within-device eye re-identification, revealing that OCT-derived features encode biometric traits. Specialist models, such as RETFound, achieved the highest intra-device re-identification rates on the Spectralis dataset (Rank-1 = 78 %). Generalist self-supervised models showed only slightly lower performance, suggesting that specialist models encode more detailed, domain-specific retinal characteristics. While this increases the risk of re-identification, it may also enhance the utility of the extracted features, which was not studied in this work.

High re-identification rates imply that, at the feature-level, OCT scans still contain personally identifiable information. For safer data sharing, methods such as differentially private data synthesis [15, 16] should be considered, which allow for the specification of the utility-privacy trade-off in advance. The substantially lower re-identification performance on the SELFF-OCT dataset compared to Spectralis could be explained by its lower image resolution and higher levels of acquisition noise and artifacts. In the cross device scenario, the feature-based re-identification performance remained close to random guessing. Possible reasons are device-specific distortions of subject-related anatomical factors such as retinal thickness [17]. More generally, our dataset does not contain scans of highly distinctive pathologies, which potentially explains the lower overall re-identification rates compared to prior work such as Nebbia et al. [7]. Further, the features from the B-scans do not cover the entirety of the OCT volume, thereby missing the fingerprint-like morphology of the retinal vessels [18].

Our study is limited by the small dataset size and number of imaging devices, which may affect the generalizability of the findings. However, the comparable performance of generalist and specialist models suggests that no domain-specific knowledge is necessary for the re-identification of healthy eyes.

References

1. Katuru A, Chung IY, Majid I, Shen LQ, Wang M. Deep learning with disc photos or OCT scans in glaucoma detection. Ophthalmol Sci. 2025;5(6).
2. Nandy Pal M, Roy S, Banerjee M. Content based retrieval of retinal OCT scans using twin CNN. Sādhanā. 2021;46(3):174.
3. Packhäuser K, Gündel S, Münster N, Syben C, Christlein V, Maier A. Deep learning-based patient re-identification is able to exploit the biometric nature of medical chest X-ray data. Sci Rep. 2022;12(1):14851.
4. Tian Y, Ji K, Zhang R, Jiang Y, Li C, Wang X et al. Towards all-in-one medical image re-identification. Proc IEEE/CVF CVPR. 2025.
5. Ueda Y, Morishita J. Patient identification based on deep metric learning for preventing human errors in follow-up X-ray examinations. J Digit Imaging. 2023;36(5):1941–53.
6. Puglisi L, Eshaghi A, Parker G, Barkhof F, Alexander DC, Ravi D. DeepBrainPrint: a novel contrastive framework for brain MRI re-identification. Proc MIDL:716–29.
7. Nebbia G, Kumar S, McNamara SM, Bridge C, Campbell JP, Chiang MF et al. Re-identification of patients from imaging features extracted by foundation models. NPJ Digit Med. 2025;8(1):469.
8. Oquab M, Darcet T, Moutakanni T, Vo H, Szafraniec M, Khalidov V et al. DINOv2: learning robust visual features without supervision. arXiv: 2304.07193. 2023.
9. Siméoni O, Vo HV, Seitzer M, Baldassarre F, Oquab M, Jose C et al. DINOv3. arXiv: 2508.10104. 2025.
10. Zhou Y, Chia MA, Wagner SK, Ayhan MS, Williamson DJ, Struyven RR et al. A foundation model for generalizable disease detection from retinal images. Nature. 2023;622(7981):156–63.
11. Kuo D, Gao Q, Patel D, Pajic M, Hadziahmetovic M. How foundational is the retina foundation model? estimating RETFound's label efficiency on binary classification of normal versus abnormal OCT images. Ophthalmol Sci. 2025;5(3):100707.

12. Sudkamp H, Koch P, Spahr H, Hillmann D, Franke G, Münst M et al. In-vivo retinal imaging with off-axis full-field time-domain optical coherence tomography. Opt Lett. 2016;41(21):4987.
13. Seibel MS, Rowedder M, Andresen J, Neumann T, Neffin R, Sudkamp H et al. Enhancing retinal SELFF-OCT image quality: a deep-learning-based pipeline. Proc SPIE MI IP. 2025;13406.
14. Chen T, Kornblith S, Norouzi M, Hinton G. A simple framework for contrastive learning of visual representations. Proc ICML:1597–607.
15. Dwork C. Differential privacy. Aut Lang Program. 2006:1–12.
16. Li K, Gong C, Li Z, Zhao Y, Hou X, Wang T. PrivImage: differentially private synthetic image generation using diffusion models with semantic-aware pretraining. Proc USENIX SEC. 2024:4837–54.
17. Nam KT, Yun C, Seo M, Ahn S, Oh J. Comparison of retinal thickness measurements among four different optical coherence tomography devices. Sci Rep. 2024;14(1):3560.
18. Köse C, İki˙baş C. A personal identification system using retinal vasculature in retinal fundus images. Expert Syst Appl. 2011;38(11):13670–81.

Quantifying Anatomical Bias in Coronary Segmentation

Why Your Model Prefers the LCA More Than the RCA

Selina Baumgart[1,2], Nikolas Deubner[2], Andreas M. Kist[1]

[1]Artificial Intelligence in Biomedical Engineering, Friedrich-Alexander-Universität Erlangen-Nürnberg (FAU), Germany
[2]Dr. Sandrock und Partner Fachärzte, Altdorf bei Nürnberg, Germany
andreas.kist@fau.de

Abstract. Deep learning-based segmentation of coronary arteries in X-ray angiography supports stenosis assessment via the Quantitative Flow Ratio. However, traditional metrics like the Dice coefficient neglect how image acquisition parameters, particularly vessel type and projection angle, affect model accuracy. This study evaluated four U-Net-based models (vanilla U-Net, nnU-Net, and U-Nets using MobileNetV2 or InceptionResNetV2 as encoders) on 599 patients covering twelve common projection angles. Results show that projection angles, including vessel overlap, have a stronger impact on segmentation quality than vessel type. InceptionResNetV2 achieved the highest overall Dice scores, while nnU-Net better captured capillaries and catheters. Distal branches remained challenging for all models. Our findings highlight the need to consider projection-angle diversity and segment-level evaluation in datasets and benchmarks to ensure clinically reliable coronary segmentation.

1 Introduction

In modern coronary artery analysis, deep learning (DL)-based segmentation methods have become a standard approach for assessing the severity of stenosis in X-ray images. The image-based measurement technique used in the context of coronary artery disease (CAD) is known as the quantitative flow ratio (QFR). It provides a quantitative assessment of stenosis severity, in addition to the doctor's visual assessment. Such quantitative methods support the decision-making process in coronary angiography, particularly when deciding whether a stent needs to be placed. Therefore, the accuracy, robustness, and reliability of these applications under different anatomical and imaging conditions are essential for clinical use. It can be assumed that the DL systems used in clinical practice adhere to current research standards and are therefore commonly evaluated using the Dice coefficient. However, these global metrics only measure the overall segmentation performance. Differences in performance depending on the vessel type or the projection angle are usually not

© Der/die Autor(en), exklusiv lizenziert an
Springer Fachmedien Wiesbaden GmbH, ein Teil von Springer Nature 2026
H. Handels et al. (Hrsg.), *Bildverarbeitung für die Medizin 2026*,
Informatik aktuell, https://doi.org/10.1007/978-3-658-51100-5_12

considered. In addition, projection-specific differences, such as different viewing angles or camera positions, are often not explicitly included in the datasets. As a result, performance differences based on vessel type or projection angle are usually not analyzed. This creates the risk that weaknesses or biases in the model's performance go unnoticed. This study focuses on DL segmentation models to investigate potential performance differences. It examines whether the left coronary artery (LCA), which consists of the left circumflex artery (LCX) and left anterior descending artery (LAD) is segmented more consistently than the right coronary artery (RCA), and whether certain projection angles, such as left anterior oblique (LAO), right anterior oblique (RAO), or cranial/caudal angles, lead to better or worse segmentation results. The insights gained from this study aim to help develop future benchmarking strategies that take anatomical and projection-related differences more clearly into account. In the long term, this should contribute to a more reliable and clinically meaningful evaluation of AI-based segmentation models in medical image analysis. In current research on the segmentation of coronary angiography images, whether derived from CT or X-ray scans, only a few studies systematically account for varying anatomical and imaging conditions within datasets. Among this already limited number of studies, even fewer explicitly analyze how such variability affects model performance, particularly with regard to different imaging modalities. Yang et al. evaluated the performance of their coronary artery segmentation approach both on a combined dataset and separately for the RCA and the LCX and LAD [1]. The results demonstrate that the vessel type has a significant impact on segmentation accuracy. In particular, the LCX exhibits high variability across angiographic projections, which poses notable challenges for model performance. Meng et al., on the other hand, divided their data set according to LAO and RAO projection angles, but did not incorporate this differentiation into the subsequent performance analysis [2]. Only a few exceptions can be found in the fields of video segmentation and IVUS analysis, where explicit bias analyses have been conducted. Research on the influence of different projection angles on the quality of coronary segmentation has been so far limited almost exclusively to 3D-reconstruction of vascular structures or has focused on identifying optimal viewing angles to support interventional procedures [3–5]. In contrast, for 2D segmentation models, a differentiated performance analysis based on vessel type or projection angle remains largely unexplored in existing research. This study aims to address this research gap by systematically investigating the projection-specific performance of segmentation models within the clinically relevant context of coronary angiography.

2 Methods

The performance of the segmentation models across different projection angle groups was evaluated using a dataset provided by Dr. Sandrock & Partner. It included 599 patients, categorized into five diagnostic groups: exclusion of CAD, artery wall changes without relevant stenosis, and 1-, 2-, and 3-vessel CAD. The data were collected between 2022 and 2024 from three cardiac catheterization laboratories in Germany. Patients with prior stent placements were excluded. The projection angle information was extracted from the metadata in each DICOM header and follows the pattern shown in Fig. 1. Twelve projection angles were identified as the most frequently used, shown in Tab. 1.

The final training set consisted of 75 grayscale angiographic images with corresponding binary segmentation masks (background: 0, vessel: 1) with mixed projection angles, covering all five diagnostic groups. The separate test datasets consisted of 25 images with corresponding segmentation masks per projection angle, also covering all five diagnostic groups, for a total of 300 annotations. Care was taken to avoid any image overlapping between the training and test datasets. All annotations were manually performed on a pixel-wise level and randomly validated by cardiology specialists from Dr. Sandrock & Partner. To evaluate and compare segmentation performance, we tested four U-Net variants: nnU-Netv2, U-Net with either a MobileNetV2 or InceptionResNetV2 backbone, and a classical vanilla U-Net architecture. The nnU-Net framework is a self-configuring deep learning framework for biomedical image segmentation. It automatically adapts its pipeline configuration, including preprocessing, network architecture, and training parameters, based on the specific characteristics of the dataset. MobileNetV2 serves as a lightweight encoder, pre-trained on ImageNet. InceptionResNetV2 is a more complex encoder model and was also pre-trained on ImageNet. Both last models were implemented using the segmentation models PyTorch (SMP) library. Grayscale input images were converted to 3-channel RGB format for compatibility with ImageNet pre-trained encoders. All images underwent ImageNet normalization. During training, extensive data augmentation was applied with the following transformations using the Albumentations library. Validation and test images received only normalization without augmentation. The vanilla U-Net architecture followed the open-source PyTorch implementation by Milesial and was trained from scratch without pre-trained weights. All images were resized to 512×512 pixels to ensure a consistent input resolution and comparability across all evaluated models. No additional normalization was applied to preserve the native intensity distributions of angiographic images. For all models, the training data were divided into 80% (60 images) for training and 20% (15 images) for validation. All four models employed identical early stopping configurations with

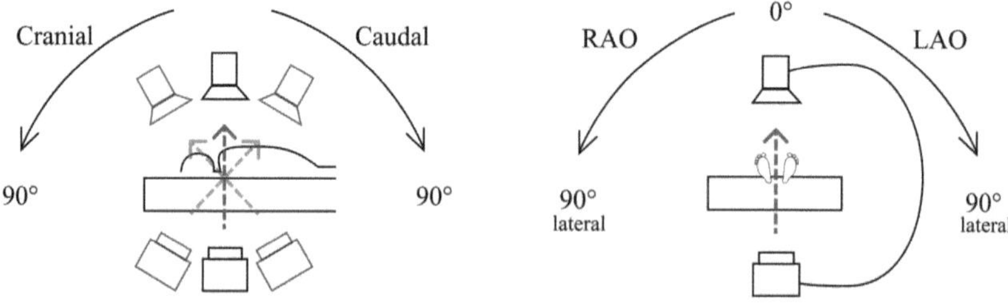

(a) Cranial and Caudal projection angle.

(b) LAO and RAO projection angle.

Fig. 1. Visual representations: LAO, RAO, Caudal, and Cranial.

a patience of 50 epochs without improvement in the validation Dice score. The differing final epoch counts (MobileNet: 291, InceptionResNetV2: 231, nnU-Net: 161, Vanilla: 168) resulted from variations in the convergence behavior of the respective architectures. The 12 test sets were used for the final performance assessment. The performance was evaluated not only using the Dice score but also by assessing a visual analysis of the segmentation of the artery, divided into its coronary segments.

3 Results

To assess model performance across all 12 test sets, the mean Dice coefficient for each model was first compared. Thereafter, individual image-level Dice scores were inspected as part of a detailed visual analysis to further evaluate segmentation quality (Tab. 1). InceptionResNetV2 achieved the highest performance in 10 out of 12 angle groups, followed by MobileNetV2, while the vanilla U-Net consistently demonstrated the lowest performance. The segmentation accuracy for LCA and RCA was highly comparable across all models, with maximum differences ranging from 0.4% to 1.5%. Overall, both arteries exhibited nearly identical Dice score ranges: LCA 0.661–0.744 and RCA 0.652–0.740. More pronounced variations were observed across different acquisition angles. The analysis indicates that the imaging angle and projection exert a stronger influence on segmentation quality than the vessel type itself. Among the four angle groups containing only LCA views, the performance difference between the best (LAO + Caudal) and the worst (RAO + Cranial) configurations ranged from 7.3% to 9.5%. In contrast, the two RCA-dominant angles (LAO 30° and LAO 40°) showed only minor variations of 1.4% to 2.1%, despite comparable vessel distribution. Consequently, the angle effect within the same vessel type (7–10% for LCA) is approximately 5–7 times greater than the vessel-type effect between LCA and RCA.

The visual analysis revealed additional insights into the differences between projection angles and angles that were not captured by the Dice scores alone (Fig. 2). Both LAO 30° and RAO 20° exhibited bimodal performance distributions, with 85–90% of cases achieving excellent segmentation results (Dice > 0.80), while 2–4 cases per model showed complete annotation failures (Dice < 0.20). In RAO 20°, these failures manifested differently across models: MobileNetV2 showed four near-complete detection errors, InceptionResNetV2 had two complete failures, whereas nnU-Net produced five segmentations with substantial annotation gaps but without total failures. In LAO 30° and LAO 40°, all models demonstrated a consistent paradox: excellent RCA segmentation performance in the dominant RCA cases, but drastic failures for the few LCA test samples within these sets (two LCAs each).

Fundamental architectural trade-offs between the models became evident. Despite its lower average performance, nnU-Net captured substantially more distal vessel structures and capillaries than the pre-trained models and exhibited superior catheter delineation in most projections. The baseline U-Net showed by far the highest frequency of catheter annotations across all angles.

All four models, regardless of their catheter delineation quality, exhibited difficulties in segment 5 (left main). InceptionResNetV2 and MobileNetV2 primarily

Tab. 1. Overview of the most frequently used angiographic angles with vessel distribution in the dataset and the average Dice scores of the models (IRNv2: InceptionResNetV2, MNV2: MobileNetV2) for each projection angle.

Projection angle	Vessel distribution	nnU-Net	IRNv2	MNV2	Vanilla
LAO 20°–30°/ Caudal 20°–30°	only LCA	0.740	**0.758**	0.757	0.651
LAO 20°–30°/ Cranial 20°–30°	mix LCA/RCA	0.741	**0.762**	0.760	0.637
LAO 30°	RCA-dominant	0.733	**0.740**	0.717	0.671
LAO 40°	RCA-dominant	0.723	**0.754**	0.733	0.667
RAO 20°–30°/ Caudal 20°–30°	only LCA	0.715	**0.730**	0.724	0.650
RAO 20°–30°/ Cranial 20°–30°	only LCA	0.670	**0.703**	0.694	0.654
RAO 20°	mix LCA/RCA	**0.800**	0.704	0.688	0.631
RAO 30°	mix LCA/RCA	0.723	0.736	**0.738**	0.675
Cranial 30°	LCA-dominant	0.734	**0.767**	0.760	0.689
Cranial 20°	LCA-dominant	0.749	**0.763**	0.752	0.691
Caudal 30°	LCA-dominant	0.722	**0.739**	0.738	0.649
Caudal 20°	only LCA	0.747	**0.766**	0.759	0.696

focused on the main branches, achieving excellent performance there, while side branches were often incomplete, and capillaries were almost entirely omitted. This was particularly pronounced around the LCA bifurcation, in the side branches of segment 11, segment 4, and the side branches of segment 3. Very distal arteries, along with segments 14 and 15, were poorly represented across nearly all projection angles. nnU-Net showed a marked decline in performance for vessels located near image borders (segments 4 and 6), whereas InceptionResNetV2 and MobileNetV2 maintained stable performance in these peripheral regions. The baseline U-Net exhibited the most severe errors in distal vessels, often omitting entire segments rather than partially capturing the anatomy. Segment 6 proved challenging for all models when overlapping with other structures, particularly in Cranial 30° and RAO + Cranial angles, angles characterized by extensive vessel overlap and high structural complexity. MobileNetV2 performed best in long segment 4 trajectories, but generally struggled more with LCX annotation compared to LAD. In LAO 40°, despite relatively straightforward RCA views, MobileNetV2 failed to annotate an entire artery and showed very poor performance in segment 4. The vanilla U-Net revealed

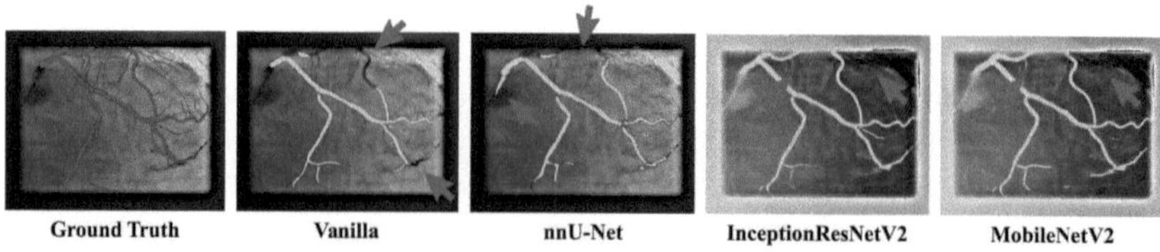

Fig. 2. Qualitative comparison caudal 30° angles across four models. Note nnU-Net failures at the image boundary in segment 6, whereas InceptionResNetV2 and MobileNetV2 show excellent delineation of the main branches but fail to capture any capillaries (red arrows).

the most pronounced qualitative deficiencies, including frequent false-positive annotations from background noise, complete omission of entire distal segments (rather than partial incompleteness as in other models), particularly in segments 14–15 and 4, and an almost complete lack of capillary detection.

4 Discussion

Here, we show that the projection angles determined by geometry and vessel overlap is the dominant factor influencing segmentation quality, rather than the anatomical identity of the vessel. Oblique angles such as LAO 30° or RAO 20° cause significant vessel overlap, making the spatial relationships between vessel structures less clear. In contrast, cranial angles provide better vessel separation and reduced overlap, resulting in consistently higher Dice scores. Analysis of individual segments revealed that distal vessel branches and side branches are particularly prone to errors, and global metrics such as the Dice score capture these differences only partially. Models like nnU-Net captured fine vessel structures and catheters more effectively, whereas InceptionResNetV2 and MobileNetV2 provided stable segmentations of the main vessel. Despite the consistent trends observed, this analysis is limited by the small amount of training data and by the use of general segmentation models rather than vessel-specific architectures. However, these findings suggest that future segmentation algorithms and evaluations should take projection-angle-specific characteristics into account and that datasets and benchmarks should include a balanced representation of challenging projection angles in addition to vessel-type diversity.

References

1. Yang S, Kweon J, Roh JH, Lee JH, Kang H, Park LJ et al. Deep learning segmentation of major vessels in X-ray coronary angiography. Sci Rep. 2019;9(1):16897.
2. Meng Y, Du Z, Zhao C, Dong M, Pienta D, Tang J et al. Automatic extraction of coronary arteries using deep learning in invasive coronary angiograms. Catheter Cardiovasc Interv. 2023;31(6):2303–17.
3. Tu S, Holm NR, Koning G, Maeng M, Reiber JHC. The impact of acquisition angle differences on three-dimensional quantitative coronary angiography. JSCI. 2011;78(2):214–22.
4. Kumari V, Kumar N, Kumar KS, Kumar A, Skandha SS, Saxena S et al. Deep learning paradigm and its bias for coronary artery wall segmentation in intravascular ultrasound scans: a closer look. J Cardiovasc Dev Dis. 2023;10(12).
5. Xia S, Zhu H, Liu X, Gong M, Huang X, Xu L et al. Vessel segmentation of X-ray coronary angiographic image sequence. IEEE Trans Biomed Eng. 2020;67(5):1338–48.

Exploring Cross-dataset Transferability in Lung Nodule Segmentation via Weak Supervision and Synthetic Anomalies

Dominik Hirsch[1], Jan Ehrhardt[1,2], Heinz Handels[1,2]

[1]Institute of Medical Informatics, University of Lübeck
[2]German Research Center for Artificial Intelligence (DFKI), Lübeck
dominik.hirsch@uni-luebeck.de

Abstract. Accurate lung nodule segmentation is critical for reliable chest CT analysis, yet current models rely heavily on large-scale, manually annotated data and often struggle to generalize to unseen datasets. This study investigates whether the transferability of an existing segmentation model can be improved without additional human-labeled lesion masks. Building on the TotalSegmentator lung-nodule task, a weakly supervised framework is proposed in which model-generated predictions serve both as pseudo-labels and as sources of synthetic anomalies, which are blended into CT volumes via 3D Poisson blending. The approach employs a two-stage DRAEM-inspired architecture, combining a pre-trained reconstruction network that captures normal-appearance priors with a discriminative network trained to localize nodular anomalies. Evaluation on the LNDb dataset shows that the proposed model improves over raw TotalSegmentator predictions on multiple metrics, increasing the Dice score from 23.87 to 26.73. However, post-processed TotalSegmentator masks still achieve higher performance (Dice 32.25), and both approaches exhibit substantial performance degradation, underscoring the challenges posed by domain shift. These findings suggest that while weak supervision with synthetic anomalies can guide feature learning, matching the accuracy and robustness of fully supervised methods remains challenging.

1 Introduction

Lung cancer accounted for approximately 1.8 million deaths in 2020, making it the leading cause of cancer-related mortality worldwide and responsible for about 18% of all cancer deaths [1]. Low-dose CT screening has been shown in large randomized trials to substantially reduce lung-cancer mortality through earlier detection of pulmonary nodules [2]. Consequently, the accurate detection and localization of pulmonary nodules is of high clinical importance. Missed nodules can delay diagnosis and worsen outcomes, motivating the development of robust automated tools to increase sensitivity and support timely clinical decisions.

Supervised deep learning models have demonstrated remarkable performance in pulmonary nodule segmentation. Nevertheless, their success critically depends on

© Der/die Autor(en), exklusiv lizenziert an
Springer Fachmedien Wiesbaden GmbH, ein Teil von Springer Nature 2026
H. Handels et al. (Hrsg.), *Bildverarbeitung für die Medizin 2026*,
Informatik aktuell, https://doi.org/10.1007/978-3-658-51100-5_13

the availability of large-scale, voxel-level annotations, which are costly and time-consuming to generate [3]. Furthermore, models trained in a supervised manner on a specific dataset often experience a considerable decline in performance when applied to external data, thereby necessitating expensive retraining or fine-tuning to maintain generalization. These limitations have intensified research efforts toward self-supervised and annotation-efficient learning paradigms that exploit large repositories of unlabeled medical images to acquire transferable and dataset-agnostic feature representations [4].

In this work, we investigate whether the transferability of an existing supervised segmentation model can be improved without relying on human-labeled lesion masks. Specifically, we build upon the TotalSegmentator lung-nodule task, which provides predicted nodule segmentation masks on chest CT volumes. By utilizing these predictions as pseudo-labels and as sources of synthetic anomalies within a weakly supervised training framework, we examine whether a model trained predominantly on weakly labeled data can achieve performance comparable-to, or even surpass, the original TotalSegmentator model. To this end, we adapt an anomaly segmentation framework to the task of pulmonary nodule segmentation by incorporating synthetic pathologies as weak supervision signals. If successful, this approach would establish a practical and scalable strategy for enhancing pretrained segmentation models and facilitate improved model generalization across heterogeneous datasets.

2 Materials and methods

2.1 Model

The proposed model follows the DRAEM framework (Discriminative joint Reconstruction-Anomaly EMbedding, Fig. 1) [5] and consists of a reconstructive and a discriminative network that jointly produce anomaly segmentation masks. The reconstructive subnetwork receives an input volume with inserted anomalies and outputs a reconstruction that more closely resembles a normal sample. The discriminative subnetwork takes the concatenation of the original and reconstructed volumes and predicts a segmentation mask highlighting anomalous regions.

Training proceeds in two stages. First, the reconstructive network is pretrained following the ModelsGenesis paradigm [4], where anomaly-free volumes are corrupted by geometric and intensity transformations and restored to their original appearance. Pretraining on normal samples allows the network to learn a prior for healthy tissue, reconstructing anomalous regions less faithfully, so that residuals between input and reconstruction provide a cue for anomaly localization. In stage two, synthetic nodules are inserted into nodule-free volumes to produce paired tuples (anomalous volume, segmentation mask). The anomalous volume is passed through the frozen reconstruction model, and the concatenated input is provided to the discriminative U-Net, which outputs the predicted segmentation. This two-stage design separates learning a normalizing reconstruction prior from the discriminative task of anomaly localization.

Contrary to the original DRAEM approach, the reconstruction network is kept frozen during the segmentation training stage. Freezing preserves the normal-appearance prior learned on curated normal data. If the reconstruction network were updated on data with diverse abnormalities, the residual signal used for detection could diminish. Empirically, freezing the reconstruction model improved segmentation performance compared with end-to-end fine-tuning.

Models were trained using the Adam optimizer on a single NVIDIA A100 GPU (40 GB) with a patch size of $[192, 168, 128]$. Both subnetworks were implemented as 3D U-Nets with approximately 2×10^7 parameters. The reconstruction model was trained for 400 epochs using mean squared error (MSE) loss, and the segmentation stage for 15 epochs with batch size 3 using focal loss ($\gamma = 2$). Early stopping was based on the validation Dice score.

2.2 Data

Model training was performed on a subset of the CT-RATE dataset [6] which consists of over 50,000 3D chest CT volumes acquired at Istanbul Medipol University Mega Hospital. Each volume is annotated with 18 binary labels for common thoracic findings, with one label corresponding to lung nodules. In addition, the TotalSegmentator lung nodule segmentation masks [7] are supplied.

A subset of CT-RATE was extracted to train the reconstruction model by selecting normal samples, defined as volumes with all 18 binary labels equal to 0. Because these labels are automatically inferred from free-text reports and may contain noise,

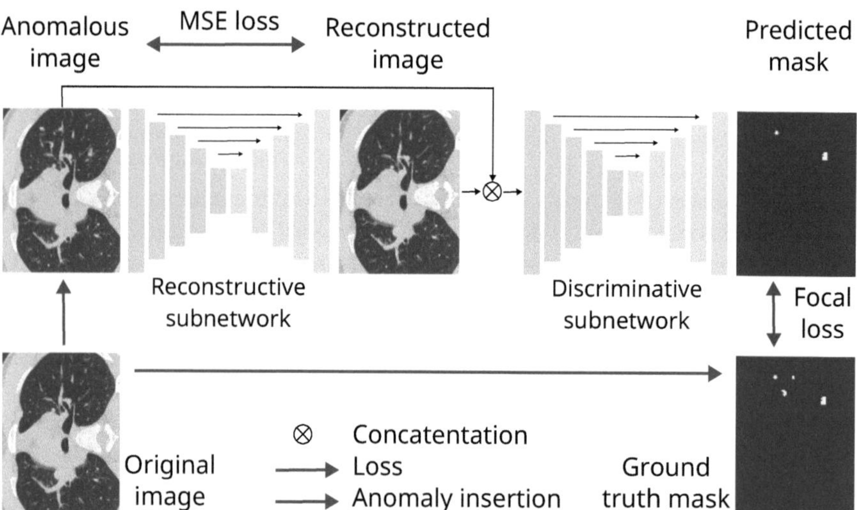

Fig. 1. Proposed model architecture following DRAEM [5]. The reconstructive network maps an anomalous volume to a reconstruction that more closely approximates a normal appearance, while the discriminative subnetwork generates a segmentation output based on the concatenation of the anomalous image and its reconstruction.

the central coronal slice of each candidate normal volume was visually inspected to exclude scans with obvious abnormalities. After this two-stage filtering procedure, 4,183 volumes met the normal criteria and were split into a training set (n = 3,983) and a held-out test set (n = 200).

Synthetic anomalies were generated from nodule masks produced by TotalSegmentator on the CT-RATE dataset. The extracted nodules were inserted into nodule-free CT volumes using 3D Poisson blending [8], with placement restricted to lung regions defined by TotalSegmentator-derived lung masks. This process yielded paired anomalous volumes and corresponding target segmentation masks. To mitigate blending artifacts, Gaussian smoothing was applied with a probability of 50% and a standard deviation of $\sigma \leq 0.5$. No human-annotated lesion masks or manual lesion labeling were used during training.

Model performance was evaluated in two experiments using publicly available chest CT collections. Firstly, 883 volumes and corresponding segmentation masks from the LIDC-IDRI dataset [9] served as an in-domain baseline. Because the TotalSegmentator lung-nodule task was partially trained on LIDC-IDRI, performance on this dataset represents a favorable reference for the pretrained TotalSegmentator model. Second, 236 volumes and masks from LNDb [10], which were not part of the training data, were employed to assess cross-dataset generalization and domain shift and thus provide a stricter test of robustness. Annotations in both LIDC-IDRI and LNDb were produced by experienced thoracic radiologists who marked all nodules with a largest diameter $\geq$ 3 mm. When multiple readers reviewed a volume, the reference standard was defined as the union of all reader annotations. Any lesion marked by at least one annotator was considered a true nodule.

2.3 Metrics

Nodule segmentation performance is evaluated using both localization- and detection-based metrics. Localization-based metrics include a volume-level Dice score to capture overall segmentation quality and to penalize missed findings. Following [6], predictions are matched to the ground truth nodules using a minimum bounding-box intersection-over-union (IoU) threshold of 0.10. The matched nodule pairs are evaluated with an instance-level Dice score ($\text{Dice}_{\text{inst}}$) and the average surface distance (ASD_{inst}) to quantify volumetric overlap and spatial accuracy for each detected lesion.

Nodule detection performance is quantified using precision, recall, and F1-score to provide an overall assessment of detection accuracy. In addition, the FROC@k metric [11] is reported, representing the fraction of ground-truth nodules correctly detected when allowing up to k false positives per volume. FROC@k thus reflects a model's clinical usefulness, with higher values indicating reliable nodule detection at an acceptable false-alarm rate.

Tab. 1. Nodule localization metrics on the LIDC-IDRI and LNDb datasets with 95% confidence intervals. Volume-level Dice score $Dice_{vol}$ reflects overall segmentation performance while instance-level metrics $Dice_{inst}$ and ASD_{inst} measure localization quality for matched ground-truth - prediction nodule pairs.

		Dil.	$Dice_{vol}$ [%] ↑	$Dice_{inst}$ [%] ↑	ASD_{inst} [mm] ↓
LIDC-IDRI	TS	0	$40.40_{[38.62,\ 42.18]}$	$59.42_{[58.57,\ 60.23]}$	$1.01_{[0.98,\ 1.05]}$
	TS	1	$\mathbf{49.27}_{[47.34,\ 51.21]}$	$\mathbf{66.94}_{[66.26,\ 67.60]}$	$\mathbf{0.70}_{[0.67,\ 0.72]}$
	Ours	1	$37.93_{[36.18,\ 39.67]}$	$62.26_{[61.55,\ 62.99]}$	$0.83_{[0.79,\ 0.87]}$
LNDb	TS	0	$23.87_{[20.74,\ 27.13]}$	$55.25_{[53.33,\ 57.21]}$	$0.85_{[0.79,\ 0.91]}$
	TS	1	$\mathbf{32.25}_{[28.47,\ 36.08]}$	$\mathbf{66.74}_{[65.32,\ 68.17]}$	$\mathbf{0.58}_{[0.53,\ 0.63]}$
	Ours	1	$26.73_{[23.51,\ 30.18]}$	$62.30_{[60.69,\ 63.86]}$	$0.68_{[0.61,\ 0.78]}$

Tab. 2. Results for nodule detection metrics on the LIDC-IDRI and LNDb datasets. FROC@k measures the percentage of correctly identified nodules when keeping the false positive budget at or below k.

		Dil.	Detection [%] ↑			FROC@k [%] ↑			
			Prec.	Rec.	F1	$k = 0$	$k = 1$	$k = 2$	$k = 4$
LIDC-IDRI	TS	0	69.65	48.67	57.30	38.19	45.12	47.44	48.47
	TS	1	**72.43**	**56.44**	**63.44**	**41.66**	**52.32**	**54.91**	**56.17**
	Ours	1	40.84	54.27	46.61	21.53	36.21	43.06	49.29
LNDb	TS	0	53.02	31.29	39.35	20.57	28.29	30.43	31.14
	TS	1	**58.84**	37.57	**45.86**	**26.29**	**33.71**	**36.29**	**37.14**
	Ours	1	32.31	**40.71**	36.03	15.14	25.86	30.57	35.14

3 Results

Tab. 1 summarizes nodule segmentation results on the LIDC-IDRI and LNDb datasets, comparing the best proposed model with the TotalSegmentator baseline. The raw TotalSegmentator masks consistently undersegment nodules, and applying a one-pixel dilation substantially improves both volume- and instance-level metrics. Because the proposed method relies on these predictions as synthetic anomalies, it exhibits a similar undersegmentation bias and achieves its highest Dice score after one-pixel dilation. On LIDC-IDRI, the proposed model attains a lower volume-level Dice than the TotalSegmentator models, which is expected given that this dataset was partially included in the TotalSegmentator training data. A clear distribution shift is observed when evaluating on LNDb. The TotalSegmentator's volume Dice decreases by 17 points, while the proposed model drops by 11. On LNDb, the proposed model achieves a volume-level Dice of 26.73%, outperforming the raw TotalSegmentator output, though it does not reach the 32.25% Dice achieved by the dilated TotalSegmentator masks.

Tab. 2 presents nodule detection metrics and similarly highlights the effect of domain shift. Both the TotalSegmentator and the proposed model exhibit markedly reduced performance across all metrics. The dilated TotalSegmentator predictions provide the strongest overall detection performance. The proposed model achieves the highest recall at 40.71%, but this sensitivity comes at the cost of a large number of false positives, resulting in the lowest precision and an F1 score of 36.03% (compared to 39.35% and 45.86% for the other methods). In terms of FROC@k, the proposed model underperforms for small false-positive budgets. Performance improves at higher thresholds but remains below that of the dilated TotalSegmentator masks.

4 Discussion

In summary, the proposed model demonstrates solid performance and outperforms the raw TotalSegmentator predictions across all segmentation metrics and several detection metrics on the LNDb data set, highlighting the potential of weakly supervised learning from pseudo-labels and synthetic anomalies. However, simple post-processing of TotalSegmentator masks, such as one-pixel dilation, still yields superior performance, emphasizing that the advantages of fully supervised training are difficult to replicate through weak supervision alone. Evaluation on LNDb reveals the impact of distribution shift. Both the baseline and the proposed model experience substantial performance drops when applied to an external dataset, underscoring the challenges of domain generalization in pulmonary nodule segmentation.

A key limitation of the proposed approach is the high false-positive rate, particularly in detection tasks. This behavior likely arises from the propagation of errors present in the TotalSegmentator predictions used for anomaly synthesis, as well as from reconstruction errors in regions with complex anatomy such as vascular structures. Future work could focus on improving the realism of synthetic anomalies, for example using GAN-based blending, or enhancing the reconstruction network to better discriminate true nodules from background structures. Such improvements may reduce false positives while preserving the benefits of weakly supervised learning.

References

1. Sung H, Ferlay J, Siegel RL, Laversanne M, Soerjomataram I, Jemal A et al. Global cancer statistics 2020: GLOBOCAN estimates of incidence and mortality worldwide for 36 cancers in 185 countries. CA Cancer J Clin. 2021;71:209–49.
2. Aberle DR, Adams AM, Berg CD, Black WC, Clapp JD, Fagerstrom RM et al. Reduced lung-cancer mortality with low-dose computed tomographic screening. N Engl J Med. 2011;365:395–409.
3. Wang S, Li C, Wang R, Liu Z, Wang M, Tan H et al. Annotation-efficient deep learning for automatic medical image segmentation. Nat Commun. 2021;12(1):5915.
4. Zhou Z, Sodha V, Pang J, Gotway MB, Liang J. Models genesis. Med Image Anal. 2021;67.
5. Zavrtanik V, Kristan M, Skočaj D. DRAEM: a discriminatively trained reconstruction embedding for surface anomaly detection. Proc IEEE ICCV. 2021:8330–9.
6. Hamamci IE, Er S et al. Developing generalist foundation models from a multimodal dataset for 3D computed tomography. arXiv: 2403.17834. 2025.
7. Wasserthal J, Breit HC, Meyer MT, Pradella M, Hinck D, Sauter AW et al. TotalSegmentator: robust segmentation of 104 anatomic structures in CT images. Radiol Artif Intell. 2023;5(5).

8. Tanaka M, Kamio R, Okutomi M. Seamless image cloning by a closed form solution of a modified Poisson problem. Proc ACM SA. 2012.
9. Armato III, Samuel G., McLennan G, Bidaut L, McNitt-Gray MF, Meyer CR, Reeves AP et al. Data from LIDC-IDRI. Cancer Imaging Arch. 2015.
10. Pedrosa J, Aresta G, Ferreira C, Rodrigues M, Leitão P, Carvalho AS et al. LNDb dataset. Version 4. Zenodo, 2023.
11. National Lung Screening Trial Research Team. Receiver operating characteristic analysis in medical imaging: contents. J ICRU. 2008;8(1):1–2.

Abstract: LesionLocator

Zero-shot Universal Tumor Segmentation and Tracking in 3D Whole-body Imaging

Maximilian Rokuss[1,2,3], Yannick Kirchhoff[1,2,3], Seval Akbal[4], Balint Kovacs[1,5], Saikat Roy[1,2], Constantin Ulrich[1,5], Tassilo Wald[1,5,6], Lukas T. Rotkopf[4], Heinz-Peter Schlemmer[4], Klaus Maier-Hein[1,5,6,7]

[1]German Cancer Research Center (DKFZ), Division of Medical Image Computing, Heidelberg, Germany
[2]Faculty of Mathematics and Computer Science, Heidelberg University, Heidelberg, Germany
[3]HIDSS4Health, Heidelberg University, Heidelberg, Germany
[4]German Cancer Research Center (DKFZ), Department of Radiology, Heidelberg, Germany
[5]Medical Faculty, Heidelberg University, Heidelberg, Germany
[6]Helmholtz Imaging, DKFZ, Heidelberg, Germany
[7]Pattern Analysis and Learning Group, Department of Radiation Oncology, Heidelberg University Hospital, Heidelberg, Germany
maximilian.rokuss@dkfz-heidelberg.de

Automated lesion segmentation and tracking in longitudinal medical imaging remain critical challenges in oncology, particularly as cancer incidence and imaging volumes continue to rise. Current promptable segmentation models are predominantly designed for 2D or single-timepoint 3D data, neglecting the temporal dimension essential for disease monitoring. We present LesionLocator, the first end-to-end framework unifying zero-shot 3D lesion segmentation and 4D tracking across longitudinal medical images, originally published in the Proceedings of CVPR 2025 [1]. Our model leverages extensive pretraining and introduces a novel synthetic longitudinal data generation technique to address the scarcity of multi-timepoint datasets. LesionLocator achieves human-level performance in universal lesion segmentation, outperforming existing promptable models by nearly 10 Dice points across diverse tumor types. Our autoregressive mask propagation achieves 86% retrieval accuracy with 79% Dice for longitudinal tracking. We provide the first open-access solution for promptable lesion tracking, releasing both synthetic 4D dataset and model weights.

References

1. Rokuss M, Kirchhoff Y, Akbal S, Kovacs B, Roy S, Ulrich C et al. LesionLocator: zero-shot universal tumor segmentation and tracking in 3D whole-body imaging. Proc IEEE/CVF CVPR. 2025:30872–85.

© Der/die Autor(en), exklusiv lizenziert an Springer Fachmedien Wiesbaden GmbH, ein Teil von Springer Nature 2026
H. Handels et al. (Hrsg.), *Bildverarbeitung für die Medizin 2026*, Informatik aktuell, https://doi.org/10.1007/978-3-658-51100-5_14

Vision-language Models for Structured Report Generation in Radiology

Towards Consistent and Reliable Chest X-ray Reporting

Md Badhon Miah, Lukas Buess, Andreas Maier

Pattern Recognition Lab, Friedrich-Alexander-Universität, Erlangen-Nürnberg, Germany
Badhon.Miah@fau.de

Abstract. Medical report generation (MRG) aims to automatically generate reports from medical images, reducing the workload on radiologists. Research in this field is progressing rapidly with large pretrained vision-language models (VLMs), but most are trained on general image-text data and fail to capture critical medical findings. Effective chest X-ray (CXR) report generation requires fine-tuning on high-quality datasets, but inconsistent reporting styles remain a key challenge. The structured radiology report generation (SRRG) approach addresses this by using large language models (LLMs) to standardize and generate consistent structured reports. In this study, we introduce SRRG-benchmark to systematically evaluate state-of-the-art LLMs for converting free-text CXR reports into structured form suitable for training VLMs. We primarily focus on assessing the medical image interpretation capabilities of VLMs across both structured and conventional free-text report generation tasks. Our results demonstrate that structured reporting improves VLMs' medical image interpretation performance compared to free-text fine-tuning, increasing MedGemma's clinical accuracy (GREEN) from 0.50 to 0.53 and RadGraph F1 from 0.27 to 0.38, with similar gains for Qwen3-VL.

1 Introduction

Chest X-ray (CXR) report generation by a radiologist is a time-consuming task, especially under limited resources and high demand. Although AI-generated draft reports can help reduce reporting time by about 25% [1], current foundational vision-language models (VLMs) still lack the clinical reliability and accuracy required for trustworthy CXR reporting. Since VLMs are primarily trained on open-source image-text data and rarely exposed to sensitive medical reports, they require fine-tuning on CXR datasets to learn clinical language and domain-specific visual interpretation. However, the wide variability in radiology reporting styles forces VLMs to learn unnecessary linguistic patterns during fine-tuning, often leading to hallucinations and making clinical evaluation of unstructured reports difficult. In contrast, structured reports provide consistency and enable organ-level evaluation by aligning generated and reference findings within predefined anatomical sections [2].

© Der/die Autor(en), exklusiv lizenziert an
Springer Fachmedien Wiesbaden GmbH, ein Teil von Springer Nature 2026
H. Handels et al. (Hrsg.), *Bildverarbeitung für die Medizin 2026*,
Informatik aktuell, https://doi.org/10.1007/978-3-658-51100-5_15

Structured reporting has evolved from the american college of radiology's 1991 guideline to the RSNA's RadLex and RadReport (2006-2007), and the ESR's 2018 white paper [3]. Despite these developments, structured reporting remains underutilized, with most studies focusing on general-purpose or OpenAI GPT-based models [3]. [4] proposed a region-guided approach where anatomical regions are detected and described using vision and Transformer-based models, and a pre-trained LLM is guided by anatomy and context-specific prompts to generate structured reports. Another study [5] explored prompt-based structuring of free-text reports but mainly relied on simple metrics such as word count and conciseness, which lack clinical depth. To enhance reporting consistency, [2] introduced structured radiology report generation (SRRG), using LLMs to convert free-text CXR reports into a structured format covering seven anatomical systems.

While prior studies have laid the foundation for SRRG, its integration with VLMs for medical image interpretation remains underexplored. The unstructured nature of most public CXR datasets further limits progress, making LLM-based structuring methods such as SRRG [2] important for preparing structured fine-tuning data. Although a recent study [6] proposed lightweight models for SRRG, we aim to further investigate reliable approaches for consistent and accurate structured reporting by evaluating diverse state-of-the-art LLMs. To this end, we introduce the SRRG-benchmark, developed to assess the capability of advanced LLMs in structuring free-text CXR reports. Furthermore, to explore whether structured reporting can improve medical image interpretation by reducing errors in CXR report generation, we formulated our primary research question: How does structured and consistent reporting influence the medical image interpretation of VLMs compared to conventional free-text reporting? As prior studies have not explored this, we fine-tuned and evaluated VLMs in both formats to assess their report generation performance. Overall, our contributions in this paper are as follows:

- We introduce the SRRG-benchmark and a novel radiology finding assignment accuracy (RadFAA) metric to evaluate structured reporting.
- We uncover that structured reporting enhances the performance of VLMs in medical image interpretation and pathology identification.

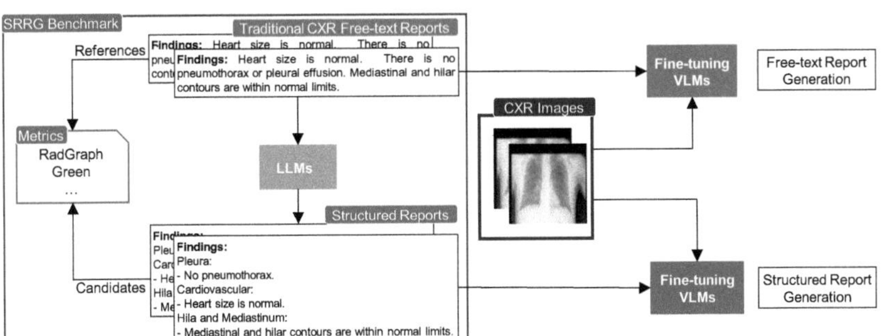

Fig. 1. SRRG benchmark (left) and structured vs. free-text VLMs fine-tuning (right).

2 Materials and methods

2.1 Dataset

We used the ReXGradient-160K dataset [7], a large public CXR collection sourced from 79 medical sites. Each study includes at least one X-ray image with a findings section and an impression summary. Since the findings section is the key part for medical report generation (MRG), we focused on this section for training and evaluation. For the experiments with VLMs, we used data from one clinical site (13,870 CXRs) due to computational constraints, split into 80% for training, 10% for validation, and 10% for testing. For the SRRG-benchmark, we randomly selected 1,000 reports from the dataset for few-shot free-text report structuring evaluation.

2.2 SRRG-benchmark

We established the SRRG-benchmark using a few-shot generation approach to assess eight state-of-the-art LLMs, based on the SRRG template proposed in [2], and added one example of a free-text report and its corresponding structured report in the prompt. We used LangExtract [8] for GPT-4.1 Mini [9] and Gemini 2.5 Flash [10], while structured outputs for the remaining models were generated locally.

2.3 VLMs fine-tuning

We fine-tuned MedGemma [11] (4B parameters) under two settings: (1) CXR images paired with free-text reports and (2) CXR images paired with structured reports generated by Gemini 2.5 Flash, the best-performing model in our SRRG-benchmark (Tab. 1). This enables a fair investigation of clinical image understanding across both reporting styles. To ensure that the observed effect was not model-specific, we also fine-tuned Qwen3-VL [12] (4B parameters) using the same settings. A parameter-efficient adapter-based fine-tuning method, LoRA [13], was used for fine-tuning.

2.4 Evaluation

Evaluating MRG requires domain-specific metrics beyond general NLP measures such as BLEU and ROUGE, which primarily assess text similarity rather than clinical accuracy [1]. In the SRRG-benchmark, LLMs converted free-text CXR reports into structured formats, and the generated structured reports were evaluated against the reference free-text reports using five standard medical report generation metrics and the proposed RadFAA score (Fig. 1). We evaluated MRG by VLMs in both structured and free-text formats in accordance with the ReXrank leaderboard [14]. Both models were assessed using four widely adopted medical report evaluation metrics, including GREEN, RadGraph, RadCliQ, and RaTEScore, using the RadEval framework [15]. Furthermore, SRRG often leads to two main issues, (1) incorrect assignment of findings to anatomical systems and (2) repetition of findings across sections. Existing medical metrics fail to capture such problems and may even reward

Tab. 1. SRRG-benchmark results for structuring free-text CXR reports into the SRRG format. Higher is better; CX-M-F1 = CheXbert Micro-F1; CX-Ma-F1 = CheXbert Macro-F1; *Bold* = best performing model on that metric; $*$ = our proposed metric.

Model	RadGraphF1	CX-M-F1	CX-Ma-F1	GREEN	F1-SRR-BERT	RadFAA*
Gemini 2.5 Flash	0.657	**0.956**	**0.939**	0.926	0.869	**0.950**
GPT-4.1 mini	**0.672**	0.939	0.918	0.913	**0.896**	0.947
MedGemma-27B	0.662	0.936	0.918	0.910	0.884	0.928
Qwen3-4B	0.653	0.942	0.919	0.881	0.887	0.917
Qwen3-14B	0.636	0.942	0.916	0.897	0.883	0.908
GPT-Oss-120B	0.603	0.936	0.908	0.889	0.885	0.934
GPT-Oss-20B	0.595	0.950	0.937	0.879	0.852	0.895
MedGemma-4B	0.517	0.917	0.892	0.917	0.854	0.785
SRR-BERT2BERT	0.594	0.903	0.868	**0.938**	0.812	0.722

duplicated outputs. To address this, we propose RadFAA, a zero shot LLM based metric that evaluates the correctness of finding to anatomy assignments in structured reports. Using a specialized prompt, an evaluating LLM (Gemma3 12B) determines whether each finding is correctly assigned, while duplicate and misplaced findings are counted as incorrect assignments. The RadFAA score is defined as

$$\text{RadFAA} = \frac{N_{\text{correct assignments}}}{N_{\text{total findings}}} \tag{1}$$

3 Results

3.1 SRRG-benchmark

To evaluate LLMs for structuring free-text CXR reports used in training VLMs, we introduced SRRG-benchmark and ranked models by the average of six clinical metrics (Tab. 1). Gemini 2.5 Flash achieved the highest performance, attaining 0.956 CheXbert-5 Micro-F1, 0.939 Macro-F1, and 95% RadFAA. GPT-4.1 Mini obtained the best RadGraph F1 (0.672) and F1-SRR-BERT (0.896). In contrast, the fine-tuned SRR-BERT2BERT [6] showed the weakest performance, with 72.2% RadFAA, where duplicated findings and organ misassignments negatively impacted structural accuracy while artificially inflating the GREEN score.

3.2 Impact of structured reporting on the performance of VLMs

A comparison of VLMs performance on free-text and SRRG-formatted CXR report generation is shown in Tab. 2. The fine-tuned MedGemma-4B achieved a higher score on 1/RadCliQ-v1, outperforming the zero-shot (no fine-tuning on ReXGradient-160K) [11] version by approximately 0.2, with minor variations observed across the other metrics. Under the SRRG setting, MedGemma-4B-FT showed higher values across all metrics compared to its free-text variants, with 1/RadCliQ-v1 increasing

Tab. 2. Performance of MedGemma and Qwen3-VL on Free-text and SRRG-formatted CXR report generation. Higher is better; *Bold* = best score for the model between Free-text and SRRG; † = best overall score for the model; N/A = not applicable ; FT= Fine-tuned.

Model	Report Type	1/RadCliQ-v1	RadGraphF1	RaTEScore	GREEN	RadFAA
MedGemma-4B-FT	SRRG	**4.483**†	**0.379**†	**0.744**†	**0.529**	0.982
MedGemma-4B-FT	Free-text	1.404	0.265	0.599	0.496	N/A
MedGemma-4B	Free-text	1.205	0.245	0.609	0.566†	N/A
Qwen3-VL-4B-FT	SRRG	**2.203**†	**0.296**†	**0.706**†	**0.482**†	0.989
Qwen3-VL-4B-FT	Free-text	1.119	0.203	0.580	0.476	N/A

from 1.404 to 4.483, RadGraph F1 from 0.265 to 0.379, RaTEScore from 0.599 to 0.744, and GREEN from 0.496 to 0.529. Additionally, Qwen3-VL model exhibited the same pattern, with SRRG-formatted outputs consistently outperforming the free-text reports across all reported metrics. In addition, both VLMs achieved approximately 99% accuracy on the RadFAA metric.

4 Discussion

In this research, we proposed SRRG-benchmark, which helps researchers select suitable LLMs for structuring free-text reports and creating high-quality training data for VLMs in CXR report generation. The benchmark covers proprietary, open-source, and lightweight models, allowing selection based on task requirements and computational resources. Our RadFAA metric aligned well with other evaluation metrics, with the top model achieving the highest RadFAA score and the lowest-performing model the lowest, demonstrating its effectiveness for evaluating structured reports.

Furthermore, our analysis shows that MedGemma fine-tuned on the CXR dataset outperforms its zero-shot (no fine-tuning on ReXGradient-160K) counterpart [11] in free-text reporting. This indicates that although MedGemma belongs to the class of medical VLMs, its performance can still be improved for specific tasks. The structured reporting setting resulted in substantially higher performance than free-text reporting across all clinically meaningful metrics for MedGemma. A similar trend observed for Qwen3-VL confirms that this advantage is not model-specific but a general benefit of structured formats. These findings suggest that structured reporting enables VLMs to generate more clinically accurate reports by reducing linguistic variability and improving medical image interpretation. This highlights the potential of structured CXR reporting as a more reliable alternative to free-text reporting. However, performance gains may be partly influenced by metric limitations, as the GREEN metric can reward duplicate findings. We therefore used multiple complementary metrics and proposed RadFAA to ensure fairer evaluation. This study used data from a single clinical site due to computational constraints. Future work may incorporate multicenter datasets and alternative structured reporting templates to improve generalizability, and explore lightweight fine-tuned LLMs for RadFAA to reduce computational overhead and potential zero-shot bias.

Acknowledgement. The authors gratefully acknowledge the scientific support and HPC resources provided by the erlangen national high performance computing center (NHR@FAU) of the Friedrich-Alexander-Universität Erlangen-Nürnberg (FAU). The hardware is funded by the german research foundation (DFG).

References

1. Buess L, Keicher M, Navab N, Maier A, Tayebi Arasteh S. From large language models to multimodal AI: a scoping review on the potential of generative AI in medicine. Biomed Eng Lett. 2025:1–19.
2. Delbrouck JB, Xu J, Moll J, Thomas A, Chen Z, Ostmeier S et al. Automated structured radiology report generation. arXiv preprint: 2505.24223. 2025.
3. Busch F, Hoffmann L, Dos Santos DP, Makowski MR, Saba L, Prucker P et al. Large language models for structured reporting in radiology: past, present, and future. Eur Radiol. 2025;35(5):2589–602.
4. Li H, Wang H, Sun X, He H, Feng J. Prompt-guided generation of structured chest X-ray report using a pre-trained LLM. Proc IEEE ICME. 2024:1–6.
5. Hartsock I, Araujo C, Folio L, Rasool G. Improving radiology report conciseness and structure via local large language models. J Imaging Inform Med. 2025:1–12.
6. Moll J, Fay L, Azhar A, Ostmeier S, Lueth T, Gatidis S et al. Structuring radiology reports: challenging LLMs with lightweight models. arXiv preprint: 2506.00200. 2025.
7. Zhang X, Acosta JN, Miller J, Huang O, Rajpurkar P. ReXGradient-160K: a large-scale publicly available dataset of chest radiographs with free-text reports. arXiv preprint: 2505.00228. 2025.
8. Google Research. LangExtract: language extraction framework. `https://github.com/google/langextract`. 2025.
9. Achiam J, Adler S, Agarwal S, Ahmad L, Akkaya I, Aleman FL et al. GPT-4 technical report. arXiv preprint: 2303.08774. 2023.
10. Comanici G, Bieber E, Schaekermann M, Pasupat I, Sachdeva N, Dhillon I et al. Gemini 2.5: pushing the frontier with advanced reasoning, multimodality, long context, and next generation agentic capabilities. arXiv preprint: 2507.06261. 2025.
11. Sellergren A, Kazemzadeh S, Jaroensri T, Kiraly A, Traverse M, Kohlberger T et al. MedGemma technical report. arXiv preprint: 2507.05201. 2025.
12. Yang A, Li A, Yang B, Zhang B, Hui B, Zheng B et al. Qwen3 technical report. arXiv preprint: 2505.09388. 2025.
13. Hu EJ, Shen Y, Wallis P, Allen-Zhu Z, Li Y, Wang S et al. LoRA: low-rank adaptation of large language models. Proc ICLR. 2022;1(2):3.
14. Zhang X, Zhou HY, Yang X, Banerjee O, Acosta JN, Miller J et al. ReXrank: A public leaderboard for AI-powered radiology report generation. arXiv preprint: 2411.15122. 2024.
15. Xu J, Zhang X, Abderezaei J, Bauml J, Boodoo R, Haghighi F et al. RadEval: a framework for radiology text evaluation. arXiv preprint: 2509.18030. 2025.

Abstract: Your other Left! Vision-language Models Fail to Understand Relative Positions in Medical Images

Daniel Wolf [1,2], Heiko Hillenhagen [2], Billurvan Taskin [2], Alex Bäuerle [3], Meinrad Beer [2], Michael Götz [2‡], Timo Ropinski [1‡]

[1]Visual Computing Group, Institute of Media Informatics, Ulm University, Germany
[2]Diagnostic and Interventional Radiology, Ulm University Medical Center, Germany
[3]Google DeepMind, France
daniel.wolf@uni-ulm.de

Imagine a radiology department where vision-language models (VLMs) assist with report generation. For such systems to be safe, they must accurately understand spatial relationships, a skill essential for radiologists, where mistakes have led to serious consequences, such as wrong-side surgeries. In our publication [1], we show that VLMs fail at this fundamental ability. Models were asked to identify the relative position of two anatomical structures in a CT slice. Even advanced VLMs, such as GPT4o, performed only at chance level, raising concerns about their reliability in clinical routine. How could they properly describe localizations in reports without this capability? We investigated potential solutions. Since segmentation models are already highly accurate, their outputs can be used to place markers on the anatomical structures. Prior work in computer vision shows that such markers can enhance spatial reasoning. While markers yielded moderate gains, accuracy remained far below results on natural images. A deeper analysis revealed the underlying cause. VLMs already possess strong prior anatomical knowledge. In other words, they "know" where organs are typically located in standard human anatomy. Instead of analyzing the actual CT image, they often fall back on this memorized knowledge when answering spatial questions. For example, if asked whether the liver is to the right of the stomach, a model may simply respond "yes" based on general anatomy, without inspecting the image at all. This shortcut is dangerous: in cases such as situs inversus, or post-surgical alterations, where organ positions deviate from the norm, the model will confidently give incorrect answers. We release MIRP, a benchmark designed to systematically test spatial reasoning. Details on https://wolfda95.github.io/your_other_left/.

[‡]These authors contributed equally to this work.

© Der/die Autor(en), exklusiv lizenziert an Springer Fachmedien Wiesbaden GmbH, ein Teil von Springer Nature 2026
H. Handels et al. (Hrsg.), *Bildverarbeitung für die Medizin 2026*, Informatik aktuell, https://doi.org/10.1007/978-3-658-51100-5_16

References

1. Wolf D, Hillenhagen H, Taskin B, Bäuerle A, Beer M, Götz M et al. Your other left! Vision-language models fail to identify relative positions in medical images. Proc MICCAI. 2025.

Abstract: Leveraging Open-source Language Models for Clinical Information Extraction

A Study in Resource-constrained Healthcare Settings

Luc Builtjes, Joeran Bosma, Mathias Prokop, Bram van Ginneken, Alessa Hering

Department of Radiology and Nuclear Medicine, Radboud University Medical Center
luc.builtjes@radboudumc.nl

Large language models (LLMs) have shown strong abilities in understanding and generating natural language, offering new opportunities for clinical text analysis. Most prior studies, however, rely on proprietary systems, raising concerns about data privacy and accessibility in healthcare. Open-source LLMs offer transparent, locally deployable, and privacy-preserving alternatives, yet their performance in low-resource languages and zero-shot medical information extraction remains underexplored. We evaluated modern open-source generative LLMs for extracting clinically relevant information from Dutch medical reports using the DRAGON 2024 benchmark. To enable this, we developed llm-extractinator [1], an open-source framework that automates structured information extraction via schema definition, dynamic prompt construction, local inference, and automatic validation. Nine multilingual models were evaluated on 28 DRAGON tasks spanning classification, regression, and named entity recognition in a strict zero-shot setup. Performance was measured using task-specific metrics (AUC, Cohen's κ, RSMAPE, F1) and aggregated into the DRAGON utility score. Llama-3.3-70B achieved the highest score ($S_{\text{DRAGON}} = 0.760$), followed by Phi-4-14B (0.751), Qwen-2.5-14B (0.748), and DeepSeek-R1-14B (0.744). These models matched or exceeded a fine-tuned RoBERTa baseline on 17 of 28 tasks. Translating Dutch input to English reduced performance ($\Delta S = -0.11$ to -0.25), emphasizing the importance of native-language inference. Our results show that open-source generative LLMs can achieve competitive performance without fine-tuning, providing a practical and privacy-preserving solution for clinical information extraction in resource-constrained settings. The llm-extractinator framework facilitates reproducible benchmarking and lowers the barrier for applying LLMs in local medical research environments.

References

1. Builtjes L, Bosma J, Prokop M, van Ginneken B, Hering A. Leveraging open-source large language models for clinical information extraction in resource-constrained settings. JAMIA Open. 2025;8(5):ooaf109.

© Der/die Autor(en), exklusiv lizenziert an
Springer Fachmedien Wiesbaden GmbH, ein Teil von Springer Nature 2026
H. Handels et al. (Hrsg.), *Bildverarbeitung für die Medizin 2026*,
Informatik aktuell, https://doi.org/10.1007/978-3-658-51100-5_17

Pathology-aware Implicit Neural Registration for Change Analysis in Retinal OCT Data

FRINR

Julia Andresen [1], Bennet Kahrs [1], Heinz Handels [1,2], Timo Kepp [2]

[1] Institute of Medical Informatics, University of Luebeck, Luebeck, Germany
[2] German Research Center for Artificial Intelligence, Luebeck, Germany
bennet.kahrs@uni-luebeck.de

Abstract. Longitudinal analysis of optical coherence tomography data is crucial for monitoring retinal disease progression. In such diseases, pathological fluid accumulations may vary considerably between examinations, causing substantial alterations in local tissue morphology. These non-correspondences challenge classical image registration methods, while convolutional registration networks typically require large datasets for training. To address this gap, we introduce FRINR, a fluid-aware registration framework based on implicit neural representations. FRINR performs pairwise registration by jointly estimating a deformation field and a residual image: the deformation aligns anatomical structures shared across time points, whereas the residual disentangles pathological changes such as newly formed fluids, guided by a sparsity constraint. In this way, FRINR enables fluid-aware registration of severely altered retinae while maintaining plausible deformation fields. Moreover, the residual images allow unsupervised detection of new pathologies without large datasets or expert annotations.

1 Introduction

Central serous chorioretinopathy (CSCR) causes fluid accumulations below and inside the retina, altering tissue morphology and impairing vision [1]. The occurrence of fluid and remissions between examinations often leads to significant structural differences between time points, which can be visualized using optical coherence tomography (OCT) but make it difficult to compare different time points. In particular, most image registration methods fail to align these images. This is because the large differences in shape are not captured and because the discrepancies caused by pathologies lead to unrealistic deformations. While pathology segmentations could be used to increase deformation realism, these need to be generated by medical experts. In addition, the annotations per time point do not directly contain information about changes, which can only be determined with pixel-level accuracy after successful registration.

© Der/die Autor(en), exklusiv lizenziert an
Springer Fachmedien Wiesbaden GmbH, ein Teil von Springer Nature 2026
H. Handels et al. (Hrsg.), *Bildverarbeitung für die Medizin 2026*,
Informatik aktuell, https://doi.org/10.1007/978-3-658-51100-5_18

Previously, we proposed FluidRegNet [2], a convolutional neural network (CNN) for fluid-aware registration of retinal OCT images. In this framework, the formation of newly emerging pathologies is modeled by small areas of altered intensities in the baseline image (the moving image), which are then extended to the fluid volume observed in the follow-up image (the fixed image). Though no manual pathology annotations are used in this method, it inherently relies on large data sets for training.

Image registration with implicit neural representations (INRs) can be applied directly to individual image pairs, as in classical image registration, but at the same time allows for the easy use of complex objective functions, as in CNN-based methods. Though still a young field of research, INRs have proven highly successful in medical image registration [3, 4]. However, in the case of medical images with pathologies, INRs face the same problems as other registration approaches. To cope with severe appearance differences between images, Byra et al. propose to use three INR networks for a single image registration task [5]. These networks generate a registration deformation field and decompose the moving image into two parts, the so-called support and residual images. The image distance between the deformed support and the fixed images is used as an additional loss term, improving registration performance and encouraging the support image to contain image features both time points have in common. This approach has been applied to healthy images only and offers limited control over which image parts are packed into the residual and which into the support image.

Inspired by the INR-based registration and image decomposition method by Byra et al. [5] (ImpRegDec) and influenced by our FluidRegNet, we propose to use two INRs for pathology-aware image registration. The first INR generates the registration deformation field, and the second produces a residual image containing the pathological deviations between moving and fixed images. To increase control of the content of the residual image, we introduce an additional sparsity loss, similar to the loss function used in [2]. The proposed fluid registration INR (FRINR) is shown to increase the plausibility of the deformation fields compared to a deformation-only INR and to be usable for the unsupervised segmentation of non-correspondences caused by disease progression.

2 Materials and methods

To enable the longitudinal registration of retinal OCT images with evolving pathologies, we propose to use two INR networks for each pair of moving image M and fixed image F, as shown in Fig. 1. Both networks receive the same input coordinates $\boldsymbol{x}$ from the image domain $\Omega \subset [-1, 1]^3$ to generate a deformation field φ that matches the anatomical features shared by the moving and fixed images, and a residual image R that captures the pathological differences between them. The deformation and residual networks are trained simultaneously using the loss function

$$\mathcal{L} = \mathcal{L}_{\text{NCC}}(F, M \circ \varphi) + \alpha \mathcal{L}_{\text{MSE}}(F, (M + R) \circ \varphi) + \beta \mathcal{L}_{\text{reg}}(\varphi) + \gamma \mathcal{L}_{\text{sparse}}(R) \quad (1)$$

where $\mathcal{L}_{\text{NCC}}$ is a combination of local and global normalized cross-correlation, as used in [5]. We regularize the deformation field using its gradient and Jacobian J_φ, i.e. $\mathcal{L}_{\text{reg}}(\varphi) = \frac{1}{|S|}\sum_{x\in S}\left(||1 - |J_\varphi(x)|| + \lambda||\nabla\varphi(x)||_2\right)$, summed over all coordinates $x \in S \subset \Omega$ passed to the networks in one iteration step. In addition to these two typical image registration objectives, the voxel-wise mean squared error is used to compare the fixed image with the appearance-adapted moving image $(M+R)$ after deformation with φ. Finally, we introduce the sparsity loss $\mathcal{L}_{\text{sparse}}(R) = \frac{1}{|S|}\sum_{x\in S}||R(x)||_1$, whose weighting controls the extent of the changes that the residual image can make to the moving image. Again, we use the baseline scan as moving image to model the formation of newly forming pathologies using deformation and intensity change with the residual.

The weighting parameters α, β, γ and λ are selected empirically and set to $\alpha = 100, \beta = 25, \gamma = 200$ and $\lambda = 0.01$. The deformation and residual networks are both SIREN networks with six SINE layers and a final linear layer [6]. As in [5], we apply Fourier encoding with six frequencies to the input coordinates, before passing them to the input and intermediate layers of the two INRs. The network weights are initialized as proposed in [5]. Both networks are trained simultaneously with AdamW optimization, an initial learning rate of 0.0001, and an exponential learning rate decay of 0.99. Network training is performed for 1,000 epochs, whereby one epoch corresponds to a run through all B-scans of the input images. The code is publicly available at `https://github.com/juliaandresen/FRINR`.

2.1 Data

For INR training and evaluation, an in-house longitudinal CSCR dataset is used, consisting of 276 image volumes (138 image pairs). Each image pair consists of two OCT volumes from subsequent visits of the same patient. The OCT images have a B-scan resolution of 496×512 voxels, with B-scan numbers of 19 or 25, and a field of view of $2 \times 6 \times 6\text{mm}^3$. For all images, the retina, intra- and subretinal fluid (IRF, SRF) and pigment epithelial detachment (PED) were segmented manually by medical experts. For INR training, the input OCT images are flattened at the Bruch's

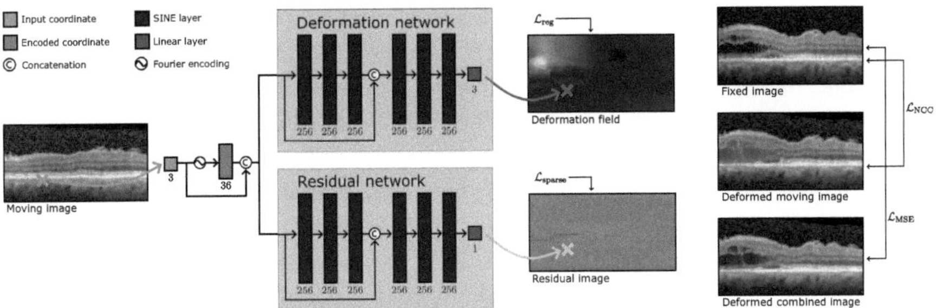

Fig. 1. Overview of the proposed INR-based image registration method. Two INRs are used to generate a residual image and deformation field. Training is performed by comparing the fixed image to the warped moving image and the warped combination of moving and residual images (exemplarily depicted on the right of the figure) and regularization terms. Numbers below layers indicate the number of output features of the respective layer.

Tab. 1. Image registration results for ANTs SyN [7], FluidRegNet [2], INR-based image registration, ImpRegDec [5] and the proposed FRINR. The Jacobian determinant of the deformation field is calculated analytically for the INR-based methods, whereas discretized approximations have to be used for ANTs SyN and FluidRegNet. ASSD stands for average symmetric surface distance and HD for Hausdorff distance of the ILM.

Method	ASSD$^{[\mu m]}\downarrow$	HD$^{[\mu m]}\downarrow$	$\lvert J_\varphi\rvert \leq 0^{[\%]}\downarrow$	$\lvert 1-\lvert J_\varphi\rvert\rvert^{\downarrow}_{\text{healthy}}$	$\lvert 1-\lvert J_\varphi\rvert\rvert^{\uparrow}_{\text{fluid}}$
Before	16.13±25.05	40.91±59.97	-	-	-
ANTs SyN	5.80±10.86	17.64±40.26	0.39±0.80	0.13±0.07	0.46±0.21
FluidRegNet	8.64±17.26	24.37±44.63	**0.04±0.10**	0.09±0.06	**0.98±0.78**
INR Reg.	5.02±2.14	12.43±7.62	0.65±0.72	0.09±0.12	0.58±0.65
ImpRegDec	5.77±8.51	14.82±24.40	0.38±0.40	0.07±0.09	0.50±0.51
FRINR	**4.95±2.09**	**12.33±8.73**	0.57±0.63	**0.06±0.10**	0.49±0.56

membrane, and B-scans are cropped to 256×496 pixels to remove confounding background, scaled to $[-1, 1]$, and downsampled to half resolution.

3 Results

In this section, first, the registration performance of FRINR is evaluated, and second, the resulting residual images are used to segment newly developing pathologies in an unsupervised manner. In Tab. 1, we report surface distances for the inner limiting membrane (ILM) before and after registration with FRINR. Additionally, we evaluate the plausibility of the deformation fields by the number of inversions and by analyzing the Jacobian determinant separately in pathology and non-pathology regions. Results are compared to ANTs SyN [7], FluidRegNet [2], ImpRegDec [5] and a registration-only INR that is trained with loss function $\mathcal{L}_{\text{INR}} = \mathcal{L}_{\text{NCC}}(F, M\circ\varphi)+\alpha\mathcal{L}_{\text{MSE}}(F, M\circ\varphi) + \beta\mathcal{L}_{\text{reg}}(\varphi)$. The settings used for ANTs SyN and FluidRegNet are the same as in our previous work [2], but results have been recalculated on the cropped images used to train the INR-based methods. For comparison to ImpRegDec [5], the code provided by the authors has been extended to 3D and adapted to grayscale images.

The results show that FRINR outperforms the other methods in terms of ILM alignment, managing to map the ILM for the extreme cases of the dataset. These extreme cases could not be handled with the CNN-based FluidRegNet, as indicated by the much higher standard deviation. Two exemplary registration results for severely altered retinae are shown in Fig. 2. A known problem of image registration with INRs, however, is the increased tendency to introduce foldings into the deformation field [4]. This can also be observed in the results here, where the INR-based approaches show an increased number of voxels with negative Jacobian.

Pathological fluids in the retina displace the surrounding tissue but typically do not introduce strong volume changes of the tissue itself. A plausible deformation should, therefore, induce stronger volume changes in pathological regions than in the surrounding tissue. All INR-based methods manage to generate such deformation fields, whereby ImpRegDec and the proposed method perform similarly well.

Tab. 2. New fluid detection and segmentation results for FRINR and FluidRegNet. We report the number of correctly identified b-scans containing new fluid (sens) and the Dice score (DSC, given in %) averaged over all B-scans that are detected as containing new fluids. Additionally, the number n_{FP} and volume V_{FP} (in pixels) of generated false positive fluids are reported.

	All fluids				IRF		SRF		PED	
Method	sens$^{\uparrow}$	DSC$^{\uparrow}$	$n_{FP}$$^{\downarrow}$	$V_{FP}$$^{\downarrow}$	sens$^{\uparrow}$	DSC$^{\uparrow}$	sens$^{\uparrow}$	DSC$^{\uparrow}$	sens$^{\uparrow}$	DSC$^{\uparrow}$
FluidRegNet	**222/293**	**59.49**	**1.09**	**91.48**	34/37	**55.95**	**179/212**	**66.57**	18/60	**50.95**
FRINR	214/293	51.57	4.57	276.42	**36/37**	55.47	169/212	62.53	**19/60**	43.69

However, the combination of support and residual image used for ImpRegDec oftentimes introduces unwanted and inconsistent behavior without clear separation of common and discriminative features, as shown in Fig. 2. Our proposed residual-only approach, in turn, offers greater control of the appearance of the residual images that primarily contain structural differences between baseline and follow-up images.

We exploit this to perform unsupervised detection of newly developed pathologies, which are segmented with $\mathcal{S} = \{x \in \Omega \mid R(\varphi(x)) < \tau_R\}$. The threshold τ_R has been found via grid search and is set to -0.15. Like this, fluids are defined as image

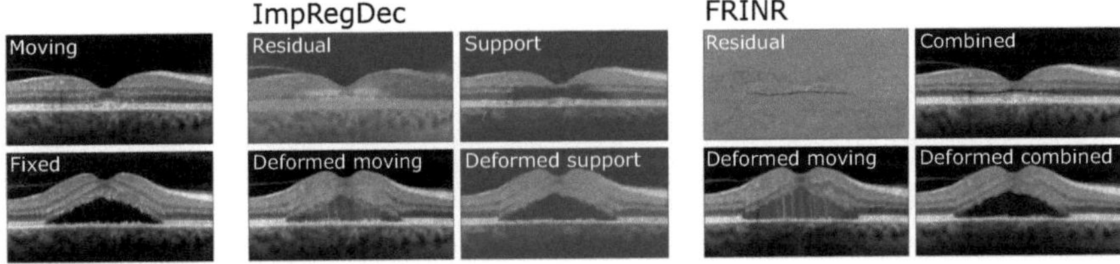

Fig. 2. Image decomposition and registration results of ImpRegDec and FRINR. The combination of residual and support images in ImpRegDec leads to an unclear separation of the tissue structures and incomplete deformations. The proposed residual-only approach, FRINR, provides more consistent results, with the residuals primarily compensating for the evolving pathologies.

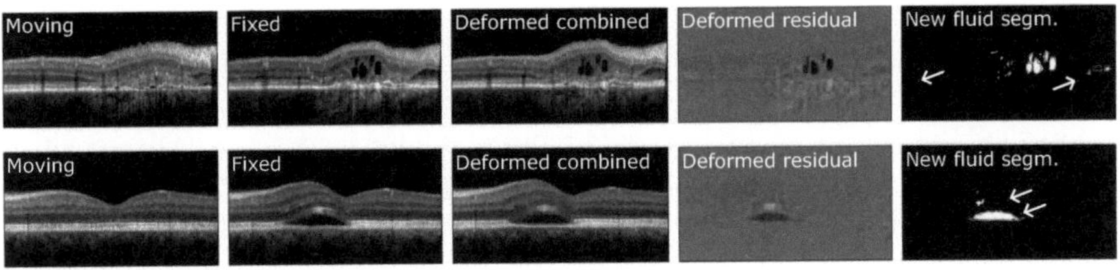

Fig. 3. Two new fluid segmentation results using thresholding on the FRINR residual images. The predicted segmentation of new pathologies is shown with the ground truth segmentation borders overlaid in green for SRF and red for IRF. Small false positive fluids are marked with arrows.

areas whose intensities have been darkened by the residual image. The deformation field extends these areas of changed intensities to the size observed in the fixed image, allowing direct comparison of $\mathcal{S}$ and the ground truth segmentation of new fluids in the fixed image. The ground truth segmentations were derived from the manual annotations by comparing baseline and follow-up b-scan images. Fluids that newly appeared in the follow-up, lesions of a fluid type not present at baseline, or dilated follow-up lesions without overlap to baseline pathologies were labeled as new. All remaining fluids in the follow-up were considered pre-existing and excluded from the new fluid ground truth. The unsupervised fluid detection and segmentation performances of FRINR are reported in Tab. 2 and compared to FluidRegNet.

Using the residual images generated by FRINR, 214 out of 293 B-scans containing newly developed fluid accumulations are detected, and detected fluids are segmented with an average Dice score of 0.5157. Given that the method is trained without using any manual annotations, the pathology delineation can be considered remarkably accurate, as further illustrated in Fig. 3. Compared to FluidRegNet, FRINR shows a slightly reduced performance both in terms of fluid detection and segmentation. Yet, FRINR performs on individual examples, while FluidRegNet is trained on an entire dataset of image pairs. As is to be expected, FRINR thus shows a higher susceptibility to small false positive results (indicated with arrows in Fig. 3), which might be reduced by a postprocessing of the resulting segmentations. Here, we kept the postprocessing consistent with [2].

4 Discussion

This paper proposed FRINR, an INR-based image registration method with increased realism of deformation fields that are pathology-aware due to the creation of a residual image that compensates for structural differences between baseline and follow-up images. Using a sparsity loss to control the appearance of these residual images, FRINR models the formation of new pathologies and successfully separates volume changes of fluids and displacement of surrounding tissue. Compared to CNN-based methods, INRs showed improved tissue mapping but more inversions. Furthermore, its lightweight design and suitability to handle anisotropic data allows adapting FRINR to 3D image volumes rather than 2D B-scans as done for FluidRegNet.

The residual images generated by FRINR were used for the unsupervised segmentation of new pathologies with promising accuracy, although a comparatively high number of false positives occur. FRINR is tailored to individual cases. Extending the method to generalizable INRs could reduce both the tendency for false-positive segmentations and inversions while improving localization in the residual image. However, this would require larger training datasets and could also degrade the ability to model severe deformations. In addition, we plan to integrate prior knowledge about the localization of pathological fluids and to speed up training times. Adapting FRINR to a pair of OCT images currently takes about one hour, compared to seven minutes for the iterative approach ANTs SyN. The present implementation offers substantial potential for runtime improvement, as it does not yet use early stopping or coordinate subsampling. However, our experiments indicate that such a subsampling leads to an overfitting to the given b-scan positions. To summarize, the proposed FRINR manages to perform fluid-aware longitudinal registration of 3D OCT images, enabling the registration of severely changed retinae and being directly applicable to individual cases without requiring manual pathology annotations.

References

1. Montero JA. Optical coherence tomography characterisation of idiopathic central serous chorioretinopathy. Br J Ophthalmol. 2005;89(5):562–4.
2. Andresen J, Ehrhardt J, von der Burchard C, Tatli A, Roider J, Handels H et al. FluidRegNet: longitudinal registration of retinal OCT images with new pathological fluids. Proc MIDL. 2024:48–60.
3. Wolterink JM, Zwienenberg JC, Brune C. Implicit neural representations for deformable image registration. Proc MIDL. 2022:1349–59.
4. Sideri-Lampretsa V, McGinnis J, Qiu H, Paschali M, Simson W, Rueckert D. SINR: spline-enhanced implicit neural representation for multi-modal registration. Proc MIDL. 2024:1462–74.
5. Byra M, Poon C, Shimogori T, Skibbe H. Implicit neural representations for joint decomposition and registration of gene expression images in the marmoset brain. Proc MICCAI. 2023:645–54.
6. Sitzmann V, Martel J, Bergman A, Lindell D, Wetzstein G. Implicit neural representations with periodic activation functions. Proc NeurIPS. 2020.
7. Avants BB, Epstein CL, Grossman M, Gee JC. Symmetric diffeomorphic image registration with cross-correlation: evaluating automated labeling of elderly and neurodegenerative brain. Med Image Anal. 2008;12(1):26–41.

Forecasting Organ Deformations in Navigated Liver Surgery using Exponential Smoothing

Michael Schwimmbeck [1,2], Christopher Auer [1], Thomas Wittenberg [2,3], Stefanie Remmele [1]

[1]Research Group Medical Technologies, University of Applied Sciences Landshut
[2]Chair for Visual Computing, Friedrich-Alexander-Universität Erlangen-Nürnberg
[3]Fraunhofer Institute for Integrated Circuits IIS, Erlangen
michael.schwimmbeck@haw-landshut.de

Abstract. Augmented reality based navigation in liver surgery requires real-time, non-rigid registration of the virtual organ model to the dynamically deforming intra-operative surface. However, computational efforts of the registration process are substantial, which motivates forecasting future deformations to minimize latency and delayed visualization. We propose a novel method to forecast liver deformations in a per-vertex manner. To meet real-time requirements, we investigate exponential smoothing to forecast anchor vertices of the organ model and propagate results to the remaining vertices. Based on a physics simulation, multiple organ model deformation series are generated to study the impact of force area, force magnitude, force direction, and the number of anchor vertices. We achieve forecasting errors in sub-millimeter precision using a Triple exponential smoothing model with 1 % anchor vertices, resulting in a computational cost of few milliseconds on standard desktop hardware. This significantly reduces latency and enables increasing process efficiency.

1 Introduction

By using augmented reality (AR) based navigation in open liver surgeries, a virtual organ model derived from pre-operative radiological data is projected directly onto the patient's liver surface. This projection yields an enhanced perception of the anatomical and vascular structures and enables surgeons to improve precision, safety, and outcomes of the intervention [1]. However, a persistent challenge is the continuous deformation of the liver, necessitating a non-rigid registration of the virtual liver model onto its in-situ counterpart. In the past, numerous non-rigid registration methods have been presented to this end; nevertheless, a significant barrier to clinical integration lies in the high computational effort and inference time of the registration step, with a duration of hundreds of milliseconds per frame [2]. This, in turn, leads to high latency and thus delayed visualization to the surgeon.

During the visual inspection stage of an open liver surgery procedure prior to the resection step, the liver undergoes periodic motion due to heartbeat and breathing,

© Der/die Autor(en), exklusiv lizenziert an
Springer Fachmedien Wiesbaden GmbH, ein Teil von Springer Nature 2026
H. Handels et al. (Hrsg.), *Bildverarbeitung für die Medizin 2026*,
Informatik aktuell, https://doi.org/10.1007/978-3-658-51100-5_19

leading to continuous deformations. Executing a complete registration pipeline for each single frame leads to high latency and reduced performance of the AR based registration [3]. Nevertheless, latency and computational resources can be improved by predicting registration results per vertex using forecasting algorithms, which are both lightweight and accurate. To our knowledge, in the case of non-rigid open liver surgery, no such approach has been studied yet.

Exponential smoothing (ES) methods are widely used in time-series forecasting and can be categorized into simple, double, and triple ES [4]. In contrast to machine learning based counterparts, ES forecasting methods are known to be fast, interpretable, adaptable, and transparent, while not requiring any training datasets. For instance, Krilavicius et al. [5] compared ES methods for tumor motion prediction during radiotherapy sessions. In our previous work [3], we applied Double ES to forecast translation vectors and rotation quaternions of rigid organ transforms.

In this study, we investigate ES for per-vertex forecasting of periodic liver deformations during open surgery. As the model deformation is directly available at the acquisition of the next frame, the delay between registration and AR visualization can be reduced, and the liver model's displacement field is pre-computed. Using the simulation open framework architecture (SOFA) physics simulation [6], which models the elastic properties of a human liver, we evaluate forecasting performance on various series of simulated deformation.

2 Materials and methods

In Fig. 1, we illustrate our approach to iteratively forecast liver deformations using single ES (SES), double ES (DES), and triple ES (TES). Forecasting is applied to the x-, y-, and z-coordinates of N_a anchor vertices. To evenly distribute anchor vertices

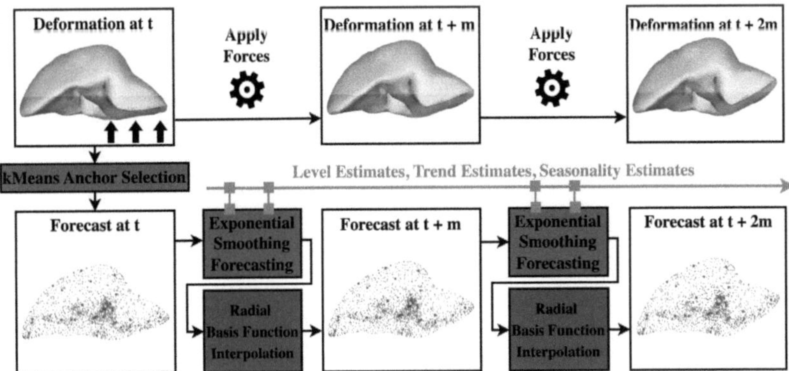

Fig. 1. Process overview. The liver surface mesh is deformed by applying forces in SOFA physics simulation [6]. Initially, N_a anchor vertices (red) are identified by kMeans clustering and subsequently forecasted m steps ahead by Exponential Smoothing. The resulting forecasts are then propagated to the remaining vertices (blue) with Radial Basis Function interpolation.

across the liver surface mesh, we initially select vertices closest to N_a k-means cluster centers. In subsequent frames, the forecasted displacement of the anchor vertices is propagated to the remaining vertices using radial basis function (RBF) interpolation [7] with a thin plate spline kernel. By setting the forecasting horizon to $m = 1$ frame, we pre-compute the deformations for the consecutive frame, ensuring direct availability at frame acquisition.

2.1 Exponential smoothing

SES [4] forecasts the observation in the next frame as $\hat{y}^{(SES)}_{t+1|t} = \alpha \cdot y_t + (1-\alpha) \cdot \hat{y}_{t|t-1}$, including the level smoothing factor $\alpha \in [0, 1]$. We set the initial forecast equal to the first observation $\hat{y}_1 = y_1$. To account for data series including a linear trend, DES [4] forecasts the observation in the next frame as $\hat{y}^{(DES)}_{t+1|t} = l_t + b_t$, comprising a level estimate $l_t = \alpha \cdot y_t + (1-\alpha) \cdot (l_{t-1} + b_{t-1})$ and a trend estimate $b_t = \beta \cdot (l_t - l_{t-1}) + (1-\beta) \cdot b_{t-1}$, supplementing the trend smoothing factor $\beta \in [0, 1]$. Initial values are set to $l_1 = y_1$ and $b_1 = y_2 - y_1$ [8]. However, if the data series includes both trend and seasonality with a period of T time steps, TES [4] introduces a seasonal estimate to approximate forecasts to seasonal patterns, which can be translated to the periodic liver deformations due to heartbeat or respiratory movements. TES supplements the seasonal smoothing factor $\gamma \in [0, 1]$ and requires a minimum of two seasons $2T$ for calibration [8]. The next frame's observation is forecasted as $\hat{y}^{(TES)}_{t+1|t} = (l_t + b_t) \cdot s_{t+1-T}$, comprising a level estimate $l_t = \alpha \cdot y_t \cdot (s_{t-T})^{-1} + (1-\alpha) \cdot (l_{t-1} + b_{t-1})$, a trend estimate $b_t = \beta \cdot (l_t - l_{t-1}) + (1-\beta) \cdot b_{t-1}$, and a multiplicative seasonal estimate $s_t = \gamma \cdot y_t \cdot (l_{t-1} + b_{t-1})^{-1} + (1-\gamma) \cdot s_{t-T}$. We compute the initial seasonality according to [4] and set the initial level and trend according to [8].

To determine optimal values α^*, β^*, and γ^*, we conduct a design-of-experiments study, in which forecasting is applied to the observations during the two calibration seasons. The smoothing factors are varied within the parameters' space $\in [0, 1]$ in increments of 0.1. We then compute the accumulated Euclidean distance $\mathrm{ED}(\alpha, \beta, \gamma)$, i.e. the forecasting error for each configuration in relation to the ground-truth observation. To stabilize the fitted curves, $\alpha = 0$ was excluded during parameter fitting. The response surface method outlined in [8] (cubic model) serves to estimate the model function $\mathrm{H}(\alpha, \beta, \gamma)$ that describes $\mathrm{ED}(\alpha, \beta, \gamma)$ w.r.t. α, β, and γ. Formally, we seek to solve $(\alpha^*, \beta^*, \gamma^*) \in \arg\min_{\alpha,\beta,\gamma \in [0,1]} \mathrm{H}(\alpha, \beta, \gamma)$ to determine the optimal parameters, which are then substituted into corresponding forecasting equations.

2.2 Data generation

We simulate various periodic liver deformations by applying forces to a tetrahedralized liver surface mesh in SOFA physics simulation [6]. To approximate the deformation properties of a liver surface, we combine a tetrahedral corotational FEM force field with an elastic model, as described by [6]. The model includes a Young's Modulus of 2 kPa and a Poisson's Ratio of 0.35, as per [2]. We use a diagonal mass of 1.5 kg, which approximates the average weight of a human liver [6].

To mimic the direction of liver lobe motion observed during clinical procedures, forces of arbitrary magnitude are applied to the lower part of each liver mesh lobe, represented by vertices in the left and right third, respectively. The inner third's lower part is constrained, simulating an anatomical fixture. We assume a frequency of 60 beats per minute (BPM) to replicate the periodic motion caused by heartbeat during surgery, representing the seasonal period length T for TES forecasting. Observations are sampled at a frame rate of 10 frames per second [3], and simulations are run ten times to model the statistical variations that occur during random scenarios.

2.3 Experiments

We examine the forecasting performance of SES, DES, and TES with respect to the force area, force magnitude, force direction, and number of anchor vertices.

The force magnitude ranges from 1 N to 5 N, as per [2]. Static scenarios apply force magnitudes in 1 N increments, while random scenarios vary between 1 N and 5 N over time. To compare the level of deformation with clinical values, we average the 3 % most deforming vertices for each static scenario.

The force direction is also applied in both static and random scenarios. In the static scenario, a unit vector is applied in upward y-direction towards the liver lobes (Fig. 1). In the random scenario, an x- and z-component $\in [-0.5, 0.5]$ is added to the vector, simulating deviations from the dominant force direction.

To determine the tradeoff between forecasting performance and time, we vary the number of anchor vertices N_a in simulation scenarios with random force magnitude and direction. Anchor vertices are selected by $N_a(p_a) = \lfloor N_v \cdot \frac{p_a}{100\,\%} \rceil$ being a random fraction of all N_v vertices with $p_a \in \{0.25\,\%, 0.5\,\%, 1\,\%, 2\,\%, 5\,\%\}$. The prediction time per frame is measured during inference on a 12th Gen Intel Core i7 CPU.

We evaluate our method on five human liver models from the 3D-IRCADb-01 dataset (patients #1 to #5) [9]. Forecasting quality is measured by the Euclidean distance (ED) between all non-static (ED > 0 mm) real and forecasted vertices. We

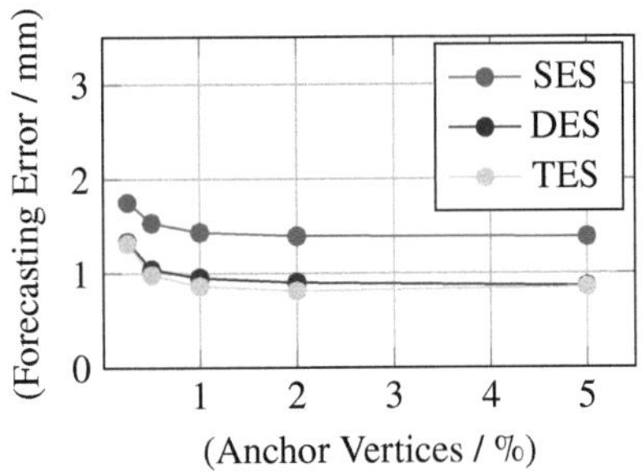

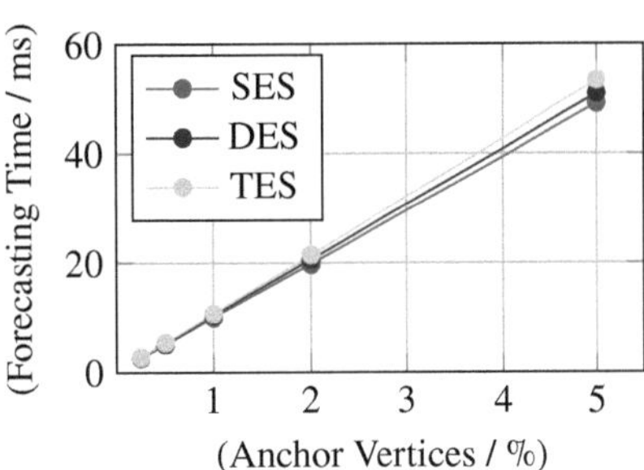

Fig. 2. Mean forecasting performance (left) and mean prediction time per frame (right) with respect to the fraction of anchor vertices from the total number of vertices. Scores were computed on standard desktop hardware for scenarios with random force direction and random force magnitude, averaged over simulation series involving five liver models.

compute metrics for the 15 test seasons following the two calibration seasons. The first three seasons are excluded to bypass the SOFA warm-up iterations.

3 Results

In Figure 2 we present the forecasting performance and prediction time of SES, DES, and TES, varying the number of anchor vertices $N_a(p_a)$. We chose $p_a = 1\,\%$ as the best tradeoff between performance and time for subsequent forecasting experiments. Forecasting results for SES, DES, and TES with respect to different simulation scenarios are depicted in Figure 3 and compared to a clinical reference [10]. TES achieves the lowest overall forecasting errors (lower than 1.27 mm in each scenario), involving a prediction time of 10.75 ms per frame on a standard desktop CPU.

4 Discussion

SES calibration results in high α-values; hence, merely prior values are propagated as future values, which demonstrates that the simulated periodic motion pattern appears to be too complex for SES forecasting. When comparing random direction scenarios with static direction scenarios, we observe that discrepancies are significantly higher for TES forecasting compared to SES and DES forecasting (Fig. 3). While TES yields smaller average errors over all experiments, it performs worse than DES once the motion becomes random in force magnitude/direction and deviates from

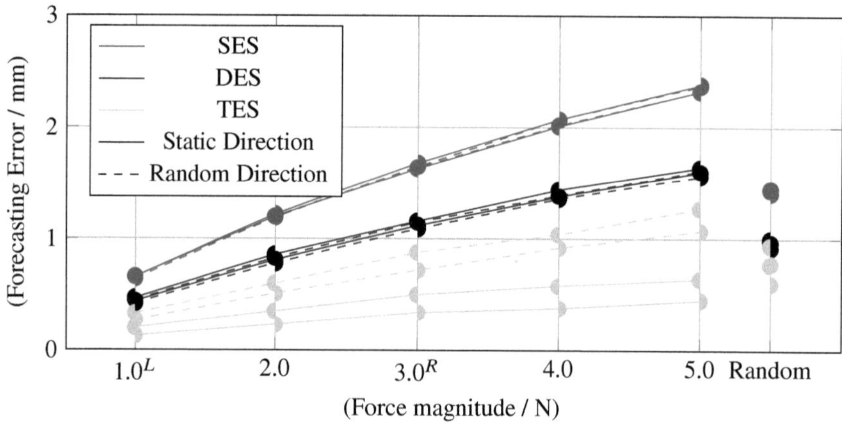

Fig. 3. Forecasting results ($p_a = 1\,\%$) for simulation scenarios including static/random force magnitude and direction (average for five liver models). Forces were applied to either the left (left semicircle) or right (right semicircle) liver lobe, and the performance was measured as the average Euclidean distance between all forecasted and ground-truth non-static vertices (ten repetitions per scenario). Force magnitudes marked with L (left lobe) and R (right lobe) resulted in maximum deformations that most closely resemble a clinical reference value [10].

the calibrated periodic pattern. In these cases, TES attempts to predict a seasonal pattern, resulting in forecasting distortions. DES, in contrast, leads to a more accurate approximation of irregular periods. However, DES overshoots at extrema during regular seasonal patterns, which is a known limitation [5]. To enhance performance and robustness in future work, effectively combining DES and TES may be beneficial to leverage their advantages while mitigating their respective limitations.

We observe higher forecasting errors when there is a substantial discrepancy in the force amplitude during calibration and inference. This could be resolved by re-calibration, triggered whenever measurement and prediction drift too far apart. Furthermore, the force frequency oscillates in practice. A sequel study could explore varying seasonalities or dampening distortions caused by the varying seasonal lengths. While uniform forces were applied to the unconstrained areas of the mesh, future work should explore more sophisticated deformation patterns derived from clinical data including organ palpation or instrument interaction.

In conclusion, our method forecasts continuous organ deformations with a per-vertex precision of less than 1.27 mm in all scenarios. Forecasting results are computed within a few milliseconds, without requiring large training datasets. We believe that this work is of value to the community as it significantly reduces latency during liver surgery navigation. Future work could further enhance accuracy, robustness, and speed by increasing forecasting horizons and combining models.

References

1. Wang X, Yang J, Zhou B et al. Integrating mixed reality, augmented reality, and artificial intelligence in complex liver surgeries: enhancing precision, safety, and outcomes. iLIVER. 2025.
2. Pfeiffer M, Riediger C, Leger S et al. Non-rigid volume to surface registration using a data-driven biomechanical model. Proc MICCAI. 2020.
3. Schwimmbeck M, Khajarian S, Auer C et al. Towards a zero-shot low-latency navigation for open surgery augmented reality applications. Int J Comput Assist Radiol Surg. 2025.
4. Hyndman RJ, Athanasopoulos G. Forecasting: principles and practice. OTexts, 2018.
5. Krilavicius T, Zliobaite I, Simonavicius H et al. Predicting respiratory motion for real-time tumour tracking in radiotherapy. Proc IEEE CBMS. 2016.
6. Faure F, Duriez C, Delingette H et al. SOFA: A multi-model framework for interactive physical simulation. Soft tissue biomechanical modeling for computer assisted surgery. Springer, 2012.
7. Fasshauer GE. Meshfree approximation methods with matlab. Vol. 6. World Scientific Publishing Company, 2007.
8. Guthrie WF. NIST/SEMATECH e-handbook of statistical methods (NIST handbook 151). Nat Inst Std Tech. 2020.
9. Soler L, Hostettler A, Agnus V et al. 3D image reconstruction for comparison of algorithm database. URL: https://www.ircad.fr/research/data-sets/liver-segmentation-3d-ircadb-01. 2010;13.
10. Clements LW, Dumpuri P, Chapman WC et al. Organ surface deformation measurement and analysis in open hepatic surgery: method and preliminary results from 12 clinical cases. IEEE Trans Biomed Eng. 2011;58(8).

Abstract: Liemorph

Transformer-based Image Registration using Flows on Lie Groups

Johannes Bostelmann, Jan Lellmann

Institute of Mathematics and Image Computing, University of Lübeck
johannes.bostelmann@uni-luebeck.de

Image registration aims to establish point correspondences between the given images $I_1, I_2 : \Omega \rightarrow \mathbb{R}^k$, typically via a deformation map $\phi : \Omega \rightarrow \Omega$ that assigns points in one image to those in the other. In our work [1], we propose to combine stationary velocity fields on Lie groups with a suitable regularization to provide fine control over the desired deformations. Specifically:

1. We parametrize ϕ using stationary velocity fields on user-specified matrix groups $G \subset \mathbb{R}^{n \times n}$ (MGSVFs). The approach is based on the flow equation adapted to matrix groups as proposed in [2].
2. We combine this parametrization with a penalty term on the velocities, which allows us to precisely select deformations that should not be penalized.
3. We integrate MGSVFs into the TransMorph [3] architecture for generating the matrix group-valued velocity fields.

Overall, this allows to improve the robustness of SVF-based registration approaches against large deformations prescribed by the chosen group – for example, against roto-translations with the choice $G = \mathrm{SE}(3)$. MGSVFs can be implemented in a fully differentiable manner, enabling easy integration into most image registration frameworks. Further advantages of the approach include inherent invertibility and trivial recovery of the inverse deformation. We validate the approach on unsupervised and weakly supervised brain MRI registration tasks on the IXI and OASIS datasets. In both cases, the proposed matrix-group extension improves performance compared to the base transformer model. Our implementation is available at `https://github.com/sennhoj321/Liemorph`.

References

1. Bostelmann J, Lellmann J. LieMorph: transformer-based image registration using flows on Lie groups. Proc BMVC. 2025.
2. Bostelmann J, Gildemeister O, Lellmann J. Stationary velocity fields on matrix groups for deformable image registration. arXiv preprint: 2410.10997. 2024.

© Der/die Autor(en), exklusiv lizenziert an
Springer Fachmedien Wiesbaden GmbH, ein Teil von Springer Nature 2026
H. Handels et al. (Hrsg.), *Bildverarbeitung für die Medizin 2026*,
Informatik aktuell, https://doi.org/10.1007/978-3-658-51100-5_20

3. Chen J, Frey EC, He Y, Segars WP, Li Y, Du Y. Transmorph: transformer for unsupervised medical image registration. Med Image Anal. 2022;82:102615.

Abstract: Synomaly Noise and Multi-stage Diffusion

A Novel Approach for Unsupervised Anomaly Detection in Medical Images

Yuan Bi [1,2†], Lucie Huang [1,2†], Ricarda Clarenbach [3], Reza Ghotbi [3], Angelos Karlas [4], Nassir Navab [1], Zhongliang Jiang [1]

[1]Computer Aided Medical Procedures, Technical University of Munich, Munich, Germany
[2]Munich Center of Machine Learning, Munich, Germany
[3]Clinic for Vascular Surgery, Helios Klinikum München West, Munich, Germany
[4]Rechts der Isar University Hospital, Technical University of Munich, Munich, Germany
yuan.bi@tum.de

Anomaly detection in medical imaging plays a crucial role in identifying pathological regions across various imaging modalities, such as brain MRI, liver CT, and carotid ultrasound (US). However, training fully supervised segmentation models is often hindered by the scarcity of expert annotations and the complexity of diverse anatomical structures. To address these issues, we propose a novel unsupervised anomaly detection framework based on a diffusion model that incorporates a synthetic anomaly (Synomaly) noise function and a multi-stage diffusion process. Synomaly noise introduces synthetic anomalies into healthy images during training, allowing the model to effectively learn anomaly removal. The multi-stage diffusion process is introduced to progressively denoise images, preserving fine details while improving the quality of anomaly-free reconstructions. The generated high-fidelity counterfactual healthy images can further enhance the interpretability of the segmentation models, as well as provide a reliable baseline for evaluating the extent of anomalies and supporting clinical decision-making. Notably, the unsupervised anomaly detection model is trained purely on healthy images, eliminating the need for anomalous training samples and pixel-level annotations. We validate the proposed approach on brain MRI, liver CT datasets, and carotid US. Ablation studies further highlight the contributions of Synomaly noise and the multi-stage diffusion process in improving anomaly segmentation [1].

References

1. Bi Y, Huang L, Clarenbach R, Ghotbi R, Karlas A, Navab N et al. Synomaly noise and multi-stage diffusion: a novel approach for unsupervised anomaly detection in medical images. Med Image Anal. 2025:103737.

[†]These authors contributed equally to this work.

© Der/die Autor(en), exklusiv lizenziert an
Springer Fachmedien Wiesbaden GmbH, ein Teil von Springer Nature 2026
H. Handels et al. (Hrsg.), *Bildverarbeitung für die Medizin 2026*,
Informatik aktuell, https://doi.org/10.1007/978-3-658-51100-5_21

Abstract: An OpenMind for 3D Medical Vision Self-supervised Learning

Constantin Ulrich[1,2†], Tassilo Wald[1,3,4†], Jonathan Suprijadi[1†], Sebastian Ziegler[1,3], Michal Nohel[5,6], Robin Peretzke[1,2], Gregor Köhler[1], Klaus Maier-Hein[1,2,3,4,7]

[1]Division of Medical Image Computing, German Cancer Research Center (DKFZ), Heidelberg, Germany
[2]Medical Faculty Heidelberg, University of Heidelberg, Germany
[3]Helmholtz Imaging, DKFZ, Heidelberg, Germany.
[4]Faculty of Mathematics and Computer Science, University of Heidelberg, Germany
[5]Faculty of Electrical Engineering and Communication, Brno University of Technology
[6]University hospital Ostrava, Department of Deputy director for science, research and education, Ostrava, Czech Republic
[7]Pattern Analysis and Learning Group, Department of Radiation Oncology, Heidelberg University Hospital, Heidelberg, Germany
constantin.ulrich@dkfz-heidelberg.de

The field of self-supervised learning (SSL) for 3D medical images lacks consistency and standardization. While many methods have been developed, it is impossible to identify the current state-of-the-art, due to i) varying and small pre-training datasets, ii) varying architectures, and iii) being evaluated on differing downstream datasets. In this paper, we bring clarity to this field and lay the foundation for further method advancements through three key contributions: We a) publish the largest publicly available pre-training dataset comprising 114k 3D brain MRI volumes, enabling all practitioners to pre-train on a large-scale dataset. We b) benchmark existing 3D self-supervised learning methods on this dataset for a state-of-the-art CNN and Transformer architecture, clarifying the state of 3D SSL pre-training. Among many findings, we show that pre-trained methods can exceed a strong from-scratch nnU-Net ResEnc-L baseline. Lastly, we c) publish the code of our pre-training and fine-tuning frameworks and provide the pre-trained models created during the benchmarking process to facilitate rapid adoption and reproduction. Available here [1].

References

1. Wald T, Ulrich C, Suprijadi J, Ziegler S, Nohel M, Peretzke R et al. An OpenMind for 3D medical vision self-supervised learning. Proc IEEE/CVF ICCV. 2025:23839–79.

†These authors contributed equally to this work.

© Der/die Autor(en), exklusiv lizenziert an
Springer Fachmedien Wiesbaden GmbH, ein Teil von Springer Nature 2026
H. Handels et al. (Hrsg.), *Bildverarbeitung für die Medizin 2026*,
Informatik aktuell, https://doi.org/10.1007/978-3-658-51100-5_22

Abstract: Faster, Self-supervised Super-resolution for Anisotropic Multi-view MRI using a Sparse Loss

Maja Schlereth [1,2], Moritz Schillinger [1], Katharina Breininger [3]

[1]Department Artificial Intelligence in Biomedical Engineering, Friedrich-Alexander-Universität Erlangen-Nürnberg, Erlangen, Germany
[2]Department of Internal Medicine 3, Universitätsklinikum Erlangen, Erlangen, Germany
[3]Center for AI and Data Science (CAIDAS), Julius-Maximilians-Universität Würzburg, Würzburg, Germany

maja.schlereth@fau.de

In medical imaging, balancing scan duration, image quality and patient comfort is crucial. Magnetic resonance (MR) imaging provides high soft-tissue contrast, but scan time increases with higher spatial resolution. Acquiring multiple low-resolution (LR) scans in different orientations can mitigate this. To enable easier downstream analysis in a unified representation, fusing these images is valuable, yet combining them remains challenging. Because high-resolution (HR) ground-truth data are largely unavailable in clinical practice, we introduce a novel fully self-supervised super-resolution (SR) approach to combine two anisotropic LR scans into one high-resolution image [1]. To train our multi-view neural network, we propose a sparse coordinate-based loss that allows the integration of arbitrarily scaled LR images. We evaluated our method on two publicly available brain MRI datasets. We simulated anisotropic LR coronal and axial scans with a slice thickness of 2, and 4 mm for the LR images. HR data was just used for evaluation purposes only and was not available during training. Our SR pipeline consists of two phases: a patient-agnostic offline phase, where the model learns cross-patient similarities, and a patient-specific online phase, where additional subject-specific information can be learned. Our results show that our approach produces SR images of equal or higher quality compared to current reference approaches. Additionally, we demonstrate that the proposed method generalizes well across different datasets. A key advantage lies in the substantial speed-up achieved in the patient-specific reconstruction, up to tenfold, while maintaining or improving image quality, making the method more applicable in clinical scenarios.

References

1. Schlereth M, Schillinger M, Breininger K. Faster, self-supervised super-resolution for anisotropic multi-view MRI using a sparse coordinate loss. Proc MICCAI. 2026:172–82.

© Der/die Autor(en), exklusiv lizenziert an Springer Fachmedien Wiesbaden GmbH, ein Teil von Springer Nature 2026
H. Handels et al. (Hrsg.), *Bildverarbeitung für die Medizin 2026*, Informatik aktuell, https://doi.org/10.1007/978-3-658-51100-5_23

Anomaly Detection in Thoracic CT
A Public Benchmark Based on CT-RATE

Franziska Weber [1], Thomas Gorges [1], Adarsh Raghunath [1,2], Andreas Maier [1]

[1]Pattern Recognition Lab, Friedrich-Alexander-Universität Erlangen-Nürnberg, Erlangen
[2]Digital Technology and Innovation, Siemens Healthineers, Erlangen
`franziska.fw.weber@fau.de`

Abstract. The workload of radiologists has grown drastically in recent years, which may lead to increased fatigue and higher risk of diagnostic oversights. Consequently, the automatic detection of anomalous scans is of high practical relevance. Conventional supervised models do not generalize reliably beyond the anomalies seen during training but covering the vast range of possible pathologies in the training data is not feasible. In other domains, anomaly detection (AD) has proven to be a viable approach for this problem. In thoracic CT, however, AD has been little explored so far with previous work relying on private data with a narrow anomaly scope. We address this gap by curating CT-RATE-AD, a public dataset for anomaly detection (AD) in thoracic CT, built on the public CT-RATE dataset. It comprises 5065 scans with 18 anomaly types in the unhealthy subset. Additionally, we evaluate several established AD methods, including training-free, reconstruction-based, and self-supervised ones, on CT-RATE-AD. These methods achieve up to 0.65 AUROC, 0.62 AP, and 16% specificity at 95% sensitivity and serve as baselines for future work. The dataset and implementation are publicly available at `https://github.com/franziskaweber/CT-RATE-AD`.

1 Introduction

In recent years, the workload of radiologists has increased significantly, leading to greater fatigue and risk of error. Missed findings, especially unexpected ones, are the most common errors [1]. For example, over 80% of experienced radiologists did not notice a gorilla image inserted into a lung CT scan when assessing lung nodules [2]. Therefore, automatically detecting abnormal scans is of high practical importance.

Supervised models reliably identify only previously seen anomalies [1]. However, acquiring enough data to cover all possible anomalies in the training set is practically infeasible. An alternative is provided by anomaly detection (AD) methods, which learn the distribution of healthy data and identify outliers as unhealthy samples.

Most AD methods are either reconstruction-based or self-supervised, with reconstruction-based methods being the most prevalent in medical AD [3]. They

© Der/die Autor(en), exklusiv lizenziert an
Springer Fachmedien Wiesbaden GmbH, ein Teil von Springer Nature 2026
H. Handels et al. (Hrsg.), *Bildverarbeitung für die Medizin 2026*,
Informatik aktuell, https://doi.org/10.1007/978-3-658-51100-5_24

train a generative model to reconstruct healthy images and use the reconstruction error as anomaly score during inference. The underlying assumption is that models trained only on healthy data cannot accurately reconstruct previously unseen abnormal regions. Self-supervised AD approaches, on the other hand, train models on proxy tasks such as the detection of synthetic anomalies inserted into the data .

Common medical applications of AD are brain MRI and chest X-ray [4]. In thoracic CT, however, AD has not yet been frequently used and no thoracic CT is included in current medical AD benchmarks [1, 3, 5]. The few previous works on AD in thoracic CT use private data and concentrate on few anomalies [6, 7], which fails to reflect the broad spectrum of pathologies encountered in clinical practice.

We address this gap by curating the public dataset CT-RATE-AD for AD on thoracic CT based on the dataset CT-RATE [8]. Our dataset contains 5065 scans covering a wide range of 18 different anomalies in the unhealthy subset. In addition, we establish a baseline for this dataset by evaluating various AD methods, including training-free, reconstruction-based, and self-supervised ones on CT-RATE-AD.

2 Materials and methods

2.1 Dataset

A dataset for benchmarking AD methods on thoracic CT scans needs to contain enough healthy cases for training and should cover a wide range of pathologies. To the best of our knowledge, the only public dataset fulfilling these conditions is CT-RATE [8]. It contains 25 692 non-contrast chest CT scans from 21 304 unique patients, reconstructed to 50 188 volumes, combined with the radiology reports and binary labels for 18 anomalies extracted from the reports using an LLM.

From CT-RATE, we construct the AD dataset CT-RATE-AD. We treat the 5505 volumes with none of the 18 anomaly labels as healthy and split the samples patient-wise into training, validation, and test set. In the training set, all available scans per patient are preserved to increase data diversity. In the validation and test data, only one scan per patient is included to avoid distorting the evaluation. This results in a training set with 3565 healthy samples from 1831 unique patients, a validation set with 500 healthy samples from 500 unique patients and a test set with 500 healthy and 500 unhealthy samples from 1000 unique patients. All volumes are resampled to 0.75 mm spacing in x- and y- and 1.5 mm spacing in z-direction and normalized to $[0, 1]$ to standardize their geometry and intensity. The frequencies of the 18 anomalies in the unhealthy test data are displayed in Fig. 1.

The training and validation set only contain healthy volumes because AD methods are developed exclusively on healthy data [1]. The unhealthy test data are sampled from CT-RATE via multi-label iterative stratification such that the anomaly-type proportions match those in the entire set of unhealthy data. The Kullback-Leibler divergence between the proportions in the full and the sampled unhealthy test data is 0.0043, indicating near equality of the distributions.

2.2 Methods

To establish a baseline, we evaluate various AD methods, including training-free, reconstruction-based, and self-supervised ones, on our dataset CT-RATE-AD.

The first training-free method is intensity-based. It computes the z-score for each voxel, where mean and standard deviation are computed locally in a cube of size $15 \times 15 \times 15$ voxels around the current voxel. The z-score measures by how many standard deviations the voxel deviates from the local mean. Voxels with z-scores above 4 are treated as potentially abnormal and grouped using 6-connectivity. Small clusters with fewer than 100 voxels are removed and the maximum z-score among all remaining potentially abnormal voxels is used as anomaly score.

The other training-free method that we consider leverages the foundation model CT-FM [9]. Foundation models are pretrained on massive amounts of data and can adapt to many different tasks. CT-FM is the first vision-centric encoder for 3D CT data and was pretrained via self-supervised contrastive learning on 148 000 CT scans covering different body parts. We use CT-FM to embed the healthy scans from the training and validation set, as no separate validation set is required for this method. Then, the distribution of these embeddings is modeled with a Gaussian mixture model. The number of components K is selected by minimizing the Bayesian information criterion over $K \in \{1, \ldots, 5\}$ which resulted in $K = 1$. For the test data, the anomaly score is obtained as the negative log-likelihood under the learned healthy distribution.

As reconstruction-based baselines, we use 2D and 3D variational auto-encoders (VAEs) [10] trained by minimizing the L_1 reconstruction error on the training set. The 2D VAE is trained slice-wise on ten random axial slices and the 3D VAE on four patches of size $128 \times 128 \times 128$ voxels per volume for 30 epochs. The model with the lowest L_1 validation error is selected for inference. At inference, the volumes are assembled from slices for the 2D VAE and with a sliding window inferer for the 3D VAE. The volume-wise L_1 reconstruction error is used as anomaly score.

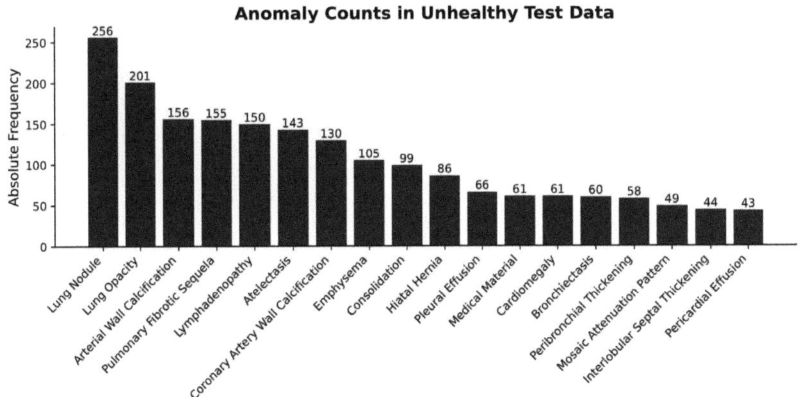

Fig. 1. Frequencies of the 18 anomalies in the unhealthy test data.

For a well-established and straightforward self-supervised approach, we follow CutPaste (CP) [11] and create synthetic anomalies by blending patches within a volume. Source and target locations are randomly selected from a central region of the volume between 25% and 75% of the volume size in all dimensions to ensure that they are likely within the body. Each patch is a cube with size randomly chosen from $\{0, 8, 16, 32, 64\}$ voxels with 0 meaning no anomaly is inserted. The anomaly is created by blending the source patch into the target region using equal weighting. An example anomaly is shown on the left in Fig. 2. Subsequently, an nnU-Net [12] is trained for anomaly segmentation. Its standard procedures are used for preprocessing, model training, and postprocessing and the available configurations 2d, 3d_fullres (3d_fr) and 3d_lowres (3d_lr) are evaluated. As the training is conducted via 5-fold cross-validation, the training and validation sets are combined for training the network. At inference, the percentage of voxels predicted as anomalous in a volume is used as anomaly score.

We adopt the most common metrics for sample-wise evaluation of AD methods, namely the area under the receiver operating characteristic curve (AUROC) and the average precision (AP). Both of these methods are threshold-independent. Additionally, we report the specificity at 95% sensitivity which measures how many scans are correctly classified as healthy when at most 5% of the unhealthy scans are missed. These 5% are below the human error rate according to most studies [13]. For the methods requiring training, we report the average metrics and their standard deviations across three independent runs to get more conclusive results.

3 Results

The results are displayed in Tab. 1. The reconstruction-based VAE approaches perform best, achieving up to 0.65 AUROC and 0.62 AP, whereas the self-supervised methods perform worse than the training-free ones with at most 0.56 AUROC (CP + 3d_fr) and 0.54 AP (CP + 2d). The two training-free methods perform simi-

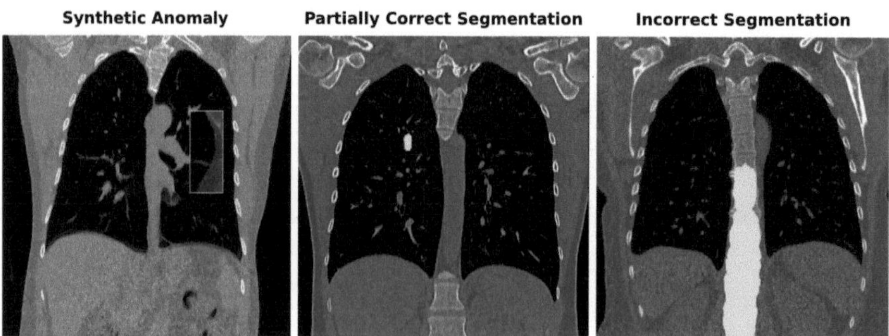

Fig. 2. Visualization of the self-supervised approach. Left: synthetic anomaly, middle: correct segmentation of lung nodule, right: erroneous segmentation of normal anatomical structure.

Tab. 1. Results of various AD methods on our CT-RATE-AD test set. For the methods requiring training, the metrics are reported in terms of their average and standard deviation across three independent runs. The best scores are highlighted in bold.

Method	AUROC	AP	Spec @ 95% Sens
Voxel Intensity	0.5830	0.5672	0.0714
CT-FM [9]	0.5707	0.5871	0.0500
2D VAE [10]	**0.6463 ± 0.0057**	**0.6212 ± 0.0035**	0.1567 ± 0.0168
3D VAE [10]	0.6455 ± 0.0212	0.6138 ± 0.0348	0.1486 ± 0.0197
CP [11] + nnU-Net 2d [12]	0.5389 ± 0.0189	0.5410 ± 0.0189	0.0000 ± 0.0000
CP [11] + nnU-Net 3d_lr [12]	0.5315 ± 0.0001	0.5100 ± 0.0004	0.0653 ± 0.0133
CP [11] + nnU-Net 3d_fr [12]	0.5623 ± 0.0088	0.5266 ± 0.0059	**0.1586 ± 0.0456**

larly with the voxel-intensity-based approach slightly surpassing the CT-FM-based one with 0.58 AUROC and 7% specificity at 95% sensitivity.

Among the reconstruction-based methods, on average, the 2D VAE yields slightly better results than the 3D version. The 3D VAE, however, has a larger standard deviation, meaning that some runs outperform the 2D model. Fig. 3 displays examples of one healthy and one unhealthy slice along with their 2D and 3D VAE reconstructions and the voxel-wise difference maps between the original and the reconstructed slices. While neither the 2D nor the 3D VAE retains fine-grained structures such as small vessels, the 2D VAE produces slightly sharper reconstructions than the 3D one. Abnormalities like lung nodules are also omitted in the reconstructions, which results in high reconstruction errors in anomalous regions.

The self-supervised methods mostly perform worst of all implemented approaches. The only exception is CP with nnU-Net 3d_fr which achieves the highest specificity of 16% at 95% sensitivity among all models. Fig. 2 illustrates that the methods capture true anomalies like lung nodules in some cases. In most cases, however, they erroneously segment normal anatomical structures such as the spine.

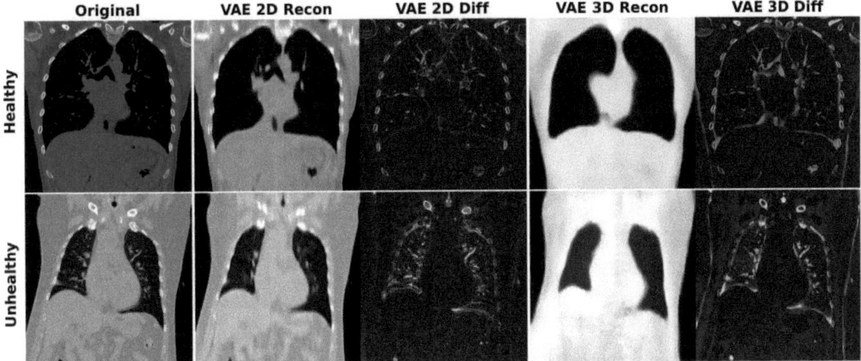

Fig. 3. One healthy and one unhealthy slice with their 2D and 3D VAE reconstructions and voxel-wise difference maps between the original and the reconstructed slices.

4 Discussion

In this paper, we evaluated various AD methods, including training-free, reconstruction-based, and self-supervised ones on our newly curated dataset CT-RATE-AD. The reconstruction-based approaches performed best, with the 2D VAE slightly surpassing the 3D one. This observation is consistent with Fig. 3, which shows that the reconstructions generated by the 3D VAE are noticeably blurrier than those of the 2D VAE. This is counterintuitive, as the 3D model should capture the volumetric anatomy better than the slice-wise version. We suspect that this observation can be explained by suboptimal parameter choices.

The self-supervised approaches performed poorly in our experiments. This is likely due to the sharp boundaries of the synthetic anomalies, which led the nnU-Net to segment clearly delimited anatomical structures such as the spine instead of the actual anomalies. Consequently, the self-supervised approaches were outperformed by two simple training-free baselines, of which one was based on voxel intensity and the other on embeddings of the pretrained foundation model CT-FM.

In summary, this paper establishes a public benchmark for AD in thoracic CT and presents results serving as a first baseline. Future work will focus on evaluating state-of-the-art reconstruction-based and self-supervised AD methods on the curated dataset.

Acknowledgement. The authors gratefully acknowledge the scientific support and HPC resources provided by the Erlangen National High Performance Computing Center (NHR@FAU) of the Friedrich-Alexander-Universität Erlangen-Nürnberg (FAU) under the NHR project b143dc. NHR funding is provided by federal and Bavarian state authorities. NHR@FAU hardware is partially funded by the German Research Foundation (DFG) – 440719683.

References

1. Zimmerer D, Full PM, Isensee F, Jäger P, Adler T, Petersen J et al. MOOD 2020: a public benchmark for out-of-distribution detection and localization on medical images. IEEE Trans Med Imaging. 2022;41(10):2728–38.
2. Drew T, Võ MLH, Wolfe JM. The invisible gorilla strikes again: sustained inattentional blindness in expert observers. Psychol Sci. 2013;24(9):1848–53.
3. Cai Y, Zhang W, Chen H, Cheng KT. MedIAnomaly: a comparative study of anomaly detection in medical images. Med Image Anal. 2025:103500.
4. Tschuchnig ME, Gadermayr M. Anomaly detection in medical imaging: a mini review. Proc iDSC. 2021:33–8.
5. Bao J, Sun H, Deng H, He Y, Zhang Z, Li X. BMAD: benchmarks for medical anomaly detection. Proc IEEE/CVF CVPR. 2024:4042–53.
6. Gao Z, Nakayama R, Hizukuri A, Kido S. Anomaly detection scheme for lung CT images using vector quantized variational auto-encoder with support vector data description. Radiol Phys Technol. 2025;18(1):17–26.

7. Lee JH, Oh SJ, Kim K, Lim CY, Choi SH, Chung MJ. Improved unsupervised 3D lung lesion detection and localization by fusing global and local features: validation in 3D low-dose computed tomography. Med Image Anal. 2025;103:103559.
8. Hamamci IE, Er S, Wang C, Almas F, Simsek AG, Esirgun SN et al. Developing generalist foundation models from a multimodal dataset for 3D computed tomography. arXiv preprint: 2403.17834. 2024.
9. Pai S, Hadzic I, Bontempi D, Bressem K, Kann BH, Fedorov A et al. Vision foundation models for computed tomography. arXiv preprint: 2501.09001. 2025.
10. Kingma DP, Welling M. Auto-encoding variational bayes. arXiv preprint: 1312.6114. 2013.
11. Li CL, Sohn K, Yoon J, Pfister T. CutPaste: self-supervised learning for anomaly detection and localization. Proc IEEE/CVF CVPR. 2021:9664–74.
12. Isensee F, Jaeger PF, Kohl SA, Petersen J, Maier-Hein KH. nnU-net: a self-configuring method for deep learning-based biomedical image segmentation. Nat Methods. 2021;18(2):203–11.
13. Brady AP. Error and discrepancy in radiology: inevitable or avoidable? Insights Imaging. 2017;8(1):171–82.

Multimodal Classification of Radiation-induced Contrast Enhancement and Tumor Recurrence using Deep Learning

Robin Peretzke[1,2,3†], Marlin Hanstein[1†], Maximilian Fischer[1,2,4,5†], Lars Wessel[6,7,8,9], Obada Alhalabi[10], Sebastian Regnery[6,7,8,9], Andreas Kudak[6,7], Maximilian Deng[6,7,8,9], Tanja Eichkorn[6,7,8,9], Philipp Hoegen-Saßmannshausen[6,7,8,9], Fabian Allmendinger[6,7,8], Jan-Hendrik Bolten[6,7,8], Philipp Schröter[6,7,8], Christine Jungk[10], Jürgen Debus[1,6,7,8,9,11], Peter Neher[1,3], Laila König[6,7,8,9], Klaus Maier-Hein[1,2,3]

[1]Deutsches Krebsforschungszentrum (DKFZ), Division of Medical Image Computing
[2]Medical Faculty, Heidelberg University, Heidelberg, Germany
[3]Pattern Analysis and Learning Group, Department of Radiation Oncology, UKHD
[4]Research Campus M[2]OLIE, Mannheim, Germany
[5]German Cancer Consortium (DKTK), DKFZ Core Center Heidelberg
[6]Universitätsklinikum Heidelberg (UKHD), Heidelberg, Germany
[7]Heidelberger Institut für Radioonkologie (HIRO), Heidelberg, Germany
[8]National Center for Tumor Diseases (NCT), NCT Heidelberg
[9]Heidelberger Ionenstrahl-Therapiezentrum (HIT), Heidelberg, Germany
[10]Universitätsklinikum Heidelberg, Neurochirurgie, Heidelberg, Germany
[11]Deutsches Krebsforschungszentrum, Clinical Cooperation Unit Radiation Oncology
maximilian.fischer@dkfz-heidelberg.de

Abstract. The differentiation between tumor recurrence and radiation-induced contrast enhancements in post-treatment glioblastoma patients remains a major clinical challenge. Existing approaches rely on clinically sparsely available diffusion MRI or do not consider radiation maps, which are gaining increasing interest in the tumor board for this differentiation. We introduce *RICE-NET*, a multimodal 3D deep learning model that integrates longitudinal MRI data with radiotherapy dose distributions for automated lesion classification, using conventional T1-weighted MRI data. Using a cohort of 92 patients, the model achieved a performance of 0.92 [F1] on an independent test set. During extensive ablation experiments, we quantified the contribution of each timepoint and modality and showed that reliable classification largely depends on the radiation map. Occlusion-based interpretability analyses further confirmed the model's focus on clinically relevant regions. These findings highlight the potential of multimodal deep learning to enhance diagnostic accuracy and support clinical decision-making in neuro-oncology.

[†]These authors contributed equally to this work.

© Der/die Autor(en), exklusiv lizenziert an
Springer Fachmedien Wiesbaden GmbH, ein Teil von Springer Nature 2026
H. Handels et al. (Hrsg.), *Bildverarbeitung für die Medizin 2026*,
Informatik aktuell, https://doi.org/10.1007/978-3-658-51100-5_25

1 Introduction

Medicine has always been an exercise in balance between benefit and harm, precision and uncertainty [1]. This tension is especially apparent in the treatment of brain tumors, where radiation also carries the potential to injure the very tissue it seeks to protect. While radiotherapy is indispensable in eliminating residual tumor cells after surgical resection, its necrotic effect is not exclusive to malignant tissue. As a result, new or progressive contrast-enhancing lesions that appear during follow-up imaging often pose a crucial diagnostic dilemma, since both malignancies are expressed via similar appearing contrast-enhanced regions in MR imaging. Thus, the differentiation between tumor recurrence and RICE remains challenging [2, 3]. Currently, the clinical differentiation between RICE and tumor recurrence is a complex and time-consuming process by an interdisciplinary tumor board, involving re-evaluation of the entire imaging trajectory. In this work, we present RICE-NET, a multimodal deep learning approach for differentiating between radiation-induced changes and glioblastoma multiforme (GBM) tumor recurrence. The network integrates longitudinal MRI data as well as radiotherapy plans to enable automated and early classification of post-treatment contrast-enhancing lesions. While several recent studies have reported promising results using advanced diffusion imaging for lesion classification [4, 5], these approaches have not yet been applied to more widely available conventional MRI sequences. Moreover, most existing studies do not incorporate dosimetric data and neglect the longitudinal evolution of imaging findings. We evaluate the contribution of each input modality to RICE-NET's classification performance. We show that radiation dosage (RD) information is critical for accurate classification, highlighting the importance of incorporating radiation dose distributions into the clinical decision-making process.

2 Materials and methods

2.1 Dataset description

RICE-Net was developed on a patient cohort, consisting of 92 GBM patients who received treatment at the University Clinic Heidelberg (UKHD), with the approval of the institutional ethics committee. For the development and evaluation, this cohort was divided into a training and validation set of 80 patients (comprising 48 with tumor recurrence and 32 with radiation-induced contrast enhancement (RICE)) and a separate, independent test set of 12 patients (7 with tumor recurrence and 5 with RICE) with a separation subject level. Within the dataset, for each subject three different imaging volumes are available. First, a post-operative, T1-weighted contrast-enhanced MRI, which is referred to as "MRI post-OP". This scan was acquired after the surgical resection and serves as a baseline image to plan the subsequent radiation therapy. Second, a follow-up T1-weighted contrast-enhanced MRI, termed the "MRI event". This scan was captured at the critical time of diagnostic uncertainty when new contrast-enhancing lesions were first detected, representing either true tumor recurrence or RICE. The indication for this scan was either a regular follow-up scan or the clarification of unclear symptoms. Third, the "RD map", a 3D map detailing the spatial distribution and cumulative dose of radiation delivered during the patient's radiotherapy treatment. The ground truth labels ("tumor recurrence" or "RICE") were confirmed and provided by clinical partners at UKHD based on biopsy results. In Figure 1 the MRI scan after resection and at the moment of the new contrast event, and the RD map for a sample subject are visualized.

All imaging volumes underwent a standardized preprocessing pipeline. The volumes were resampled to an isometric spacing and co-registered using the advanced normalization tools (ANTS) [6]. The brain was extracted from the skull using HD-BET [7], and intensities were normalized via z-scoring. Finally, the volumes were cropped to a consistent size of 224x224x224 voxels centered on the brain. For those patients, whom only a single fraction of the radiation treatment was available, the total RD was calculated by scaling a single-fraction dose map with the number of fractions, assuming consistent radiation delivery.

2.2 Deep learning architecture

A 3D residual network (ResNet18) architecture, adapted for volumetric medical image classification, was implemented using the MONAI[2] framework [8]. The network extends the original 2D ResNet design [9] to three dimensions, enabling the extraction of spatially coherent features across MRI volumes. Residual connections facilitate efficient gradient flow, improving stability and representational capacity. The model comprises an initial 3D conv. layer followed by four res. blocks with batch norm. and ReLU, concluding with global avg. pooling and a fully connected classification layer. ResNet18 was chosen for its balance between expressiveness and computational efficiency.

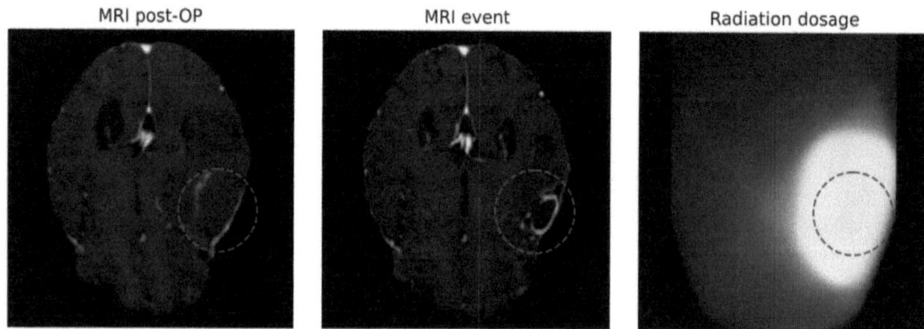

Fig. 1. Axial slice of sample subject with tumor recurrence. On the left, the post-operative MRI with the resection area highlighted with a red circle. The middle image shows the new progression, which is to be classified as recurrence or RICE. On the right, the radiation treatment plan is displayed, with the isocenter positioned in the region of the resection cavity.

[2] https://monai.io/

2.3 Experimental setup

To assess the contribution of each data modality, we conducted a series of ablation experiments with a fixed network architecture. In these experiments, we varied the input modalities and their combinations, data folds were kept fix across all experiments with a subject level split. The following input datapoints were considered: (1) MRI post-OP, (2) MRI event, (3) RD followed by various combinations of the individual data points: (4) MRI post-OP + MRI event, (5) MRI post-OP + RD, (6) MRI event + RD, and (7) all available data points combined. For each different scenario, an individual model was trained. For experiments involving multiple modalities, the inputs were concatenated along the channel dimension. All models were trained for 800 epochs using a five-fold cross-validation on the 80-patient training set. For training, the Adam optimizer and cross-entropy loss are implemented, along with a weighted random sampler to ensure equal representation of both classes during training. As augmentations, we used elastic deformations, rotations, scaling, Gaussian noise, and brightness and gamma adjustments. We selected the macro F1-score as evaluation metric, representing the unweighted average of the F1-scores computed for each class. The F1-score, the harmonic mean of precision and recall, provides a balanced measure that remains robust under class imbalance. For model interpretability, occlusion sensitivity maps are evaluated to identify critical input regions by systematically masking image parts and observing the effect on the output [10]. We occluded small cubic 3D regions synchronously across all co-registered volumes and measured the resulting change in output probability, highlighting regions most influential for distinguishing RICE from tumor recurrence. The maps provide an intuitive view of model attention that aids clinical interpretation.

3 Results

The performance of the model architecture on our dataset was evaluated with a series of ablation studies designed to assess the relative contribution of each input modality. The results of these experiments, summarized in Figure 2, report model performance in terms of the F1-score. Metrics were obtained from five-fold cross-validation and from majority voting on an independent hold-out test set to evaluate generalization performance. In the single-modality experiments, the radiation dosage map served as the most informative input, resulting in a macro F1-score of 0.78 on the validation set. The post-operative MRI and contrast event MRI result in lower F1 scores of 0.70 and 0.58, respectively. Performance was evaluated across multiple modality combinations. Integrating MRI with the radiation dose (RD) map yielded the best validation results, with the contrast-event MRI + RD model reaching an F1-score of 0.83 and the post-operative MRI + RD model achieving 0.828. Using all three inputs produced a validation F1-score of 0.804. On the independent test cohort, an ensemble of cross-validated models achieved an F1-score of 0.916. Figure 2 shows an example occlusion map for a correctly classified RICE case, highlighting the spatial regions within the input volumes that most strongly contributed to the model's prediction.

4 Discussion

We present RICE-Net, a multichannel 3D ResNet-18 for differentiating RICE from tumor recurrence using MRI and radiotherapy data. The model was trained on post-operative and contrast-event MRI volumes together with radiation dose distributions, and ablation studies quantified the contribution of each modality. Combining MRI with dose maps further improved results, with the best performance achieved when all modalities were integrated, confirming their complementary value. Notably, combining the radiation plan with event MRI did not outperform the combination with post-operative MRI, reflecting the clinical challenge of distinguishing true progression from treatment effects using MRI alone. Post-operative MRI and dose information may already encode early markers of RICE risk, enabling earlier prediction. A pronounced performance gap between cross-validation and test F1-scores, especially in MRI-only experiments (≈ 0.35 lower on test), highlights statistical uncertainty from limited cohort size. The main limitations are the small cohort size, lack of

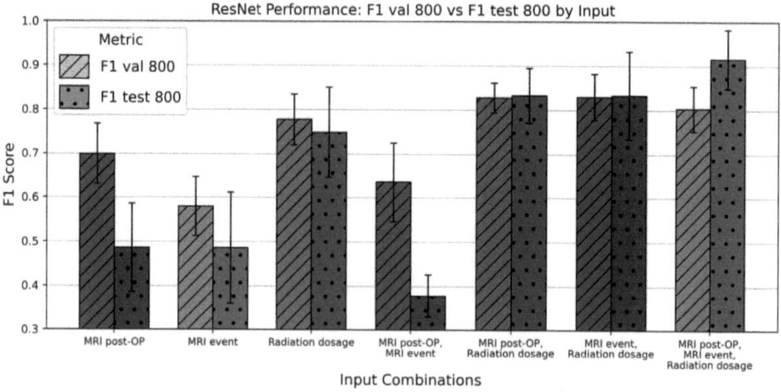

Fig. 2. F1 Macro after 800 training epochs on validation data (striped) aggregated across all folds and majority vote on the test data (dotted) by input volume combinations with cross validation standard deviation as error bars.

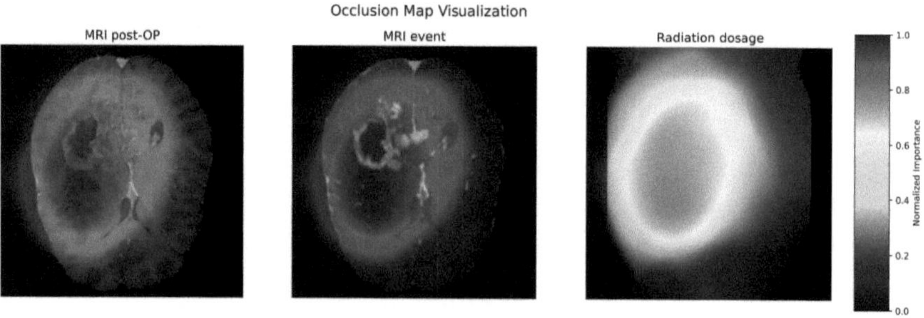

Fig. 3. Occlusion visualization with RICE overlaid over all three inputs.

unaffected subjects, and the simple channel-wise fusion, which may miss complex MRI-dose interactions. Future work should expand the dataset, include non-recurrent cases, and explore advanced fusion and clinical variable integration.

Acknowledgement. This work was supported in part by the DKTK Joint Funding upgrade SUBPAN, by the DFG grant 410981386 and by the Research Campus M2OLIE under the funding code 13GW0388A.

References

1. Haanen J, Obeid M, Spain L, Carbonnel F, Wang Y, Robert C et al. Management of toxicities from immunotherapy: ESMO clinical practice guideline for diagnosis, treatment and follow-up. Ann Oncol. 2022;33(12):1217–38.
2. Eichkorn T, Lischalk JW, Schwarz R, Bauer L, Deng M, Regnery S et al. Radiation-induced cerebral contrast enhancements strongly share ischemic stroke risk factors. Int J Radiat Oncol Biol Phys. 2024;118(5):1192–205.
3. Eichkorn T, Lischalk JW, Hörner-Rieber J, Deng M, Meixner E, Krämer A et al. Analysis of safety and efficacy of proton radiotherapy for IDH-mutated glioma WHO grade 2 and 3. J Neurooncol. 2023;162(3):489–501.
4. Bernhardt D, König L, Grosu AL, Rieken S, Krieg SM, Wick W et al. DEGRO practical guideline for central nervous system radiation necrosis part 2: treatment. Strahlenther Onkol. 2022;198(11):971–80.
5. Wang S, Martinez-Lage M, Sakai Y, Chawla S, Kim S, Alonso-Basanta M et al. Differentiating tumor progression from pseudoprogression in patients with glioblastomas using diffusion tensor imaging and dynamic susceptibility contrast MRI. Am J Neuroradiol. 2016;37(1):28–36.
6. Tustison NJ, Cook PA, Holbrook AJ, Johnson HJ, Muschelli J, Devenyi GA et al. The ANTsX ecosystem for quantitative biological and medical imaging. Sci Rep. 2021;11(1):9068.
7. Isensee F, Schell M, Pflueger I, Brugnara G, Bonekamp D, Neuberger U et al. Automated brain extraction of multisequence MRI using artificial neural networks. Hum Brain Mapp. 2019;40(17):4952–64.
8. Cardoso MJ, Li W, Brown R, Ma N, Kerfoot E, Wang Y et al. Monai: an open-source framework for deep learning in healthcare. arXiv preprint: 2211.02701. 2022.
9. He K, Zhang X, Ren S, Sun J. Deep residual learning for image recognition. Proc IEEE CVPR. 2016:770–8.
10. Zeiler MD, Fergus R. Visualizing and understanding convolutional networks. Proc ECCV. 2014:818–33.

Comparative Analysis of Machine Learning Models for 3-month Survival Prediction in Aneurysmal Subarachnoid Hemorrhage

Alexia Rizoudis[1], Santiago Cepeda[2], Frank Kramer[1], Dominik Müller[1]

[1]IT-Infrastructure for Translational Medical Research, Faculty of Applied Computer Science, University of Augsburg, Germany

[2]Specialized Group in Biomedical Imaging and Computational Analysis (GEIBAC), Instituto de Investigación Biosanitaria de Valladolid (IBioVALL), Valladolid, Spain

dominik.mueller@informatik.uni-augsburg.de

Abstract. Accurate outcome prediction after aneurysmal subarachnoid hemorrhage (aSAH) remains challenging due to the heterogeneity of clinical and imaging data. This study compares four machine learning approaches for three-month survival prediction using volumetric CT data and clinical metadata from 733 patients across nine Spanish centers. Using the AUCMEDI framework, we implemented: (1) an image-only 3D DenseNet121 CNN, (2) a CNN with metadata integration via feature-level late fusion, (3) a metadata-only XGBoost model, and (4) a fusion XGBoost model combining CNN predictions with metadata. The image-only CNN achieved the best performance (F1-score = 0.78, AUC = 0.84), confirming the strong prognostic value of CT imaging. Adding metadata slightly reduced performance, while the fusion XGBoost reached a competitive F1-score (0.76) and improved interpretability. These results demonstrate that CT-based deep learning enables reliable survival prediction in aSAH, and that model-level fusion provides an interpretable alternative.

1 Introduction

Subarachnoid hemorrhage (SAH) is a severe and often devastating form of hemorrhagic stroke, typically resulting from the rupture of an intracranial aneurysm, referred to as aneurysmal SAH (aSAH) [1]. Although relatively rare compared to ischemic stroke, aSAH carries high mortality and morbidity rates [2]. Survivors frequently experience lasting cognitive and psychosocial consequences, including fatigue, anxiety, and impaired social functioning [2].

Despite advances in treatment, including surgical clipping or endovascular coiling, outcomes remain difficult to predict and have only marginally improved over recent decades [2]. Prognosis varies widely with hemorrhage severity, neurological status at admission, and complications such as rebleeding or delayed cerebral ischemia [2]. Traditional risk scores, such as the World Federation of Neurological

© Der/die Autor(en), exklusiv lizenziert an
Springer Fachmedien Wiesbaden GmbH, ein Teil von Springer Nature 2026
H. Handels et al. (Hrsg.), *Bildverarbeitung für die Medizin 2026*,
Informatik aktuell, https://doi.org/10.1007/978-3-658-51100-5_26

Surgeons (WFNS) scale [3], and clinical judgment are routinely used to estimate prognosis. However, reliance on clinical judgement alone may be limited for accurate outcome prediction [1]. Furthermore, most prediction models have seen limited adoption in clinical practice due to methodological shortcomings and poor integration into workflows [1]. Recent advances in artificial intelligence, particularly convolutional neural networks (CNNs), have shown strong performance in various medical imaging tasks and are capable of identifying subtle imaging features not apparent to human observers [4]. In aSAH, initial CT scans already capture key features such as aneurysm size, edema, or intraventricular hemorrhage, making them a promising basis for automated outcome prediction [2, 5].

This study investigates whether three-month mortality in aSAH can be predicted directly from CT images and how performance changes when structured clinical metadata are incorporated.

2 Materials and methods

This study predicts three-month survival in aSAH using four machine learning pipelines: an image-only CNN, a CNN with metadata integration, a metadata-only XGBoost model, and a hybrid fusion XGBoost combining both inputs. Figure 1 provides an overview of all workflows. All deep learning models were implemented using the in-house framework AUCMEDI [6], which enables efficient training and evaluation and has been publicly released on GitHub to ensure reproducibility: `https://github.com/rizoudal/aSAH-mortality-prediction.git`.

2.1 Dataset and volume preprocessing

Patients with aSAH treated between 2022 and 2025 were retrospectively included. Inclusion criteria comprised a confirmed aneurysm on CT angiography or digital

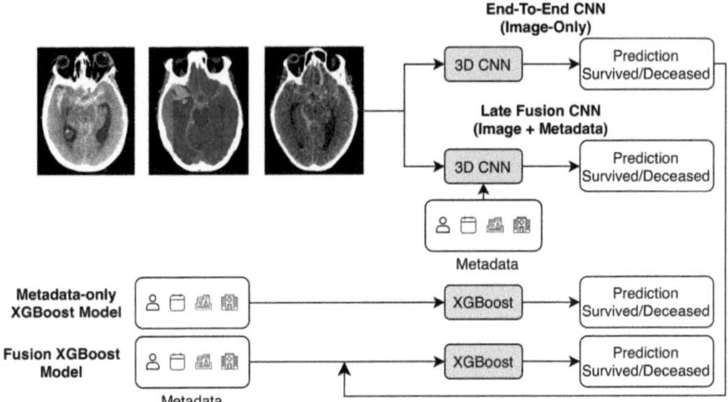

Fig. 1. Workflows of the four classification pipelines: (a) image-only CNN, (b) CNN with metadata (feature-level late fusion), (c) metadata-only XGBoost, and (d) fusion XGBoost combining CNN predictions with metadata.

subtraction angiography, an admission non-contrast CT scan prior to treatment, and a known three-month outcome. Cases with idiopathic SAH, insufficient image quality, or missing follow-up were excluded. The dataset included 733 patients from nine Spanish centers: 206 from Río Hortega University Hospital, 39 from Hospital Clínic de Barcelona, 49 from Basurto University Hospital, 67 from Vigo University Hospital, 73 from Central University Hospital of Asturias, 67 from Hospital del Mar, 102 from Miguel Servet University Hospital, 115 from Vall d'Hebron University Hospital, and 15 from Canary Islands University Hospital. Clinical parameters comprised age, sex, WFNS scale [3], modified Fisher (mF) scale [7], aneurysm location and size according to the Subarachnoid Hemorrhage International Trialists study [1], and three-month mortality.

The dataset was split into 80% training and 20% testing. Stratified splitting by three-month survival and hospital ensured balanced representation of centers and outcome classes, supporting fair and generalizable evaluation. All CT volumes were converted from DICOM to NifTI format, intensity values were clipped to 0-100 Hounsfield units to suppress outliers, and images were nonlinearly registered to a standard CT template (1mm^3 isotropic, 256 x 256 x 256 voxels). Finally, non-brain tissue was removed using automated skull stripping to isolate intracranial structures for analysis. The resulting preprocessed volumes were visually inspected to confirm accurate alignment, orientation, and skull removal.

2.2 Model architectures

2.2.1 End-to-end CNN model. As part of preprocessing, all CT images were resampled to a uniform voxel spacing, normalized to 0–255, cropped to 100 x 120 x 100 voxels, and converted to three RGB channels. During training, extensive data augmentation was applied, including geometric, photometric, and elastic transformations to enhance model robustness and mitigate overfitting. Z-score normalization was applied using the mean and standard deviation from the ImageNet dataset. Model training was performed using a 3D DenseNet121 architecture [8] with ImageNet-pretrained weights [9] and five-fold cross-validation to create an ensemble. Early stopping halted training if validation loss did not improve for 30 epochs, and a dynamic learning rate scheduler reduced the rate by 0.1 after eight stagnant epochs, down to a minimum of 1e^{-7}. Training used a batch size of 45 and the weighted focal loss [10] to address class imbalance. The model with the lowest validation loss was saved, and final predictions were obtained by aggregating the five cross-validation outputs using the median strategy.

2.2.2 CNN with metadata integration. A second pipeline combined image data with clinical metadata (Sec. 2.1). The image branch used the same 3D DenseNet121 backbone with ImageNet-pretrained weights (Sec. 2.2.1). Metadata were integrated via feature-level late fusion, concatenating the numerical metadata vector with image-derived features before the final fully connected layers. Models were selected according to the lowest validation loss, and predictions were aggregated via the mean of cross-validation outputs.

2.2.3 Metadata-only XGBoost model. As a third approach, a gradient boosting model (XGBoost [11]) was trained solely on the structured clinical features from Sec. 2.1. The same five-fold cross-validation scheme as for the CNN models ensured consistency. Class imbalance was addressed by weighting the minority class according to its fold-specific frequencies, and early stopping was applied based on validation loss. Final predictions were computed from the five cross-validation models by taking their median, and feature importance values were extracted to assess the contribution of individual metadata variables.

2.2.4 Fusion XGBoost model. The fourth approach combined image-based predictions with clinical metadata. An XGBoost classifier was trained on feature vectors containing six metadata variables and two class probabilities from the image-only CNN (Sec. 2.2.1). Out-of-fold CNN predictions from five-fold cross-validation provided unbiased probabilities for all training samples. The model was trained using the same strategy as in Sec. 2.2.3. Final test predictions were obtained by aggregating the outputs of the five models via the median of predicted probabilities, leveraging complementary information from both imaging and non-imaging data.

3 Results

All models were evaluated on the independent test set using accuracy, area under the receiver operating characteristic curve (AUC), sensitivity, specificity, and F1-score. Each model was implemented as an ensemble of five submodels trained via five-fold cross-validation. All reported metrics represent macro-averaged values across both outcome classes.

The image-only CNN achieved the highest performance, with an accuracy of 0.82, an AUC of 0.84, sensitivity and specificity of 0.81, and a macro F1-score of 0.78. Adding clinical metadata slightly reduced performance (accuracy = 0.76, AUC = 0.84, F1-score = 0.73). Softmax-based aggregation instead of mean produced identical results.

The metadata-only XGBoost model reached an accuracy of 0.77, an AUC of 0.83, and an F1-score of 0.74. The fusion XGBoost model, combining CNN-based predictions with clinical metadata, achieved an accuracy of 0.79, an AUC of 0.88, and an F1-score of 0.76.

Across all approaches, the image-only model performed best overall, except for the AUC, where the fusion-based XGBoost ranked second across all metrics and reached the highest AUC score. Fig. 2 additionally reports class-specific results for the non-survival outcome.

4 Discussion

This study compared four machine learning strategies for predicting three-month survival in aSAH using volumetric and clinical metadata. The image-only CNN achieved the best overall performance, except for the AUC, confirming the prognostic value of CT imaging and aligning with prior work on deep learning-based feature extraction from medical images [4, 12].

Previous AI-based studies in aSAH have used either clinical or imaging data. Early approaches relied on handcrafted features such as aneurysm location or WFNS grading [1]. More recent deep learning models operate directly on CT scans. For example, Hu et al. quantified bleeding volume to predict mortality [13], and Yuan et al. used automated segmentation of intracranial bleeding compartments to predict delayed cerebral ischemia [14]. Together, these studies confirm the potential of end-to-end image-based prediction.

Integrating clinical metadata into the CNN did not improve performance, with a slight decrease in accuracy and F1-score. While most prior studies report gains from combining imaging and clinical data [15], this discrepancy may stem from redundancy between modalities. Many variables, such as WFNS or mF grade, are proxies of image-derived information already captured by the CNN, and integrating this additional information may introduce bias [16]. The strong performance of the image-only model underscores the rich prognostic information embedded in CT scans, consistent with evidence that intraventricular hemorrhage, aneurysm size, and edema are key predictors of poor outcomes [2, 5]. Moreover, image-only approaches are easier to generalize and deploy, as they are independent of clinical data quality [12]. The best-performing alternative was the XGBoost-based fusion model, combining CNN-predicted probabilities with clinical metadata. It ranked second across metrics and illustrated the potential of model-level (late) fusion. Feature importance identified age, WFNS, and mF grade as the dominant predictors, consistent with established risk factors. In the fusion model, however, the CNN-derived probability was among the top-ranked features, surpassing most clinical variables except age, further emphasizing the dominant role of imaging information.

Future work should focus on validating these models in larger datasets, integrating uncertainty estimation, and improving model interpretability. The strong

Approach	Dead				
	Acc	AUC	Sens	Spec	F1
CNN	**0.82**	0.84	0.78	**0.84**	**0.70**
CNN+Metadata	0.76	0.84	0.83	0.73	0.65
XGB	0.77	0.83	**0.85**	0.74	0.67
XGB+CNN	0.79	**0.88**	**0.85**	0.77	0.69

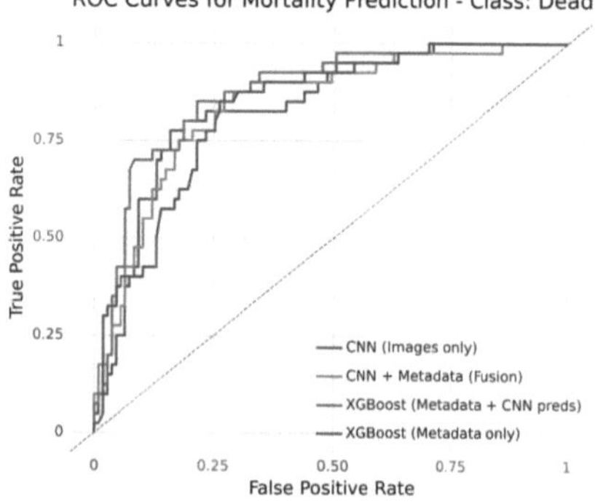

Fig. 2. Evaluation results for predicting non-survival on the independent test set. Left: classification metrics for all evaluated models. Right: ROC curves illustrating model performance for the non-survival class.

performance of the image-only model emphasizes that routine CT data alone may suffice for accurate prognostication after SAH, enabling fast, automated risk assessment at admission. Meanwhile, the consistent results of the XGBoost fusion approach illustrate how combining interpretable classifiers with deep feature extractors can provide an effective and transparent alternative.

Acknowledgement. We thank the participating Neurosurgery Departments for their valuable collaboration: University Hospital Miguel Servet (Juan Casado Pellejero, Laura Beatriz López), University Hospital Central de Asturias (Julio Gutiérrez, José Ignacio Gimeno Calabuig), Hospital del Mar (Alberto Pérez Giraldo, David Rodríguez Benítez), Vigo University Hospital (Adolfo de la Lama, David Rodríguez Bangueses), Basurto University Hospital (José Undabeitia Huertas), Canarias University Hospital (Julio Plata), Vall d'Hebron University Hospital (Fuat Arikan, Silvia Vásquez, Helena Calvo Rubio), and Hospital Clinic of Barcelona (Ramón Torné, Alejandra Mosteiro).

References

1. Jaja BNR, Saposnik G, Lingsma HF, Macdonald E, Thorpe KE, Mamdani M et al. Development and validation of outcome prediction models for aneurysmal subarachnoid haemorrhage: the SAHIT multinational cohort study. BMJ. 2018;360:j5745.
2. Connolly ES, Rabinstein AA, Carhuapoma JR, Derdeyn CP, Dion J, Higashida RT et al. Guidelines for the management of aneurysmal subarachnoid hemorrhage. Stroke. 2012;43(6):1711–37.
3. Teasdale GM, Drake CG, Hunt W, Kassell N, Sano K, Pertuiset B et al. A universal subarachnoid hemorrhage scale: report of a committee of the world federation of neurosurgical societies. J Neurol Neurosurg Psychiatry. 1988;51(11):1457.
4. García-García S, Cepeda S, Müller D, Mosteiro A, Torné R, Agudo S et al. Mortality prediction of patients with subarachnoid hemorrhage using a deep learning model based on an initial brain CT scan. Brain Sci. 2024;14(1):10.
5. Rosengart AJ, Schultheiss KE, Tolentino J, Macdonald RL. Prognostic factors for outcome in patients with aneurysmal subarachnoid hemorrhage. Stroke. 2007;38(8):2315–21.
6. Mayer S, Müller D, Kramer F. Standardized medical image classification across medical disciplines. arXiv: 2210.11091v1. 2022.
7. Frontera JA, Claassen J, Schmidt JM, Wartenberg KE, Temes R, Connolly ES et al. Prediction of symptomatic vasospasm after subarachnoid hemorrhage: the modified Fisher scale. Neurosurgery. 2006;59(1):21.
8. Huang G, Liu Z, van der Maaten L, Weinberger KQ. Densely connected convolutional networks. Proc IEEE CVPR. 2017.
9. Russakovsky O, Deng J, Su H, Krause J, Satheesh S, Ma S et al. ImageNet large scale visual recognition challenge. Int J Comput Vis. 2015;115(3):211–52.
10. Lin TY, Goyal P, Girshick R, He K, Dollar P. Focal loss for dense object detection. Proc IEEE ICCV. 2017:2980–8.
11. Chen T, Guestrin C. XGBoost: A scalable tree boosting system. Proc KDD. 2016:785–94.

12. Wang X, Shen T, Yang S, Lan J, Xu Y, Wang M et al. A deep learning algorithm for automatic detection and classification of acute intracranial hemorrhages in head CT scans. Neuroimage Clin. 2021;32:102785.
13. Hu P, Wu Y, Yan T, Shu L, Liu F, Xiao B et al. Deep learning-based quantification of total bleeding volume and its association with complications, disability, and death in patients with aneurysmal subarachnoid hemorrhage. J Neurosurg. 2024;141(2):343–54.
14. Yuan JY, Chen Y, Jayaraman K, Kumar A, Zlepper Z, Allen ML et al. Automated quantification of compartmental blood volumes enables prediction of delayed cerebral ischemia and outcomes after aneurysmal subarachnoid hemorrhage. World Neurosurg. 2023;170:e214–e222.
15. Holste G, Partridge SC, Rahbar H, Biswas D, Lee CI, Alessio AM. End-to-end learning of fused image and non-image features for improved breast cancer classification from MRI. Proc IEEE/CVF ICCV. 2021:3287–96.
16. Cui C, Yang H, Wang Y, Zhao S, Asad Z, Coburn LA et al. Deep multimodal fusion of image and non-image data in disease diagnosis and prognosis: a review. Prog Biomed Eng. 2023;5(2):022001.

Abstract: DIY Challenge Blueprint

From Organization to Technical Implementation in Biomedical Image Analysis

Leonard Klausmann [1,2†], Tobias Rueckert [1,3†], David Rauber [1], Raphaela Maerkl [1], Suemeyye R. Yildiran[1], Max Gutbrod [1], Christoph Palm [1,2]

[1]Regensburg Medical Image Computing (ReMIC), OTH Regensburg
[2]Regensburg Center of Health Sciences and Technology (RCHST), OTH Regensburg
[3]AKTORmed Robotic Surgery, Neutraubling
leonard.klausmann@oth-regensburg.de

The high cost of challenge platforms prevents many people from organizing their own competitions. The do-it-yourself (DIY) challenge blueprint [1] allows you to host your own biomedical AI benchmark challenge. Our DIY approach circumvents the current constraints of commercial challenge platforms. A sovereign, extensible and cost-efficient deployment is provided via containerised, identity-managed and reproducible pipelines. Focus lies on GDPR-compliant hosting via infrastructure-as-code, automated evaluation, modular orchestration, and role-based identity and access management. The framework integrates Docker-based execution and standardised interfaces for task definitions, dataset curation and evaluation. All in all it is designed to be flexible and modular, as demonstrated in the MICCAI 2024 PhaKIR challenge [2, 3]. In this case study, different medical tasks on a multicentre laparoscopic dataset with framewise labels for phases and spatial annotations for instruments across full-length videos were supported. This case study empirically validates the DIY challenge blueprint as a reproducible and customizable challenge-hosting infrastructure. The full code can be found at `https://github.com/remic-othr/PhaKIR_DIY`.

References

1. Klausmann L, Rueckert T et al. Diy challenge blueprint: from organization to technical realization in biomedical image analysis. Proc MICCAI. 2025:85–95.
2. Rueckert T et al. Comparative validation of surgical phase recognition, instrument keypoint estimation, and instrument instance segmentation in endoscopy: results of the Phakir 2024 challenge. arXiv: 2507.16559. 2025.
3. Rueckert T et al. Phakir dataset: surgical procedure phase, keypoint, and instrument recognition. Version 1.0. Zenodo, 2025.

[†]These authors contributed equally to this work.

© Der/die Autor(en), exklusiv lizenziert an
Springer Fachmedien Wiesbaden GmbH, ein Teil von Springer Nature 2026
H. Handels et al. (Hrsg.), *Bildverarbeitung für die Medizin 2026*,
Informatik aktuell, https://doi.org/10.1007/978-3-658-51100-5_27

Abstract: Minimum Data, Maximum Impact
20 Annotated Samples for Explainable Lung Nodule Classification

Luisa Gallée [1,2,3], Catharina S. Lisson [2], Christoph G. Lisson[2], Daniela Drees[2], Felix Weig[2], Daniel Vogele [2], Meinrad Beer [2,3], Michael Götz [1,2,3]

[1]Experimental Radiology, Ulm University Medical Center
[2]Department of Diagnostic and Interventional Radiology, Ulm University Medical Center
[3]XAIRAD - Cooperation for Artificial Intelligence in Experimental Radiology
Ulm, Germany
luisa.gallee@uni-ulm.de

Classification models with human-interpretable explanations improve clinicians' trust and diagnostic usability. A promising approach is to integrate pathology-related visual attributes used by radiologists, aligning AI decisions with clinical reasoning. Radiologists use attributes such as shape and texture as established diagnostic criteria, and mirroring these in AI decision-making enhances transparency and enables explicit validation of model outputs. However, progress is limited by the scarcity of large medical image datasets annotated with such attributes. To address this, we propose generating attribute-annotated images using an attribute-conditional diffusion model [1]. Applied to the LIDC-IDRI dataset, which contains lung nodule images with malignancy and attribute labels the model produces realistic, high-quality images, validated through a radiologist user study. Nevertheless, the data-demanding nature of diffusion models leads to substantial performance degradation when only limited annotated data are available, especially with 20 images. We therefore introduce a semi-conditional training strategy that also leverages unlabeled images by dynamically enabling conditioning. This reduces annotation effort while maintaining reasonable image quality. The second step of this work is to incorporate the generated images into the training of explainable models, such as HierViT [2]. This improves attribute prediction accuracy by 13.4% and malignancy prediction accuracy by 1.8% compared with using only the small annotated dataset. These results demonstrate that domain-driven synthetic augmentation can meaningfully reduce annotation burden and make explainable medical image classifiers more applicable.

References

1. Gallée L, Lisson CS, Lisson CG et al. Minimum data, maximum impact: 20 annotated samples for explainable lung nodule classification. iMIMIC Workshop at MICCAI. 2025.
2. Gallée L, Lisson CS, Beer M, Götz M. Hierarchical vision transformer with prototypes for interpretable medical image classification. arXiv preprint: 2502.08997. 2025.

© Der/die Autor(en), exklusiv lizenziert an
Springer Fachmedien Wiesbaden GmbH, ein Teil von Springer Nature 2026
H. Handels et al. (Hrsg.), *Bildverarbeitung für die Medizin 2026*,
Informatik aktuell, https://doi.org/10.1007/978-3-658-51100-5_28

Impact of Preprocessing Methods on Racial Encoding and Model Robustness in CXR Diagnosis

Dishantkumar Sutariya, Eike Petersen

Fraunhofer Institute for Digital Medicine MEVIS
eike.petersen@mevis.fraunhofer.de

Abstract. Deep learning models can identify racial identity with high accuracy from chest X-ray (CXR) recordings. Thus, there is widespread concern about the potential for racial shortcut learning, where a model inadvertently learns to systematically bias its diagnostic predictions as a function of racial identity. Such racial biases threaten healthcare equity and model reliability, as models may systematically misdiagnose certain demographic groups. Since racial shortcuts are diffuse – non-localized and distributed throughout the whole CXR recording – image preprocessing methods may influence racial shortcut learning, yet the potential of such methods for reducing biases remains underexplored. Here, we investigate the effects of image preprocessing methods including lung masking, lung cropping, and contrast limited adaptive histogram equalization (CLAHE). These approaches aim to suppress spurious cues encoding racial information while preserving diagnostic accuracy. Our experiments reveal that simple bounding box-based lung cropping can be an effective strategy for reducing racial shortcut learning while maintaining diagnostic model performance, bypassing frequently postulated fairness-accuracy trade-offs.

1 Introduction

The integration of artificial intelligence (AI) into medical imaging holds transformative promise. However, the deployment of these systems in real-world healthcare settings has revealed critical concerns about their fairness and reliability across diverse patient populations. One alarming finding concerns the potential for racial bias in AI models for chest X-ray (CXR) disease diagnosis [1–3]. These models have been shown to be capable of inferring race from standard CXR recordings with very high accuracy [2] – despite race being imperceptible to human radiologists. This raises the potential for racial shortcut learning, where a model trained for disease classification might inadvertently exploit racial correlations for disease classification [2, 4, 5]. While it is generally challenging to assess whether a potential racial shortcut is indeed exploited [4, 5], such disparities threaten to undermine the trust and safety of AI in clinical practice [1].

Racial shortcuts are particularly challenging to assess and mitigate because of their diffuse nature: racial prediction does not rely on localized features but rather

© Der/die Autor(en), exklusiv lizenziert an
Springer Fachmedien Wiesbaden GmbH, ein Teil von Springer Nature 2026
H. Handels et al. (Hrsg.), *Bildverarbeitung für die Medizin 2026*,
Informatik aktuell, https://doi.org/10.1007/978-3-658-51100-5_29

depends on image features distributed throughout the whole recording [2], with race classification feasible even based on just the grayscale histogram of a recording [3]. Image preprocessing techniques may therefore have an effect on the potential for demographic (racial) shortcut learning, but the extent to which such methods can help reduce biases remains underexplored.

To address this gap, we here investigate the potential of three generic CXR preprocessing methods to alleviate biases while maintaining diagnostic performance. We implement and evaluate two lung masking strategies as well as contrast-limited adaptive histogram equalization (CLAHE) to restrict and enhance model focus to clinically relevant regions, thereby potentially suppressing demographic confounders embedded in the imaging data. We evaluate (internally and externally) racial encoding as well as diagnostic performance in models trained and evaluated on such preprocessed recordings. Among other findings, we show that simple bounding box-based lung cropping can reduce racial encoding while maintaining overall diagnostic accuracy.

2 Materials and methods

2.1 Related work

Gichoya et al. [2] demonstrated that AI models can infer patients' racial or ethnic identity from chest radiographs with high accuracy, even when clinicians cannot. This ability to predict self-reported race with high AUROC scores across multiple modalities, imaging vendors, and clinical tasks is concerning, as it suggests that AI models may be relying on non-clinical, demographically linked signals rather than focusing on medically meaningful patterns [3, 4]. Gichoya et al. [2] already demonstrated that racial shortcuts are non-localized and diffuse, and Burns et al. [3] showed that racial identity can even be identified from grayscale intensity histograms alone, disregarding all structural information. Technical recording parameters such as the view positioning have been found to be major contributors to race detection capability [6], and Wang et al. [7] showed that generic data augmentation can substantially reduce the potential for demographic shortcut learning in CXR diagnosis.

That models *can* learn to identify racial identity does not necessarily imply that they *do* exploit this potential shortcut. Glocker et al. [4, 5] investigated demographic encoding in CXR diagnosis models, observing small but statistically significant differences in latent embeddings between racial groups after accounting for various confounding factors. These differences were more pronounced in a foundation model compared to a single-disease model [5]. Still, racial 'encoding' in diagnostic (single-disease) models was similar to an ImageNet-trained baseline model, indicating that racial shortcut learning occurred only to a minor degree, if at all. Seyyed-Kalantari et al. [1] demonstrated that standard CXR diagnosis models exhibit systematic underdiagnosis for Black patients across multiple disease labels, but such disparities tend to disappear after controlling for confounding factors such as age, sex, and disease distribution [4]. Nevertheless, due to the gravity of concerns about potential racial biases, the need for generic methods that can reduce the potential for demographic biases while maintaining or potentially even improving diagnostic accuracy remains.

2.2 Datasets

2.2.1 MIMIC-CXR. The MIMIC-CXR-JPG dataset [8, 9] comprises 377,110 images across 227,835 studies, covering 65,379 patients. Following the findings of Lotter [6], we exclude lateral views and retain only frontal (AP/PA) recordings. Following Weng et al. [10], we discard multiple recordings for the same patient and keep just one out of the set with the most disease labels provided to minimize the risk of label errors. From the resulting 41,168 recordings, we construct a test set by randomly sampling 35 positive instances for each of the 11 disease labels for each of the top-4 racial/ethnic groups (White, Black, Asian, Hispanic), resulting in a total test-set size of 1,430 samples. The remaining data are randomly split into a training and validation set of 34,400 (95%) and 1,811 (5%) samples, respectively. We ensure that there is no patient overlap between any of the three sets.

2.2.2 CheXpert. The CheXpert dataset [11] comprises 224,316 CXR recordings and diagnostic labels from 65,240 patients. We use the same sampling strategies (frontal views, one recording per patient) and racial/ethnic groups as in MIMIC-CXR. The entire resulting set of 51,627 samples is used for external evaluation only.

2.3 Experimental setup

We finetune an ImageNet-pretrained DenseNet-121 for multi-label disease classification on MIMIC-CXR and evaluate diagnostic performance as well as racial encoding on the MIMIC-CXR test set and externally on CheXpert. For all purposes, recordings were downscaled to 224×224. For optimization, we use AdamW, label smoothing (0.1), batch size 8, initial learning rate (LR) 10^{-4}, cosine annealing over 30 epochs (decreasing to a minimum LR of 10^{-6}), and early stopping (patience 5) on validation AUROC. We use standard image augmentations (random rotations by $\pm 10°$ and random horizontal / vertical flips). Racial encoding is evaluated by freezing the image encoder and training a race classification head. We rerun all experiments with 5 different seeds. All experiments were implemented using PyTorch and executed on NVIDIA A100 GPUs. Our full code is available at `https://github.com/dishant24/BVM_Chest_X-Ray_Fair_AI`.

2.4 Preprocessing methods

To reduce race-correlated pixel-level signals in CXR recordings and prevent models from learning demographic shortcuts, we investigate different preprocessing methods. The aim is to suppress racial encoding while preserving clinical features, thereby potentially improving fairness, robustness, and generalization across racial groups. These methods are selected here because they represent simple preprocessing methods that are trivial to implement but might affect the degree of racial encoding in model inputs without removing (or even enhancing) diagnostically relevant information.

2.4.1 Contrast limited adaptive histogram equalization (CLAHE). Unlike standard histogram equalization that operates on the entire image, CLAHE [12] processes images in small, non-overlapping (8×8) tiles. For each tile, it computes a local intensity histogram, clips it to a specified limit (to prevent over-amplification of noise, we use 2) and redistributes the clipped portion to ensure better contrast across the entire intensity range. The cumulative distribution function (CDF) is computed for each tile to create a local mapping function. The per-tile mappings are then recombined using bilinear interpolation, yielding the enhanced output image. CLAHE boosts local contrast without causing the over-amplification of noise often seen with global histogram equalization, emphasizing fine details and potentially aiding the model's ability to discern pathological patterns.

2.4.2 Lung masking. To mitigate the influence of confounding factors and potentially enhance model fairness and generalizability by restricting model attention to clinically relevant image regions, we implement lung masking as a preprocessing step similar to the approaches taken by Aslani et al. [13] and Sourget et al. [14]. We utilize lung segmentation masks from CheXmask [15], a high-quality lung segmentation mask dataset for CXR recordings. The dataset includes reliability scores (RCA) for each segmentation, ensuring mask quality. We filtered samples to include only those with an average Dice RCA greater than 0.7. A morphological dilation with a 60-pixel margin (on the original mask resolution of 1024×1024) was applied to preserve diagnostically relevant contextual features near lung and heart boundaries.

2.4.3 Lung cropping. As an alternative to lung masking, we cropped the image to a bounding box containing the whole lung mask. This approach avoids the introduction of abrupt, high-intensity transitions at mask edges and reduces the risk of models exploiting artificial boundaries and intensity fluctuations as shortcuts.

3 Results

Table 1 presents the main results of our experiments. Diagnostic performance on the internal (MIMIC) test set is consistent across preprocessing methods and comparable to the baseline model without preprocessing, with a small disadvantage for the lung masking approach. On the external (CheXpert) evaluation set, this disadvantage is more pronounced (lung masking AUROC 0.696 vs. 0.742 for the baseline), with the other two methods (CLAHE and lung cropping) performing similarly to the baseline.

In terms of racial encoding, all models enable race prediction with above-chance accuracy, as expected [2, 4, 5]. On the internal (MIMIC) test set, all methods yield similar race identification performance. Externally (on CheXpert), however, both lung masking and lung cropping show reduced race identification performance compared to the baseline (AUROC 0.566 and 0.593, respectively, vs. 0.623 for the baseline), indicating reduced racial encoding. CLAHE yields a similar degree of racial encoding compared to the baseline.

Tab. 1. Comparison of preprocessing methods on racial and diagnostic AUROC, mean ± standard deviation across repetitions.

Method	Race AUROC Internal	External	Diagnostic AUROC Internal	External
Baseline	0.639 ± 0.003	0.623 ± 0.004	0.764 ± 0.003	0.742 ± 0.001
Masking	0.630 ± 0.005	0.566 ± 0.013	0.759 ± 0.002	0.696 ± 0.005
Cropping	0.641 ± 0.006	0.593 ± 0.007	0.763 ± 0.003	0.738 ± 0.004
CLAHE	0.642 ± 0.007	0.624 ± 0.024	0.765 ± 0.004	0.738 ± 0.005

We also evaluated average inter-racial differences in diagnostic model performance across all disease labels. The average diagnostic AUROC differences on the internal test set are 0.0325 (Baseline), 0.0282 (CLAHE), 0.0352 (Cropping), and 0.0316 (Masking), and 0.0781 (Baseline), 0.0706 (CLAHE), 0.0678 (Cropping), and 0.0792 (Masking) on the external test set.

4 Discussion

In this study, we evaluated whether simple preprocessing can improve the generalization and robustness of chest X-ray classifiers while mitigating racial bias. We compared four pipelines – a baseline approach with no additional preprocessing, lung masking, lung cropping, and CLAHE – across internal and external evaluation datasets. Our findings indicate that simple lung cropping can yield reduced racial encoding (and, thus, reduced risk for racial biases) while maintaining high diagnostic performance. Lung masking, while reducing racial encoding, resulted in a notable drop in external diagnostic performance as also reported by Sourget et al. [14], while CLAHE had no notable effect on either racial encoding or diagnostic performance. Our study contributes to a growing body of evidence showing that there are no inherent fairness-accuracy trade-offs but that model fairness and diagnostic performance can be improved in tandem [16].

For correctly interpreting our results, it is notable that our baseline is strong and implements various best practices emerging from prior research, including a limitation to frontal CXR recordings [6], preferential sampling of images with the maximum number of diseases labeled to reduce the risk of label bias [10] and data augmentation [7], all of which have been shown to reduce the risk of bias. It is conceivable that the impact of preprocessing methods such as the ones investigated here might differ in a more basic setting with higher risk of bias.

Future research should systematically study the effect of CLAHE hyperparameters – particularly the clip limit and grid tile size – on model generalization, assessing whether principled tuning can yield gains in model fairness and robustness. In addition, advanced masking strategies, such as inpainting or gated or partial convolutions that natively handle missing data [17], could reduce information loss and boundary artifacts, potentially resulting in better performance of the lung masking approach.

References

1. Seyyed-Kalantari L, Zhang H, McDermott MBA, Chen IY, Ghassemi M. Underdiagnosis bias of artificial intelligence algorithms applied to chest radiographs in under-served patient populations. Lancet Digit Health. 2021;27(12):2176–82.
2. Gichoya JW et al. AI recognition of patient race in medical imaging: a modelling study. Lancet Digit Health. 2022;4(6):e406–e414.
3. Burns JL et al. Ability of artificial intelligence to identify self-reported race in chest X-ray using pixel intensity counts. J Med Imaging. 2023;10(6):061106.
4. Glocker B, Jones C, Bernhardt M, Winzeck S. Algorithmic encoding of protected characteristics in chest X-ray disease detection models. EBioMedicine. 2023;89:104467.
5. Glocker B, Jones C, Roschewitz M, Winzeck S. Risk of bias in chest radiography deep learning foundation models. Radiol Artif Intell. 2023;5(6).
6. Lotter W. Acquisition parameters influence AI recognition of race in chest X-rays and mitigating these factors reduces underdiagnosis bias. Nat Commun. 2024;15(1):7465.
7. Wang R, Kuo PC, Chen LC, Seastedt KP, Gichoya JW, Celi LA. Drop the shortcuts: image augmentation improves fairness and decreases AI detection of race and other demographics from medical images. EBioMedicine. 2024;102:105047.
8. Johnson AEW, Pollard TJ, Berkowitz SJ, Greenbaum NR, Lungren MP et al. MIMIC-CXR: a de-identified publicly available database of chest radiographs with free-text reports. Sci Data. 2019;6(1):317.
9. Johnson A, Lungren M, Peng Y, Lu Z, Mark R, Berkowitz S et al. MIMIC-CXR-JPG: chest radiographs with structured labels. PhysioNet, 2024.
10. Weng N, Bigdeli S, Petersen E, Feragen A. Are sex-based physiological differences the cause of gender bias for chest X-ray diagnosis? Proc FAIMI. 2023:142–52.
11. Irvin J, Rajpurkar P, Ko M, Yu Y, Ciurea-Ilcus S, Chute C et al. CheXpert: a large chest radiograph dataset with uncertainty labels and expert comparison. Proc AAAI CAI. 2019;33(1):590–7.
12. Zuiderveld KJ et al. Contrast limited adaptive histogram equalization. Graph Gems. 1994;4(1):474–85.
13. Aslani S, Lilaonitkul W, Gnananthan V, Raj D et al. Optimising chest X-rays for image analysis by identifying and removing confounding factors. Proc MICAD. 2022:245–54.
14. Sourget T, Hestbek-Møller M, Jiménez-Sánchez A, Junchi Xu J, Cheplygina V. Mask of truth: model sensitivity to unexpected regions of medical images. J Imaging Inform Med. 2025.
15. Gaggion N, Mosquera C, Mansilla L, Saidman JM, Aineseder M, Milone DH et al. CheXmask: a large-scale dataset of anatomical segmentation masks for multi-center chest X-ray images. Sci Data. 2024;11(1):511.
16. Petersen E, Holm S, Ganz M, Feragen A. The path toward equal performance in medical machine learning. Patterns. 2023;4(7).
17. Liu G, Reda FA, Shih KJ, Wang TC, Tao A, Catanzaro B. Image inpainting for irregular holes using partial convolutions. Proc ECCV. 2018:85–100.

AI-based Automated Framework for Quantitative PET/CT Image Analysis

Sonja Adomeit [1,2†], Lukas Förner [1,2,3†], Elisabeth Scheurer[4], Jan Bäßler [4], Elina Gastreich de Llanes [1,2], Jonas Böhringer[1,2], Ralph A. Bundschuh [5], Constantin Lapa [4,6], Kartikay Tehlan [1,2,3], Thomas Wendler [1,2,3,6,7]

[1]Department of Diagnostic and Interventional Radiology and Neuroradiology, University Hospital Augsburg
[2]Digital Medicine, University Hospital Augsburg
[3]Computer-Aided Medical Procedures and Augmented Reality, Technical University of Munich
[4]Department of Nuclear Medicine, University Hospital Augsburg
[5]Department of Nuclear Medicine, University Hospital Carl Gustav Carus
[6]Bavarian Cancer Research Center (BZKF) Augsburg
[7]Center of Advanced Analytics and Predictive Sciences, University of Augsburg
sonja.adomeit@med.uni-augsburg.de

Abstract. Radiomics extracts quantitative features from medical images, offering biomarkers for diagnosis, prognosis, and evaluation of treatment response. Yet, its broader application in research is limited by the absence of standardized, end-to-end workflows for multimodal imaging. We present an open-source Python-based pipeline that allows for interactive studies and series selection, as well as automated conversion, segmentation, and quantitative analysis of positron emission tomography (PET) / computed tomography (CT) DICOM images. Leveraging widely adopted segmentation models for PET analysis and CT organ delineation, the pipeline computes key radiomics, producing structured outputs for analysis. Its modular design facilitates reproducible, scalable, and clinically relevant radiomics studies, addressing a critical gap in medical image analysis infrastructure. The code is available under: https://github.com/Clinical-Computational-Medical-Imaging/MUSIQ

1 Introduction

The digitization of medical imaging and the rise of artificial intelligence (AI) have transformed clinical research and are increasingly supporting daily practice [1]. Within this broader context, radiomics computationally derives quantitative descriptors from medical images, capturing intensity patterns, spatial relationships, and structural properties beyond visual assessment [2, 3]. These feature sets are applied

[†]These authors contributed equally to this work.

© Der/die Autor(en), exklusiv lizenziert an Springer Fachmedien Wiesbaden GmbH, ein Teil von Springer Nature 2026
H. Handels et al. (Hrsg.), *Bildverarbeitung für die Medizin 2026*, Informatik aktuell, https://doi.org/10.1007/978-3-658-51100-5_30

across imaging modalities and diseases, showing promise for linking image data with disease biology and clinical outcomes [4, 5].

Despite its potential, the adoption of radiomics in clinical data science is hindered by the lack of standardized, end-to-end workflows [6, 7]. Conventional workflows depend on separate tools for data handling, preprocessing, segmentation, and feature extraction, each with distinct dependencies and formats. The lack of integration increases manual effort, variability, and limits reproducibility. Although tools like matRadiomics [8], LIFEx [9], and CERR [10] particularly aid non-programmers in radiomics extraction and analysis, their focus on graphical user interfaces makes them less suited for seamless integration into deep learning pipelines for advanced data science.

By integrating complementary anatomical and functional data, PET/CT is particularly well-suited for combined quantitative analysis [11]. Therefore, we present an open-source, Python-based pipeline for PET/CT radiomics extraction to address a critical gap in reproducible, scalable, and extensible radiomics research infrastructure.

2 Materials and methods

The following section outlines each step of the proposed pipeline (Fig. 1).

2.1 Data preparation and initialization

Relevant imaging series are selected from the digital imaging and communications in medicine (DICOM) directory using user-defined keywords or via manual selection. Alignment of PET and CT images is required. DICOM files are converted to neuroimaging informatics technology initiative (NIfTI) format. For PET data, voxel intensities are expressed as standardized uptake value (SUV) normalized by injected dose, physical decay, and patient body weight. Patient data are parsed from DICOM metadata and structured in JSON format.

2.2 Segmentation

The pipeline supports automated segmentation for functional and anatomical imaging using widely adopted open-source models. PET lesion masks are generated from SUV-normalized PET volumes with autoPET3 [12]. Anatomical segmentation of CT data is performed with TotalSegmentator [13] and Moose [14, 15], enabling organ and skeletal delineation. Outputs are stored as NIfTI masks with accompanying metadata, including model, software version, and execution parameters.

2.3 Radiomics extraction

Computed radiomics metrics cover lesion-wise PET intensity, whole-body tumor burden, morphological and dissemination descriptors, as well as CT-based measurements.

For each patient, we first derive conventional SUV-based PET metrics: SUV_{max} (highest voxel intensity), SUV_{mean} (mean SUV), and SUV_{peak}, which we define as the median SUV in a fixed 1 cm^3 cubic region centered on the hottest voxel (peak-ROI definitions vary across studies) [16, 17]. Lesion metabolic tumor volume (MTV) is obtained as the volume of all voxels exceeding either an absolute SUV threshold (2.5–4.0) [18] or a relative threshold (30–50% of SUV_{max}) [19].

To capture whole-body disease burden, we aggregate lesion-wise metrics. The total metabolic tumor volume (TMTV) is defined as the combined volume of all segmented lesions [20]. Total lesion activity (TLA) is computed as SUV_{mean} multiplied by the corresponding lesion volume and summed over all lesions [21].

Morphological descriptors are derived from the binary lesion mask. The lesion count equals the number of spatially distinct connected components. Individual and total lesion volumes are computed by summing the physical voxel volumes of the respective components. Surface area is estimated from the isosurface of the binary mask using a marching-cubes approach with correct voxel spacing [22]. Tumor dissemination (D_{max}) is quantified as the maximum 3D Euclidean distance between any two lesion voxels and can be standardized by patient anthropometrics (SD_{max}) [23]. Organ overlap ratios are obtained by intersecting the lesion mask with predefined organ segmentations [7].

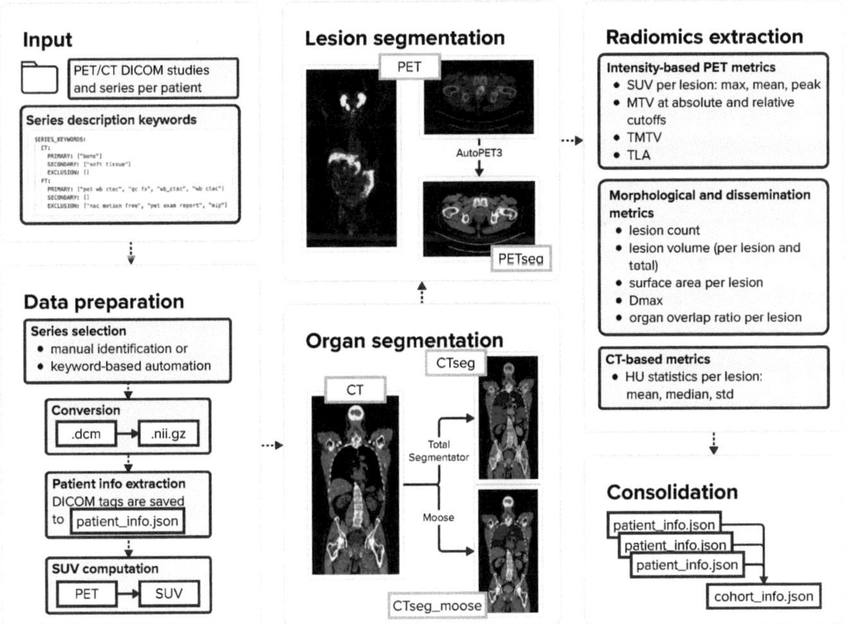

Fig. 1. Workflow visualization from data input to result consolidation. Dotted lines indicate workflow order, solid lines denote conversion/computation. Turquoise boxes describe the data modality of example images.

Finally, for each PET-defined lesion, we extract CT-based intensity statistics (mean, median, standard deviation of Hounsfield units) from the corresponding CT region to enable joint PET/CT analyses.

3 Results

The following case studies illustrate practical applications of the presented pipeline.

3.1 Automated PSMA-PET-based tumor quantification in prostate cancer and its association with Gleason score

We retrospectively analyzed in-house prostate-specific membrane antigen (PSMA) PET/CT scans from 369 patients with histologically confirmed prostate cancer to evaluate the relationship between PET-derived metrics and histopathological aggressiveness. The median and mean Gleason scores were 7.0 and 7.63, respectively. Spearman correlation analysis between Gleason scores and all pipeline-computed radiomics revealed that MTV at thresholds 4.0 (ρ = 0.416), 3.5 (ρ = 0.406), 3.0 (ρ = 0.399), 2.5 (ρ = 0.397), and TLA (ρ = 0.403) showed the strongest positive correlations ($p < 0.001$), suggesting a significant positive association between metabolic tumor burden and aggressiveness (Fig. 2).

3.2 AI-based FDG PET/CT analysis for immunotherapy response in metastatic melanoma

The pipeline was evaluated on 76 patients with metastatic melanoma undergoing immunotherapy. Baseline and follow-up fluorodeoxyglucose (FDG) PET/CT images were processed automatically and compared with manual segmentations by a nuclear

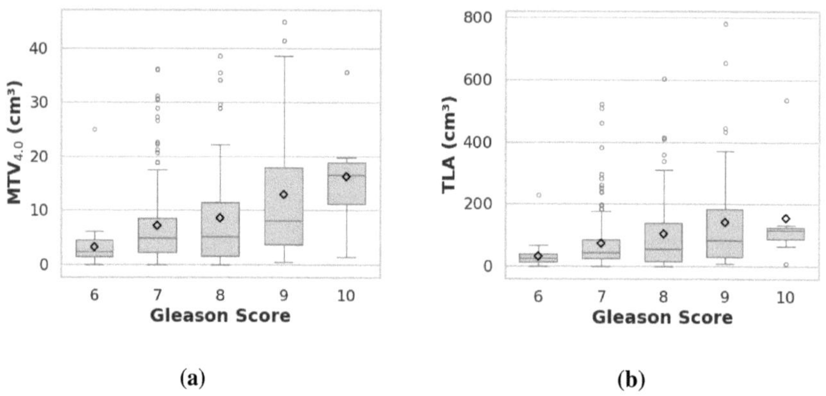

(a) (b)

Fig. 2. $MTV_{4.0}$ (a) and TLA (b) across Gleason scores, with ◇ indicating mean values. Data points exceeding 1.5 times the interquartile range were excluded for visual clarity.

medicine expert. AI segmentations showed good agreement with manual annotations, particularly for SUV_{max}, TMTV, and TLA (R^2 = 0.86–0.89), while discrepancies in D_{max} reflected methodological differences: manual measurements were taken on coronal maximum intensity projection images, while AI calculated 3D maximal distance between tumor voxels. Changes in automatically derived metrics between baseline and follow-up images corresponded well with clinical outcomes (stable disease, partial metabolic response, mixed response, progressive disease) and were consistent with lymph node dissection results [24].

4 Discussion

We present an open-source, Python-based pipeline for standardized PET/CT radiomics analysis, addressing the current lack of integrated workflows for radiomics computation in advanced data science. The pipeline is evaluated in two case studies using different tracers (PSMA, FDG), yielding results deemed clinically plausible.

Future developments will focus on expanding functionality, improving interoperability, and facilitating research adoption, as well as evaluating the robustness on further real-world clinical datasets. Planned enhancements include the incorporation of additional radiomics feature sets – such as PERCIST [16] metrics, texture features, and multiorgan-derived markers – and expanded segmentation models for both functional and anatomical imaging, along with meaningful visualizations. Beyond PET/CT, the pipeline's modular design allows extension to other imaging modalities, including MRI and alternative PET tracers beyond FDG and PSMA, enabling more comprehensive multi-parametric analyses. To facilitate community use and collaboration, the framework will be released as an open-source Python package. Together, these improvements will strengthen the pipeline's role as a scalable and extensible framework for radiomics research and its translation into clinical practice.

By combining robust processing, flexible integration, and a pathway for continuous expansion, this pipeline lays the foundation for reproducible, multimodal radiomics analyses that can accelerate digital medicine.

Acknowledgement. This research was partially funded by the Intramural Research Funding "MultiPro" of the Faculty of Medicine, University of Augsburg, the Bavarian Center for Cancer Research as part of the Lighthouse "Local Therapies", as well as by the Bavarian Ministry of Economic Affairs, Regional Development and Energy (StMWi) under grant number DIK-2310-0004// DIK0556/02.

References

1. Alowais SA, Alghamdi SS, Alsuhebany N, Alqahtani T, Alshaya AI, Almohareb SN et al. Revolutionizing healthcare: the role of artificial intelligence in clinical practice. BMC Med Educ. 2023;23(1):689.

2. Lambin P, Rios-Velazquez E, Leijenaar R, Carvalho S, van Stiphout RGPM, Granton P et al. Radiomics: extracting more information from medical images using advanced feature analysis. Eur J Cancer. 2012;48(4):441–6.
3. Gillies RJ, Kinahan PE, Hricak H. Radiomics: images are more than pictures, they are data. Radiology. 2016;278(2):563–77.
4. Aerts HJWL, Velazquez ER, Leijenaar RTH, Parmar C, Grossmann P, Carvalho S et al. Decoding tumour phenotype by noninvasive imaging using a quantitative radiomics approach. Nat Commun. 2014;5(1):4006.
5. van Timmeren JE, Cester D, Tanadini-Lang S, Alkadhi H, Baessler B. Radiomics in medical imaging: "how-to" guide and critical reflection. Insights Imaging. 2020;11(1):91.
6. Traverso A, Wee L, Dekker A, Gillies R. Repeatability and reproducibility of radiomic features: a systematic review. Int J Radiat Oncol Biol Phys. 2018;102(4):1143–58.
7. Zwanenburg A, Vallières M, Abdalah MA, Aerts HJWL, Andrearczyk V, Apte A et al. The image biomarker standardization initiative: standardized quantitative radiomics for high-throughput image-based phenotyping. Radiology. 2020;295(2):328–38.
8. Camastra C, Pasini G, Stefano A, Russo G, Vescio B, Bini F et al. Development and implementation of an innovative framework for automated radiomics analysis in neuroimaging. J Imaging. 2024;10(4):96.
9. Nioche C, Orlhac F, Boughdad S, Reuzé S, Goya-Outi J, Robert C et al. LIFEx: a freeware for radiomic feature calculation in multimodality imaging to accelerate advances in the characterization of tumor heterogeneity. Cancer Res. 2018;78(16):4786–9.
10. Deasy JO, Blanco AI, Clark VH. CERR: a computational environment for radiotherapy research. Med Phys. 2003;30(5):979–85.
11. Hatt M, Cheze Le Rest C, Antonorsi N, Tixier F, Tankyevych O, Jaouen V et al. Radiomics in PET/CT: current status and future AI-based evolutions. Semin Nucl Med. 2021;51(2):126–33.
12. Rokuss M, Kovacs B, Kirchhoff Y, Xiao S, Ulrich C, Maier-Hein KH et al. From FDG to PSMA: a hitchhiker's guide to multitracer, multicenter lesion segmentation in PET/CT imaging. arXiv: 2409.09478. 2024.
13. Wasserthal J, Breit HC, Meyer MT, Pradella M, Hinck D, Sauter AW et al. TotalSegmentator: robust segmentation of 104 anatomic structures in CT images. Radiol Artif Intell. 2023;5(5):e230024.
14. Ferrara D, Pires M, Gutschmayer S, Yu J, Abdelhafez YG, Abenavoli E et al. Sharing a whole-/total-body [18F]FDG-PET/CT dataset with CT-derived segmentations: an ENHANCE.PET initiative. Res Sq. 2025:rs.3.rs–7169062.
15. Sundar LKS, Yu J, Muzik O, Kulterer OC, Fueger B, Kifjak D et al. Fully automated, semantic segmentation of whole-body 18F-FDG PET/CT images based on data-centric artificial intelligence. J Nucl Med. 2022;63(12):1941–8.
16. Wahl RL, Jacene H, Kasamon Y, Lodge MA. From RECIST to PERCIST: evolving considerations for PET response criteria in solid tumors. J Nucl Med. 2009;50:122S–150S.
17. Vanderhoek M, Perlman SB, Jeraj R. Impact of the definition of peak standardized uptake value on quantification of treatment response. J Nucl Med. 2012;53(1):4–11.
18. Kido H, Kato S, Funahashi K, Shibuya K, Sasaki Y, Urita Y et al. The metabolic parameters based on volume in PET/CT are associated with clinicopathological N stage of colorectal cancer and can predict prognosis. EJNMMI Res. 2021;11(1):87.
19. Du S, Sun H, Gao S, Xin J, Lu Z. Metabolic parameters with different thresholds for evaluating tumor recurrence and their correlations with hematological parameters in

locally advanced squamous cell cervical carcinoma: an observational 18F-FDG PET/CT study. Quant Imaging Med Surg. 2019;9(3):440–52.

20. Im HJ, Bradshaw T, Solaiyappan M, Cho SY. Current methods to define metabolic tumor volume in positron emission tomography: which one is better? Nucl Med Mol Imaging. 2018;52(1):5–15.
21. Boellaard R, Delgado-Bolton R, Oyen WJG, Giammarile F, Tatsch K, Eschner W et al. FDG PET/CT: EANM procedure guidelines for tumour imaging: version 2.0. Eur J Nucl Med Mol Imaging. 2015;42(2):328–54.
22. Lorensen WE, Cline HE. Marching cubes: a high resolution 3D surface construction algorithm. SIGGRAPH Comput Graph. 1987;21(4):163–9.
23. Cottereau AS, Nioche C, Dirand AS, Clerc J, Morschhauser F, Casasnovas O et al. ^{18}F-FDG PET dissemination features in diffuse large B-cell lymphoma are predictive of outcome. J Nucl Med. 2020;61(1):40–5.
24. Förner L, Bäßler J, Sulski C, Enke J, Lapa C, Wendler T. Automated AI-based PET/CT analysis for monitoring immunotherapy response in metastatic melanoma. Proc EANM. 1:100004.

This chapter is published under the Creative Commons Attribution 4.0 International License (http://creativecommons.org/licenses/by/4.0/deed.en).

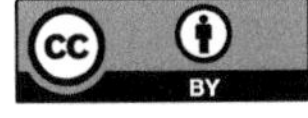

Master Class on Reproducibility
A Student Hackathon on Advanced MRI Reconstruction Methods

Lina Felsner[1,2,3†], Sevgi G. Kafali[1†], Hannah Eichhorn[1,2], Agnes A. J. Leth[1], Aidas Batvinskas[1], André Datchev[1], Fabian Klemm[1], Jan Aulich[1], Puntika Leepagorn[1], Ruben Klinger[1], Daniel Rueckert[1,3,4,5], Julia A. Schnabel[1,2,3,6]

[1]School of Computation, Information & Technology, Technical University of Munich (TUM), Germany
[2]Institute of Machine Learning in Biomedical Imaging, Helmholtz Munich, Germany
[3]Munich Center for Machine Learning (MCML), Germany
[4]School of Medicine and Health, TUM University Hospital Rechts der Isar, Germany
[5]Department of Computing, Imperial College London, UK
[6]School of Biomedical Engineering and Imaging Sciences, King's College London, UK
{lina.felsner,s.kafali}@tum.de

Abstract. We report the design, protocol, and outcomes of a *student reproducibility hackathon* focused on replicating the results of three influential MRI reconstruction papers: (a) MoDL, an unrolled model-based network with learned denoising [1]; (b) HUMUS-Net, a hybrid unrolled multi-scale CNN+Transformer architecture [2]; and (c) an untrained, physics-regularized dynamic MRI method that uses a quantitative MR model for early stopping [3]. We describe the setup of the hackathon and present reproduction outcomes alongside additional experiments, and we detail fundamental practices for building reproducible codebases.

1 Introduction

Magnetic resonance imaging (MRI) is known for its strong soft-tissue contrast and can be used to diagnose several diseases from tumors to strokes and joint injuries. One of the biggest challenges in MRI is the long scan time, which is why accelerated MRI reconstruction has been extensively studied over the last few decades. This is done by using sophisticated algorithms which can mitigate acceleration artifacts. Deep learning has transformed accelerated MRI reconstruction by casting it as a learned regularized inverse problem. A standard approach for high-quality reconstructions with strong physics grounding are unrolled neural networks, which explicitly interleave *data-consistency* with learned *priors*. The model-based deep

†These authors contributed equally to this work.

© Der/die Autor(en), exklusiv lizenziert an
Springer Fachmedien Wiesbaden GmbH, ein Teil von Springer Nature 2026
H. Handels et al. (Hrsg.), *Bildverarbeitung für die Medizin 2026*,
Informatik aktuell, https://doi.org/10.1007/978-3-658-51100-5_31

learning architecture for inverse problems (MoDL) [1] introduces a supervised unrolled network that integrates a variational framework with a data-consistency term and a learned CNN to capture image redundancy. Another unrolled network, called HUMUS-Net [2] is a hybrid architecture that leverages transformers to model long-range dependencies while retaining the efficiency and inductive bias of convolutions. Following the growing interest in unsupervised approaches, Slavkova *et al.* [3] proposed an untrained, i.e., self-supervised network that exploits the architectural bias and scan-specific optimization, while benefiting from physics-based regularization to reduce reliance on fully sampled ground truth. Even at higher acceleration rates, these previous studies all yield extraordinary image reconstruction quality, validated by extensive evaluations and experiments.

However, complex and intricate deep learning frameworks, specialized data acquisition protocols, and sophisticated training regimens, can make it challenging to verify reported results. Additional challenges might arise while reproducing the results due to varying software dependencies, hardware configurations, random seeds, and subtle differences in pre-processing or hyperparameter tuning. Therefore, best practices emphasize the use of version-controlled code, standardized computing environments, and fully executable pipelines. These practices are supported by pragmatic checklists and further reinforced by the findable, accessible, interoperable, and reusable (FAIR) principles [4], which extend the scope from data to also models and workflows. Beyond FAIR, the FUTURE-AI [5] principles offer a concise, consensus framework for trustworthy medical AI across the full lifecycle considering: fairness, universality, traceability, usability, robustness, and explainability. The guideline translates these six pillars into actionable recommendations for data curation, model development, validation, deployment, and monitoring. Following these principles alongside open code and defined environments could also strengthen both the credibility and reproducibility of reported results.

For computational research reproducibility has become an essential component [6]. In the medical imaging community, two main conferences have been holding hackathons focusing on reproducibility: the annual meeting of international society of magnetic resonance in medicine (ISMRM) [7] and medical image computing and computer assisted interventions (MICCAI) [8]. In addition, educational hackathons specifically focusing on reproducibility have emerged as a valuable tool for promoting best practices in a teaching environment. Initiatives such as the 'reproduced papers' series [9] or classroom setting type hackathons [10] highlight the growing recognition of reproducibility challenges. Particularly, the 'reproduce CVPR Hackathon' [10], organized at Friedrich-Alexander-Universität Erlangen-Nürnberg (FAU) has aimed to reproduce papers from CVPR 2024. The FAU hackathon contained three stages: automated detection of code availability, a PhD hackathon to evaluate reproducibility effort, and a master's course to reproduce CVPR papers.

This work documents a student hackathon organized to reproduce three selected works in the context of accelerated MRI reconstruction: HUMUS-Net, MoDL, and untrained+physics model. The hackathon has been designed to (1) help students connect theory and practice in inverse problems applied to MRI reconstruction; and (2) emphasize reproducibility and responsible use of MRI data.

2 Methods

In this section we describe the setup of our reproducibility hackathon. This hackathon has been an integral component of the 'deep learning for inverse problems in medical imaging' master seminar at Technical University of Munich (TUM). Its primary objective has been to transition students from paper reading (i.e., theoretical understanding) to practical application with a hands-on experience.

The hackathon spanned a total of four hours, divided across three sessions. Paper selection was done by the seminar course instructors. During this selection, instructors ensured code and data availability including MR images and the respective raw data, as well as pre-trained model weights. Seven students from the School of computation, information and technology at TUM, originating from diverse master's programs, formed three teams. Each team selected one out of six possible papers. The task was to recreate one of the figures in the result section of the chosen scientific paper. The students were asked to utilize the provided pre-trained weights, thus bypassing the need for training models from scratch to avoid differences in code or training set-up. If the students could complete the task before the deadline, they were asked to show additional out-of-distribution (i.e., cross-domain) results in a test dataset for bonus credit.

- *Team A:* The first team consisted of two students and focused on reproducing MoDL's results [1] utilizing its corresponding codebase [11] and dataset [12]. The model was trained with a variable density (VD) k-space sampling mask with an acceleration rate of R=6. The students additionally tested on self-generated VD mask following a Gaussian distribution and GRAPPA-style sampling masks, with results reported for R=4 and R=14.
- *Team B:* Team B, comprising three students, tackled HUMUS-Net [2] using its codebase [13] and single- and multi-coil data (fastMRI knee dataset [14]) with an acceleration rate of R=8. Since this team had an additional student it was challenged to also evaluate the model on the brain multi-coil fastMRI dataset [12]. The students also compared the results to a Zero-filled approach.
- *Team C:* The third team consisted of two students and focused on an "untrained+physics" model by Slavkova *et al.* [3] utilizing its corresponding codebase [15] and dataset [16].

For all models, error maps were calculated as the difference between the reconstructed image and the fully sampled ground truth image. The evaluation metrics included structural similarity (SSIM) and peak signal-to-noise ratio (PSNR).

All experiments were performed on a workstation featuring Ubuntu 24.04 LTS, an Intel Xeon W-2133 CPU, 30 GB RAM, and a single NVIDIA GeForce GTX 1080 GPU.

The hackathon concluded with student teams presenting both the original papers and their reproduced results via posters within the seminar.

3 Results

The results for the reproducibility hackathon for each team/paper are reported below.

Tab. 1. Results for MoDL using in-domain and out-of-distribution (cross-domain) sampling masks. Image quality metrics for Acc. rate: acceleration rate. SSIM: structural similarity. PSNR: peak signal-to-noise ratio.

Mask	Acc. rate	SSIM	PSNR [dB]
Original VD	R=6	0.92 ± 0.00	38.51 ± 0.75
Self-gen. VD	R=4	0.93 ± 0.00	40.06 ± 0.88
Self-gen. VD	R=14	0.85 ± 0.01	30.59 ± 1.01
GRAPPA-style	R=4	0.87 ± 0.01	30.56 ± 0.78
GRAPPA-style	R=14	0.52 ± 0.02	18.30 ± 0.82

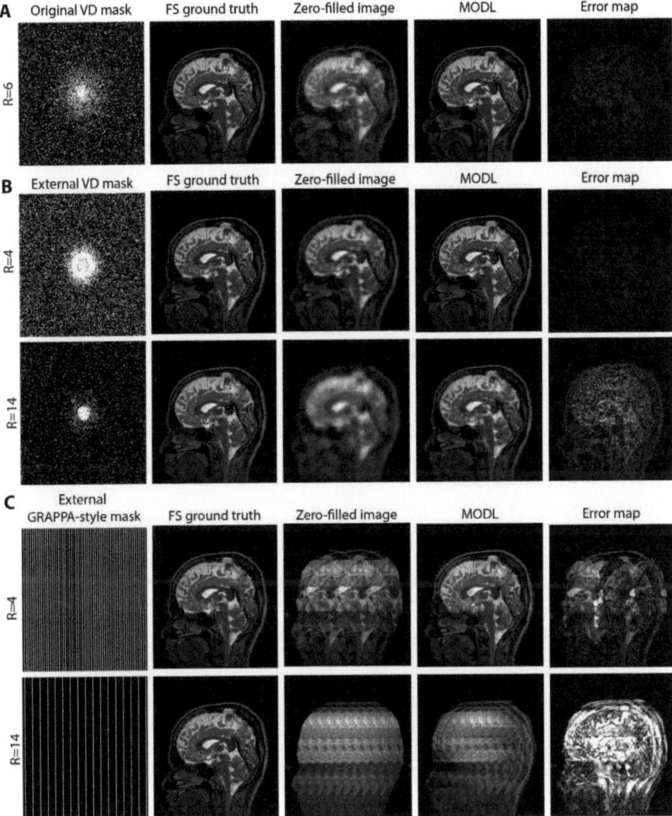

Fig. 1. Results for MoDL using in-domain and out-of-distribution (cross-domain) sampling masks. Fully-sampled (FS) ground truth, zero-filled image as well as MoDL reconstruction. (A) Same-domain results with an acceleration rate of R=6. (B) Cross-domain results, tested in a self-generated variable density (VD) sampling mask, with acceleration rates of R=4 and R=14. (C) Cross-domain results, tested in a self-generated GRAPPA-style sampling mask, with acceleration rates of R=4 and R=14.

Tab. 2. Results for HUMUS-Net using in-domain (knee) and out-of-distribution, i.e., cross-domain (brain) target organs. Image quality metrics. PSNR: peak signal-to-noise ratio. SSIM: structural similarity.

Dataset	Model	SSIM	PSNR [dB]
Knee	HUMUS-Net (Train)	0.8870	36.28
Knee	HUMUS-Net-L (Train+val)	0.8912	36.71
Brain	HUMUS-Net	0.8871	31.9
Brain	Zero-filled	0.6832	25.9

3.1 Team A: MoDL

Team A could sucessfully reproduce the results from the MoDL paper. Figure 1A shows representative images consisting of original VD mask, fully sampled ground truth, zero-filled image, MODL reconstructed image as well as the error map. Figure 1B and C demonstrate results from out-of-distribution cases, where the model was tested on a self-generated VD sampling mask, and a GRAPPA-style sampling mask. Table 1 illustrates the image quality metrics involving PSNR and SSIM across in-domain acceleration rate of R=6, and out-of-distribution (i.e., cross-domain) results from self-generated VD and GRAPPA-style sampling masks at R=4 and R=14. The image quality metrics with self-generated VD masks were comparable to those from the model trained and tested with original VD mask across R=4 and R=14. When MoDL was tested on a self-generated GRAPPA-style mask, the PSNR and SSIM values decreased.

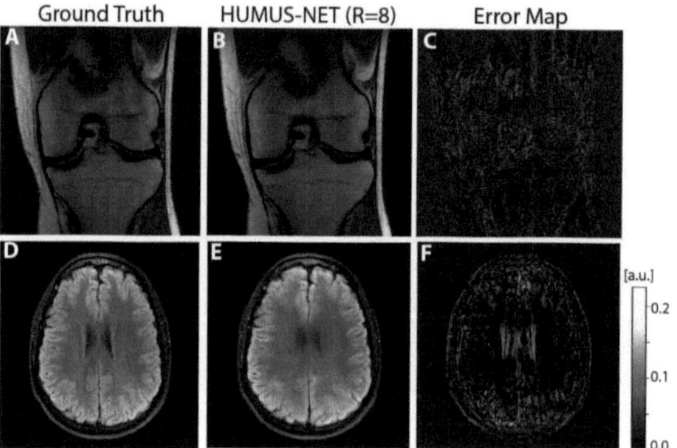

Fig. 2. Results for HUMUS-Net using in-domain (knee) and out-of-distribution, i.e., cross-domain (brain) target organs. HUMUS-Net results together with the corresponding ground truth and error map. (A-C): same-domain reconstructions. (D-F): cross-domain brain MRI reconstructions.

3.2 Team B: HUMUS-Net

Other than suggested in the README files, the HUMUS-Net implementation did not support single-coil data. However, the reproduction of the results for the multi-coil data was successful. The reconstruction results together with the corresponding fully-sampled ground truth images are shown in Figure 2. Table 2 shows PSNR and SSIM results for in-domain (i.e., knee) and out-of-distribution (cross-domain) results. Interestingly, the SSIM values for the brain (out-of-distribution) data, was as good as for the in-domain trained knee data.

3.3 Team C: Untrained+Physics

Unfortunately, the students were not able to reproduce the results. While the paper presents promising results in untrained deep learning for dynamic MR image reconstruction, the code lacked several components necessary for robust and reproducible implementation.

Documentation was insufficient: the README provided little guidance, and the requirements file omitted package versions, leading to execution failures due to deprecated methods. Critical elements, such as complex-valued loss handling, were missing, and the codebase contained numerous commented-out sections and non-functional placeholders that obscured the intended logic.

Reported expectations in the original work [3] stated training times around 3–5 hours over 9,999 epochs with a gradually decreasing loss and convergence. In our experiments, after 11 hours of training, only 5,050 epochs were completed and loss values remained high (e.g., loss 639,949 at epoch 5,049).

The authors were contacted for clarification and indicated that the codebase is no longer actively maintained. The implementation relies on a previous version of PyTorch predating built-in support for complex numbers, which clarifies the handling of imaginary components as two separate channels. The authors recommended to create a Conda environment that uses previous versions of the packages, and added that they were happy to help in that regard. This was out-of-scope for this project.

4 Discussion and conclusion

In the reproducibility study, students were requested to mimic a realistic scenario of using pre-trained weights to evaluate the models and recreate one of the figures in the original study (i.e. no further training). When time permitted, students were asked to include additional out-of-distribution results. Out of three studies, two of them could be reproduced. For MoDL and HUMUS-Net, results are in accordance with the published results. For the out-of-distribution task it was found that the MoDL approach generalizes well to varying VD sampling patterns with different acceleration rates, which is in accordance with the authors theory behind weight sharing. The model performance suffered for self-generated GRAPPA-style sampling masks, possibly requiring training from scratch. HUMUS-Net yielded good generalization among out-of-distribution target organs (e.g., brain). The Untrained+Physics model could not be reproduced.

There were a few reasons as to why the teams could complete the task and do further testing with the first two studies. The studies that could be reproduced had: (i) proper documentation with clear guidance on their README files; (ii) complete dependency list of required libraries and Python versions. The third study could not be reproduced due to an outdated codebase and README, insufficient information on training configurations, inadequately commented code, and missing training checkpoints. This highlights the importance of the FAIR and FUTURE-AI principles and commitment to reproducibility.

The main limitation of the hackathon was the strict four-hour time constraint, as it was conducted as part of a seminar. Future work could involve a full seminar course on reproducibility with more students, including model training and extended time for implementation and experiments. While more challenging to organize, a full reproducibility study would be more informative.

Overall, this work demonstrates a reproducibility hackathon on MR image reconstruction in a teaching environment. We conclude that clean, well-documented, and reproducible code should be a prerequisite for publication to ensure transparency and to fight the reproducibility crisis [6].

Acknowledgement. This work is supported by the Konrad Zuse School of Excellence in Reliable AI (relAI). Dr. Sevgi Gokce Kafali is sponsored by Alexander von Humboldt Foundation in Germany.

References

1. Aggarwal HK, Mani MP, Jacob M. MoDL: model-based deep learning architecture for inverse problems. IEEE Trans Med Imaging. 2019;38(2):394–405.
2. Fabian Z, Tinaz B, Soltanolkotabi M. HUMUS-net: hybrid unrolled multi-scale network architecture for accelerated MRI reconstruction. Proc NeurIPS. 2022.
3. Slavkova KP, DiCarlo JC, Wadhwa V, Wu C, Virostko J, Kumar S et al. An untrained deep learning method for reconstructing dynamic MR images from accelerated model-based data. Magn Reson Med. 2023.
4. Wilkinson MD, Dumontier M, Aalbersberg IJ, Appleton G, Axton M, Baak A et al. The FAIR guiding principles for scientific data management and stewardship. Sci Data. 2016;3(1):1–9.
5. Lekadir K, Frangi AF, Porras AR, Glocker B, Cintas C, Langlotz CP et al. FUTURE-AI: international consensus guideline for trustworthy and deployable artificial intelligence in healthcare. BMJ. 2025;388.
6. Stupple A, Singerman D, Celi LA. The reproducibility crisis in the age of digital medicine. NPJ Digit Med. 2019;2:2.
7. Maier O, Baete SH, Fyrdahl A, Hammernik K, Harrevelt S, Kasper L et al. CG-SENSE revisited: results from the first ISMRM reproducibility challenge. Magn Reson Med. 2021;85(4):1821–39.

8. Balsiger F, Jungo A, Chen J, Ezhov I, Liu S, Ma J et al. The MICCAI hackathon on reproducibility, diversity, and selection of papers at the MICCAI conference. arXiv preprint: 2103.05437. 2021.
9. ReproducedPapers.org. a hub for reproduced deep learning papers and their reproductions. https://reproducedpapers.org/. 2020.
10. Let's reproduce CVPR (FAU). reproducibility project at FAU. https://www.reproducecvpr.tf.fau.eu/. 2024.
11. Aggarwal HK, Mani MP, Jacob M. Code for model-based deep learning architecture for inverse problems. https://github.com/hkaggarwal/modl. 2018.
12. Aggarwal HK. MoDL: model-based deep learning dataset. Zenodo, 2019.
13. Zalan Fabian, Berk Tinaz, and Mahdi Soltanolkotabi. Code for transformer-convolutional hybrid unrolled multiscale network for accelerated MRI reconstruction. https://github.com/z-fabian/HUMUS-Net. 2022.
14. Zbontar J, Knoll F, Sriram A, Murrell T, Huang Z, Muckley MJ et al. fastMRI: an open dataset and benchmarks for accelerated MRI. arXiv preprint: 1811.08839. 2018.
15. Slavkova K et al. Code for ConvDecoder with physics-based regularization (CD+r) for MRI. https://github.com/kslav/cdr_mri. 2022.
16. Slavkova K et al. Dataset for ConvDecoder with physics-based regularization (CD+r) for MRI. https://utexas.box.com/s/ynm4g740x3rrtiuzdsqma9bweqmonk6v. 2022.

Abstract: Adding the Temporal Dimension in Image Reconstruction for Proton Therapy Verification

Julius Werner [1], Veronica Ferrero [2,3], Francesco Pennazio [2], Elisa Fiorina [2], Jona Kasprzak [1], Jorge Roser [1], Magdalena Rafecas [1]

[1]Institut für Medizintechnik, Universität zu Lübeck, Lübeck, Germany
[2]Istituto Nazionale di Fisica Nucleare, Sezione di Torino, Turin, Italy
[3]Department of Physics, Università degli Studi di Torino, Turin, Italy
friedemann.werner@uni-luebeck.de

Proton therapy is a tumor treatment technique that uses the unique dose profile of protons to deliver high doses to the tumor while sparing surrounding tissue. This precision creates a need to actively verify the delivered dose during treatment. Many techniques for dose verification have been proposed; most focus on the spatial distribution of secondary particle emissions caused by proton-matter interactions. Among them are prompt gamma's (PGs), i.e. high-energy photons emitted within 10 ps after a proton interacts with the tissue. Therefore, their emission is linked to the proton in time and space. Using a specialized measurement procedure – prompt gamma timing – and a tomographic-like reconstruction we can retrieve the PGs spatial and temporal distribution [1]. The combination of time and space enables the study of proton motion. Through non-linear regression with proton motion models, we then estimate the stopping power – a crucial material parameter to accurately plan and execute the treatment [2, 3]. Several challenges in instrumentation, reconstruction, modeling and postprocessing must be overcome to implement this unique approach. Still, we have used this novel combination of image computation techniques to estimate the stopping power of a homogeneous phantom with an accuracy of 2 % [4].

References

1. Pennazio F, Ferrero V, D'Onghia G, Garbolino S, Fiorina E, Villarreal OAM et al. Proton therapy monitoring: spatiotemporal emission reconstruction with prompt gamma timing and implementation with PET detectors. Phys Med Biol. 2022;67(6):065005.
2. Ferrero V, Werner J, Cerello P, Fiorina E, Vignati A, Pennazio F et al. Estimating the stopping power distribution during proton therapy: a proof of concept. Front Phys. 2022;10.
3. Werner J, Pennazio F, Schmid N, Fiorina E, Bersani D, Cerello P et al. Stopping power and range estimations in proton therapy based on prompt gamma timing: motion models and automated parameter optimization. Phys Med Biol. 2024.

© Der/die Autor(en), exklusiv lizenziert an
Springer Fachmedien Wiesbaden GmbH, ein Teil von Springer Nature 2026
H. Handels et al. (Hrsg.), *Bildverarbeitung für die Medizin 2026*,
Informatik aktuell, https://doi.org/10.1007/978-3-658-51100-5_32

4. Werner J, Ferrero V, Aglietta M, Cerello P, Fiorina E, Kasprzak J et al. In-beam measurement of stopping power using multi-detector prompt gamma timing in proton therapy. Phys Med. 2024;125:103890.

Reversible Image Augmentations for Unsupervised Deep Learning in Computed Tomography

Laura Hellwege [1,2], Johann C. Engster [2], Moritz Schaar [2], Thorsten M. Buzug [1,2], Maik Stille [2]

[1]Institute of Medical Engineering, University of Lübeck, Lübeck, Germany
[2]Fraunhofer Research Institution for Individualized Medical Technology and Engineering (IMTE), Lübeck, Germany
l.hellwege@uni-luebeck.de

Abstract. We propose a physically consistent, reversible image augmentation approach for an unsupervised computed tomography (CT) reconstruction deep learning framework. The framework has the unique property of calculating the loss in the projection domain, so no image-domain ground truth is required. Even though previous evaluation proved feasibility of unsupervised deep learning for inverse problems like CT reconstruction, it also showed frail behavior after data alterations. To increase training diversity without violating projection-image fidelity, we apply reversible image augmentations that preserve non-zero image pixels, record the sampled parameters, and invert the transforms on the U-Net++ output. We describe implementation details, parameter sampling schemes and practical constraints for CT data, and discuss how the approach permits richer, physically consistent augmentation for improving performance in unsupervised reconstruction.

1 Introduction

Computed tomography is an important imaging modality in medical diagnostics, providing detailed cross-sectional images of the human body. Recently, it was shown that unsupervised reconstruction via deep learning is feasible for the inverse imaging problem in computed tomography [1]. The approach opens up the possibility of solving arbitrary continuous inverse problems in an unsupervised manner for later application to unseen data, which is highly beneficial in many imaging disciplines. Exemplarily, the paper proposed to show feasibility for the filter step in CT reconstruction, since ground-truth FBP reconstructions for evaluation are easily accessible. However, large, diverse datasets are often difficult to obtain due to ethical considerations [2]. Hence, effective image augmentation techniques are essential for enhancing model performance. Traditional image augmentations are not reversed in the training process since the ground-truth image (used for loss calculation) is processed accordingly. In unsupervised learning with CT data, however, the image-domain deep-learning model's loss is calculated in the projection data domain. In

© Der/die Autor(en), exklusiv lizenziert an
Springer Fachmedien Wiesbaden GmbH, ein Teil von Springer Nature 2026
H. Handels et al. (Hrsg.), *Bildverarbeitung für die Medizin 2026*,
Informatik aktuell, https://doi.org/10.1007/978-3-658-51100-5_33

this domain, arbitrary data augmentation leads to meaningless reconstructed images. Vice versa, arbitrary image augmentation after reconstruction without inversion also compromises the geometrical and physical adherence of images to the underlying projection data. To solve this problem, we introduce reversible image augmentations for CT images by allowing transformations to be undone. This approach enables the generation of diverse training samples for the image processing deep-learning model while preserving physical correspondences between image and projection data.

2 Material and methods

2.1 Including image augmentations in unsupervised network training

Recently, an unsupervised training approach for CT imaging was proposed [1] that is visualized in Figure 1. The forward pass input is the projection data, which is mapped to the image domain by a backprojection layer, yielding a blurred image. This image is processed by a U-Net++ with a ResNeXt-101 (32×16d) encoder [3], which predicts the image reconstruction $\hat{f}$. For unsupervised training a forward projection layer is applied to obtain the predicted projection data $\hat{p}$. Including image augmentations modifies the training pipeline (indicated by additions in orange). Before the input is passed to the network, augmentations are applied with their respective parameters θ. The augmentations are inverted after network prediction to restore the original physical properties. The resulting predicted sinogram is compared pixel-wise with the original sinogram to compute the loss $\mathcal{L}_2(p, \hat{p})$ in the projection domain. Gradients propagate through $\hat{p}$, the backprojection layer and $\hat{f}$ back into the U-Net++.

For training, validation and testing, the 2DeteCT dataset [4] is employed, which includes over 5,000 CT reconstructed 2D filtered backprojection (FBP) slices and their respective 2D projection data. We utilize 2,800 slices and the corresponding

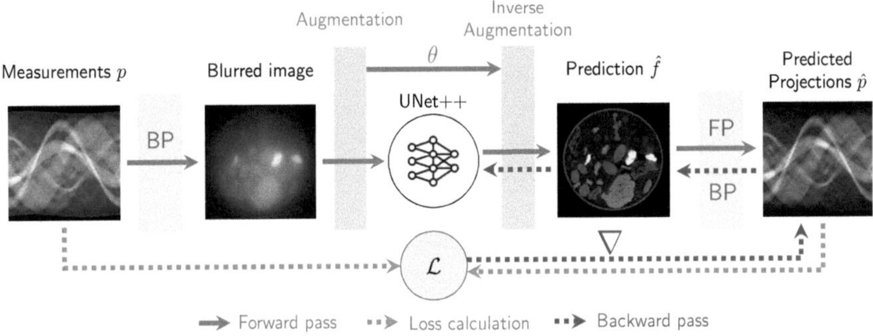

Fig. 1. Adapted unsupervised training scheme from [1] including proposed image augmentation approach. Domain transform is indicated by forward (FP) or backward (BP) projection layers. Image augmentations are inserted before UNet++ input, the augmentation parameters θ are stored, and inverse augmentations are applied on the respective network output.

Tab. 1. Augmentation categories and example transforms from *Albumentations* package [5].

Category	Example transforms
Geometric	HorizontalFlip, VerticalFlip, Affine, Perspective
Crop / Patch / Pad	RandomCrop, CenterCrop, PadIfNeeded
Resize / Rescale	Resize, SmallestMaxSize, LongestMaxSize
Photometric	RandomBrightnessContrast, HueSaturationValue, RGBShift
Blur / Sharpen / Noise	GaussianBlur, MedianBlur, MotionBlur, GaussNoise
Non-linear distortions	ElasticTransform, GridDistortion, OpticalDistortion

projections, as differences in geometry have been reported for the other measurements, which is critical for the reconstruction network. To keep validation times during training short, 100 projection datasets for validation between epochs, 2,400 for training and 300 test datasets for evaluation are used. Training employed the ADAM optimizer with learning rate 10^{-4} on a single NVIDIA RTX A6000 (48 GB VRAM) for 500 epochs. After training, the network's predicted image from unseen projection data yields the desired reconstruction.

2.2 Determination of reversible augmentations

The neural network processes CT images. To ensures consistency with the data in the projection domain, it is critical to preserve all pixels that lie within the field of view (FOV) and represent non-zero attenuation. Hence, we define an augmentation as reversible only if it does not substantially alter or remove non-zero pixels inside the FOV. For general image augmentations, *Albumentations* [5] is a powerful toolbox. Categories and examples of the provided augmentations are shown in Table 1.

Operations that irreversibly discard too much image information are unsuitable for inversion. Cropping permanently removes pixels outside the crop box and cannot be recovered even with exact crop coordinates. Random downsampling and resizing lose information through interpolation. Photometric adjustments such as contrast changes or gamma correction as well as blur or sharpen operations are typically non-bijective and thus not reversible. In general, RGB color transform are not applicable for grayscale CT data. Moderate additive noise is generally acceptable for CT augmentation. It becomes reversible if the exact noise image is stored. Non-linear spatial distortions are reversible when dense displacement fields are saved and exact inverse resampling is applied. Storing noise images or displacement fields is memory-expensive, which is why both were not considered in this work. The geometric category contains the most suitable transforms for reversible augmentation. Spatial flips are self-inverse and preserve all pixels inside the original image. The boolean flip parameters are sampled by the Bernoulli distribution $\mathcal{B}(p)$ with probability $p \in [0, 1]$ as

$$\text{flip}_x \sim \mathcal{B}(p = 0.5), \text{flip}_y \sim \mathcal{B}(p = 0.5)$$

Affine-type transforms including rotation, scaling, translation and shear are acceptable provided cropping is moderate and the transform parameters are recorded so an exact reverse application is possible. We choose the parameters sampled from the uniform distribution $\mathcal{U}(I)$ in the interval I as

$$\text{rotation} \sim \mathcal{U}([-90°, +90°]) \qquad \text{scale} \sim \mathcal{U}([0.8, 1.2])$$
$$\text{shear}_x \sim \mathcal{U}([-10°, +10°]) \qquad \text{shear}_y \sim \mathcal{U}([-10°, +10°])$$
$$\text{translation}_x \sim \mathcal{U}([-10\%, +10\%]) \qquad \text{translation}_y \sim \mathcal{U}([-10\%, +10\%])$$

Here, the shear parameters refer to the corner angles of the sheared image border, and the translation parameters refer to the relative translation w.r.t the image size.

3 Results

We show the effect of the chosen augmentations in Figure 2. The difference images in Figure 2d indicate that the images that underwent augmentation following reverse augmentation underlie a small systematic error from interpolation operations. Figure 2 also shows the distribution of this systematic error for 100 exemplary images. It should be noted here, that in the network training the augmentation will be applied on images generated from simple backprojection. However, this distribution provides a baseline difference that we can expect to observe in the final reconstructions.

In Figure 3, the distributions of mean squared error (MSE) and the structural similarity index (SSIM) relative to the FBP image are shown. Close agreement with the ground-truth image corresponds to low MSE and high SSIM. A direct comparison of training with and without the proposed augmentations shows that

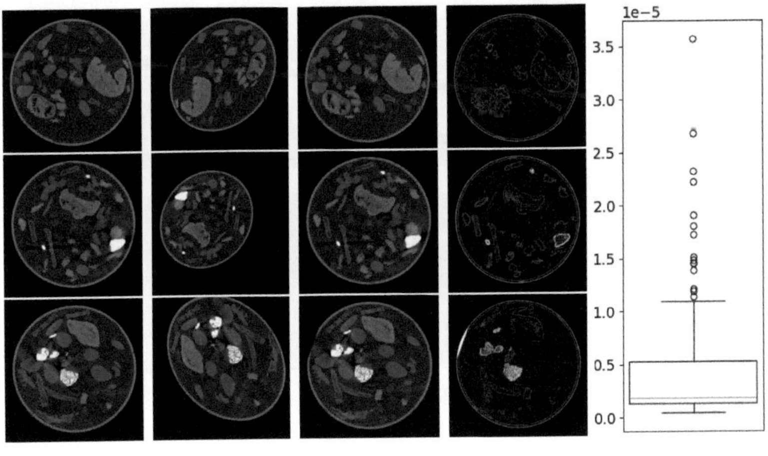

Fig. 2. Visualization of systematic error from image augmentation. (a) CT images in value range $[0, 0.1]\ \frac{1}{\text{cm}}$, (b) after augmentation, (c) after reverse augmentation, and (d) the absolute difference to the original image in $[0, 0.01]\ \frac{1}{\text{cm}}$. The last subfigure shows the MSE distribution of the difference images for 100 randomly augmented CT images.

training with augmentations achieves higher average performance. Figure 4 shows the networks' performance on an example dataset whose BP image was augmented. Reverse augmentations were applied on the network predictions and are compared to the FBP ground truth. Higher overall agreement on image values for most image parts is observable. Merely fewer, small regions surrounding higher density objects show a higher discrepancy compared to the prediction without augmented training. The MSE value for this example drops from $\mathrm{MSE}_{\mathrm{w/o}} = 6.77 \cdot 10^{-5} \frac{1}{\mathrm{cm}^2}$ to $\mathrm{MSE}_{\mathrm{with}} = 2.40 \cdot 10^{-5} \frac{1}{\mathrm{cm}^2}$.

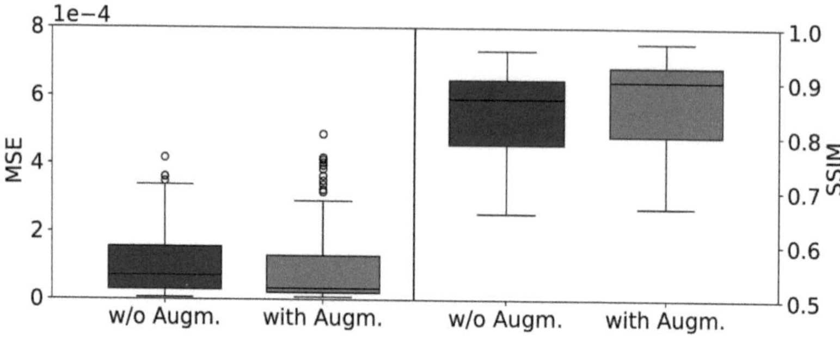

Fig. 3. Boxplots of MSE and SSIM distribution for predicted test datasets from networks trained without and with proposed augmentations w.r.t. FBP image.

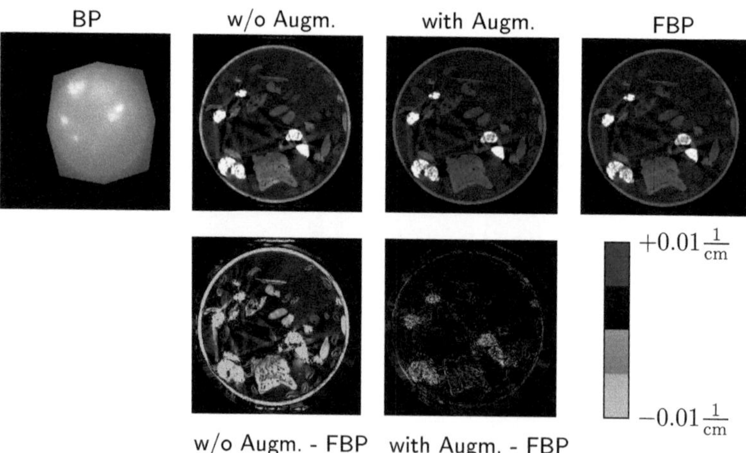

Fig. 4. Examplary prediction of the networks trained without and with image augmentations from augmented simple backprojection (BP) following image augmentation inversion. The predictions and FBP are shown in the value range [0.0, 0.1] $\frac{1}{\mathrm{cm}}$. The second row shows their difference to the FBP reconstruction.

4 Discussion

In this work, we introduced reversible image augmentations to an unsupervised deep learning framework for CT image reconstruction. During the implementation, several interesting aspects emerged that call for further discussion. It is important to note that the introduction of image augmentations can potentially introduce bias into the model as was shown in Figure 2. Even though the augmentations are designed to be reversible, they influence the relationship between image data and the projection domain which could lead to inconsistent modeling. To circumvent this, the consideration of augmenting projection data instead of image data arises. We hypothesize that since the model effectively learns a deconvolution step, the content of the reconstructed images might not be as important as the accuracy of corresponding projection data. Our results indicate improvement of performance on average. Still, severe outliers in terms of MSE values were observed in Figure 2 and Figure 3. A closer look at the outliers showed that these are extreme cases in which higher cropping occurred. These transformations will be further restricted in future and are included in this paper for reasons of transparency. To further improve performance, it is advisable to integrate an additional model operating in the projection domain, since backprojection from unprocessed data may cause significant information loss due to blurring. A projection-domain model could better capture the data's physical properties and enhance reconstruction quality. Additionally, including noise and elastic deformations in the augmentation process may further improve model robustness and generalization. Overall, reversible image augmentations show promise for advancing unsupervised CT reconstruction.

Disclaimer. This work was partially funded by the state of Schleswig-Holstein through the project "Individualisierte Medizintechnik für bildgestützte, robotische interventionen (IMTE 2)", project number: 125 24 009.

References

1. Hellwege L, Engster JC, Schaar M, Buzug TM, Stille M. Unsupervised learning for inverse problems in computed tomography. arXiv preprint: 2508.05321. 2025.
2. Wang S, Cao G, Wang Y, Liao S, Wang Q, Shi J et al. Review and prospect: artificial intelligence in advanced medical imaging. Front Radiol. 2021;1.
3. Iakubovskii P. Segmentation models PyTorch. `https://github.com/qubvel/segmentation_models.pytorch`. v0.3.3. 2019.
4. Kiss MB, Coban SB, Batenburg KJ, van Leeuwen T, Lucka F. 2DeteCT: a large 2D expandable, trainable, experimental computed tomography dataset for machine learning. Sci Data. 2023;10(1):576.
5. Buslaev A, Iglovikov VI, Khvedchenya E, Parinov A, Druzhinin M, Kalinin AA. Albumentations: fast and flexible image augmentations. Inf. 2020;11(2):125.

Automatic Patient Positioning Control and Correction on MRI Localizer Images

Zeineb Azouzi[1,2], Linda Vorberg[1,3], Rainer Schneider[2], Andreas Maier[1], Fabian Wagner[2]

[1]Pattern Recognition Lab, Friedrich-Alexander-Universität, Erlangen-Nürnberg, Germany
[2]Magnetic Resonance, Siemens Healthineers AG, Erlangen, Germany
[3]Computed Tomography, Siemens Healthineers AG, Forchheim, Germany
zeineb.azouzi@fau.de

Abstract. Accurate anatomical positioning is essential in magnetic resonance imaging (MRI) to ensure the acquisition of diagnostically useful images. In high-throughput clinical workflows, MRI technicians must position patients rapidly, increasing the likelihood of off-isocenter placements that may necessitate manual repositioning. This study introduces an anatomy-specific, automatic patient positioning control algorithm that predicts required positioning corrections. To support this, we developed and evaluated a segmentation and post-processing pipeline designed to provide actionable feedback to the user. Two annotation strategies – morphological and abstract – were employed. Experimental results show a mean error of 0.35 ± 1.27 mm on the shoulder using morphological annotations and 0.50 ± 1.10 mm on the wrist using abstract annotations. These results suggest that the proposed approach achieves sufficient accuracy for integration into clinical MRI workflows based on the evaluated datasets.

1 Introduction

Magnetic resonance imaging (MRI) offers a non-invasive view into the human body revealing fine anatomical structures. Currently, MRI technologists manually plan sequences based on localizer images, which provide an anatomical overview over the field of view (FOV). Positioning the examined patient's anatomy accurately in the isocenter of the MRI scanner is therefore critical for the imaging procedure. This manual workflow is time-consuming and repetitive and gets particularly challenging for young or less-experienced practitioners. In high-throughput clinical workflows, where complex anatomies have to be scanned and interpreted in just minutes, the pressure to work quickly magnifies the chance for human errors. Those risk patient safety and undermine reproducibility across follow-up scans [1]. Additionally, it is important to position the region of interest as close as possible to the isocenter, where field homogeneity is highest, to achieve clinically optimal image quality. Consequently, automated planning of magnetic resonance scans has gained increasing

© Der/die Autor(en), exklusiv lizenziert an
Springer Fachmedien Wiesbaden GmbH, ein Teil von Springer Nature 2026
H. Handels et al. (Hrsg.), *Bildverarbeitung für die Medizin 2026*,
Informatik aktuell, https://doi.org/10.1007/978-3-658-51100-5_34

attention, aiming to reduce variability and standardize acquisition. Recently, machine learning-based image processing has allowed for automatic, accurate, and fast analysis of unseen anatomies, including patient positioning in localizer images [2, 3]. In [4], the performance of a deep learning-based pipeline for automated MRI scan positioning was evaluated. This algorithm includes two major steps, namely a region proposal step that extracts a volume of interest followed by an orientation plane segmentation.

The objective of this proof-of-concept study is twofold. First, we segmented 3D scout images using a prototype deep learning-based pipeline to extract morphological regions. For this purpose, we trained nnU-Net [5], which is a self-configuring framework for medical image segmentation, to generate segmentation masks. We ultimately tested our end-to-end pipeline on real-world MRI scans and evaluated it using pre-defined evaluation metrics. Second, we exploited the predicted segmentation masks in a post-processing step to assess the patient positioning in the FOV. Our method aims to automatically validate the correct patient positioning and give feedback to the technologist. Fig. 1 shows our proposed pipeline. The following sections detail our methodology, from data segmentation to post-processing, and discuss the results obtained from testing on clinical MR data. In summary, the main contributions of this paper are:

1. We implemented a deep learning image processing pipeline that segments MR localizer scans and post-processes the predicted segmentation masks to correct positioning of the patient. In addition, we used two different annotation strategies, namely morphological and abstract annotations.
2. We conducted a thorough evaluation of the employed segmentation model and further predicted anatomy positionings on two human anatomies.

2 Materials and methods

2.1 Data acquisition

In this study, the automated slice planning is based on segmenting anatomies of interest on MR scouts and postprocessing the predicted landmarks. We examined two human body regions: the shoulder and the wrist. We trained our model using 3D full-resolution MR localizer volumes. All scans were acquired using a scout sequence with a repetition time (TR) of 3.4 ms and an echo time (TE) of 1.29 ms. For the shoulder, the data had a resolution of (288 × 176 × 120) and a median slice thickness of 1.57 mm. For the wrist, the resolution was (224 × 224 × 80) with a slice thickness of 2.0 mm. The dataset comprised 34 shoulder and 29 wrist scans for training, and 14 cases of each anatomy were reserved for testing. Data were acquired using MRI scanners spanning 0.55 T, 1.5 T and 3 T (Siemens Healthineers scanner models) to mirror clinical variability. To increase robustness, the training set included both correctly centered scans and scans deliberately translated along the z-axis by 50–15 mm. This range was a design choice, to emulate off-center positioning observed in routine clinical workflows.

2.2 Annotation strategies

For this study, we adopted two labeling strategies (Fig. 2). For the shoulder, three different bones were delineated: scapula, humerus, and clavicula following a detailed morphological annotation. For the wrist, we adapted a geometrical segmentation approach, using spheres to mark approximate regions of the forearm, carpus, meta carpus, and thumb. Our purpose for the wrist annotation is to locate the overall position of the anatomies rather than the detailed anatomical boundaries.

2.3 Model training

Our approach builds upon nnU-Net [5], a framework that automatically configures segmentation pipelines. We employed the 3D full-resolution configuration for both anatomies, following the framework's standard self-configuring pipeline without architectural or hyperparameter modifications. We trained each anatomy separately, as their morphology and label definitions differ. For every dataset, nnU-Net automatically determined preprocessing parameters such as resampling, normalization, and patch size. The training was performed for 1000 epochs using a five-fold cross-validation scheme as recommended by the nnU-Net baseline.

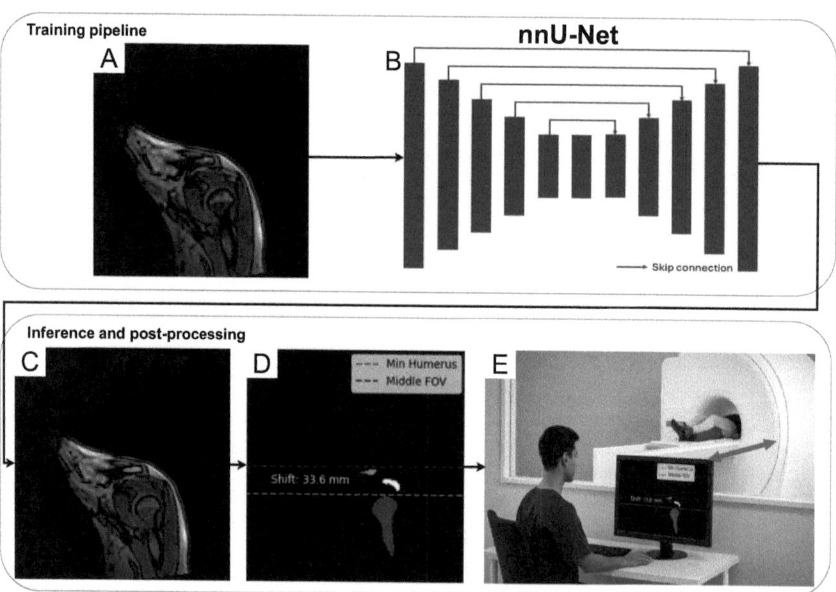

Fig. 1. Proposed pipeline for acquisition planning. During model development, raw MR scout scans (A) are manually annotated to construct the training dataset and used to train the nnU-Net framework (B). During inference, the trained model predicts 3D segmentation masks from raw localizer images (C), which are subsequently post-processed to define reference structures and estimate an anatomical shift along the z-axis (D). This shift is provided as a recommendation for patient table translation during scan planning (E).

2.4 Post-processing

After inference, we post-process the predicted segmentation masks to calculate the optimal patient positioning along the z-axis (Fig. 3). For this step, we define landmarks for shoulder and wrist: the upper point of the humerus mask and the center of mass of the central reference sphere, respectively. For each landmark, we calculate the shift to the midline in z-direction of the scan in mm. This shift serves as a feedback for the technologist indicating how to shift the patient to be centered in the field of view. An overview of the implemented pipeline is illustrated in Fig. 1.

2.5 Evaluation

To assess the anatomical localization accuracy, we used the Dice similarity coefficient (DSC), a widely used metric for medical image segmentation tasks [6]. It is calculated per test case at the anatomy level to quantify how well the predicted segmentation aligned with the expected annotations [6]. In addition to the DSC, we defined an error shift, which is calculated as the signed difference between the predicted and the ground truth landmarks defined in the previous section. It reflects in the magnitude and direction of the anatomical repositioning required to ensure proper placement within the field of view (FoV).

3 Results

We present quantitative results for the proposed anatomical positioning pipeline based on nnU-Net segmentation, evaluated across two anatomies (shoulder and

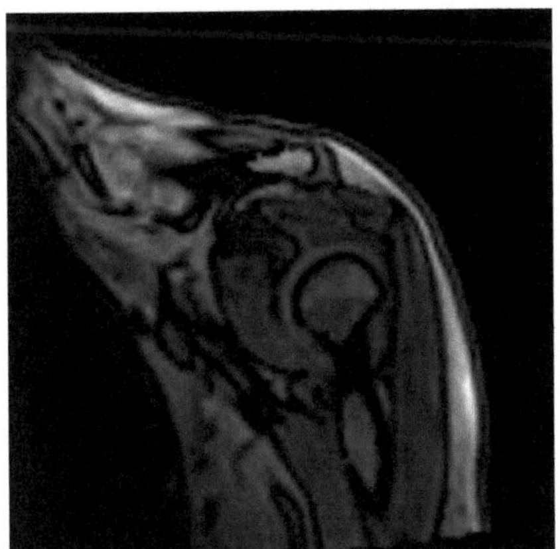

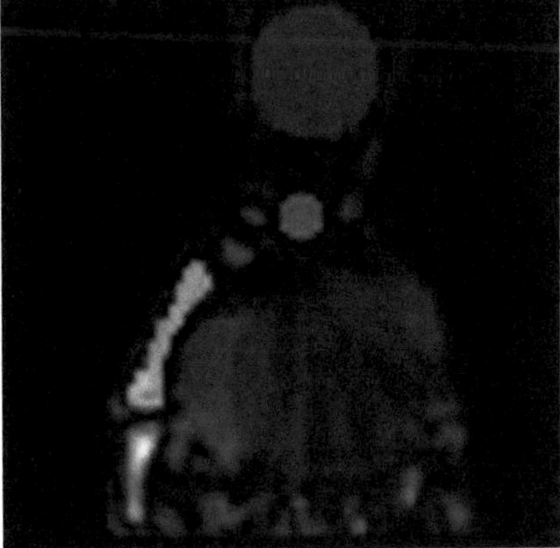

Fig. 2. Annotation techniques. Shoulder morphological annotation: humerus in red, clavicle in green, and scapula in blue. Wrist abstract annotation: forearm in red, carpus in green, metacarpus in blue, and thumb in yellow. Both figures are slices taken from a 3D localizer volume.

Anatomy	Error Shift (mm)	Dice Scores
Shoulder	0.35 ± 1.27	Humerus: 0.95 ± 0.01 Clavicle: 0.51 ± 0.15 Scapula: 0.77 ± 0.03
Wrist	0.50 ± 1.10	Forearm: 0.79 ± 0.09 Carpus: 0.85 ± 0.06 Metacarpus: 0.89 ± 0.05 Thumb: 0.78 ± 0.05

Tab. 1. Mean and standard deviation (std dev) of the z-axis error shift and Dice scores for both anatomies using both labeling techniques.

wrist). Predicted segmentations were evaluated using the DSC label-wise. In addition, we introduced another metric to assess the performance of our entire pipeline: the difference in anatomical shift (in mm) between the ground truth and inferred masks. The shift quantifies the predicted structure's position along the z-axis, which is critical for guiding optimal MRI slice positioning. A summary of all results is presented in Tab. 1.

For the shoulder, nnU-Net demonstrated a mean DSC of 0.95 ± 0.01 for the humerus. The evaluation of clavicle and scapula showed DSC performances of 0.77 ± 0.03 and 0.51 ± 0.15, respectively. For the wrist, nnU-Net demonstrated consistent performance across all four labels (Tab. 1).

In addition to segmentation accuracy, we assessed how precisely the predicted segmentations enabled estimation of the anatomical z-shift. For the shoulder, the mean difference in the shift between the prediction and the ground truth was 0.35 ± 1.27 mm. For the wrist, the shift error was comparable to the shoulder (0.50 ± 1.10 mm).

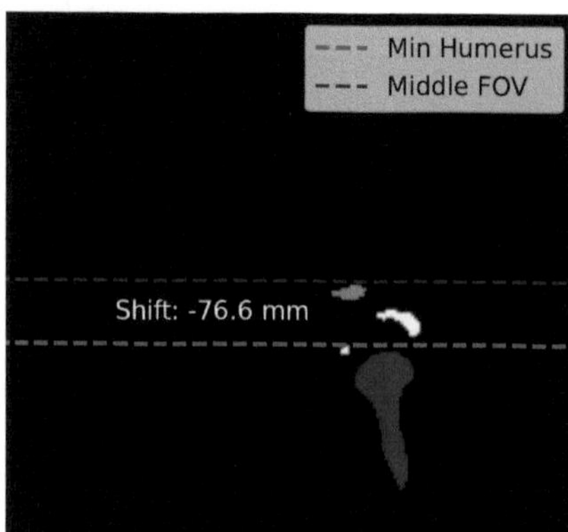

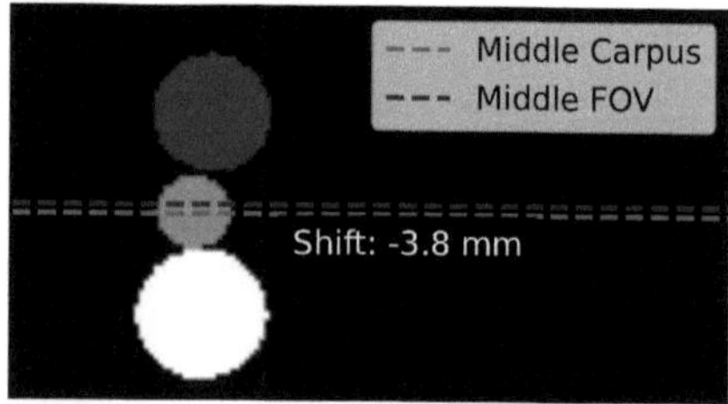

Fig. 3. Shift calculation for the shoulder (left) and the wrist (right). For the shoulder, we used the upper point of the humerus as a landmark whereas for the wrist we considered the center of mass of the carpus. For both landmarks, we calculated the distance to the middle FOV.

4 Discussion

The quantitative results demonstrate that nnU-Net achieves strong and consistent segmentation across both anatomies. In fact, the high Dice scores, particularly for the humerus and wrist bones, translate into robustness in segmenting anatomies with sub-millimeter error in the estimated anatomical shift. The lower scapula score may be attributed to anatomical complexity and lower contrast in the MRI images, leading to occasional false negatives or missed boundaries. However, these limitations did not substantially affect downstream positioning estimation.

The low standard deviations on the wrist labels highlight the generalizability of the model in various test cases. Even though the shoulder segmentation showed slightly lower DSC for some labels (e.g., scapula), the predicted position of the humerus, used as a primary reference, was sufficiently accurate to successfully reposition the anatomy.

Although the abstract annotation does not capture detailed anatomical boundaries, it showed consistent shift estimation, which suggests that precise annotation is not required for z-direction centering. Even though the z-shift is derived from a single reference region, predicting multiple labels in both annotation strategies provides additional spatial context. This reduces sensitivity to cropped anatomy within the FOV and enables the use of complementary reference structures for more-advanced repositioning tasks.

Overall, our proposed pipeline demonstrated strong and consistent segmentation across both anatomies, providing sub-millimeter accuracy in predicting anatomical shifts. Such precision ensures that the numeric shift vector can be trusted to adjust the patient table without requiring a repeat scout. From a technical perspective, vendor guidelines recommend a rescan by a detected shift exceeding 30 mm in z-direction, which indicates a mis-centering within the FOV. However, this threshold remains anatomy- and protocol-specific. The proposed system therefore serves as a proof-of-concept for a quantitative aid, offering objective feedback while leaving the final decision to the technologist's or radiologist's expertise.

The proposed end-to-end deep learning-based pipeline, trained and evaluated on labeled shoulder and wrist localizer scans using both morphological and abstract annotations, thus offers a practical solution for automatic anatomical localization in 3D MR localizer scans. By computing an anatomical shift along the z-axis that can be directly communicated to the technologist, the method might support efficient and standardized patient positioning in the future, reducing workflow time, minimizing unnecessary rescans, and improving reproducibility and quality of MRI examinations.

References

1. Lecouvet FE, Claus J, Schmitz P, Denolin V, Bos C, Vande Berg BC. Clinical evaluation of automated scan prescription of knee MR images. J Magn Reson Imaging. 2009;29(1):141–5.

2. Hornegger J. AI makes medicine more efficient, individual and preventive. Work and AI 2030. Ed. by Knappertsbusch I, Gondlach K. Springer, 2023:297–304.
3. Li C, Bhatia P, Zhao Y. Knee orientation detection in MR scout scans using 3D U-net. Proc SPIE MI CAD. 2020;11314:869–75.
4. Zhao Y, Zeng K, Zhao Y, Bhatia P, Ranganath M, Kozhikkavil ML et al. Deep learning solution for medical image localization and orientation detection. Med Image Anal. 2022;81:102529.
5. Isensee F, Jaeger PF, Kohl SA, Petersen J, Maier-Hein KH. nnU-net: a self-configuring method for deep learning-based biomedical image segmentation. Nat Methods. 2021;18(2):203–11.
6. Müller D, Soto-Rey I, Kramer F. Towards a guideline for evaluation metrics in medical image segmentation. BMC Res Notes. 2022;15(1):210.

Abstract: Speckle2Self

Self-supervised Ultrasound Speckle Reduction Without Clean Data

Xuesong Li [1,2], Nassir Navab [1,2], Zhongliang Jiang [1,2]

[1]Computer Aided Medical Procedures (CAMP), Technical University of Munich, Munich, Germany

[2]Munich Center for Machine Learning (MCML), Munich, Germany

zl.jiang@tum.de

Image denoising is a fundamental task in computer vision, particularly in medical ultrasound (US) imaging, where speckle noise significantly degrades image quality. Although recent advancements in deep neural networks have led to substantial improvements in denoising for natural images, these methods cannot be directly applied to US speckle noise, as it is not purely random. Instead, US speckle arises from complex wave interference within the body microstructure, making it tissue-dependent. This dependency means that obtaining two independent noisy observations of the same scene, as required by pioneering Noise2Noise, is not feasible. Additionally, blind-spot networks also cannot handle US speckle noise due to its high spatial dependency. To address this challenge, we introduce Speckle2Self [1], a novel self-supervised algorithm for speckle reduction using only single noisy observations. The key insight is that applying a multi-scale perturbation (MSP) operation introduces tissue-dependent variations in the speckle pattern across different scales, while preserving the shared anatomical structure. This enables effective speckle suppression by modeling the clean image as a low-rank signal and isolating the sparse noise component. To demonstrate its effectiveness, Speckle2Self is comprehensively compared with conventional filter-based denoising algorithms and SOTA learning-based methods, using both realistic simulated US images and human carotid US images. Additionally, data from multiple US machines are employed to evaluate model generalization and adaptability to images from unseen domains. Project page: https://noseefood.github.io/us-speckle2self/

References

1. Li X, Navab N, Jiang Z. Speckle2Self: self-supervised ultrasound speckle reduction without clean data. Med Image Anal. 2025;106:103755.

© Der/die Autor(en), exklusiv lizenziert an
Springer Fachmedien Wiesbaden GmbH, ein Teil von Springer Nature 2026
H. Handels et al. (Hrsg.), *Bildverarbeitung für die Medizin 2026*,
Informatik aktuell, https://doi.org/10.1007/978-3-658-51100-5_35

Distil or Cluster?
Data-efficient Learning for Ultrasound in Practice

Jennifer Ochmann[1†], Johanna P. Müller [1†], Franciskus X. Erick [1], Bernhard Kainz [1,2]

[1]Department of Artificial Intelligence in Biomedical Engineering, Friedrich-Alexander-Universität Erlangen-Nürnberg, DE
[2]Department of Computing, Imperial College London, UK
johanna.paula.mueller@fau.de

Abstract. Training deep learning models on ultrasound videos is like drinking from a firehose, most frames are redundant or noisy, yet drive high computational cost. We ask: can we learn just as well from less? We benchmark coreset construction, clustering, dataset distillation, and random sampling on large-scale echocardiography datasets. Clustering-based coresets, especially those using CNN embeddings, Wasserstein distance, and two-pass DBSCAN, match or surpass full-data training while reducing cost by up to 15×. They also rival dataset distillation in accuracy but are up to 30× faster. Surprisingly, random subsets sometimes outperform engineered coresets, with macro-F1 peaking at just 5% of the data. These results show that *less can be more*, offering a scalable path to efficient, fair training in medical video analysis.

1 Introduction

Deep learning has transformed medical image analysis, enabling classification, segmentation, and motion tracking [1]. Ultrasound video, particularly echocardiography, illustrates both promise and challenges: each study has thousands of often redundant frames [2], making full-dataset training costly and potentially harmful to generalisation. Deep networks can automate interpretation, predicting ejection fraction at cardiologist-level accuracy [2] and detecting hypertrophy [3], but rely on large, often redundant datasets. Coreset construction (CC) selects small, representative subsets to preserve performance while reducing cost [4], typically via clustering or embedding-space sampling for diversity and class balance [5], yet remains underused in video-based medical AI. Dataset distillation (DD) creates synthetic samples approximating the training distribution [6, 7], refined by gradient matching or last-layer Laplace and Wasserstein regularisation [8]. DD is effective on CIFAR and ImageNet but costly and largely unexplored for high-dimensional temporal data. Random sampling offers a simple baseline [9], competitive when redundancy is

[†]These authors contributed equally to this work.

© Der/die Autor(en), exklusiv lizenziert an Springer Fachmedien Wiesbaden GmbH, ein Teil von Springer Nature 2026
H. Handels et al. (Hrsg.), *Bildverarbeitung für die Medizin 2026*, Informatik aktuell, https://doi.org/10.1007/978-3-658-51100-5_36

high but prone to class imbalance in small subsets. Video datasets such as EchoNet-Dynamic [2] and EchoNet-LVH [3] feature temporal redundancy, frame imbalance, and high computational costs, making them ideal for data-efficient evaluation. Methods like EchoDFKD [10], latent dynamic diffusion models [11], and uncertainty-aware coreset-distillation hybrids [12] demonstrate structured, efficient training. We systematically benchmark clustering-based coresets, dataset distillation, and random sampling for echocardiography classification, analysing accuracy, macro-F1, subset size, and runtime. Our contributions are: (1) benchmarking coreset strategies across multiple datasets, (2) showing CNN-embedding clustering coresets match or surpass DD while 10–30× faster, (3) demonstrating $\sim 5\,\%$ of data suffices for near-full performance, with random subsets competitive at moderate compression, and (4) providing practical guidance for scalable, fair medical AI. By showing that *less can be more*, we establish coreset construction as a practical tool for efficient, scalable, and fair medical video training.

2 Methodology

We consider CC for video datasets, where each video has n frames $x_i \in \mathbb{R}^{H\times W}$, aiming to select $\mathcal{S} \subset \mathcal{X}$ such that a model f_θ trained on $\mathcal{S}$ performs comparably to one trained on $\mathcal{X}$

$$\mathcal{S} = \arg \min_{\mathcal{S}\subset\mathcal{X},|\mathcal{S}|\ll|\mathcal{X}|} \mathcal{L}_{\text{val}}(f_\theta(\mathcal{S}), y) \tag{1}$$

with $\mathcal{L}_{\text{val}}$ the validation loss. Frames are embedded via PCA, proper orthogonal decomposition (POD), or CNN features $\phi(x)$ (CNNFE), capturing linear or semantic structure. Pairwise similarity between embeddings $\mathbf{z}_i$ and $\mathbf{z}_j$ is measured using vector-space distances

$$d_{\text{Euclidean}} = ||\mathbf{z}_i - \mathbf{z}_j||_2 \tag{2}$$

$$d_{\text{spherical}} = \arccos \frac{\mathbf{z}_i^\top \mathbf{z}_j}{||\mathbf{z}_i||\,||\mathbf{z}_j||} \tag{3}$$

or probability-space divergences (after softmax normalisation $\mathbf{P}_i = \text{softmax}(\mathbf{z}_i)$) such as Jensen-Shannon divergence (JS), Total variation distance of probability measures (TVD), and Wasserstein W_1. Frames are clustered using k-medoids (KM) or density-based spatial clustering of applications with noise (DB1/DB2). In DB1, ϵ is set to the mean nearest-neighbour distance; DB2 re-applies clustering to noise points. K-medoids selects medoids $\{m_1, \ldots, m_k\}$ by minimising the sum of distances

$$\{m_1, \ldots, m_k\} = \arg \min_{\mathcal{M}\subset\mathcal{X}} \sum_{x_i\in\mathcal{X}} \min_{m_l\in\mathcal{M}} d(z_i, m_l) \tag{4}$$

Coresets are formed by sampling proportionally from each cluster, with at least one frame per cluster, $n_l = \max\left(1, \lfloor |C_l||\mathcal{S}|/n \rfloor\right)$, and noise points are included in DB-based methods.

DD generates a synthetic set $\mathcal{S}$ approximating the feature distribution of $\mathcal{X}$ via MMD:

$$\mathcal{L}_{\text{MMD}} = \left\| \frac{1}{|\mathcal{X}|} \sum_{x_i} \phi_\theta(x_i) - \frac{1}{|\mathcal{S}|} \sum_{s_j} \phi_\theta(s_j) \right\|^2 \tag{5}$$

optimised by gradient descent, and the final coreset comprises real frames closest to the distilled samples in feature space. Combining three feature embeddings, five distance measures, and three clustering strategies yields forty-five coreset variants for comprehensive evaluation.

3 Results

3.1 Datasets and Metrics

We evaluate three echocardiography video datasets: EchoNet-Dynamic (EN-D) [2] with 10,030 apical-4-chamber videos annotated for ejection fraction and volumes; EchoNet-Paediatric (EN-P) [2] with similar paediatric data; and EchoNet-LVH (EN-LVH) [3] with 12,000 parasternal long-axis videos annotated for septal and wall thickness. In addition, we include the ImageNet Video Visual Relation (VidVRD) dataset [13], a large-scale natural video benchmark for visual relation detection, containing object trajectories and spatiotemporal relationship annotations across diverse action-centric scenes. Datasets are frame-extracted for embedding, clustering, and coreset construction. Performance is evaluated via accuracy (Acc), macro-F1 (mF1), subset size, and construction time, reflecting predictive and computational efficiency.

3.2 Results

Tab. 1 presents Acc and mF1 for ResNet18 models trained on IN and EN-D coresets. On IN, Wasserstein CNNFE achieves the highest Acc on DB2 (21.19 %) and the highest mF1 on KM (9.05 %, Euclidean CNNFE (ResNet18 [14])). For EchoNet-Dynamic, Wasserstein CNNFE attains the highest Acc and mF1 on DB2 (79.86 % and 47.18 %). Euclidean and Spherical coresets produce competitive results across sub-datasets, with CNNFE and PCA variants often reaching top mF1. JS and TVD metrics show more variable performance. DD achieves 21.93 % Acc and 8.11 % mF1 on IN, and 78.70 % Acc and 43.22 % mF1 on EN-D.

Fig. 1 shows Acc and mF1 for ResNet18 models trained on EchoNet-Dynamic coresets of varying sizes (1%, 5%, 10%, 20%). Clustering-based coresets achieve the highest Acc at 20% (79.86 %) and highest mF1 at 10% (44.54 %). DD coresets reach 78.70 % Acc and 43.22 % mF1 at 10%. Random selection performs lower or comparably (Acc 67.23–77.43 %, mF1 34.27–45.62 %). All models are benchmarked against the full dataset (horizontal lines: Acc 76.76 %, mF1 41.09 %).

Fig. 2 shows Acc versus runtime for EN-D, EN-P, and EN-LVH across All Frames, DD, Clustering (CNNFE-DB2 with Wasserstein distance), and Random. DD has the highest runtime (EN-D: 214.10h; EN-P: 45.71h; EN-LVH: 216.01h), followed by Clustering, All Frames, and Random. For EN-D, All Frames achieves the highest accuracy (78.97 %) and mF1 (45.21 %) in 3.18h, while Random is lowest

Tab. 1. Classification accuracy (Acc) and macro F1 (mF1) (%) of ResNet18 [14] models trained on ImageNet Video Visual Relation and EchoNet-Dynamic coresets. *1st-ranked.*

		ImageNet Video Visual Relation						EchoNet-Dynamic					
		DB2		DB1		KM		DB2		DB1		KM	
Method	Variant	Acc	mF1	Acc	mF1	Acc	mF1	Acc	mF1	Acc	mF1	Acc	mF1
All	–		-	16.99	6.54	-			-	78.97	45.21	-	
Rand.	–		-	18.74	7.22	-			-	76.76	41.09	-	
Wasserst.	POD	21.19	7.96	20.15	7.93	18.55	7.24	77.84	45.74	76.62	46.03	63.35	42.63
	PCA	19.94	8.54	19.54	6.94	16.08	5.66	78.22	46.11	58.29	42.11	67.87	45.57
	CNNFE	20.65	7.22	10.95	5.02	12.07	5.74	**79.86**	41.67	76.27	46.18	70.97	**47.18**
Euclid.	POD	18.45	7.18	21.11	8.13	20.02	7.79	73.20	43.84	77.61	46.28	78.74	46.16
	PCA	19.64	7.21	19.48	7.53	20.49	7.62	78.69	42.49	78.24	46.11	67.81	44.96
	CNNFE	19.96	6.80	20.20	7.54	21.88	**9.05**	77.84	44.62	71.67	44.46	68.19	42.51
Spherical	POD	20.23	7.93	19.86	7.54	17.54	6.71	78.86	45.93	70.62	45.32	77.96	43.91
	PCA	19.91	7.12	15.76	6.07	20.81	8.27	74.35	46.22	68.18	42.19	74.66	46.62
	CNNFE	18.34	7.81	19.91	6.80	19.32	7.42	77.91	45.83	72.41	47.09	78.01	45.61
JS	POD	15.28	5.91	15.31	5.95	18.50	6.76	72.61	46.94	75.64	44.38	77.94	44.30
	PCA	19.06	7.26	20.33	7.40	19.75	6.56	70.17	45.65	75.16	44.32	76.88	45.39
	CNNFE	20.97	7.6	13.24	5.95	21.69	8.56	76.61	46.53	77.52	45.01	71.32	46.67
TVD	POD	20.36	7.10	17.76	6.52	11.11	4.82	72.15	45.42	75.41	45.45	76.33	46.71
	PCA	19.62	6.79	20.28	7.87	20.52	7.12	73.35	42.08	74.92	46.44	75.92	45.91
	CNNFE	19.25	6.50	**22.06**	8.44	19.91	7.99	68.10	44.01	72.52	42.47	75.15	44.49
DD	–		-	21.93	8.11	-			-	78.70	43.22	-	

(Acc 66.61 %, mF1 41.89 %, 0.18h) and DD slightly lower (Acc 78.70 %, mF1 43.22 %, 214.10h). For EN-P, All Frames has highest accuracy (84.72 %, 0.01h) and DD highest mF1 (42.71 %, 45.71h). For EN-LVH, Random reaches top accuracy

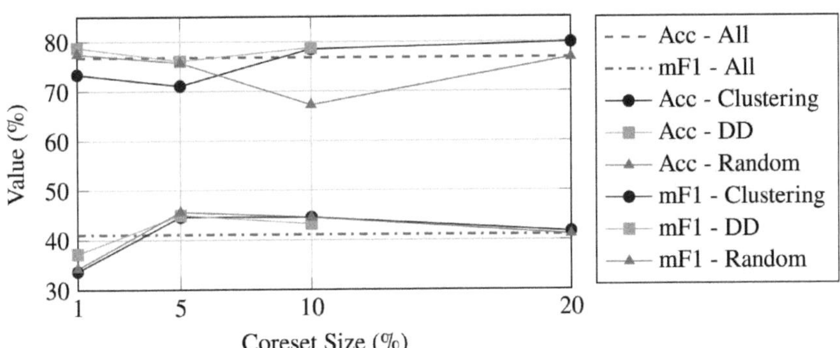

Fig. 1. Classification accuracy (Acc) and macro F1 score (mF1) of ResNet18 models trained on coresets of varying sizes (1%, 5%, 10%, 20%) from the EchoNet-Dynamic dataset. Lines correspond to different coreset selection methods: Clustering, DD, and Random.

(94.50 %) and mF1 (50.65 %, 0.01h), with DD similar (Acc 94.38 %, mF1 48.98 %, 216.01h).

4 Discussion

4.1 Dataset Distillation

DD produces compact synthetic sets approximating the full data distribution (e.g., 78.70 % Acc, 43.22 % mF1 on EN-D) but is computationally expensive, often exceeding 200h (Fig. 2). Clustering-based coresets achieve similar or better performance (CNNFE-Wasserstein on EN-D: 79.86 % Acc, 47.18 % mF1) at a fraction of the runtime. Trends on IR suggest DD's marginal gains rarely justify its cost.

4.1.1 Coresets for Ultrasound. Ultrasound datasets, with low signal-to-noise ratios and high intra-class variability, benefit from clustering-based coresets over linear methods or random sampling. CNN embeddings with Wasserstein or Euclidean distances capture clinically relevant dynamics, and small coresets (5–10 %) retain near-full performance. IN confirms these principles generalise beyond medical imaging.

4.1.2 Coresets vs Random Subsets. Random 10–20 % subsets sometimes match mF1 of clustering coresets, suggesting class coverage and temporal diversity suffice for moderate compression. Clustering coresets outperform random selection under extreme compression (1–5 %), capturing rare patterns, a trend consistent on IN.

4.1.3 Distance Metrics and Embeddings. CNN embeddings consistently outperform linear embeddings. Wasserstein distances favour representative frames, especially in ultrasound sequences with subtle motion; JS and TVD metrics vary, while Euclidean and spherical distances remain competitive, balancing quality and runtime.

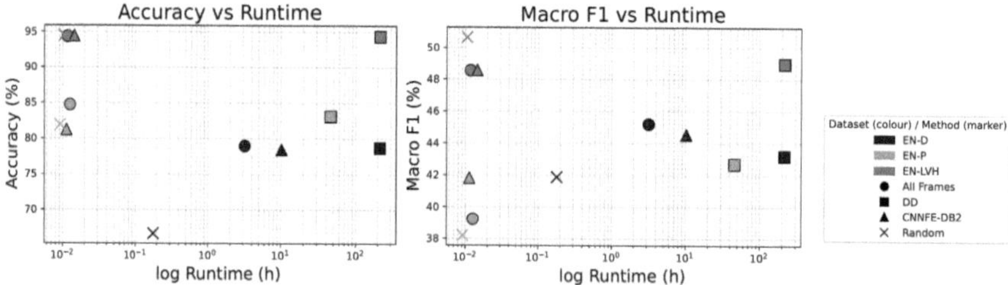

Fig. 2. Comparison of performance metrics (Accuracy / MF1) versus runtime for different coreset construction methods across datasets. Methods are DD, CNNFE DB2 Wasserstein, Random subset.

4.2 Practical Guidelines

Fig. 3 summarises recommendations: for high compression in ultrasound data, use clustering-based coresets with CNN embeddings, particularly for rare patterns. Random subsets suffice for moderate compression or limited resources and should be included as baselines. DD is generally not cost-effective for high-dimensional medical videos. Wasserstein or Euclidean distances with CNN embeddings balance selection quality and runtime; linear embeddings are useful in low-resource settings but less performant. Integrating uncertainty-aware regularisation (e.g., Laplace last-layer calibration, ensemble consistency) produces efficient, well-calibrated, class-balanced coresets.

5 Conclusion

We evaluated data-efficient strategies for ultrasound video classification, including coreset construction, dataset distillation, and random sampling. Clustering-based coresets with CNN embeddings and distributional distances provide the most practical, efficient solution, matching or surpassing distillation performance at a fraction of the cost. As little as $\sim 5\,\%$ of the data often achieves near-full accuracy, with random subsets remaining competitive at moderate compression. Future work may integrate lightweight distillation, temporal redundancy, and uncertainty-aware objectives for efficient, calibrated pseudocoresets. Overall, our findings show that *less can be more*, establishing coreset construction as a scalable and fair approach for clinical AI.

Acknowledgement. The authors gratefully acknowledge the scientific support and HPC resources provided by the Erlangen National High Performance Computing Center (NHR@FAU) under the NHR projects b143dc and b180dc. NHR funding is provided by federal and Bavarian state authorities. NHR@FAU hardware is partially funded by the German Research Foundation (DFG) – 440719683. Additional support

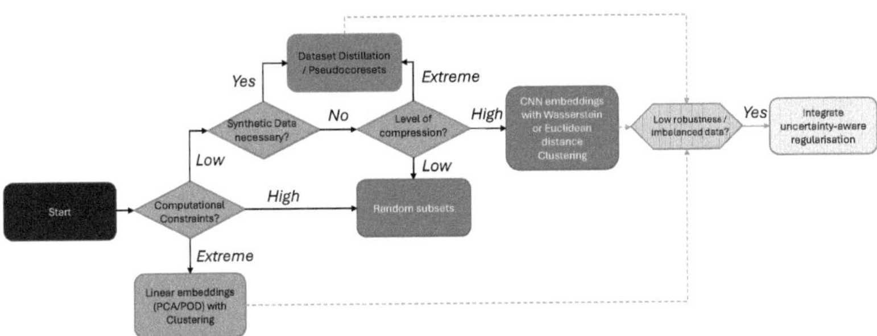

Fig. 3. Decision diagram for selecting data-efficient training strategies in medical video analysis. Choices depend on compression level, computational constraints, and robustness needs.

was also received by the ERC – project MIA-NORMAL 101083647, DFG KA 5801/2-1, INST 90/1351-1 and by the state of Bavaria.

References

1. Litjens G, Kooi T, Bejnordi BE, Setio AAA, Ciompi F, Ghafoorian M et al. A survey on deep learning in medical image analysis. Med Image Anal. 2017;42:60–88.
2. Ouyang D, He B, Ghorbani A, Lungren MP, Ashley EA, Liang DH et al. Video-based AI for beat-to-beat assessment of cardiac function. Nature. 2020;580(7802):252–6.
3. Zhang J, Ghorbani A, Ouyang D, He B, Takeda A, al. et. EchoNet-LVH: detecting left ventricular hypertrophy using echocardiography videos. NPJ Digit Med. 2021;4(1):1–8.
4. Bachem O, Lucic M, Krause A. Practical coreset constructions for machine learning. arXiv: 1703.06476. 2017.
5. Sener O, Savarese S. Active learning for convolutional neural networks: a core-set approach. Proc ICLR. 2018.
6. Wang T, Zhu JY, Torralba A, Efros AA. Dataset distillation. Proc ICLR. 2018:519–28.
7. Zhao B, Bilen H. Dataset condensation with gradient matching. Proc ICLR. 2021.
8. Erick FX, Müller JP, Li Z, Kainz B. Last layer Laplacian pseudocoresets for robust medical image analysis. Proc MICCAI. 2025.
9. Toneva M, Sordoni A, Combes RT des, Trischler A, Bengio Y. An empirical study of example forgetting during deep neural network learning. Proc ICLR. 2019.
10. Petit G, Palluau N, Bauer A, Dlaska C. EchoDFKD: data-free knowledge distillation for cardiac ultrasound segmentation using synthetic data. Proc IEEE/CVF WACV. 2025.
11. Chen T, Shi Y, Zheng Z, Yan B, Hu J, Zhu XX et al. Ultrasound image-to-video synthesis via latent dynamic diffusion models. Proc MICCAI. 2024.
12. Xiong Y, Xu Y, Zhang Y, Du B. Distilling OCT cervical dataset with evidential uncertainty proxy. Image Vis Comput. 2024;151:105250.
13. Shang X, Ren T, Guo J, Zhang H, Chua TS. Video visual relation detection. Proc ACM MM. 2017.
14. He K, Zhang X, Ren S, Sun J. Deep residual learning for image recognition. Proc IEEE CVPR. 2016:770–8.

Scanliner with Integrated Fiducial Markers for 3D-reconstruction of Residual Limbs using Ultrasound Imaging

Anna-Lisa Allgaier[1†], Katrin Volk[1†], Anja Zillner[1†], Luise Robra[1], Jonas Bornmann[2], Andreas Leiniger[2], Rainer Brucher[1], Alfred M. Franz[1,3]

[1]Institute for Mechatronics and Medical Engineering, Ulm University of Applied Sciences
[2]Ottobock SE and Co. KGaA
[3]Institute for Computer Science, Ulm University of Applied Sciences
alfred.franz@thu.de

Abstract. The loss of a lower limb severely affects mobility and quality of life, with the fit of the prosthesis being essential for user comfort and functionality. Techniques for manufacturing prosthetic sockets, such as plaster casting, are time-consuming and dependent on the prosthetist's expertise, while advanced imaging modalities like computed tomography (CT) and magnetic resonance imaging (MRI) are costly and introduce positioning-related inaccuracies. Ultrasound (US) presents a promising alternative for capturing both external and internal limb structures in a non-invasive manner, though mostly limited to 2D. This study investigates a novel approach for 3D reconstruction of US scans using a N-shaped fiducial pattern integrated into a liner applied to the limb. The fiducials facilitate registration of US images to reconstruct a 3D model. Validation on a limb phantom yielded an average reconstruction accuracy of 1.5 mm for bone and 1.7 mm for skin on a partial volume. While our findings demonstrate feasibility of the method, future work aims to enhance reconstruction accuracy by refining image alignment techniques and expanding the scanning approach to the whole limb.

1 Introduction

Limb loss severely impacts quality of life, with estimated 4 million individuals worldwide living with an amputation [1]. In Germany, approximately 150,000 people rely on a prosthetic leg, with 57 % experiencing moderate to severe pain, often due to insufficient prosthesis fit. Poor fit not only affects physical comfort but also reduces prosthesis usage and overall mobility [2]. To achieve an optimal fit between the residual limb and the prosthetic socket, accurate measurement of the limb geometry is essential. Conventional measurement techniques, such as plaster casting, are labor-intensive, time-consuming, and dependent on the prosthetist's expertise [1]. Optical three-dimensional (3D) scanning provides an objective alternative for capturing

[†]These authors contributed equally to this work.

© Der/die Autor(en), exklusiv lizenziert an
Springer Fachmedien Wiesbaden GmbH, ein Teil von Springer Nature 2026
H. Handels et al. (Hrsg.), *Bildverarbeitung für die Medizin 2026*,
Informatik aktuell, https://doi.org/10.1007/978-3-658-51100-5_37

external limb geometry but does not provide visualization of internal structures such as bones and soft tissues [2]. Advanced imaging modalities like computed tomography (CT) and magnetic resonance imaging (MRI) enable detailed assessment of internal anatomy. CT involves radiation exposure, and both CT and MRI are associated with high costs and long examination times. Additionally, the supine positioning required for these imaging modalities alters the natural shape of the limb, potentially reducing measurement accuracy [2, 3].

Ultrasound (US) presents a promising alternative, offering non-invasive imaging of both external and internal structures without the limitations of other methods [2]. A common approach for generating 3D volumes from 2D US images is tracked US, in which the probe pose is recorded by external tracking systems [4]. While this method offers high accuracy, it also introduces a much more complex setup compared to conventional US. Consequently, alternative approaches for trackerless 3D US are being explored. Prevost et al [5] replace traditional speckle decorrelation techniques by a convolutional neural network (CNN) to estimate motion between consecutive US frames. While this approach is promising and has already been adopted in some work outside the field of prosthetics, it only works reliably for uniform movement of the US probe.

Therefore, aids such as skin pads have already been discussed to improve the reconstruction process. For example, Dai et al. [6] introduced a coupling pad with embedded N-shaped lines to improve sensorless freehand 3D US reconstruction. Kingma et al. [7] investigated near-field fiducials to register CT and 3D US data. The objective of our study is applying the idea of these concepts to prosthetics by using a fiducial pattern integrated into a liner (*Scanliner*) that is pulled over the residual limb for the scanning process. These fiducials, consisting of air-filled silicone tubes arranged in a predefined configuration, facilitate registration of US images enabling reconstruction of a 3D model.

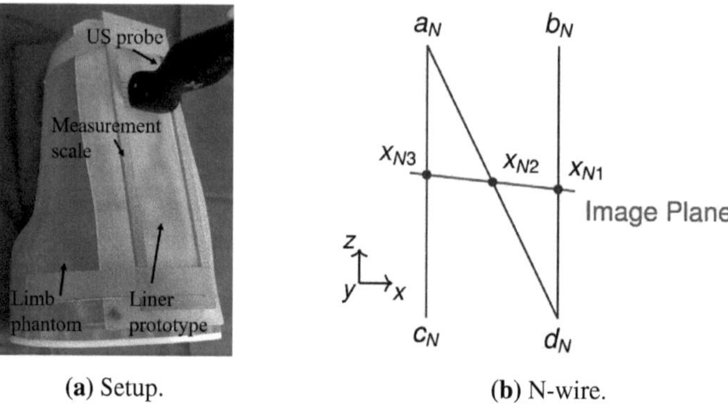

(a) Setup. **(b)** N-wire.

Fig. 1. (a) Setup for the scanning process of the residual limb phantom. (b) Geometry of the N-wire inside the liner.

2 Materials and methods

2.1 Scanliner and reconstruction method

As fiducial markers for alignment of US images we use a N-shaped fiducial pattern. It is included in a liner that is used between the skin and the US device for the scanning process. Our prototype used in this study is a rectangular section of the liner with the N-shaped fiducial pattern (Fig. 1a). The pattern is inspired by N-wire calibration dummies [8], which are also used to estimate the position of an US image. The prototype was manufactured using polyurethane and the wires are air-filled silicone cords with a diameter of 1 mm.

Automatic detection of these silicone cords involves several image analysis functions and two iterations (Fig. 2). The first iteration calculates the approximate position of each fiducial. The important parts of the image are separated from the background with a threshold value that is calculated based on the overall brightness of the area where the fiducials appear in the image (*Initial state 1*). Then the regions where the fiducials could not appear are set to black (*Result 1*). After that, the remaining white areas inside the image are labeled and the MATLAB function "regionprops" is used to identify adjacent white pixels. The identified regions are filtered by comparing the eccentricity with the ratio of 0.97 between the width and length of the adjacent pixels. The remaining regions are then improved by a rectangular (8 x 3 px) closing function followed by an opening function that removes connected pixels with less than 10 pixels. The second iteration now calculates the exact position by using only a preselected area from the first iteration, despite variations in brightness and small artifacts removed as described above. The remaining areas are counted and the three largest areas are selected (*Initial state* 2). A 10 x 10 px rectangle is drawn around these fiducials, the center of each is calculated and the three points are sorted from left to right. Then the weighted middle of these areas is calculated by determining a threshold for each fiducial. This is necessary because each fiducial appears in a different brightness. Each fiducial is extracted from the original image with the individual threshold and setting the area around the fiducial to black. Then the weighted

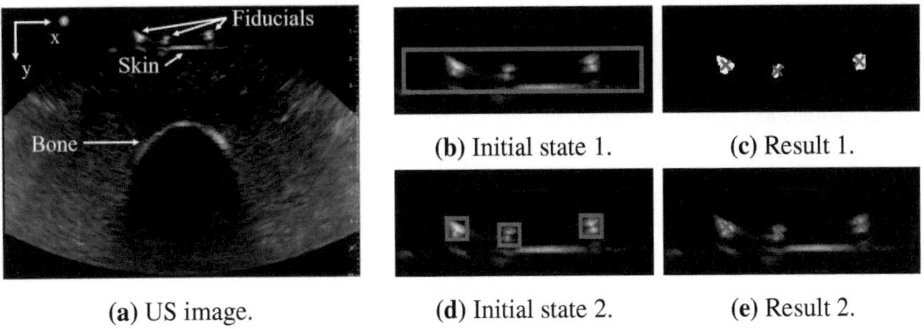

(a) US image. (b) Initial state 1. (c) Result 1. (d) Initial state 2. (e) Result 2.

Fig. 2. (a) US image of the residual limb phantom. (b-e) Initial states and results of the two iterations of the detection algorithm, where the area inside the red rectangles is analyzed.

middle point of the remaining area is calculated and used as the final fiducial point (*Result* 2).

The N-wire approach [8] is then used to calculate the position of an US image in the liner coordinate system from the detected fiducial positions. For using the equation

$$x_{N2} = a_N + \frac{||x_{I1} - x_{I2}||}{||x_{I1} - x_{I3}||}(d_N - a_N) \tag{1}$$

the N-wire geometry and the wire intersection positions in the US image plane must be known (Fig. 1b). The parameters a_N and d_N are the end points of the N-wire and the points x_{I1}, x_{I2}, and x_{I3} describe the fiducial points extracted from the image. The length of the N-wire is described by the direction z, while the width is described by the direction x. The utilization of a single N-wire limited the calculation to three degrees of freedom (DOF) based on the established pattern. Consequently, the test setup requires the probe to be positioned perpendicular to the N-wire, without any rotational deviation.

2.2 Experimental hardware and software setup

As US system, the iQ+ scanner (Butterfly Network, Inc., Burlington, Massachusetts, US) in the 'bladder' mode with a depth of 10 cm was used. The scanner was connected to a Galaxy Tab S6 (Samsung Electronics Co., Ltd., Suweon, South Korea) using a multiport adapter EE-P3200 (also from Samsung), which allows both the US probe to be connected via USB-C and a HDMI output to be used. The HDMI output was connected to a DVI2USB video grabber (Epiphan Systems Inc., Ottawa, Ontario, Canada) to transfer the live US image stream, in this case the tablet screen content, to a PC for further processing. The software used on the PC includes MATLAB (version 24.2.0.2712019 (R2024b)), the Public Software Library for Ultrasound Toolkit (PLUS, version Plus-2.8.0.62873a16), 3D Slicer (version 5.4.0) and the Medical Imaging Interaction Toolkit (MITK, version 2021.10). The MATLAB Code includes our algorithm for detection of fiducials in US images, the calculation of the transformation matrices, an optimization of the transformation matrices, and the calculation of the image spacing from known distances inside the US image. For the aforementioned optimization, we use the approach of Dai et al for compensating manufacturing inaccuracies in N-wire structures [6].

Our approach for freehand 3D reconstruction involves recording 2D B-mode US images with the liner for position calculation. After that, the position of each fiducial is determined in the US images and used to calculate the transformations as described above. We used the MetaImage (MHA) file format for storing the images together with their transformation matrices in 3D Slicer. With PLUS we reconstructed the 3D volume based on the MHA file. The same parameters as in [4] were set for the reconstruction algorithm: *Interpolation*: linear, *Compounding mode*: maximum, *Optimization*: partial and *Hole filling*: on. The structures of interest (skin and bone) were then manually segmented in the 3D US volume applying 3D Slicer. MITK was used to quantitatively evaluate the reconstruction accuracy by measuring the distances between CT reference and 3D US volume after registering them as described in the following.

2.3 Data recording and evaluation

For evaluation we used a phantom, which replicates anatomical and acoustic properties of a residual limb [4]. Markers are embedded into the phantom for registration between the reconstructed 3D model and a reference CT scan (Fig. 3). We recorded a series of 40 images with a distance of 5 mm between each image. Care was taken to ensure that all three fiducials were clearly visible and separated from each other. Liner and measurement scale were fixed at the lateral and proximal ends of the phantom, and the femur was scanned from proximal to distal. In addition, we recorded a continuous video of an additional sweep, similar to what one would expect in realistic use of the method, but this does not have a reference distance between the individual frames.

To assess the accuracy of fiducial detection in the image series, the distances between the reference positions and the positions calculated using the reconstruction method were determined. For evaluation of the video recording, skin and bone surfaces of the reconstructed 3D model and the surfaces of the CT reference were compared. The two data sets were registered by using the marker 1–4 (Fig. 3a). For both skin and bone, a point set consisting of eleven layers at equal intervals was defined (Fig. 3b). This resulted in a point set with $3 \cdot 11 = 33$ points for the skin and $5 \cdot 11 = 55$ points for the bone. For each pair of point sets, the average Euclidean distance was calculated.

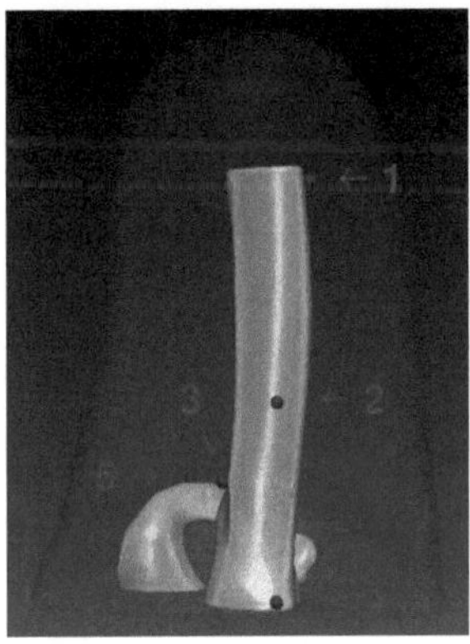

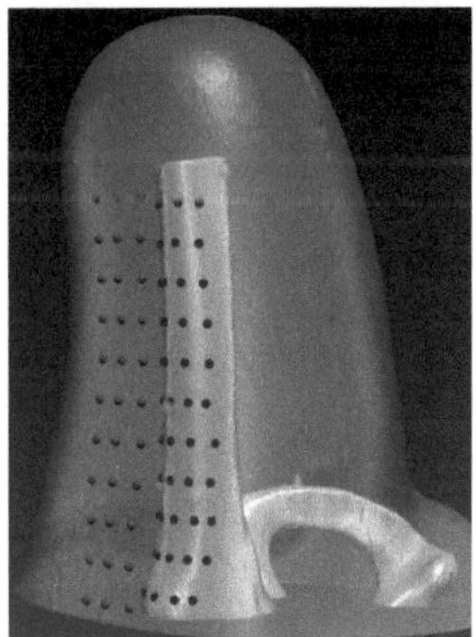

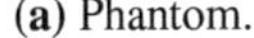

(a) Phantom.

(b) Point sets.

Fig. 3. (a) Residual limb phantom with registration markers in red. (b) Reference point sets on the bone (purple) and on the skin (green).

3 Results

The deviation from the reference position of the image series to the position calculated by our reconstruction method is 1.3 ± 1.0 mm ($\mu \pm \sigma$) on average. All values are visualized in Fig. 4a, where the x-axis shows the reference position on the liner, while the y-axis shows the deviation. The visual appearance of the registered models from the video recording with 301 frames of the residual limb phantom and the CT reference are shown in Fig. 5. The average distance of the 55 points on the bone is 1.5 ± 1.0 mm. For the 33 points on the skin the distance is 1.7 ± 1.7 mm.

4 Discussion and conclusion

The results of the 3D reconstruction are influenced by several factors. First, the image series indicate that the deviation is greater at both ends of the liner. This may be caused by the shape of the N-wire where two of the fiducials are positioned closer at the ends (Fig. 4a), leading to reflections in the US images. Second, the assumption that the N-wire inside the liner is a flat plane misses the deformation of the flexible liner, that deforms due to the adaption to the anatomic shape of the residual limb, i.e. the phantom. The shape of the liner could also be affected by not applying constant contact pressure when using the US probe. Another factor that affects our measurements is that US probes rely on constant speed of sound, typically 1540 m/s. Our phantom has a slightly different speed of sound, which leads to an offset of 6 % when comparing the CT scan to our results [4].

Despite the influencing factors that cause deviations, we consider our results promising as deviation errors for the image series of 1.3 ± 1.0 mm and segmentations from video-based reconstruction (skin: 1.7 ± 1.7 mm, bone: 1.5 ± 1.0 mm) are small. Compared to electromagnetic tracking-based ultrasound reconstructions over larger scan volumes by Heine et al. [4], the higher accuracy achieved in this work is expected due to the use of a linear transducer and a locally constrained scan region.

The N-shaped fiducial pattern used in this study does not allow for the determination of all DOF. In the current setup, this limitation was addressed by positioning

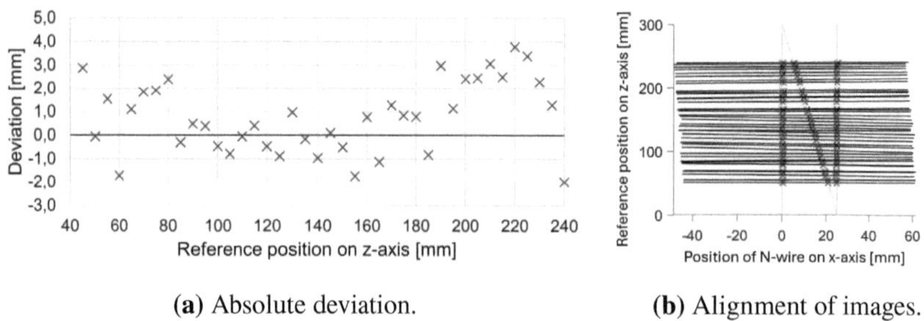

(a) Absolute deviation. **(b)** Alignment of images.

Fig. 4. (a) Absolute deviation from the calculated position to the reference position for the images of the residual limb phantom. (b) Aligned images along the N-wire with a 5 mm distance.

the US probe perpendicularly to the skin, which proved sufficient for the conducted experiments. Future work may extend the fiducial pattern into a third dimension to enable the definition of all six DOF. However, this extension would introduce new challenges, including increased liner thickness, resulting in higher weight and potentially reduced image quality.

While this study demonstrates the feasibility of partial 3D reconstruction using the proposed Scanliner approach, achieving a full reconstruction of a residual limb will require additional scanning sweeps and the development of methods for accurate alignment of multiple image sequences. Regarding the transfer of the method to real anatomy, it should be noted that reduced bone contrast in amputees has been reported in previous studies [9]. Furthermore, soft tissue mobility caused by movement and changes in amputee posture represents an additional challenge, as it can influence the shape of the residual limb.

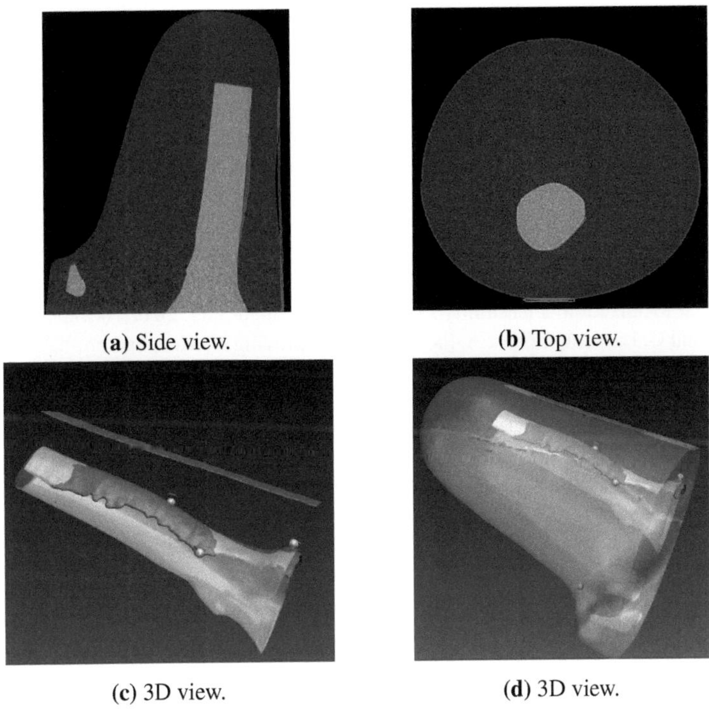

(a) Side view. **(b)** Top view.

(c) 3D view. **(d)** 3D view.

Fig. 5. (a) Side and (b) Top view of CT reference with overlayed segmentations from the US-based reconstruction in orange. (c) 3D view of reconstructed bone surface in orange with bone from CT in white and (d) additionally with skin from CT.

Acknowledgements

We would like to thank Verena Schweinstetter for her excellent preliminary work in the area of fiducial integration during her master thesis.

References

1. Paternò L, Ibrahimi M, Gruppioni E, Menciassi A, Ricotti L. Sockets for limb prostheses: a review of existing technologies and open challenges. IEEE Trans Biomed Eng. 2018;65(9):1996–2010.
2. Ranger BJ, Feigin M, Zhang X, Moerman KM, Herr H, Anthony BW. 3D ultrasound imaging of residual limbs with camera-based motion compensation. IEEE Trans Neural Syst Rehabil Eng. 2019;27(2):207–17.
3. Colombo G, Bertetti M, Bonacini D, Magrassi G. Reverse engineering and rapid prototyping techniques to innovate prosthesis socket design. Proc SPIE TDICA. 2006;6056:60560P.
4. Heine P, Robra L, Komposch J, Börsig J, Bornmann J, Leiniger A et al. Ultrasound-based 3D reconstruction of residual limbs using electromagnetic tracking. Proc BVM. 2025:89–94.
5. Prevost R, Salehi M, Jagoda S, Kumar N, Sprung J, Ladikos A et al. 3D freehand ultrasound without external tracking using deep learning. Med Image Anal. 2018;48:187–202.
6. Dai L, Zhao K, Li Z, Zhu J, Liang L. Advancing sensorless freehand 3D ultrasound reconstruction with a novel coupling pad. Proc MICCAI. 2024;15004:559–69.
7. Kingma R, Rohling RN, Nguan C. Registration of CT to 3D ultrasound using near-field fiducial localization: a feasibility study. Comput Aided Surg. 2011;16(2):54–70.
8. Carbajal G, Lasso A, Gómez Á, Fichtinger G. Improving N-wire phantom-based freehand ultrasound calibration. Int J Comput Assist Radiol Surg. 2013;8(6):1063–72.
9. Pröbsting E, Blumentritt S, Kannenberg A. Veränderungen am Bewegungsapparat als Folge von Amputationen an der unteren Extremität. Z Orthop Unfall. 2017;12(1):77–91.

Anatomy-informed 3D Reconstruction of Tracked Ultrasound Sweeps

A Proof of Concept

Alexander Furtner [1,2], Zoe Reinke [1,2], Thomas Wendler [1,2,3,4,5]

[1]Department of Diagnostic and Interventional Radiology and Neuroradiology, University Hospital Augsburg, Germany
[2]Digital Medicine, University Hospital Augsburg
[3]Computer-Aided Medical Procedures and Augmented Reality, Technical University of Munich, Germany
[4]Bavarian Cancer Research Center (BZKF) Augsburg, Germany
[5]Center of Advanced Analytics and Predictive Sciences, University of Augsburg, Germany
zoe.reinke@uni-a.de

Abstract. Ultrasound is a widely used imaging technique that typically produces a sequence of 2D images. However, tracked ultrasound is an increasingly popular method of converting 2D sweeps into 3D. The tracker provides data that enables subsequent reconstruction of an ultrasound volume. However, due to factors such as measurement inaccuracy, synchronization issues, and other disruptive influences, this tracking data may not accurately provide pose with exactitude. Here, we demonstrate that modifying the tracking data using anatomical knowledge can improve the compounded volume. This was achieved using a gradient descent approach to detect and correct potential errors in the tracking data. Validating against an MRI scan and comparing metrics – such as the Dice-Sørensen coefficient, Hausdorff distance, as well as volume and surface area change – demonstrates that improvements can be achieved.

1 Introduction

Ultrasound (US) is an imaging modality that is frequently used in clinics due to its low cost, non-invasiveness, and real-time visualisation capabilities. Conventional US techniques yield a series of 2D images or videos. However, it is also possible to obtain 3D volumes in real-time using special 3D US probes. Nevertheless, these systems are very cost-intensive, and are not widely available. Therefore, the utilisation of tracked US (TUS) as means of extending 2D US to 3D US is gaining popularity. Such devices combine a conventional 2D US probe with a position tracker (typically electromagnetic, optical, or inertial), whose data subsequently allows the 2D US frames ("sweep") to be reconstructed into a 3D US volume. However, tracking may contain errors due to measurement noise, synchronization issues, or interference

© Der/die Autor(en), exklusiv lizenziert an
Springer Fachmedien Wiesbaden GmbH, ein Teil von Springer Nature 2026
H. Handels et al. (Hrsg.), *Bildverarbeitung für die Medizin 2026*,
Informatik aktuell, https://doi.org/10.1007/978-3-658-51100-5_38

factors such as metallic objects for electromagnetic tracking (EMT), and occlusions for optical tracking. Consequently, here, an effort is made to optimise the obtained tracking data based on anatomical knowledge and the acquired 2D US frames.

1.1 Related work

The acquisition of 3D volumetric data from US imaging has been an active research area, driven by clinical demand for improved visualization and quantitative assessment of complex anatomical structures.

Barratt et al. provide an example of EMT device optimization in their study on carotid artery imaging. An EMT device's measurement rate and filter settings were tuned to reduce mean positional and rotational deviations, achieving sub-millimetre accuracy suitable for freehand 3D reconstruction [1]. Another significant class of work focuses on tracking and field calibration to dynamically reduce EMT errors. One method combines sensor motion models with redundant electromagnetic field measurements to perform real-time localization and field distortion mapping [2].

Beyond calibration methods, machine learning-based error compensation has gained traction. In particular, artificial neural networks have been employed to learn systematic distortion patterns from EMT data and correct them after the acquisition [3]. Moreover, advances in deep learning enable 3D freehand ultrasound acquisition without the need for external tracking systems, allowing the spatial relationship between successive frames to be inferred directly from the image data [4, 5].

Yet, to the best of our knowledge, no efforts have been made to use anatomical knowledge and the ultrasound frames to directly correct the tracked poses.

2 Materials and methods

The analysis was conducted using the SegThy dataset [6], a public dataset consisting of 3D US reconstructions of the neck with a focus on the thyroid gland, recorded in a total of 28 healthy volunteers. The US was acquired with a linear 12 MHz probe tracked using the TUS system by PIUR Imaging GmbH (Vienna, Austria). In addition to the US, the data set for each patient includes an MRI using a T1-weighted VIBE (volumetric interpolated breath-hold) sequence. In 16 of the 28 volunteers, both modalities have the structures thyroid gland, left and right carotid artery, and left and right jugular vein as segmented labels, annotated by an expert on the 3D US.

For 15 of the 16 patients, we additionally had access to two US sweeps (left and right), along with tracking data provided as a time series of 4×4 rigid transformation matrices. In this work, the tracking data was then matched to each frame using the timestamps on the frames and in the tracking data recordings.

2.1 Preprocessing of the data

The labels of the vena jugularis were excluded due to deformations by transducer pressure. As the corresponding US images exclusively display the carotid arteries in the region of the thyroid gland, the field of view of the MRI on both sides was cropped at the level of the thyroid gland.

2.2 Segmentation and reconstruction

On the 2D US frames, AI-supported segmentation of the carotid arteries and thyroid lobes was performed bilaterally for each patient. To this end, a prompt-based approach employing the MedSAM2 [7, 8] model was adopted. Initially, the prompts were set on the middle frame for each US sweeps. In accordance with the provided prompts, the automatic segmentation process was executed and propagated bi-directionally. The carotid artery and thyroid lobes were both primarily segmented using bounding box prompts, but also using additional negative prompts to finetune the segmentation (Fig. 1). Notably, the prompts were manually defined for each patient to ensure optimal segmentation results, reflecting our best interpretation of the corresponding US scans.

The reconstruction of the 3D volume from transformation matrices and binary segmentation frames was performed using a voxel-based approach. First, the physical size of the volume and the corresponding bounding box were determined. For this purpose, the corner points of all US frames containing relevant image information were transformed into tracking coordinates using their respective transformation matrices.

Subsequently, a 3D bounding box was filled with voxels, employing the same voxel spacing as given in the MRI (0.65 mm × 0.65 mm × 1 mm). The frames were then transformed into their place in the volume. To minimise the gaps between the slices, a Gaussian weighting was applied in the direction of insertion. The standard deviation σ of this Gaussian was set to half the slice thickness, ensuring smooth interpolation between adjacent frames.

2.3 Optimisation of the tracking data

The optimisation of tracking data refers to the modification of individual transformation matrices targeting a more precise mapping of the anatomy.

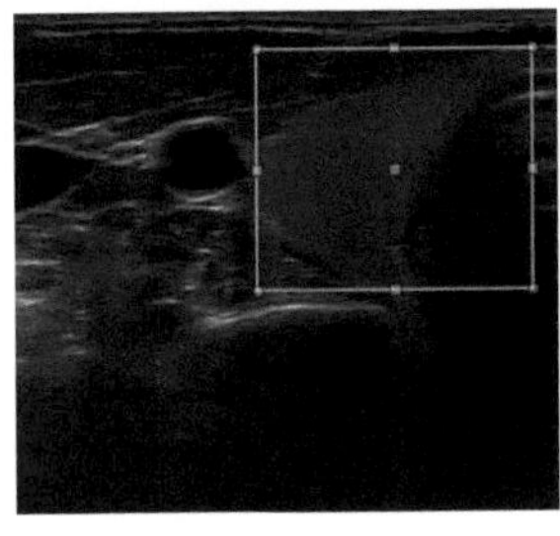

(a) Bounding box prompt to specify that the largest coherent structure within this area is to be segmented.

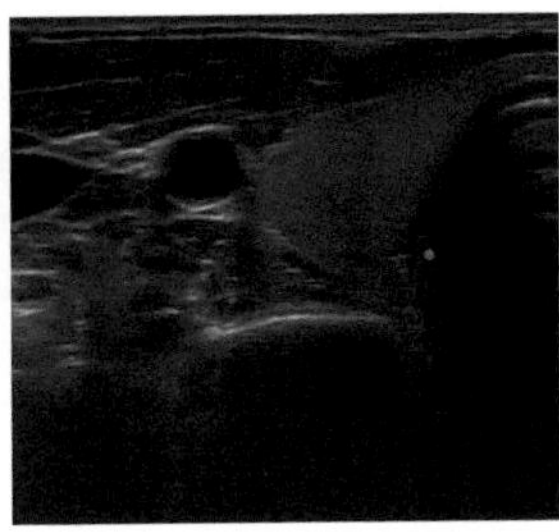

(b) Additional negative prompt to ensure that this area is excluded from the segmentation.

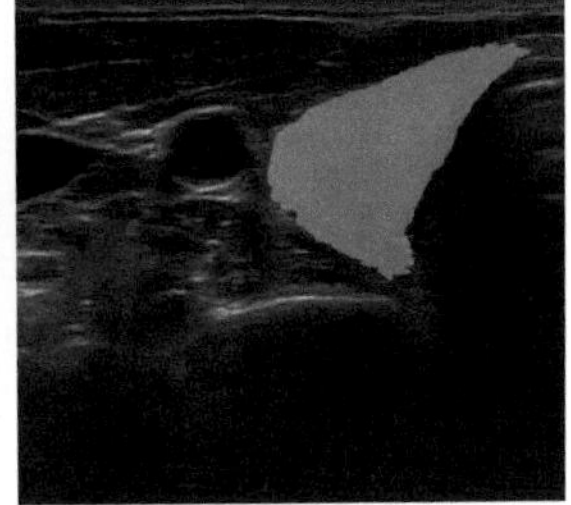

(c) Predicted segmentation mask on the prompted frame.

Fig. 1. Example of MedSAM2 prompts used for segmentation of the right thyroid lobe and the resulting segmentation mask on the center frame of a US sweep.

Alg. 1 Optimisation of pose parameters for US reconstruction.

procedure OPTIMISATION(frames, $\text{poses}_{\text{base}}, \lambda_R, \lambda_t$, iterations, lr, ϵ)
  $\delta_{\text{rot}} \leftarrow \begin{bmatrix}1 & 0 & 0 & 0\end{bmatrix}^\top$ ▹ identity quaternion
  $\delta_t \leftarrow \begin{bmatrix}0 & 0 & 0\end{bmatrix}^\top$ ▹ zero translation vector
  Init ADAM with learning rate lr
  for $i = 1$ to iterations **do**
    Reset gradients
    $\Delta T \leftarrow$ convert δ_{rot} and δ_t to 4x4 transformation matrices
    $\text{poses}_{\text{new}} \leftarrow \text{poses}_{\text{base}} \times \Delta T$ ▹ Apply error transformation
    Reconstruct 3D volume from frames and $\text{poses}_{\text{new}}$
    Compute SDF from volume
    Compute loss L_{total}
    Backpropagate L_{total}
    Update parameters using ADAM
    Normalize δ_{rot} quaternions
  end for
  $\Delta T \leftarrow$ convert δ_{rot} and δ_t to 4x4 transformation matrices
  $\text{poses}_{\text{final}} \leftarrow \text{poses}_{\text{base}} \times \Delta T$
  return $\text{poses}_{\text{final}}$
end procedure

As demonstrated in the pseudocode (Alg. 1), this is achieved through the utilisation of gradient descent, in conjunction with a differentiable loss function that penalises anatomically non-plausible edges from the segmentation masks and "jumps" in the rotation and translation of the tracking data. The optimiser was ADAM [9]. In particular, two vectors are optimised: a quaternion rotation vector and a translation vector.

After optimisation, the quaternion vector is converted into a rotation matrix and combined with the translation vector to form a transformation matrix, as in the original tracking data. The resulting matrix is then multiplied by the actual transformation matrix, thus functioning as an error correction matrix. In each iteration of the optimisation process, the volume is reconstructed using the adjusted data. Converting the volume into a signed distance field (SDF) emphasizes the morphology of the thyroid and carotids, revealing edges and discontinuities, while simultaneously providing a representation of the surface geometry of the anatomical structures.

The specific loss function employed in this optimisation is a Charbonnier loss, which is applied to the gradients of the SDF in the x-, y-, and z-directions. This approach is designed to promote spatial smoothness in the reconstructed 3D volume by penalising substantial local alterations in the SDF.

Similar loss functions, including L1, L2, and Huber loss, were considered but showed no significant advantages.

The loss is given by

Tab. 1. Aggregated mean ± standard deviation per modality, averaged bilaterally, for ΔSurface and ΔVolume relative to MRI, with Mann-Whitney U-test p-values relative to the optimized tracking method.

Modality	ΔSurface [%]	p-value	ΔVolume [%]	p-value
Original	28.987 ± 18.117	0.202	33.126 ± 23.619	0.106
Optimised	36.475 ± 20.607	–	18.980 ± 21.736	–
Label	-2.352 ± 8.759	<0.001	1.258 ± 11.083	0.01

Tab. 2. Aggregated mean ± standard deviation per modality, averaged bilaterally, for DSC and HD95 relative to MRI, with Mann-Whitney U-test p-values relative to the optimized tracking method.

Modality	DSC	p-value	HD95 [mm]	p-value
Original	0.619 ± 0.084	0.775	6.191 ± 2.291	0.902
Optimised	0.608 ± 0.106	–	6.748 ± 3.863	–
Label	0.717 ± 0.066	0.001	3.889 ± 1.473	0.007

$$L_{\text{Charb}} = \frac{1}{N} \sum_{x,y,z} \sqrt{\left(\frac{\partial \text{SDF}}{\partial x}\right)^2 + \left(\frac{\partial \text{SDF}}{\partial y}\right)^2 + \left(\frac{\partial \text{SDF}}{\partial z}\right)^2 + \epsilon^2} \tag{1}$$

where N is the total number of voxels, used for normalization, and ϵ is a constant for numerical stability.

Furthermore, the optimisation of translation and rotation parameters is regularised by two weighting terms, λ_R and λ_t, with the objective of preventing excessive deviation from the initial tracking data. This is achieved by incorporating quadratic penalty terms into the overall loss calculation.

The total composite loss is

$$L_{\text{total}} = L_{\text{Charb}} + \lambda_{\text{rot}} \, ||\mathbf{q}_{\text{vec}}||^2 + \lambda_{\text{t}} \, ||\mathbf{t}||^2 \tag{2}$$

where $\mathbf{q}_{\text{vec}} = (x, y, z)$ is the vector part of the quaternion representing the rotation correction, $\mathbf{t} = (t_x, t_y, t_z)$ is the translation correction vector, λ_{R} and λ_{t} are weighting factors both fixed to 10^{-5} following a grid search between 10^{-6} and 0.5.

2.4 Validation

To evaluate the effect of the optimisation on the tracking data, the results were validated against MRI in a bilateral analysis. The right thyroid lobe and carotid artery were treated as a single volume, with the left side assessed accordingly. For this purpose, ImFusion Suite (Imfusion GmbH, Munich, Germany) is utilised to rigidly register the individual structure (as a labelmap) against its equivalent from the MRI and calculate the dice-sørensen coefficients (DSC), the 95th percentile of the Hausdorff distance (HD95 [mm]), and the percentage change in volume and surface area relative to the MRI (ΔV [%]). The metrics were calculated for the following three US volumes: (a) reconstruction with original tracking data, (b) reconstruction with optimised tracking data, and (c) US labels provided within SegThy – which were labeled manually in the compounded 3D US without any correction.

3 Results

The structures were evaluated bilaterally for all 15 patients, and the mean of both sides was used to obtain a patient-level quantification. The proposed tracking optimisation improved ΔV (Tab. 1, Fig. 2) compared to reconstruction using the original tracking data. Yet, the difference was not statistically significant. However, no improvement was observed for the remaining metrics using our approach (Tab. 2, Fig. 3).

When compared to the 3D US label maps, the optimized images showed statistically significant differences in all metrics.

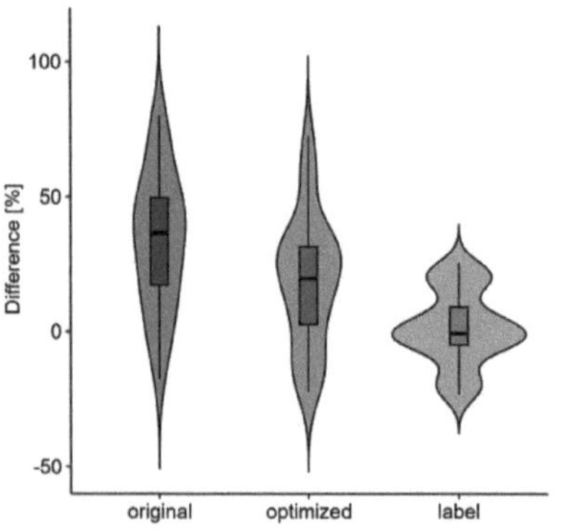

(a) Violin plots of percentage differences in volume relative to MRI.

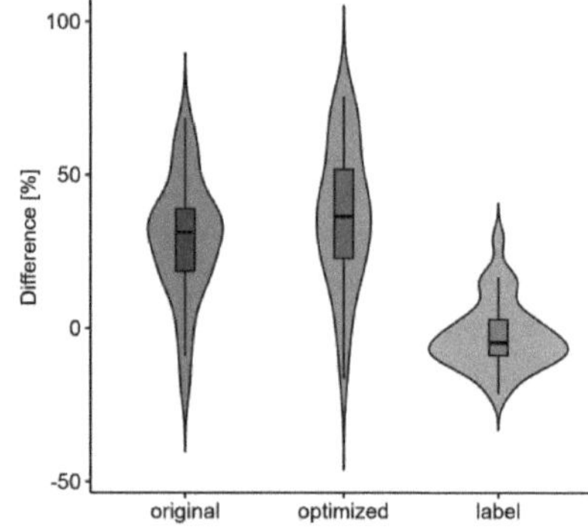

(b) Violin plots of percentage differences in surface area relative to MRI.

Fig. 2. Violin plots of reconstruction accuracy using ΔVolume and ΔSurface.

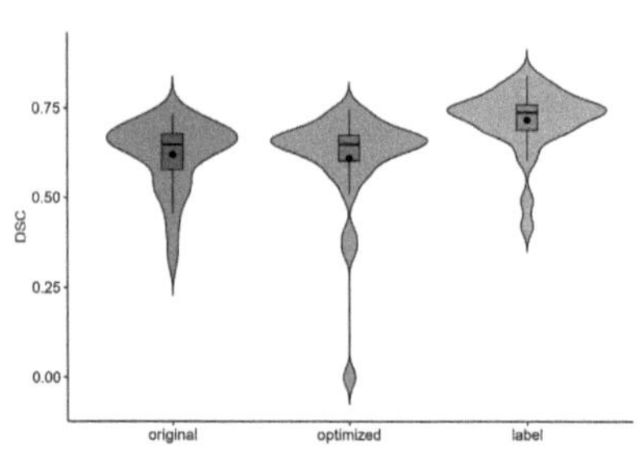

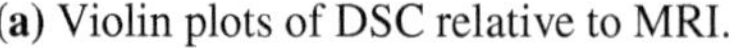

(a) Violin plots of DSC relative to MRI.

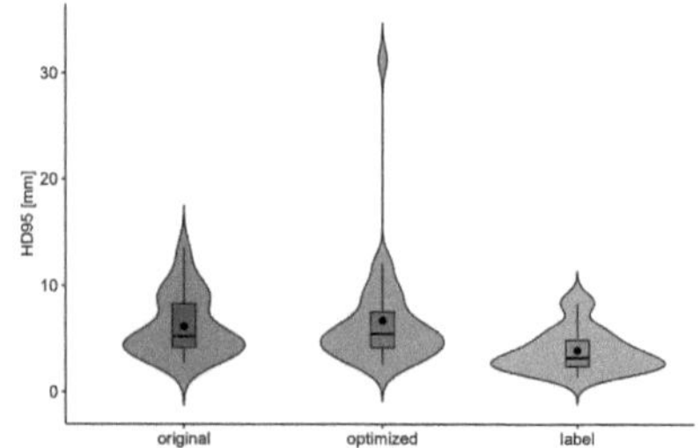

(b) Violin plots of HD95 relative to MRI.

Fig. 3. Violin plots of reconstruction accuracy using DSC and HD95.

Qualitatively, the reconstructed images look smoother and lack the aforementioned anatomically non-plausible "jumps" (Fig. 4). Visual comparison with MRI masks is also satisfactory.

4 Discussion

In this work, we introduced a method for correcting tracking data in TUS guided by anatomical plausibility. We evaluated our approach on a fifteen-patient subset of the SegThy dataset by comparing segmentation masks of the carotid arteries and thyroid lobes between 3D US and MRI.

Our results indicate that improving the recorded tracking data by incorporating anatomical knowledge can enhance the correspondence between 3D US and MRI. Although the observed improvements were not statistically significant, the validation results point towards a potential positive change, providing an indicative proof of concept. The tracking data exhibited minimal noise and no outliers, which may explain why the optimisation had only a limited effect. The discrepancies observed between the publicly provided SegThy masks and our reconstructions suggest possible inaccuracies in the public dataset, or alternatively, that the segmentation masks of 3D US and MRI collaboratively generated by an expert and MedSAM2 are inherently more consistent.

The statistically significant difference between the proposed approach and the label maps provided by SegThy may point at differences in the interpretation of the US images by the experts in the current evaluation and the ones labeling the SegThy dataset. Potentially, the annotators of SegThy "corrected" errors in tracking, resulting in smoother structures that deviate from the underlying images.

The study is limited by the small number of evaluated patients. Moreover, the employed validation is error-prone, as MRI masks may contain inaccuracies due to the low contrast of the thyroid in the used sequences. MRI was employed as a surrogate for the ground truth, although its accuracy may be inherently limited. Also,

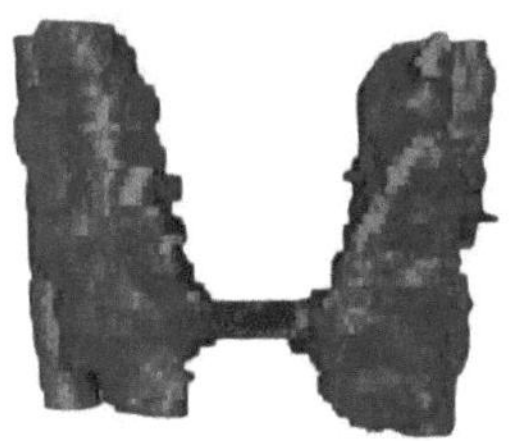

(a) Segmentation of the MRI volume of the thyroid and carotid arteries.

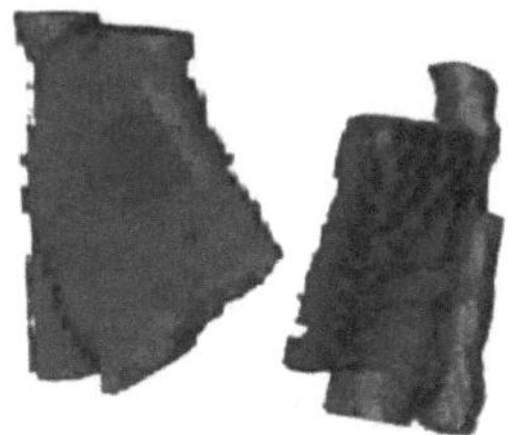

(b) Non-optimised reconstruction of the thyroid and carotid arteries.

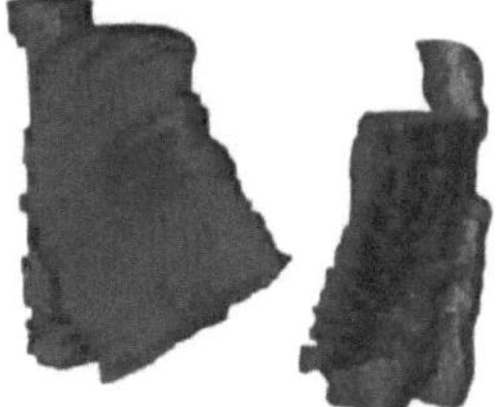

(c) Optimised reconstruction of the thyroid and carotid arteries.

Fig. 4. Exemplary reconstructions of segmentation masks for thyroid and carotid for different modalities, including the optimised result.

perfect registration is infeasible due to motion and swallowing artifacts in both 3D US and MRI, as well as the non-rigid deformations that were not modeled here.

Future extensions of this work could focus on improving segmentation quality and incorporating deformable registration techniques to achieve better alignment between 3D US and MRI. Robustness to noise typical for EMT tracking could also be investigated to validate the optimisation for noisy data.

Extension of the evaluation to as many patients of SegThy as possible and inclusion of more organs (muscles, trachea, etc) would also be possible, as well as validation using other public datasets.

In summary, this study provides a proof-of-concept that anatomically informed correction of tracking data can enhance the reliability and internal consistency of tracked ultrasound, paving the way towards more robust and reproducible 3D US imaging.

Acknowledgement. This research was partially funded by the Bavarian Ministry of Economic Affairs, Regional Development and Energy (StMWi) under grant number LSM-2403-0017.

References

1. Barratt DC, Davies AH, Hughes AD, Thom SA, Humphries KN. Optimisation and evaluation of an electromagnetic tracking device for high-accuracy three-dimensional ultrasound imaging of the carotid arteries. Ultrasound Med Biol. 2001;27(7):957–68.
2. Sadjadi H, Hashtrudi-Zaad K, Fichtinger G. Simultaneous electromagnetic tracking and calibration for dynamic field distortion compensation. IEEE Trans Biomed Eng. 2016;63(8):1771–81.
3. Krumb H, Hofmann S, Kügler D, Ghazy A, Dorweiler B, Bredemann J et al. Leveraging spatial uncertainty for online error compensation in EMT. Int J Comput Assist Radiol Surg. 2020;15(6):1043–51.
4. Luo M, Yang X, Wang H, Du L, Ni D. Deep motion network for freehand 3D ultrasound reconstruction. Proc MICCAI. 2022.
5. Prevost R, Salehi M, Jagoda S, Kumar N, Sprung J, Ladikos A et al. 3D freehand ultrasound without external tracking using deep learning. Med Image Anal. 2018;48:187–202.
6. Krönke M, Eilers C, Dimova D, Köhler M, Buschner G, Schweiger L et al. Tracked 3D ultrasound and deep neural network-based thyroid segmentation reduce interobserver variability in thyroid volumetry. PLoS One. 2022;17(7):e0268550.
7. Ma J, Yang Z, Kim S, Chen B, Baharoon M, Fallahpour A et al. MedSAM2: segment anything in 3D medical images and videos. arXiv: 2504.03600. 2025.
8. Ravi N, Gabeur V, Hu YT, Hu R, Ryali C, Ma T et al. SAM 2: segment anything in images and videos. Proc ICLR. 2025.
9. Kingma DP, Ba J. Adam: a method for stochastic optimization. arXiv: 1412.6980. 2017.

This chapter is published under the Creative Commons Attribution 4.0 International License (http://creativecommons.org/licenses/by/4.0/deed.en).

Abstract: When Two Wrongs Don't Make a Right

Examining Confirmation Bias and the Role of Time Pressure During Human-AI Collaboration in Computational Pathology

Emely Rosbach [1], Jonas Ammeling [1], Christof A. Bertram [2], Andreas Riener [1], Marc Aubreville [3]

[1]Technische Hochschule Ingolstadt, Ingolstadt, Germany
[2]Institute of Pathology, University of Veterinary Medicine Vienna, Vienna, Austria
[3]Flensburg University of Applied Sciences, Flensburg, Germany
emely.rosbach@thi.de

Artificial intelligence (AI)-based decision support systems hold the potential to enhance diagnostic accuracy and boost efficiency in computational pathology. However, human-AI collaboration can also give rise to new cognitive biases or intensify existing ones, such as confirmation bias driven by false confirmation, where erroneous human judgments are reinforced by inaccurate AI outputs. This effect may be exacerbated under time pressure, a pervasive factor in routine pathology that places strain on medical experts' cognitive resources. In this study [1], we quantified confirmation bias arising from false confirmation through AI suggestions and examined the moderating influence of time constraints in a web-based experiment involving pathology experts (n = 28) estimating tumor cell percentages. Our results indicate that AI integration fuels confirmation bias, as evidenced by a statistically significant positive linear mixed-effects model coefficient showing that greater alignment between AI recommendations and erroneous human estimates subsequently increases agreement with system advice. Conversely, time pressure appeared to mitigate this dynamic. These findings highlight potential pitfalls of medical AI and contribute to establishing a foundation for the safe implementation of AI-based decision support systems into clinical practice.

References

1. Rosbach E, Ammeling J, Krügel S, Kießig A, Fritz A, Ganz J et al. When two wrongs don't make a right: examining confirmation bias and the role of time pressure during human-AI collaboration in computational pathology. Proc NYSDS. 2025.

© Der/die Autor(en), exklusiv lizenziert an
Springer Fachmedien Wiesbaden GmbH, ein Teil von Springer Nature 2026
H. Handels et al. (Hrsg.), *Bildverarbeitung für die Medizin 2026*,
Informatik aktuell, https://doi.org/10.1007/978-3-658-51100-5_39

Abstract: Unlocking the Potential of Digital Pathology

Novel Baselines for Compression

Maximilian Fischer[1,2], Peter Neher[1], Peter Schüffler[3,4], Sebastian Ziegler[1], Shuhan Xiao[1], Robin Peretzke[1,2], David Clunie[5], Constantin Ulrich[1,2], Michael Baumgartner[1], Alexander Muckenhuber[3], Silvia Dias Almeida[1,2], Michael Götz[6], Jens Kleesiek[7], Marco Nolden[1], Rickmer Braren[8], Klaus Maier-Hein[1,2]

[1]German Cancer Research Center Heidelberg, Division of Medical Image Computing
[2]Medical Faculty Heidelberg, University of Heidelberg, Germany
[3]TUM School of Medicine, Institute of Pathology, Technical University of Munich
[4]TUM School of Computation, Technical University of Munich, Munich, Germany
[5]PixelMed Publishing, Bangor, Pennsylvania, United States
[6]Clinic of Diagnostics and Interventional Radiology, Ulm University Clinic, Ulm, Germany
[7]Institute for AI in Medicine (IKIM), University Medicine Essen, Essen, Germany
[8]Department of Diagnostic and Interventional Radiology, Faculty of Medicine, Technical University of Munich, Munich, Germany
maximilian.fischer@dkfz-heidelberg.de

Digital pathology offers the opportunity to transform clinical practice in histopathological image analysis, yet faces a significant hurdle: the substantial file sizes of pathological WSIs. Whereas current digital pathology solutions rely on lossy JPEG compression to address this issue, lossy compression can introduce color and texture disparities, potentially impacting clinical decision-making. Prior research addresses perceptual image quality and downstream performance independently of each other, we jointly evaluate compression schemes for perceptual and downstream task quality on four different datasets. In addition, we collect an initially uncompressed dataset for an unbiased perceptual evaluation of compression schemes. Our results show that deep learning models fine-tuned for perceptual quality outperform conventional compression schemes like JPEG-XL or WebP for further compression of WSI. We introduce a novel evaluation metric based on feature similarity between original files and compressed files that aligns with the downstream performance on the compressed WSI. Our study provides novel insights for the assessment of lossy compression schemes for WSI and encourages a unified evaluation of lossy compression schemes to accelerate the clinical uptake of digital pathology [1].

References

1. Fischer M, et al. Unlocking the potential of digital pathology: novel baselines for compression. J Pathol Inform. 2025;17:100421.

© Der/die Autor(en), exklusiv lizenziert an
Springer Fachmedien Wiesbaden GmbH, ein Teil von Springer Nature 2026
H. Handels et al. (Hrsg.), *Bildverarbeitung für die Medizin 2026*,
Informatik aktuell, https://doi.org/10.1007/978-3-658-51100-5_40

Towards a Visual Distinction of Benign and Tumorous Wound Surface in Epidermolysis Bullosa

Ding Xin[1], Verena Wally[2,3], Chrstina Guttmann-Gruber[4], Bernadette Liemberger[4], Johann Bauer[2,3], Andreas Uhl[1]

[1]Department of Artificial Intelligence and Human Computer Interfaces, University of Salzburg, Austria
[2]Department of Dermatology and Allergology, University Hospital of the Paracelsus Medical University Salzburg, Austria
[3]EB House Austria, Research Program for Molecular Therapy of Genodermatoses, Department of Dermatology and Allergology, University Hospital of the Paracelsus Medical University Salzburg, Austria
[4]EB Research Institute GmbH, Salzburg, Austria
andreas.uhl@plus.ac.at

Abstract. It is investigated if a purely vision-based approach might be able to conduct a discrimination of benign and tumorous Epidermolysis bullosa wound surfaces. Although being based on a critically small dataset, best results obtained are above 0.9 in specificity and precision/recall for the two class discrimination. Results encourage further work in this direction, in particular to continue training data collection to further enhance classification.

1 Introduction

Epidermolysis bullosa (EB) is a genetic skin disease caused by mutations in either one of 16 currently known genes that all play a role in conferring stability to the epidermal-dermal junction of the skin. EB subtypes differ significantly in severity, which is reflected by the extent of involvement of epithelial tissues (e.g., only skin or also mucous membranes), as well as complications and secondary manifestations associated with the distinct EB-subtypes [1].

Patients suffering from the junctional (JEB) or the recessive-dystrophic type of EB (RDEB) are particularly prone to skin wounding upon minor friction. Due to mutation, the partial or complete absence of proteins important for maintaining skin integrity leads to the development of wounds, which often become chronic and are characterized by infections and persistent inflammation. Such wound environments promote the development of squamous cell carcinomas (SCC) that are associated with a particularly high rate of early deaths of affected patients [2].

Therefore, early diagnostics of EB-SCCs is of high clinical significance, but appears impaired against the background of chronic, non-healing wounds or exuberant granulation tissue, rendering them hard to detect by visual inspection only. Currently,

© Der/die Autor(en), exklusiv lizenziert an
Springer Fachmedien Wiesbaden GmbH, ein Teil von Springer Nature 2026
H. Handels et al. (Hrsg.), *Bildverarbeitung für die Medizin 2026*,
Informatik aktuell, https://doi.org/10.1007/978-3-658-51100-5_41

management guidelines for EB-SCCs recommend regular whole-body monitoring from as early as 10 years on, and punch biopsies that are painful and again damage the skin, are required for histological evaluation of suspicious lesions. As patients frequently develop multiple primary tumours, multiple sites need to be analysed, which is often only possible under local or general anaesthesia. Subsequent tumor excision requires radical surgery and sometimes even amputation, resulting in severe issues regarding wound closure [3]. As also currently available non-surgical treatments lack good efficacy, early tumor detection and early classification of EB-wounds for assessing the risk of developing an SCC in the future, without causing additional harm by invasive procedures are urgently needed and awaited [2, 3].

In this work we aim to get an idea if a purely vision-based approach might be able to conduct a discrimination of benign and tumorous wound surfaces, with the long-term goal of avoiding invasive punch biopsies. Given the critically small dataset resulting from disease rarity, we implemented feature subset selection evaluated in a strict two-level leave-one-out cross-validation (LOOCV) and leave-one-patient-out cross-validation (LOPOCV) [4] (Sec. 3). The obtained results as suggest continuing the data collection effort to further increase classification results (Sec. 3).

2 Materials and methods

2.1 Dataset and preprocessing

This study utilised a dataset comprising 49 clinical skin images (29 tumor images and 20 no-tumor images), extracted from JPEG imagery taken from the later biopsy location during patient wound documentation (iPad mini). Fig. 1 illustrates the distribution of patient-level image patches grouped by diagnostic category (histologically confirmed). During preprocessing, all images were rescaled proportionally and padded with mirrored content to match the network's input dimensions. Fig. 2 provides representative examples from the dataset, without exhibiting obvious category-specific visual characteristics, questioning a purely vision-based approach.

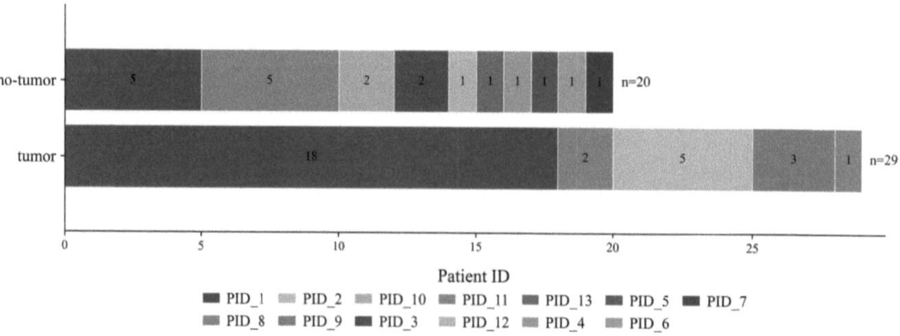

Fig. 1. Patient-wise distribution of image patches across diagnostic categories.

2.2 Feature selection

The mismatch of low sample number and high dimensionality of current classification network models is often termed "curse of dimensionality" and causes overfitting and classifier misbehaviour. To address this, we apply a two-stage process, in which the network embeddings most suited to be fed into the classifiers are selected.

The feature pre-selection strategy aims at rapidly identifying a discriminative and low-redundancy embeddings feature subset (inspired from [5]). The procedure iterates through features in descending order of X-variance. A candidate feature is only included in the pre-selected set if the absolute value of its Spearman correlation coefficient with all features in the existing selected set is below the threshold $\tau = 0.5$, the top 100 features are kept.

To address the optimisation problem of feature combinations following pre-screening, this study employs the classical ant colony optimisation (ACO) algorithm [6]. Let the pre-selected feature set be $F = f_1, f_2, ..., f_M$. Each ant probabilistically constructs a feature subset $S \subseteq F$ where $|S| \in [3, 15]$. The heuristic information used in the algorithm fuses Relief-F and mutual information (MI) with equal weighting to balance the local discriminative capability and global statistical dependency of features. The fitness function is customized as follows

$$\text{Fitness}(S) = \text{AUC-PR}_{\text{avg}}(S) - \lambda_{\text{size}} \cdot \frac{|S|}{M} + \lambda_{\text{stab}} \cdot \text{Stability}(S) \quad (1)$$

To compute AUC-PR$_{\text{avg}}$, we calculate the area under the precision-recall curve based on the sample-level out-of-fold probabilities from the outer LOOCV/LOPOCV. To take the small sized dataset into account, the study introduces a subset size penalty term $\lambda_{\text{size}} \cdot |S|/M$ (where $\lambda_{\text{size}} = 0.5$, $|S|$ denotes the feature subset size, and M represents the total number of features after pre-selection) into the feature selection fitness function to regulate model complexity. Building upon [7] (linking feature selection stability to model robustness), a stability reward term Stability(S), weighted by $\lambda_{\text{stab}} = 0.15$, is further incorporated. This term quantifies

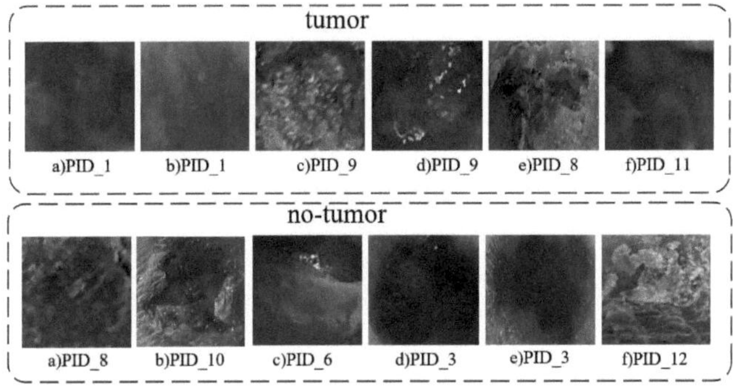

Fig. 2. Example of skin tumor and no-tumor image patches.

the robustness of the feature subset to data perturbations by calculating the selection frequency of each feature through iterative subsampling and feature screening [8].

3 Results

3.1 Experimental setup and evaluation criteria

This study employs feature extraction using various deep neural network models including CNNs as well as tranformer-based architectures with results being presented from the best only: ConvNeXt, ViT, and DeiT [9] and CoAtNet [10]. All networks use either ImageNet pre-trained weights, or domain-specific weights fine-tuned on the ISIC 2019 skin image dataset (see [11] for fine-tuning training parameters). For feature extraction, embeddings were extracted from the layer preceding the classification layer. Four machine learning algorithms were employed for classification experiments: CatBoost, Logistic Regression, Support Vector Machines, and Linear Support Vector Classification. Given the limited sample size and to mitigate patient-related bias, this study employed both LOOCV and LOPOCV to estimate classification results. Performance evaluation utilized two core metrics: AUC-PR and specificity. The AUC-PR is insensitive to class distribution and aligns with medical diagnostics' requirement for reliable positive sample identification. Specificity is directly reflecting the critical ability to avoid false-positive diagnoses in clinical practice.

3.2 LOOCV experimental results

After deep feature extraction, the dimensionality of features generated by each network ranged between 768 and 1024 dimensions. In Figs. 3 and 4 we compare classification performance of the full feature set (patterned bars) against the pre-selected 100-dimensional subset (solid bars), aiming to validate whether pre-selection can achieve dimensionality optimisation while maintaining classification efficacy. Further, results of networks trained on ImageNet data are compared to those fine-tuned on ISIC2019 data.

Analysis indicates ConvNeXt provides the most balanced AUC-PR and specificity among pre-training variants. ImageNet-pre-trained ConvNeXt with CatBoost shows marked gains after pre-screening. Dimensionality reduction has heterogeneous effects, but more often improves specificity across configurations. The comprehensive pre-screening results reveal that, excluding ViT, ImageNet-pre-trained models generally yield specificity higher than or comparable to ISIC2019 across most classifier combinations, and AUC-PR is superior in most cases. Consequently, subsequent ACO feature selection will focus on ImageNet-pre-trained models, prioritising the optimisation of feature combinations to further enhance overall discriminative capability.

Based on the ACO feature selection results depicted (Fig. 5), the following conclusions may be drawn: Features extracted by the ConvNeXt network demonstrated optimal and most stable performance across both AUC-PR and specificity metrics.

Compared to the results in Fig. 3 and Fig. 4, the specificity of nearly all models shows a slight improvement. Notably, the ConvNeXt model achieves specificity above 0.9 across all four classifiers, demonstrating excellent negative sample recognition capability. Regarding AUC-PR, except for the DeiT model, the remaining models show improvements over the full feature subset and pre-screening stage on most classifiers, again ConvNeXt results exceed 0.9. This outcome demonstrates that, besides the superiority of the ConvNeXt architecture, the ACO feature selection phase can

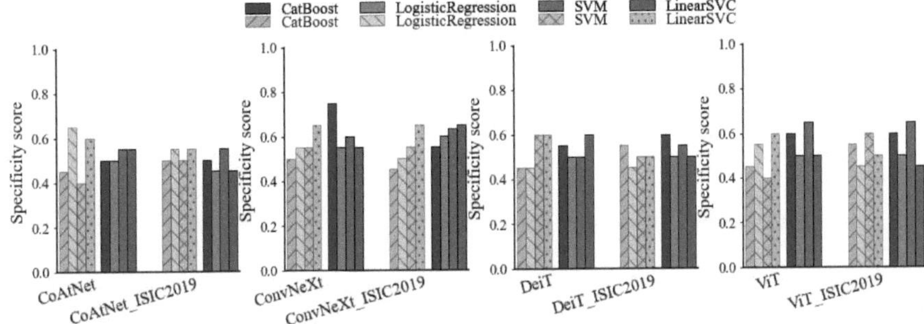

Fig. 3. Specificity Comparison of Full Feature Set vs. Pre-screened Feature Set.

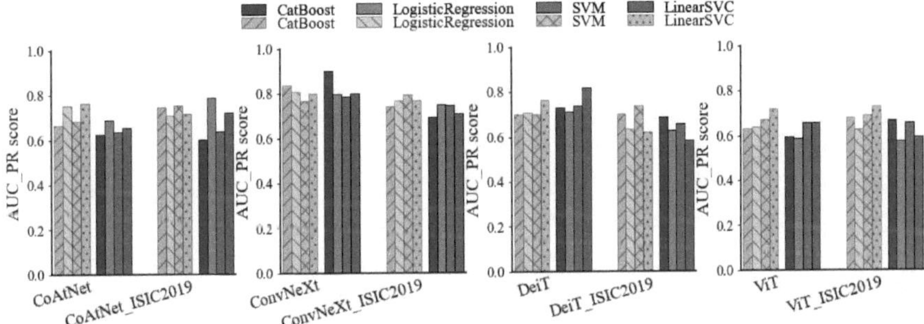

Fig. 4. AUC-PR Comparison of Full Feature Set and Pre-screened Feature Set.

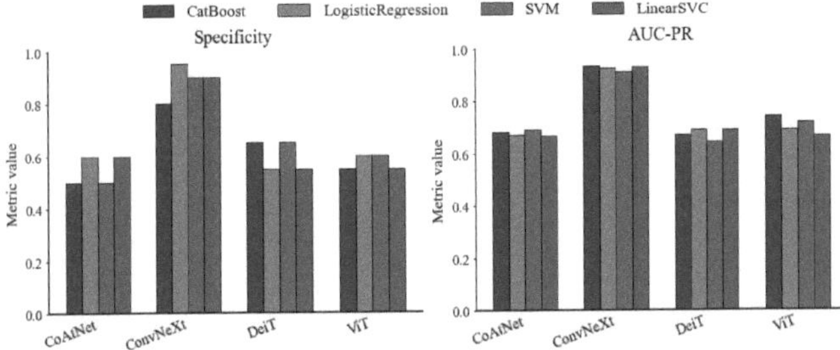

Fig. 5. Performance Comparison of Feature Selection Methods Based on ACO.

systematically identify highly discriminative and robust feature combinations while effectively controlling the size of the feature subset.

As demonstrated in Fig. 6 (showing the distribution of incorrectly classified patches among patients), the ConvNeXt model exhibits stable performance across all four classifiers, indicating that the features extracted by this network architecture possess strong generalization capabilities and can effectively adapt to variations between patients. In particular, even in patients with low patch numbers, for LR and LinearSVC there is not a single patient with all patches being misclassified.

Further analysis of misclassified cases reveals a high degree of consistency in the error patterns across classifiers. Within tumor samples, cases a, f, d, and e (as annotated in Fig. 2) were misclassified as non-tumorous by all classifiers. In contrast, only cases b and g exhibited misclassification in two of the classification models. Among the no-tumor samples, cases a, c, and d were misclassified only by some of the classifiers.

3.3 LOPOCV experimental results

In LOOCV, both training and test sets may simultaneously contain samples from the same patient, potentially causing patient-level information leakage and introducing optimistic bias in cross-patient generalization performance. Thus, this paper further employs LOPOCV: The results described in this subsection are consistent with the LOOCV results (Sec. 3.2) in that both were calculated at sample level (image/lesion level) to ensure comparability.

Within the LOPOCV framework, Figs. 7 and 8 demonstrate that feature preselection consistently yields stable improvements in specificity and AUC-PR. Overall, ConvNeXt maintains best performance across both metrics, reflecting superior cross-patient generalization capabilities.

Based on the results of ACO feature selection using LOPOCV (Fig. 9) , compared to the pre-screening stage (Figs. 7 and 8), the specificity of most backbone-classifier combinations improved further, with AUC-PR also increasing (except for DeiT). Among the positive results, ConvNeXt continued to demonstrate the most balanced performance, consistent with the LOOCV findings. Comparing to LOOCV results (Fig.5): In terms of specificity, all networks except ConvNeXt surprisingly improved

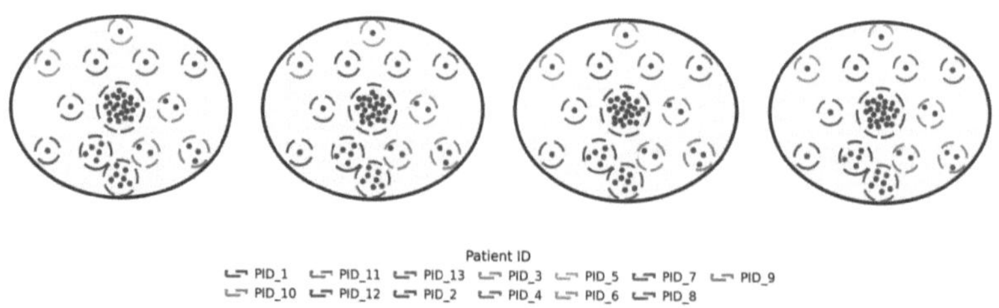

Fig. 6. Patient-level Patch Classification by ConvNeXt (Red: Correct, Grey: Incorrect; Left to Right: CatBoost, LR, SVM, LinearSVC).

under the LOPOCV protocol. Although a few ConvNeXt combinations showed slight declines, the magnitude was negligible, and ConvNeXt results remained leading overall. On the other hand, the AUC-PR of applying LOPOCV is generally lower than that of LOOCV.

4 Conclusion

This study investigates the classification of rare cutaneous tumors within epidermolytic bullous lesions under conditions of extremely small sample sizes. By combining rigorous cross-validation with multi-stage feature selection, we validated that

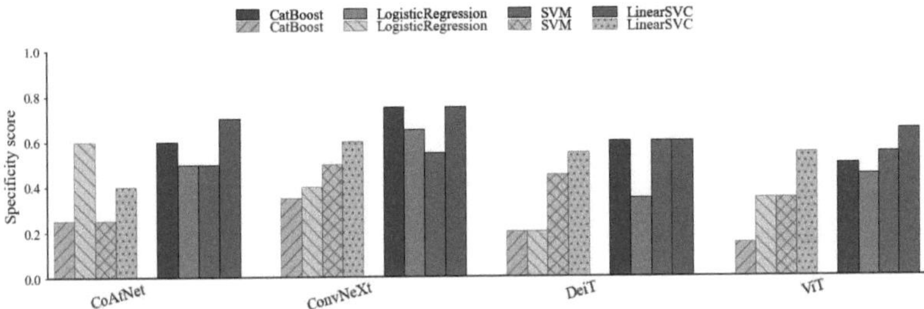

Fig. 7. Specificity Comparison of Full Feature Set vs. Pre-screened Feature Set.

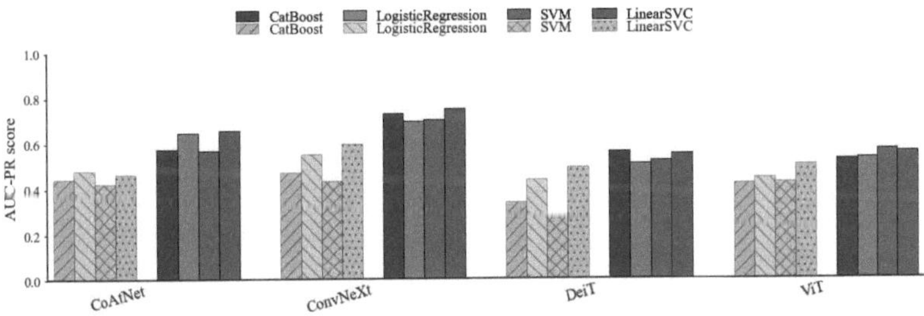

Fig. 8. AUC-PR Comparison of Full Feature Set and Pre-screened Feature Set.

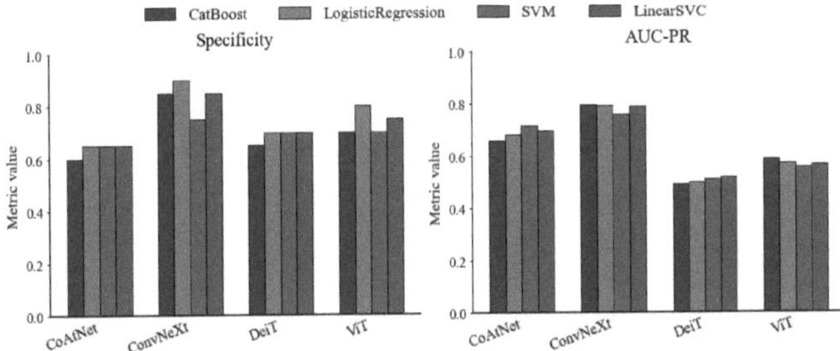

Fig. 9. Performance Comparison of Feature Selection Methods Based on ACO.

a pure vision-based workflow yields discriminative results. Among the evaluated models, ConvNeXt demonstrated the strongest and most balanced performance – likely due to its convolutional inductive bias aligning well with the statistical characteristics of medical images in this study, enabling robust feature extraction even under data scarcity.

To ensure estimation reliability, we concurrently reported LOOCV and LOPOCV estimates. Reduced AUC-PR under the LOPOVC protocol (while specificity was even increased) may indicate patient level bias in LOOCV results, but could also be caused by the intrinsic reduced training set size in LOPOCV. Continued data sample collection is imperative to further confirm results.

Acknowledgement. The data and samples for this project have been provided by the EB Biobank of the EB Research Institute GmbH, Salzburg, Austria. This work has been partially supported by the WISS 2025 project "ServEB" (20102/F2300645-FPR).

References

1. Has C, Bauer JW, Bodemer C, Bolling MC, Bruckner-Tuderman L, Diem A et al. Consensus reclassification of inherited epidermolysis bullosa and other disorders with skin fragility. Br J Dermatol. 2020;183(4):614–27.
2. Niltem E, Rujimethapass N, Sukhneewat C, Limpongsanurak W, Singalavanija S. Clinical features and outcomes of epidermolysis bullosa in thai children: a 20-year review from a tertiary care center. Arch Community Med Public Health. 2022;8(4):140–6.
3. Lucky AW, Pope E, Crawford S. Dystrophic epidermolysis bullosa. GeneReviews. Ed. by Adam MP, Feldman J, Mirzaa GM et al. Updated 2025 Aug 7. Seattle (WA): University of Washington, 2006.
4. Hegenbart S, Uhl A, Vécsei A. Systematic assessment of performance prediction techniques in medical image classification: a case study on celiac disease. Proc IPMI. 2011;6801:498–509.
5. Alirezanejad M, Enayatifar R, Motameni H, Nematzadeh H. Heuristic filter feature selection methods for medical datasets. Genomics. 2020;112(2):1173–81.
6. Dorigo M, Maniezzo V, Colorni A. Ant system: optimization by a colony of cooperating agents. IEEE Trans Syst Man Cybern B Cybern. 1996;26(1):29–41.
7. Kalousis A, Prados J, Hilario M. Stability of feature selection algorithms: a study on high-dimensional spaces. Knowl Inf Syst. 2007;12(1):95–116.
8. Meinshausen N, Buehlmann P. Stability selection. J R Stat Soc Series B Stat Methodol. 2010;72(4):417–73.
9. George AB, Bathini S, R NS. Deep learning for oral health: benchmarking ViT, DeiT, BEiT, ConvNeXt, and swin transformer. arXiv: 2509.23100. 2025.
10. Dai Z, Liu H, Le QV, Tan M. CoAtNet: marrying convolution and attention for all data sizes. Proc NeurIPS. 2021;34:3965–77.
11. Pacal I, Ozdemir B, Zeynalov J, Gasimov H, Pacal N. A novel CNN-ViT-based deep learning model for early skin cancer diagnosis. Biomed Signal Process Control. 2025;104:107627.

Enabling Fast and Mobile Histopathology Image Annotation through Swipeable Interfaces
SWAN

Sweta Banerjee[1†], Timo Gosch[1†], Sara Hester[1†], Viktoria Weiss[2], Thomas Conrad[3], Taryn A. Donovan[4], Nils Porsche[1], Jonas Ammeling[5], Christoph Stroblberger[6], Robert Klopfleisch[3], Christopher Kaltenecker[6], Christof A. Bertram[2], Katharina Breininger[7], Marc Aubreville[1]

[1]Flensburg University of Applied Sciences, Flensburg, Germany
[2]University of Veterinary Medicine, Vienna, Austria
[3]Freie Universität Berlin, Berlin, Germany
[4]Schwarzman Animal Medical Center, New York, USA
[5]Technische Hochschule Ingolstadt, Ingolstadt, Germany
[6]Medical University of Vienna, Vienna, Austria
[7]Julius-Maximilians-Universität Würzburg, Würzburg, Germany
sweta.banerjee@hs-flensburg.de

Abstract. The annotation of large-scale histopathology image datasets remains a major bottleneck in developing robust deep learning models for clinically relevant tasks, such as mitotic figure classification. Folder-based annotation workflows are usually slow, fatiguing, and difficult to scale. To address these challenges, we introduce swipeable annotations (SWAN), an open-source, MIT-licensed web application that enables intuitive image patch classification using a swiping gesture. SWAN supports both desktop and mobile platforms, offers real-time metadata capture, and allows flexible mapping of swipe gestures to class labels. In a pilot study with four pathologists annotating 600 mitotic figure image patches, we compared SWAN against a traditional folder-sorting workflow. SWAN enabled rapid annotations with pairwise percent agreement ranging from 86.52 % to 93.68 % (Cohen's κ = 0.61–0.80), while for the folder-based method, the pairwise percent agreement ranged from 86.98 % to 91.32 % (Cohen's κ = 0.63–0.75) for the task of classifying atypical versus normal mitotic figures, demonstrating high consistency between annotators and comparable performance. Participants rated the tool as highly usable and appreciated the ability to annotate on mobile devices. These results suggest that SWAN can accelerate image annotation while maintaining annotation quality, offering a scalable and user-friendly alternative to conventional workflows. The full codebase of the SWAN project, including analyses, can be found here: https://github.com/DeepMicroscopy/SWAN.

[†]These authors contributed equally to this work.

© Der/die Autor(en), exklusiv lizenziert an
Springer Fachmedien Wiesbaden GmbH, ein Teil von Springer Nature 2026
H. Handels et al. (Hrsg.), *Bildverarbeitung für die Medizin 2026*,
Informatik aktuell, https://doi.org/10.1007/978-3-658-51100-5_42

1 Introduction

The digitization of whole slide images (WSIs) has enabled the development of deep learning models for automating clinically relevant tasks. However, these models are dependent on accurate annotations by domain experts. In medical imaging, and particularly in histopathology, generating high-quality labels is often a major bottleneck, as it requires domain experts to inspect thousands of images, a process that is time-intensive, tiring, and subject to inter-observer variability. In digital histopathology research, a common annotation workflow involves manually sorting image patches into different folders. While simple, this approach is not optimized for speed, scalability, completeness, or user engagement. Although a wide range of annotation tools have been developed in other domains [1, 2], many of which are commercial, most are tailored for desktop computer environments, limiting flexibility and accessibility. Recent advances in mobile computing and cloud-based data management offer new opportunities to rethink how expert annotation is performed. Mobile-enabled interfaces can allow domain experts to contribute annotations conveniently, even outside the traditional laboratory environment, streamlining collaborative labeling.

In this work, we present swipeable annotations (SWAN), a MIT-licensed, mobile-friendly annotation platform designed to streamline patch-level labeling in digital histopathology. The system supports rapid, scalable, and user-friendly workflows, enabling efficient annotation directly from smartphones or tablets. We describe the platform's design principles, implementation, and user interface (UI), and evaluate its usability, annotation consistency and speed compared to conventional desktop-based methods. Our results demonstrate that mobile-enabled annotation can significantly enhance flexibility and engagement in expert-driven image labeling, addressing a key barrier to scalable dataset generation in computational pathology.

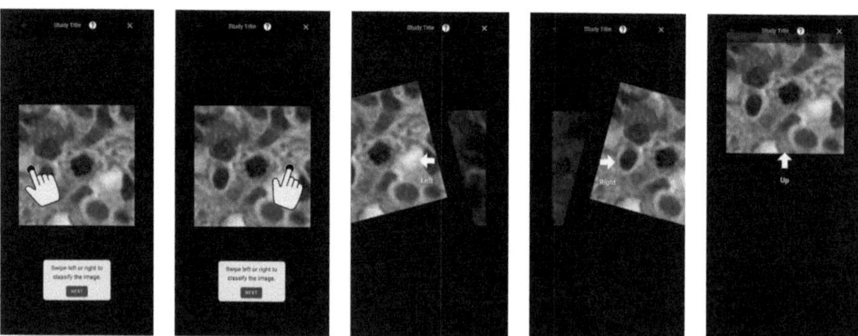

Fig. 1. Swipe interactions in SWAN (mobile version): left, right, and up for classification or postponing, and corresponding thumb icons from the help intro.

2 Materials and methods

Using a swipe-based interaction, popularized for the use-case of binary decision making by dating apps, our tool makes the annotation process more efficient and engaging. Users can label image patches with ease by simply swiping left, right, up, or down. Mistakes can be corrected by going back. The interface can also be used on a tablet or on a desktop computer with a mouse. The tool records timestamped user input and metadata, which enables smooth integration with current annotation pipelines and quantitative analyses. We envision two major use cases for this tool:

- *Annotation*: For annotation of images patches into up to four categories, by swiping left, right, up and down (Fig. 1).
- *Pathologist education*: Training pathologists by displaying the correct option after they swipe their choice (Fig. 2).

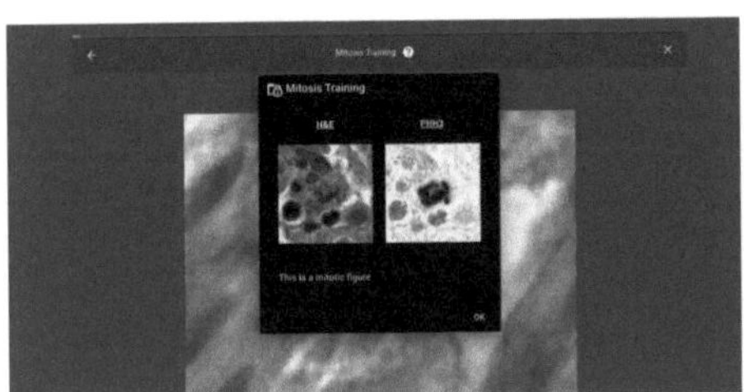

Fig. 2. Application of SWAN for pathologist training (desktop version).

2.1 Software architecture and workflow design

SWAN, which is available on our github repository[2], is implemented using a Django-based backend and a Vuetify-based frontend. It has two main UI:

- *Administrator:* Enables study definition, dataset management, and user-management. Annotation classes for each direction and UI-related settings can be configured here.
- *Participant:* Provides access to assigned studies for annotation and training.

A typical annotation workflow then involves the following steps:

1. The admin creates a project group and assigns the existing experts to it.
2. The admin uploads the data set as an image archive (`.zip` or `.tar` format).
3. The admin creates the study, selects the dataset and defines the UI configuration.
4. Participants log in and open an assigned study from the overview. New users are greeted with an onboarding sequence.
5. Participants annotate by swiping left, right, up, or down, and can resume from their last position in subsequent sessions.
6. The annotations and associated metadata can be exported to a CSV file.

The order of the data set is randomized for each participant.

[2]`https://github.com/DeepMicroscopy/SWAN`

2.2 User study

To demonstrate the practical use of SWAN, we conducted a pilot user study, evaluating the usability and efficiency of SWAN's swipe-based interface for a classification annotation workflow and to compare it against the routine desktop folder-based annotation workflow. We chose the task of subclassification of mitotic figures (MFs) into typical and atypical MFs. This task is particularly well-suited for evaluating the impact of different annotation strategies because it is an emerging topic of research and has shown only moderate inter-rater variability in prior studies [3]. We chose a random subset of 600 mitotic figure image patches that were cropped from the canine cutaneous mast cell tumor (CCMCT) dataset [4]. All images were in the `.png` format with dimensions of 128×128 pixels.

Four pathologists participated in this user study. To minimize recall bias, a washout period of at least two weeks was implemented before each phase. The user study was conducted in three phases:

2.2.1 SWAN (Initial). In the first of three phases, participants were provided with login credentials to access the SWAN platform and annotate the assigned image set. For this study, the left swipe was mapped to the *normal* class and the right swipe to the *atypical* class. These annotations, including timestamp information, were then exported as CSV files for downstream quantitative analyses.

After completing the annotations, each participant was asked to fill in a post-study questionnaire that collected information about their professional background, experience in histopathology, familiarity with atypical mitotic figures (AMFs) classification, and device used. Usability aspects like responsiveness, ease of use, intuitiveness of the swipe mechanism, perceived image quality, confidence, engagement, and willingness to reuse, were assessed using 5-point Likert scales. Additional open-ended questions addressed uncertainty during classification, technical issues, and suggestions for improvement.

2.2.2 SWAN (Enhanced). In the second study phase, we incorporated feedback from pathologists and updated the SWAN app as follows:

- To address the pixelation reported in the first phase, we introduced two features: an image-scaling option to display images at partial screen size and a toggle for image interpolation.
- We introduced a feature allowing to assign a swiping direction, e.g., upwards, with a postpone functionality, enabling revisiting difficult or confusing images at the end of the trial.

Upon finishing the annotations, each participant was asked to complete the post-study questionnaire again, where they were additionally asked focused questions regarding factors related to new functionality in this phase.

Tab. 1. Average annotation times in seconds per participant per image across all three phases.

Participant	SWAN(Initial)	SWAN(Enhanced)	Folder-Based
expert 1	1.58	1.67	1.83
expert 2	2.83	2.41	4.30
expert 3	2.72	2.60	2.25
expert 4	1.67	2.18	2.90

Tab. 2. Pairwise inter-observer agreement across participants for SWAN (Initial), SWAN (Enhanced), and folder-based annotation modes. Percent agreement and Cohen's κ are reported separately for each mode.

Participant Pair	SWAN(Initial)		SWAN(Enhanced)		Folder-Based Method	
	Agreement	Cohen's κ	Agreement	Cohen's κ	Agreement	Cohen's κ
expert 1 vs expert 2	87.98 %	0.66	86.52 %	0.61	90.15 %	0.69
expert 1 vs expert 3	85.64 %	0.61	87.67 %	0.66	87.15 %	0.63
expert 1 vs expert 4	87.81 %	0.67	93.68 %	0.80	91.49 %	0.73
expert 2 vs expert 3	82.30 %	0.55	87.83 %	0.69	86.98 %	0.66
expert 2 vs expert 4	85.14 %	0.63	87.52 %	0.66	91.32 %	0.75
expert 3 vs expert 4	81.47 %	0.55	87.67 %	0.67	89.65 %	0.72

2.2.3 Folder-based method. In this phase, the same participants were asked to annotate the same image set using their routine desktop folder-based method, where they put the images into two different folders according to normal or atypical MFs and to manually record their annotation times.

3 Results

Across participants, mean annotation time per image was 1.58–2.83 s for the initial SWAN phase and 1.67–2.60 s for the enhanced SWAN phase, while the folder-based method was generally slower (1.83–4.30 s; Tab. 1). Pairwise percent agreement was 81.47–87.98% (Cohen's κ=0.55–0.67) for the initial phase of SWAN, 86.52–93.68% (Cohen's κ=0.61–0.80) for the enhanced version of SWAN (Tab. 2), and 86.98–91.49% (κ=0.63–0.75) for the folder-based method, which was comparable to enhanced SWAN. Fleiss' κ across all four participants was 0.610, 0.680, and 0.695 for SWAN (Initial), SWAN (Enhanced), and the folder-based phase, respectively.

In addition to the quantitative analyses, participants provided post-study questionnaire feedback after each SWAN iteration, and the questionnaires are available in our GitHub repository. Usability ratings were high in both phases (SWAN (Initial): Mean = 5.00; SWAN (Enhanced): Mean = 5.00), and responsiveness of the smartphone swipe interactions was rated similarly highly (SWAN (Initial): Mean = 4.75; SWAN (Enhanced): Mean = 5.00). Perceived image quality improved from Mean = 4.00 in SWAN (Initial) to Mean = 4.75 in SWAN (Enhanced), which participants attributed to the adjustable image scaling feature (Mean = 4.00). The enhanced questionnaire additionally assessed the image scaling option and the upward swipe to postpone unclassified cases. No significant technical issues were reported, and participants indicated they would likely use the platform for larger studies and recommend it to colleagues, reflecting strong acceptance and usability.

4 Discussion

Annotation can be a repetitive and mentally fatiguing task, and finding ways to make it more engaging is an important step toward scaling annotation efforts. The concept behind SWAN is to provide an annotation experience that is more intuitive, lightweight, and accessible, allowing users to label data not only at a desktop PC but also on mobile devices, in more flexible settings.

Our pilot study demonstrates that this idea has strong potential. The app received positive feedback for its usability and convenience, with improved ratings in the second phase of the study, particularly for image quality and responsiveness. After introducing image scaling and upward swipe functionality in the enhanced version of SWAN, the inter-rater agreement (Cohen's κ 0.61–0.80, Fleiss' κ 0.680) was comparable to the folder-based method (Cohen's κ 0.63–0.75, Fleiss' κ 0.695), as shown in Tab. 2.

While these small differences could well be explained by measurement error, other factors might also be involved: for one, there was a lower familiarization with the SWAN interface. Furthermore, since the SWAN tool presents one image at a time, unlike folder-based workflows that provide more contextual overview, a limited comparability between samples might be involved that could reduce discrimination. Future versions of SWAN can directly address these limitations by incorporating enhanced navigation options or hybrid viewing modes.

Overall, these results point to a promising starting point – an annotation platform that can make annotation for classification tasks more enjoyable and flexible without compromising the quality. Continued development and larger user studies will help determine how best to balance engagement, efficiency, and annotation quality.

Acknowledgement. The authors would like to acknowledge support by the German Research Foundation (DFG, Project No.s 520330054, 460333672 CRC1540 EBM and 545049923), the Austrian Science Fund (FWF, Project No. I 6555) and the Bavarian State Ministry of the Sciences and the Arts (project FOKUS-TML).

References

1. Marée R, Rollus L, Stévens B, Hoyoux R, Louppe G, Vandaele R et al. Collaborative analysis of multi-gigapixel imaging data using cytomine. Bioinformatics. 2016;32(9):1395–401.
2. Bankhead P, Loughrey MB, Fernández JA, Dombrowski Y, McArt DG, Dunne PD et al. QuPath: open source software for digital pathology image analysis. Sci Rep. 2017;7(1):1–7.

3. Bertram CA, Weiss V, Donovan TA, Banerjee S, Conrad T, Ammeling J et al. Histologic dataset of normal and atypical mitotic figures on human breast cancer (AMi-Br). Proc BVM. 2025:113–8.
4. Bertram CA, Aubreville M, Marzahl C, Maier A, Klopfleisch R. A large-scale dataset for mitotic figure assessment on whole slide images of canine cutaneous mast cell tumor. Sci Data. 2019;6(1):274.

Prediction of Patient and Mobile C-arm Orientation in Orthopedic Trauma Procedures

Joshua Scheuplein [1,2], Björn Kreher [2], Andreas Maier [1]

[1]Pattern Recognition Lab, Department of Computer Science,
Friedrich-Alexander-Universität Erlangen-Nürnberg, Erlangen, Germany
[2]Advanced Therapies, Siemens Healthineers AG, Forchheim, Germany
joshua.scheuplein@fau.de

Abstract. Accurate knowledge of patient and mobile C-arm system orientation is essential for intraoperative 3D scan acquisition, yet this information is currently entered manually by operating room staff, making the process time-consuming and error-prone. We propose a deep learning approach for the joint classification of patient and C-arm orientation using only a pair of anterior-posterior and lateral projection images. The method builds on frozen DAX foundation model embeddings, combined with a task-specific head network trained on 633 clinical 3D scans. The developed model achieved a weighted mean F1-score of 89.9% (±1.3%). It can be seamlessly incorporated into the clinical 3D workflow to automatically infer orientation from pre-existing scout views, thus reducing the need for manual intervention and enhancing intraoperative efficiency.

1 Introduction

Intraoperative imaging with mobile C-arm systems has become a cornerstone of modern orthopedic trauma procedures, enabling three-dimensional visualization of patient anatomy and assisting in precise implant placement [1]. Before acquiring a 3D scan, the operating room (OR) staff must manually set both the patient orientation on the operating table and the relative position of the C-arm system, as depicted in Fig1 1. This procedure is not only time-intensive but also susceptible to human error, which poses a significant risk for surgical flow disruption [2]. Automated estimation of patient and C-arm orientation from projection images could therefore streamline the 3D workflow and reduce intraoperative delays.

Previous studies have investigated various aspects of intraoperative pose estimation using deep learning (DL). Esfandiari et al. demonstrated that deep neural networks can predict the C-arm position relative to the CT volume from a single X-ray image [3]. Similarly, Kausch et al. proposed an automated approach for C-arm positioning to obtain standard projections during spinal surgery, employing a sequential pipeline for pose regression [4]. While these studies primarily focused on C-arm pose estimation, Fang et al. further examined the retrieval of orientation metadata

© Der/die Autor(en), exklusiv lizenziert an
Springer Fachmedien Wiesbaden GmbH, ein Teil von Springer Nature 2026
H. Handels et al. (Hrsg.), *Bildverarbeitung für die Medizin 2026*,
Informatik aktuell, https://doi.org/10.1007/978-3-658-51100-5_43

w.r.t. the patient anatomy, such as laterality [5]. Moreover, Ravi et al. demonstrated that DL-based orientation and structure classification can also facilitate autonomous protocol selection in angiography [6].

However, a gap remains in jointly classifying patient and C-arm system orientation within a single DL model. To overcome this limitation, we present an efficient approach that builds on foundational feature extractors pre-trained with the DINO adapted to X-ray (DAX) method [7]. Leveraging these rich, transferable representations, we demonstrate that a compact and lightweight task-specific head network can be effectively trained on a dataset of only 633 clinical 3D scans to accurately classify both patient and C-arm orientation from just two projection scout images, which are typically acquired during iso-center positioning of the C-arm system.

2 Materials and methods

2.1 Dataset

A custom dataset was collected in collaboration with a clinical partner, comprising 3D scans from various anatomical regions. In total, 633 scans from 392 individual patients were included. The ground truth orientation labels were extracted from the DICOM headers, which record the manual inputs provided by the OR staff prior to the actual 3D acquisition step. Fig. 2a illustrates all possible combinations of patient and C-arm orientations, while Fig. 2b shows their distribution.

From each scan, 100 image pairs were sampled, with each pair consisting of one anterior-posterior (AP) and one lateral (LAT) image. This resulted in a final dataset containing 63,300 samples in total. The AP images were randomly selected from each set of projection images covering an orbital angle range of $\theta \in [-45°, +45°]$, whereas the LAT views were randomly sampled from the remaining projections.

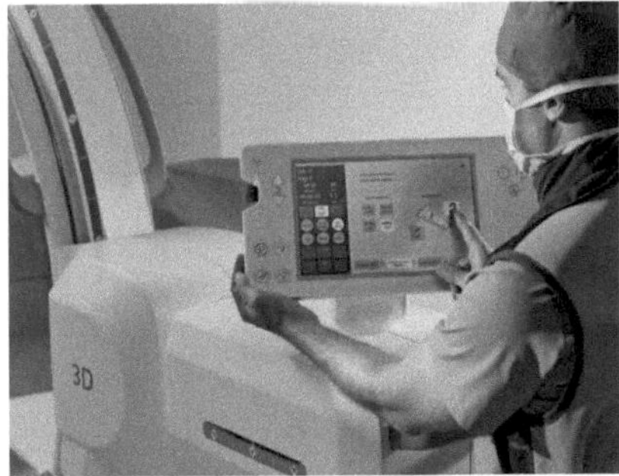

Fig. 1. User interface (UI) of a mobile C-arm system from Siemens Healthineers [8]. Prior to each 3D scan, the OR staff manually enters orientation information via buttons on the touch display. Patient orientation is categorized into four classes (prone, supine, or lateral decubitus right/left), while the C-arm orientation is differentiated into two classes (head first or feet first).

To reliably evaluate the model performance independent of a specific train-test split, we employed k-fold cross-validation, dividing the original dataset into distinct subsets. The maximum number of folds was constrained by the orientation category with the fewest available scans. For the class HFDL, only six scans from three individual patients were collected, and to ensure that samples from the same patient appeared in only one fold, k was set to three consequently.

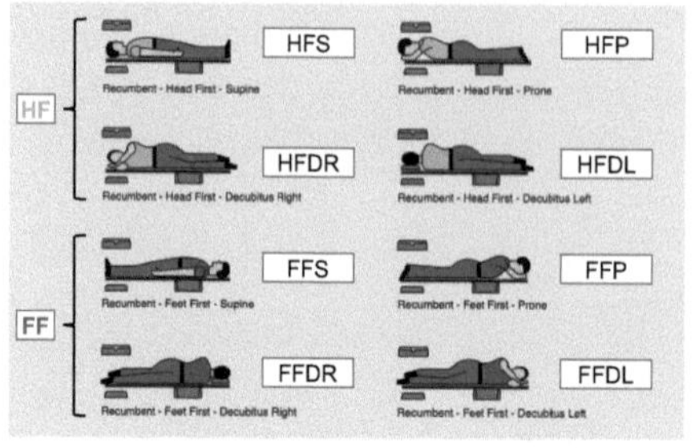

(**a**) Possible orientation setups [9].

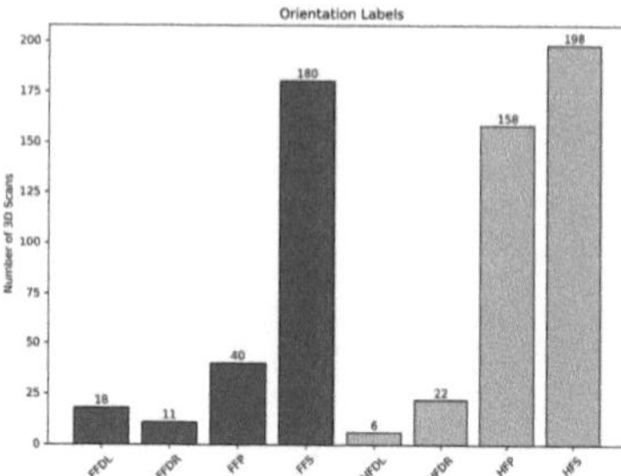

(**b**) Histogram of orientation labels.

Fig. 2. Summary of the dataset used in this study. (a) Eight distinct combinations of patient and C-arm system orientation can occur during clinical routine. (b) Because patient orientation correlates with the type of surgical procedure, the dataset is highly imbalanced across the different categories.

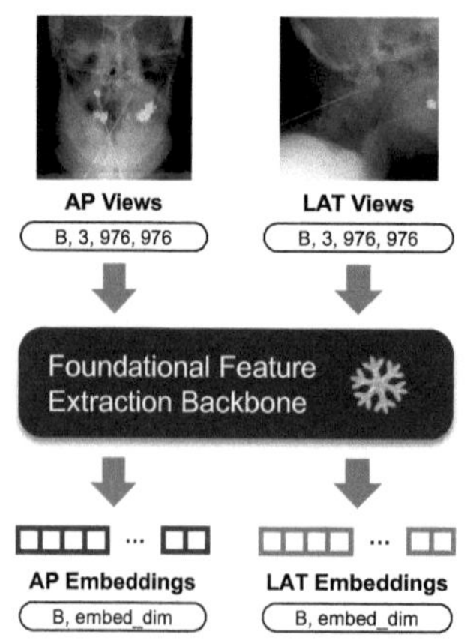

(**a**) Feature extraction using frozen DAX foundation model.

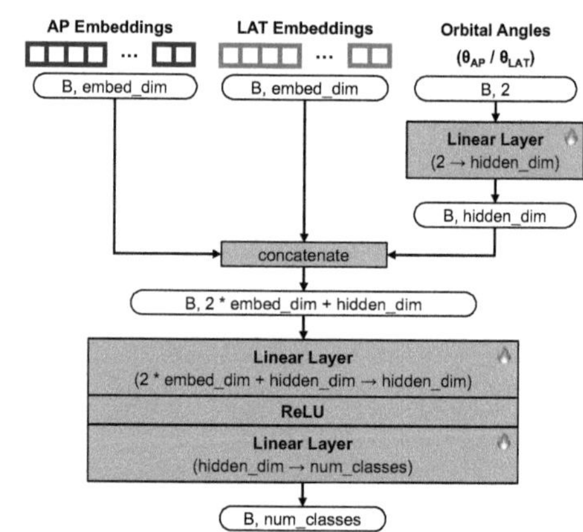

(**b**) Head network architecture used for predicting orientation categories.

Fig. 3. High-level processing pipeline. Based on frozen feature embeddings for both AP and LAT images (a) as well as information about the corresponding orbital angles of the mobile C-arm system, a lightweight head network (b) is implemented for solving the given classification problem.

2.2 Model training

Fig. 3 illustrates our two-step approach. First, the class tokens from the last five layers of a DAX ViT-S-16 backbone with an embedding dimension of 384 are extracted as frozen feature encodings. Second, a trainable head network, with hidden dimension of 512, concatenates the AP and LAT image embeddings along with the additionally encoded orbital angles to predict the given orientation setup. Less than 10% of the 24 million total model parameters are contained in the head network.

The model was trained using cross-entropy loss (CEL) and optimized based on stochastic gradient descent (SGD) with momentum set to 0.9 and a weight decay of 1×10^{-4}. The learning rate was fixed to 2×10^{-5} throughout training, i.e., no learning rate scheduling was applied. Model training was conducted with a batch size of 512 on a single NVIDIA A100 GPU for 1000 epochs.

3 Results

In order to better understand the model's learned representations, we first analyzed the backbone feature space using UMAP embeddings as shown in Fig. 4. Distinct clusters emerge for different orientation categories, indicating that the frozen DAX embeddings already encode discriminative information relevant to this task. Clusters of similar patient orientations, such as right and left decubitus or prone and supine, appear close to each other, while separation between head-first (HF) and feet-first (FF) classes, reflecting differences in C-arm orientation, can still be observed.

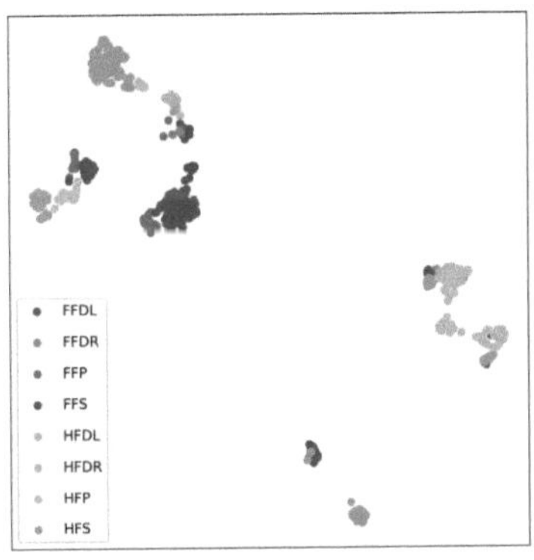

Fig. 4. UMAP visualization illustrating the discriminative properties of the frozen DAX embeddings. Each point in the scatter plot represents one 3D scan from the dataset described in Section 2.1. To obtain the UMAP representation for each sample, the backbone embeddings of the two projection images closest to orbital angles of 0° and 90° were concatenated. The color coding indicates the corresponding orientation class: lighter shades indicate HF categories, while darker shades represent FF categories.

Tab. 1 delineates the quantitative performance of the proposed model across all eight orientation categories, assessed through 3-fold cross-validation. The weighted mean precision and recall achieve values of 89.9% (±1.2%) and 90.5% (±1.2%), respectively, demonstrating solid overall consistency. The model exhibits exceptional performance in prone and supine orientations, where F1-scores surpass 85% with small variability across folds. Conversely, the decubitus classes display significantly lower and more variable performance metrics, reflecting the limited number of available training samples for these orientations.

Tab. 1. Quantitative results based on a 3-fold cross-validation experiment.

	Accuracy	Precision	Recall	F1-Score
FFDL	98.8 ± 0.6	77.1 ± 16.6	94.4 ± 6.70	83.2 ± 6.70
FFDR	98.8 ± 0.6	45.7 ± 33.2	46.0 ± 35.9	45.6 ± 34.2
FFP	98.4 ± 0.5	93.6 ± 3.80	79.5 ± 11.2	85.5 ± 6.50
FFS	96.0 ± 0.4	92.8 ± 1.50	93.2 ± 1.80	93.0 ± 0.70
HFDL	99.1 ± 0.3	33.6 ± 34.8	22.2 ± 24.0	26.7 ± 28.4
HFDR	99.3 ± 0.6	91.8 ± 1.30	86.7 ± 18.8	88.1 ± 11.3
HFP	95.9 ± 1.2	92.6 ± 0.60	90.7 ± 6.10	91.5 ± 2.90
HFS	94.7 ± 1.3	89.7 ± 3.90	94.3 ± 2.70	91.8 ± 1.90
Weighted Mean	96.0 ± 0.5	89.9 ± 1.20	90.5 ± 1.20	89.9 ± 1.30

As a final evaluation, we present confusion matrices in Fig. 5 to further characterize the model's errors, indicating which classes are most frequently confused. Consistent with the metrics reported in Tab. 1, the classes FFDR and HFDL exhibit the lowest performance and highest misclassification rates. When considering patient and C-arm orientation categories separately, the matrices reveal that the model reliably distinguishes FF from HF C-arm orientations, as well as prone and supine patient positions, whereas the highest confusion occurs between right and left decubitus cases.

4 Discussion

We presented a DL approach for joint classification of patient and mobile C-arm system orientation using only a single pair of AP and LAT projection images. By leveraging frozen DAX embeddings together with a lightweight task-specific head network, the model achieved a weighted mean F1-score of 89.9% (±1.3%). The current limitations include diminished performance for underrepresented classes and evaluation on data from a single clinical site and imaging modality, which may limit generalizability. Moreover, ground truth labels were directly obtained from manual input by OR staff without additional verification. Given the time constraints

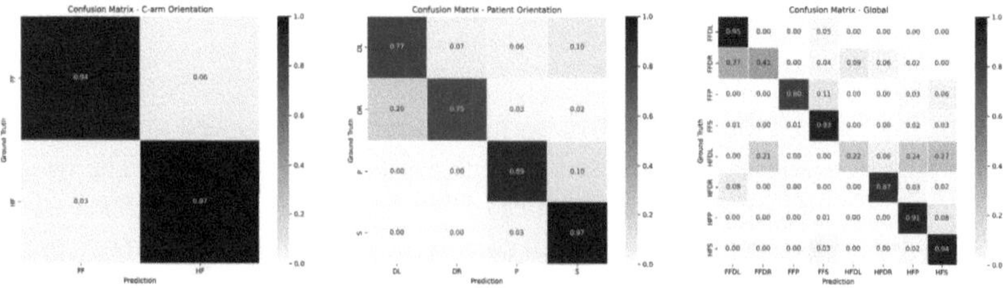

Fig. 5. Confusion matrices for C-arm (left), patient (center), and combined (right) orientation labels. Each cell shows the class-wise score averaged over all three test folds.

of interventional procedures, this may introduce errors and associated label noise, suggesting the incorporation of a rigorous label validation strategy.

Future work will comprise the collection of an expanded, multi-institutional dataset and the use of data augmentation strategies, such as advanced sampling of image pairs, to mitigate class imbalance. For example, augmented decubitus cases can be generated from scans originally acquired in prone or supine positions by rotating the AP/LAT sampling intervals by ±90° w.r.t. the original source 3D scan. In addition, incorporating geometric constraints such as epipolar consistency [10] during feature sampling from the two scout images could further enhance the robustness and spatial coherence of the learned representations.

The proposed solution can be seamlessly integrated into the standard workflow for 3D scan acquisition. Since surgeons routinely acquire AP and LAT scout images to verify correct iso-center positioning of the mobile C-arm system, these projections are inherently available as input without requiring additional radiation exposure to the patient. Once the 3D workflow is initiated by the OR staff, the model can perform inference on the most recent AP and LAT images to automatically pre-select the corresponding UI options, thereby reducing manual input, saving time, and enhancing overall workflow efficiency.

References

1. Tonetti J, Boudissa M, Kerschbaumer G, Seurat O. Role of 3D intraoperative imaging in orthopedic and trauma surgery. Orthop Traumatol Surg Res. 2020;106(1, Supplement):S19–S25.
2. Khan A, Shappell SA, Boquet AJ. Characterization of surgical flow disruptions in orthopedic surgery using a human factors approach. Perioper Care Oper Room Manag. 2025;39:100488.
3. Esfandiari H, Andreß S, Herold M, Böcker W, Weidert S, Hodgson AJ. A deep learning approach for single shot c-arm pose estimation. Proc CAOS/TAMIS. 2020;4:69–73.
4. Kausch L, Thomas S, Kunze H, Norajitra T, Klein A, Ayala L et al. C-arm positioning for standard projections during spinal implant placement. Med Image Anal. 2022;81:102557.
5. Fang X, Harris L, Zhou W, Huo D. Generalized radiographic view identification with deep learning. J Digit Imaging. 2021;34(1):66–74.
6. Ravi A, Bernhardt P, Hoffmann M, Kordon F, Bayer S, Achenbach S et al. Deep learning-based classification of coronary arteries and left ventricle using multimodal data for autonomous protocol selection or adjustment in angiography. Sci Rep. 2025;15(1):15186.
7. Scheuplein J, Rohleder M, Maier A, Kreher B. DINO adapted to X-ray (DAX): foundation models for intraoperative X-ray imaging. Proc MICCAI. 2026:138–48.
8. User interface of the cios spin. Siemens Healthineers AG. 2025. URL: https://marketing.webassets.siemens-healthineers.com/1800000004349706/1cc13970ee5d/v/6629c5aebf67/AT_Internet_Productimage_Cios_Spin_More_Efficiency_1800000004349706.jpg (visited on 10/13/2025).
9. Digital imaging and communications in medicine (DICOM) standard. National Electrical Manufacturers Association (NEMA). 2024. URL: http://dicom.nema.org/medical/dicom/current/output/html/figures/PS3.3_C.7.3.1.1.2-1.svg (visited on 10/13/2025).

10. Aichert A, Wang J, Schaffert R, Dörfler A, Hornegger J, Maier AK. Epipolar consistency in fluoroscopy for image-based tracking. Proc BMVC. 2015:82–1.

Abstract: DINO Adapted to X-ray (DAX)

Foundation Models for Intraoperative X-ray Imaging

Joshua Scheuplein [1,2], Maximilian Rohleder [1,2], Andreas Maier [1], Björn Kreher [2]

[1] Pattern Recognition Lab, Department of Computer Science, Friedrich-Alexander-Universität Erlangen-Nürnberg, Erlangen, Germany
[2] Advanced Therapies, Siemens Healthineers AG, Forchheim, Germany
joshua.scheuplein@fau.de

Intraoperative X-ray imaging represents a key technology for guiding orthopedic interventions. Recent advancements in deep learning have enabled automated image analysis in this field, thereby streamlining clinical workflows and enhancing patient outcomes. However, many existing approaches depend on task-specific models and are constrained by the limited availability of annotated data. In contrast, self-supervised foundation models have exhibited remarkable potential to learn robust feature representations without label annotations. In this work, we introduce DINO adapted to X-ray (DAX), a novel framework that adapts DINO for training foundational feature extraction backbones tailored to intraoperative X-ray imaging. Our approach involves pre-training on a dataset comprising over 632,000 image samples, which surpasses other publicly available datasets in both size and feature diversity. To validate the successful incorporation of relevant domain knowledge into our DAX models, we conduct an extensive evaluation of all backbones on three distinct downstream tasks and demonstrate that small head networks can be trained on top of our frozen foundation models to successfully solve applications regarding (1) body region classification, (2) metal implant segmentation, and (3) screw object detection. The results of our study underscore the potential of the DAX framework to facilitate the development of robust, scalable, and clinically impactful deep learning solutions for intraoperative X-ray image analysis. Source code and model checkpoints are publicly available at `https://github.com/JoshuaScheuplein/DAX` [1].

References

1. Scheuplein J, Rohleder M, Maier A, Kreher B. DINO adapted to X-ray (DAX): foundation models for intraoperative X-ray imaging. Proc MICCAI. 2026:138–48.

© Der/die Autor(en), exklusiv lizenziert an
Springer Fachmedien Wiesbaden GmbH, ein Teil von Springer Nature 2026
H. Handels et al. (Hrsg.), *Bildverarbeitung für die Medizin 2026*,
Informatik aktuell, https://doi.org/10.1007/978-3-658-51100-5_44

Abstract: Automated Multimodel Segmentation and Tracking for AR-guided Open Liver Surgery using Scene-aware Self-prompting

Serouj Khajarian [1,2], Michael Schwimmbeck [1,3], Konstantin Holzapfel[4], Johannes Schmidt[4], Christopher Auer [1], Stefanie Remmele [1], Oliver Amft [2,5]

[1]Research Group Medical Technolgies, University of Applied Sciences Landshut
[2]Intelligent Embedded Systems Lab., University of Freiburg
[3]Chair for Visual Computing, Friedrich-Alexander-Universität Erlangen-Nürnberg
[4]LAKUMED Kliniken, Landshut
[5]Hahn-Schickard, Freiburg
serouj.khajarian@haw-landshut.de

In open liver surgery, augmented reality (AR) guidance requires continuous segmentation and tracking of the liver surface to achieve the necessary alignment between the preoperative model and its corresponding intraoperative state. In this work [1], we present a multimodel approach for semantic segmentation and tracking in AR-assisted open liver surgery. Our method combines a domain-specific RGBD model, a foundational semantic segmentation model, and a semi-supervised video object segmentation (VOS) model. The models were integrated into an auto-promptable pipeline, using a scene-aware re-prompting algorithm that adapts to changes in the surgical scene. We tested our method using intraoperative RGBD videos from ten open liver surgeries, collected from a head-mounted AR device. We evaluated the segmentation accuracy (IoU) and temporal resolution (FPS) of our method for different re-prompting strategies, comparing them against the performance of the individual models. Our multimodel approach attained a median IoU of 71 % at 13.2 FPS without re-prompting. It outperformed individual models, enhancing segmentation accuracy beyond the stand-alone RGBD model and offering better temporal resolution than the foundation model. With scene-aware reprompting, the multimodel pipeline reaches the upper-bound setting of the semi-supervised VOS model (initialized by an optimal reference frame), achieving 74.7 % IoU at 11.5 FPS. Our scene-aware re-prompting strategy offers a balance between segmentation accuracy and temporal resolution, thus addressing the demands of real-time AR-guided open liver surgery.

References

1. Khajarian S, Schwimmbeck M, Holzapfel K, Schmidt J, Auer C, Remmele S et al. Automated multimodel segmentation and tracking for AR-guided open liver surgery using scene-aware self-prompting. Int J Comput Assist Radiol Surg. 2025:1–9.

© Der/die Autor(en), exklusiv lizenziert an
Springer Fachmedien Wiesbaden GmbH, ein Teil von Springer Nature 2026
H. Handels et al. (Hrsg.), *Bildverarbeitung für die Medizin 2026*,
Informatik aktuell, https://doi.org/10.1007/978-3-658-51100-5_45

Perfusion-aware Surgical Planning

Simulating the Effects on Planned Hepatic Resection Zones using Graph-based Vessel Modeling

Janine Rothert [1,2,3], Judith L. Salz[2], Joy Rakshit[1], Viola Ehses[4], Florentine Huettl[4], Tobias Huber[4], Hauke Lang[4], Georg Rose[2,3], Sylvia Saalfeld[1], Georg Hille[1]

[1]Institute for Medical Informatics and Statistics, University Hospital Schleswig-Holstein Campus Kiel

[2]Institute for Medical Engineering, Otto von Guericke University Magdeburg

[3]Research Campus Stimulate Magdeburg

[4]Clinic for General, Visceral, and Transplant Surgery, University Medical Center Mainz

janine.rothert@ovgu.de

Abstract. Accurate estimation of the functional liver remnant is essential for planning safe liver resections. Unintended vessel transections and subsequent perfusion loss may compromise the functional liver remnant and increase the post-operative risk. We present an approach that models portal and hepatic veins as directed graphs to simulate blood flow and predict downstream perfusion loss by cut vessels. Quantitative metrics, including perfused functional liver remnant and spatial mismatch to the planned resection zone, are automatically computed and visualized. We demonstrated on 22 patients and 31 resections zones that in most cases non-perfused regions extended beyond the planned resection zone, indicating potential risk areas for risk stratification. In conclusion, graph-based perfusion modeling provides quantitative and visual feedback to support pre-operative planning of complex liver resections. This approach may aid in identifying high-risk territories and optimizing resection strategies, demonstrating promising value for surgical decision support.

1 Introduction

Hepatic resection remains the definitive curative option for many patients with primary and secondary liver malignancies, yet the procedure balances two critical imperatives: oncologic completeness and preservation of sufficient functional liver remnant (FLR). Accurate pre-operative planning of the resection zone is thus indispensable, owing to the highly variable intra-hepatic vascular anatomy and the non-trivial relationship between anatomical volume and functional viability. While contemporary computer-assisted planning platforms for hepatic resection routinely offer 3D segmentation of the liver parenchyma and intrahepatic vascular trees, enabling volumetric and geometric evaluation of resection proposals, the consideration

© Der/die Autor(en), exklusiv lizenziert an Springer Fachmedien Wiesbaden GmbH, ein Teil von Springer Nature 2026
H. Handels et al. (Hrsg.), *Bildverarbeitung für die Medizin 2026*, Informatik aktuell, https://doi.org/10.1007/978-3-658-51100-5_46

of functional consequences of vessel transection (i.e., resulting perfusion deficits) in the remnant parenchyma, although an evermore relevant research question [1, 2], still remains to see the transfer of current research work to implementation in commercial planning systems.

Transection of portal inflow or hepatic venous outflow during resection may result in regions of non-perfused parenchyma, which can compromise post-operative liver function or predispose to ischemia, necrosis, or bile leakage. Computational haemodynamic models of liver perfusion have shown promise in predicting acute changes following partial resections [2]. Building upon these advances, simulating and visualizing the resulting perfused versus non-perfused liver tissue, based on planned cut-planes and vascular connectivity, may provide surgical planners with critical functional insight beyond mere volumetry. Integrating perfusion-aware simulation into hepatic resection planning offers several potential benefits: improved estimation of the effective FLR (rather than anatomical volume alone), early identification of possible ischemic or congested zones, optimization of alternative resection strategies with maximal perfusion preservation, and ultimately reduction of post-operative complications and improved outcomes. Indeed, the advent of vessel-guided parenchyma-sparing hepatectomies underscores the importance of functional vascular territories in planning [3].

By coupling anatomical visualization with physiologically meaningful modeling, the proposed approach strengthens the bridge between morphological pre-operative planning and functional post-operative prognosis.

2 Materials and methods

We present a graph-based modeling of hepatic vessels to simulate vessel transections and predict downstream perfusion loss for pre-operative planning.

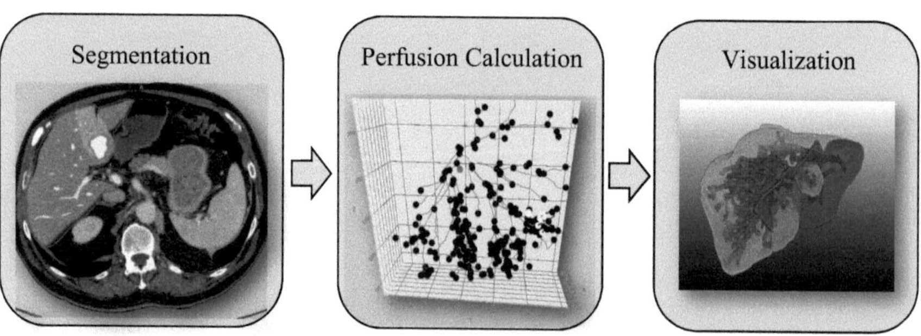

Fig. 1. The figure shows the pipeline for determining potential perfusion loss in liver parenchyma by planned resection zones. The segmentation masks are generated (left) within a surgical planning software serving as the input for the main perfusion calculation (middle), where the vessel systems are represented as directed graphs. The analysis and visualization (right) is then based on these calculations.

The pipeline consists of three major components (Fig. 1). First, segmentations of the liver, portal vein, and hepatic vein, along with an initial resection zone planning, serve as input data for the algorithm. Because the arterial vascular system was imaged at a different time during contrast administration and runs parallel to the portal venous system, its effects are assumed to be sufficiently captured by the portal vein assessment and are therefore not considered further in subsequent stages of the study.

Second, downstream perfusion loss is calculated using directed graph representations of both vessel systems. The graphs are generated by skeletonizing the vessel segmentations to obtain centerlines, followed by adding nodes at vessel intersections and defining edges between them. Graph directionality, representing blood flow, is determined by identifying the node with the largest vessel radius, which is assumed to represent the entry point to the liver. Intersections between the resection zone and vessel centerlines were assumed as transections points and therefore label downstream branches as non-perfused and upstream branches as perfused according to the graph direction. A Nearest Neighbor Segment Approximation based on the minimal Euclidean distance is used to assign each voxel of the liver parenchyma with its closest perfused or non-perfused vessel, following the approach described by Selle et al. [4]. This divides the liver into perfused remnant and non-perfused regions for subsequent analysis and visualization.

Third, the analysis and visualization phase quantifies the non-perfused area relative to the planned resection zone. Key metrics include the planned FLR and the calculated perfused FLR. For comparing both, an area-based overlap metric (Dice similarity coefficient (DSC)) with higher scores reflecting less additional non-perfused areas beyond the planned resection zone and a distance-based metric, the maximum Hausdorff distance (HD), highlights spatial discrepancies where particular caution may be required during surgery to perfusion loss; higher values indicate more extensive non-perfused regions.

We demonstrated the method on 22 patient cases with 31 planned resection zones treated at the University Hospital of Mainz . The input segmentations were obtained semi-automatically from the surgical planning software (© FUJIFILM Healthcare), while the resection zone was manually and retrospectively defined by a surgeon based on the surgery protocol. However, in clinical routine the software is used for the pre-operative intervention planning.

3 Results

Tab. 1 represents treatment related metrics for the planned resection zones in comparison to the determined non-perfused liver parenchyma from resection-related transections. While the liver volume (LV), planned FLR and the resection zone volume (ResV) can be directly derived from the initial data input, the perfused FLR, the non-perfused volume per resection zone (non-PV) and the overlap metrics are calculated based on our algorithm.

Tab. 1. The table shows treatment related parameter for every patient and planned resection zone. While the liver volume (LV), planned functional liver remnant (planned FLR) and the likely perfused functional liver remnant (perfused FLR) are calculated patient wise (P-ID), the resection zone volume (ResV), the non-perfused volume due to intersections with vessels from one resection zone (non-PV) and the overlap between the resections zones and additional non-perfused areas are determined for each individual resection zone. No intersection with vessels are indicated by (-) for the overlap calculation. The Dice similarity coefficient (DSC) represent the overlap between the planned resection zone and the non-perfused area, while the maximum Hausdorff distance (HD) indicates spatial discrepancies.

P-ID	LV [cm³]	Planned FLR [%]	Perfused FLR [%]	ResV [cm³]	Non-PV [cm³]	DSC [%]	HD [mm]
Typical resection zone planning (Fig. 2a)							
1	2996.51	78.17	35.63	220.84	1391.27	27.40	123.26
				93.60	136.67	81.30	21.19
				260.70	510.08	67.65	66.07
				78.96	139.47	72.30	46.86
2	3672.30	96.97	94.89	111.34	187.83	74.43	44.04
3	1954.66	96.83	93.53	14.77	34.04	81.06	13.95
				12.20	23.20	77.79	22.65
				24.09	69.22	51.63	31.01
4	2103.94	80.17	33.31	417.24	1403.12	45.84	98.57
5	2234.22	93.85	85.07	114.78	177.59	78.52	29.12
				22.69	169.39	23.63	79.23
6	2372.02	66.92	61.49	784.71	913.58	92.41	35.72
7	1988.17	50.25	23.64	942.09	1496.08	77.28	53.55
				8.94	22.07	57.65	18.21
				38.00	441.48	15.85	115.65
8	2544.60	96.46	96.21	90.02	96.55	96.50	14.82
9	1861.83	98.44	97.51	29.01	46.41	76.94	21.50
10	2097.59	85.59	84.41	302.26	327.1	96.05	13.79
11	2154.21	38.69	33.52	1320.79	1432.11	95.96	37.16
12	1581.91	83.78	72.68	256.59	432.22	74.50	53.33
13	3019.8	91.91	91.17	244.33	266.67	95.63	26.82
14	2041.39	95.31	91.99	95.70	163.52	73.84	26.04
∅	2330.23 ± 557.10	82.38 ± 18.57	71.08 ± 27.81	249.36 ± 341.59	449.08 ± 515.95	69.73 ± 23.63	45.12 ± 32.53
No vessel transection (Fig. 2b)							
15	1982.22	98.44	98.44	18.69	-	-	-
				12.24	-	-	-
16	1761.12	99.39	99.39	10.76	-	-	-
∅	1871.67 ± 156.34	98.92 ± 0.67	98.92 ± 0.67	13.90 ± 4.22	-	-	-
Transection with hepatic or portal vein entry (Fig. 2c)							
17	4824.75	42.04	0.00	2796.52	4824.74	73.39	120.66
18	2808.66	43.21	0.00	1595.15	2808.66	72.44	121.71
19	3090.65	27.97	0.00	2226.16	3090.64	83.74	85.31
20	1918.25	69.47	0.00	585.61	1918.25	46.78	107.56
21	2535.75	50.89	0.02	1245.23	2535.35	65.87	104.35
22	2245.29	33.64	0.00	1490.02	2245.23	79.78	135.01
∅	2903.89 ± 1027.08	44.34 ± 14.58	0.00 ± 0.01	1656.45 ± 770.92	2903.83 ± 1027.10	70.33 ± 13.10	112.43 ± 17.25

4 Discussion

The described work determines the possible perfusion loss for planned resection zones based on the hepatic and portal veins represented as directed graphs. Further evaluation and visualization enables the surgeons to optimize the planning of resection zones by integrating physiological modeling to identify unintended vessel transections due to visual coverage by other relevant anatomical structures. This relationship becomes particularly evident when examining individual patient outcomes.

In two patients with three resection zones (Tab. 1, no vessel transections), the calculated non-perfused region shows a complete overlap with the defined resection zone indicated by (-). This typically occurs when the resection zone does not intersect with any segmented vessel branches, resulting in no additional non-perfused parenchyma outside the intended resection mask. From a surgical planning perspective, this may indicate that critical vascular structures are intentionally preserved, or that these cases are associated with lower imaging resolution and suboptimal vessel segmentations, which likely contributed to a simplified vascular model and less sensitive downstream detection. However, since the non-visualized vessels are primarily small, the impact on perfusion is expected to be less significant. Owing to the redundancy and connectivity of the microvascular network, some of these territories may still receive perfusion, which should be considered when interpreting the results. Therefore, rather than viewing the non-perfused areas as absolute boundaries, these visualizations should be interpreted as regions with a higher probability of insufficient perfusion and an associated increase in risks of liver failure and localized ischemia or congested areas [1].

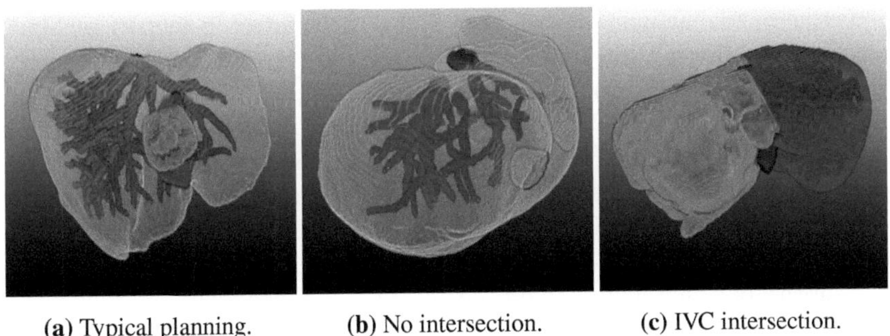

(a) Typical planning. **(b)** No intersection. **(c)** IVC intersection.

Fig. 2. Visualization of the algorithm's results regarding the downstream loss due to vascular transections. The FLR is visualized in white, while the planned resection zone is visualized in green and the calculated non-perfused parenchyma beyond the resection zone in red. Hepatic vein in blue and portal vein in purple are visible inside the liver. Image (a) shows a typical result where additional perfusion loss is visible within small distance to the initial resection zone. Subfigure (b) shows no intersection with segmented vessles at all leading to no additional perfusion loss, while subfigure (c) shows an intersection with the IVC and complete perfusion loss.

In contrast, for six patients (Tab. 1, transection with hepatic or portal vein entry), a complete loss of liver perfusion was calculated, with the algorithm reporting a perfused volume of 0%. In these cases, either the inferior vena cava (IVC) was partially contained within the planned resection zone or the beginning of the hepatic or portal vein. Two of these scenarios reflect patients with complex oncologic cases and vessel invasion by an hepatocellular carcinoma and intrahepatic cholangiocarcinoma. Subsequent vessel reconstruction was performed which was not represented in the input data. In the remaining cases, the planned resection planes partially encompassed portions of the IVC as well as hepatic or portal venous structures. These inclusions are most likely attributable to subtle discrepancies in segmentation or the graphical rendering of the resection planes within the software and do not correspond to the actual surgical approach. Our algorithm enables to the surgical planner to easily detect cases where major vessels are unintentionally transected and could therefore be corrected directly during the planning stage. This aligns with previous findings by Lang et al. who demonstrated that computer-assisted risk analysis can lead to substantial corrections for larger discrepancies in major hepatectomies compared to traditional planar 2D CT-based FLR assessment [5].

Building on this, our work distinguishes itself from related research by addressing more complex planning scenarios. In contrast to Li et al. [1], who focused primarily on clinical risks of perfusion loss in the context of planar transection surfaces, our approach also evaluates complex, irregularly shaped resection zones for parenchyma-sparing hepatectomies represented in our dataset. Besides this, while Christ et al. [6, 7] reviewed various strategies for modeling metabolism in liver remnants (partially including perfusion modeling) and discussed how such models may be integrated into clinical workflows, our method enables identification of unintended vessel transections and supports direct correction during virtual planning.

Furthermore, our approach can be extended in the future to support anatomical resections by allowing surgeons to select a specific vessel branch as the point of transection. The resulting non-perfused territory can then serve as an initial guidance resection mask, which can be iteratively adapted based on individual surgical expertise and intraoperative considerations. This capability could enhance the planning of segment-oriented resections in addition to the provision of intuitive feedback on vascular consequences. Overall, these observations demonstrate both the potential and the current limitations of graph-based perfusion simulation in pre-operative liver surgery planning. Future improvements in image quality, vessel segmentation accuracy, and interactive surgical interfaces may further increase the robustness and clinical utility of this method.

In conclusion, our approach demonstrates that graph-based modeling of hepatic vessels can estimate perfusion loss of planned liver resections and highlights regions at increased risk of insufficient perfusion, providing valuable guidance for planning complex liver resection that may ultimately enhance patient outcomes.

Acknowledgement. This work was partially supported by the German Federal Ministry of Research, Technology and Space within the Research Campus STIMULATE under the grant number '13GW0473A' and the German Research Foundation under the grant number '547369510'. The authors declare no competing interests.

References

1. Li XL, Xu B, Zhu XD, Huang C, Shi GM, Shen YH et al. Simulation of portal/hepatic vein associated remnant liver ischemia/congestion by three-dimensional visualization technology based on preoperative CT scan. Ann Transl Med. 2021;9(9):756.
2. Tithof J, Pruett TL, Rao JS. Lumped parameter liver simulation to predict acute haemodynamic alterations following partial resections. J R Soc Interface. 2023;20(207):20230444.
3. Torzilli G. Parenchyma-sparing vessel-guided major hepatectomy: nonsense or new paradigm in liver surgery? Br J Surg. 2021;108(2):109–11.
4. Selle D, Spindler W, Preim B, Peitgen HO. Mathematical methods in medical imaging: analysis of vascular structures for liver surgery planning. Mathematics unlimited: 2001 and beyond. Springer, 2001:1039–59.
5. Lang H, Radtke A, Hindennach M, Schroeder T, Frühauf NR, Malagó M et al. Impact of virtual tumor resection and computer-assisted risk analysis on operation planning and intraoperative strategy in major hepatic resection. Arch Surg. 2005;140(7):629–38.
6. Christ B, Dahmen U, Herrmann KH, König M, Reichenbach JR, Ricken T et al. Computational modeling in liver surgery. Front Physiol. 2017;8:906.
7. Christ B, Collatz M, Dahmen U, Herrmann KH, Höpfl S, König M et al. Hepatectomy-induced alterations in hepatic perfusion and function-toward multi-scale computational modeling for a better prediction of post-hepatectomy liver function. Front Physiol. 2021;12:733868.

Software Prototyping in Java

Examples on Automatic Annotation and AI-based Instrument Tracking for Stroke Treatment

Mohamed Tababi[1], Timo Baumgärtner[1,2], Charissa Morales[1], Jan Komposch[1], Johannes Roßkopf[3], Till Malzacher[3], Michael Braun[3], Bernd Schmitz[3], Alfred M. Franz[1,4]

[1]Department of Computer Science, Ulm University of Applied Sciences (THU)
[2]Institute for AI Safety and Security, German Aerospace Center (DLR)
[3]Neuroradiology Section, District Hospital Guenzburg
[4]Division of Intelligent Medical Systems, German Cancer Research Center (DKFZ) Heidelberg

alfred.franz@thu.de

Abstract. Software prototypes for image-guided therapy (IGT) are complex to implement. In this paper, we present an easy-to-compile Java software that communicates with existing toolkits to process tracking and image data in real time. As an application example, we used an electromagnetic tracking system to automatically annotate 815 fluoroscopic images with catheters and guidewires for stroke treatment. Building on this, we trained a you only look once (YOLO) model for image-based tracking of these instruments. In our test data, the instrument was correctly detected in 87% of the frames. We further demonstrated usage of the model by exporting it to the open neural network exchange (ONNX) format and loading it into our Java software prototype for live instrument detection.

1 Introduction

Image-guided therapy (IGT) aims to provide physicians with additional information, such as overlays of anatomical details, medical instruments and/or guidance information during medical procedures [1]. Many approaches were presented in the past, e.g. for percutaneous (e.g., [2]), catheter-based (e.g., [3]) or endoscopic (e.g., [4]) interventions. If such approaches are to be researched, it is necessary to set up not only complex hardware but also software that establishes a real-time connection to the hardware and provides algorithms, e.g. for the fusion of coordinate spaces (registration [1]).

Fortunately, open-source libraries and toolkits with a powerful range of features have been developed for this purpose (e.g. Slicer IGT (www.slicerigt.org), PLUS (plustoolkit.org), CustusX (www.custusx.org), MITK-IGT (github.com/IMSY-DKFZ/MITK-IGT), IGSTK (github.com/Kitware/IGSTK)), which can communicate

© Der/die Autor(en), exklusiv lizenziert an
Springer Fachmedien Wiesbaden GmbH, ein Teil von Springer Nature 2026
H. Handels et al. (Hrsg.), *Bildverarbeitung für die Medizin 2026*,
Informatik aktuell, https://doi.org/10.1007/978-3-658-51100-5_47

with each other using the OpenIGTLink [5] protocol. These libraries and toolkits offer a wide range of functions including hardware communication and are usually implemented in C++. Compiling them is relatively complex and time-consuming, which is why the barrier to entry for creating new research prototypes on this codebase is relatively high. However, it seems feasible to connect instances of existing software via OpenIGTLink to another simple application that can easily be expanded with new prototypical features. Java seems suitable for this purpose because it is widely used, can be easily compiled in the right setup, and also offers functionalities for graphical user interfaces (GUI), including real-time visualization of 2D and 3D graphics. Java further offers static typing which is beneficial for a stable and predictable software behavior as required by IGT systems with hardware connection and real-time visualization.

Therefore, the main objective of this work is a Java software prototype for IGT research that communicates with other toolkits via OpenIGTLink and is easy to compile and extend. To demonstrate its applicability, we use our prototype for training and demonstration of an artificial intelligence (AI) model for instrument detection in stroke treatment. Our use case is motivated by the idea to simplify the setup of IGT systems. For this purpose, we use tracking hardware to automatically annotate data for machine learning so that it is subsequently possible to work purely image-based. In preliminary work, the required instruments were already equipped with electromagnetic (EM) sensors to track them [3]. We use these instruments to automatically annotate a fluoroscopic dataset for training a neural network on instrument localization. While the training was conducted in Python, we extend the Java prototype with real-time tracking functionality using the trained neural network. This motivates our selection for the YOLO model, specifically YOLO-v8 [6], which supports real-time capability while maintaining an acceptable tradeoff between speed and accuracy in detecting small objects, such as the tip of a medical instrument.

2 Methods

2.1 Software prototype

To enable research in IGT, various aspects need to be considered for a software prototype. It should include capabilities to connect to tracking hardware, visualize instruments together with patient data, perform a registration of the trackers with the patient and offer the possibility to include video streams. As motivated above, we decided to use Java as a programming language. Fig. 1 shows the basic structure and a screenshot of our prototype. We selected JavaFX (openjfx.io) as GUI framework and Gradle (gradle.org) as build tool. The repository is hosted on GitHub, which allows the use of GitHub Actions for continuous integration. The source code was divided into several packages. The most important of these are `inputOutput` for connecting to data sources via OpenIGTLink or from files, `algorithm` for program logic, and `controller` for user interface controller code. The views for this are in FX Markup Language (FXML) format under `resources`. Connection to hardware is established in classes like `OIGTImageSource` or `OIGTTrackingDataSource` of the package `inputOutput` using an OpenIGTLink connection to existing tools such as MITK-IGT or PLUS.

In the following two sections, we illustrate possible applications of the software by using it first for automatic annotation of fluoroscopic data in stroke treatment, and second for real-time tracking of instruments with the trained model. Our sample applications focus on researching assistance systems for thrombectomy. Thrombectomy, a method of mechanical stroke treatment, requires the physician to navigate through the vessel tree in order to reach the location of an occlusion by using fluoroscopy. In order to enable IGT assistance, tracked instruments can be used [3]. However, as already discussed, the setup of tracking hardware can be challenging. Ramadani et al. summarized alternative AI-driven image-based tracking methods [7]. Inspired by the idea of AI-based tracking, we trained a network for instrument tracking using fluoroscopic vision only and used our software for automatic annotation (Sec. 2.2) as well as AI-based tracking (Sec. 2.3).

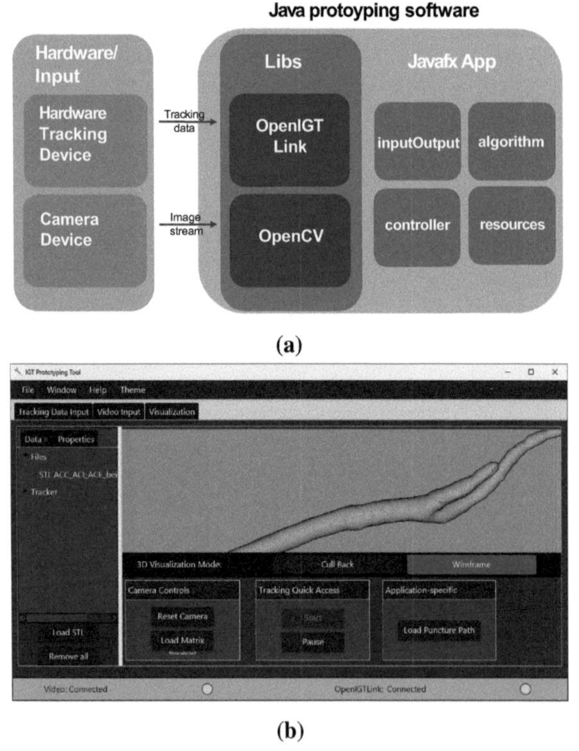

Fig. 1. (a) The main components of the software prototype. (b) Screenshot showing the 3D view of a part of a segmented vessel tree for stroke treatment (arteria carotis interna (ACI) and externa (ACE)). Video stream and tracking are active but visualized in tabs in the background.

2.2 Application for annotating fluoroscopy data

Using a simplified vessel phantom made from glued tubes, we simulated stroke treatment in a clinical environment using a fluoroscopy device of type siemens ARTIS icono biplane. As instruments, we used a tracked guidewire prototype (GW) and a tracked probing catheter prototype (PC), from previous work [3] both equipped with EM sensors, as well as a NDI Aurora 6DOF FlexTube (SR, NDI product no. 610060) and an Asahi Fubuki 8F straight catheter (AC). To localize the AC, the sensor SR was inserted until the tip of the sensor and catheter are aligned. Registering tracking and image coordinates using point-based registration of the OpenCV method `estimateAffine2D`, we end up with images that are annotated with the instrument's position. Hence, we recorded automatically annotated data and acquired 17 image sequences consisting of 815 (GW:199, PC:217, SR:310, AC:89) single frames with annotated tips using five different paths and 685 background frames without visible instrument tip. Due to the diameter and stiffness of the AC, we could not access some smaller tubes of our phantom, leading to a lower frame number. There were also problems with the guidewire in one tube branch, which is why this path was omitted for the GW. After data recording, we applied geometric, brightness, and contrast augmentation, resulting in 7335 additional images. The dataset was split into 6991 training, 1023 validation and 821 test images, ensuring that images of one sequence do not spread between the sets.

We then fine-tuned the YOLO model [6] using our fluoroscopy dataset. We tested two different YOLO variants: `8n[ano]` and `8l[arge]`. We trained with stochastic gradient descent, a learning rate of 0.01 and a momentum of 0.9. Both model variants were trained until they no longer improve significantly on the validation data. This procedure, also known as early stopping, helps to prevent overfitting. This results in the `8n` variant being trained for effectively 187, and the `8l` variant for 184 epochs. Note also that the `8l` model has more than 13 times the capacity of the nano variant in terms of the number of trainable parameters. The mean average precision was used as a loss function for training. However, this metric is not meaningful for assessing the detection on the test data. Since the actual tip of the instrument is a single point rather than a larger object with outer boundaries, we decided to measure the distance from this point to the center of the predicted bounding box. As a final result, we report if the actual tip is inside a circle with a radius of 3.9 mm (10 pixels) or 7.8 mm (20 pixels) around the predicted tip. The thresholds of 3.9 mm for high-precision localization and 7.8 mm for lower-precision localization were chosen to provide interpretable measures of accuracy. We further consider only predictions with a confidence of 0.25 or higher as decision threshold to reduce the number of candidates.

2.3 Application for real-time instrument tracking

Based on our experience with the fluoroscopy dataset, we aim to demonstrate the usage of our Java prototype with a real-time instrument tracking module working purely on an image stream. As a simple example for assistance in navigating a vessel tree, we further equipped the tracking module with an interactive interface (Fig. 2). It allows users to define a path for the catheter via point-and-click and obtain distance measurements from a marked target (thrombus). Since this use case is intended more for demonstrations outside the clinic, we fine-tuned an additional image-based localization model on simulated lab conditions using a light board and a webcam in grayscale mode for imaging. With a transparent vessel dummy, this leads to quite similar images as in fluoroscopy. We refer to the data recorded in this way as webcam dataset.

We opted to integrate the YOLO model directly into the Java application. This design eliminates the need for an external server. To achieve this, we perform the following steps: First, we export the model to the Open Neural Network Exchange (ONNX) format. We use the ONNX Runtime library to load the model in Java. Video frames are captured, converted to grayscale, and preprocessed by resizing and normalizing them to fit the model's input requirements. Subsequently, we convert these frames into tensors and pass them to the ONNX model for inference. After the model predicts objects in a frame, results are filtered based on confidence scores and refined through non-maximum suppression to eliminate overlapping detections. Frames are converted back to their original color and format. Finally, the catheter tip is detected and tracked using a bounding box overlaid on the video (Fig. 2). The ONNX format is agnostic to the framework used for training, and in principle, the same processing pipeline could be adapted to other network models. Furthermore, ONNX runtime is well-optimized for both CPU and GPU, enabling inference without compromising detection speed.

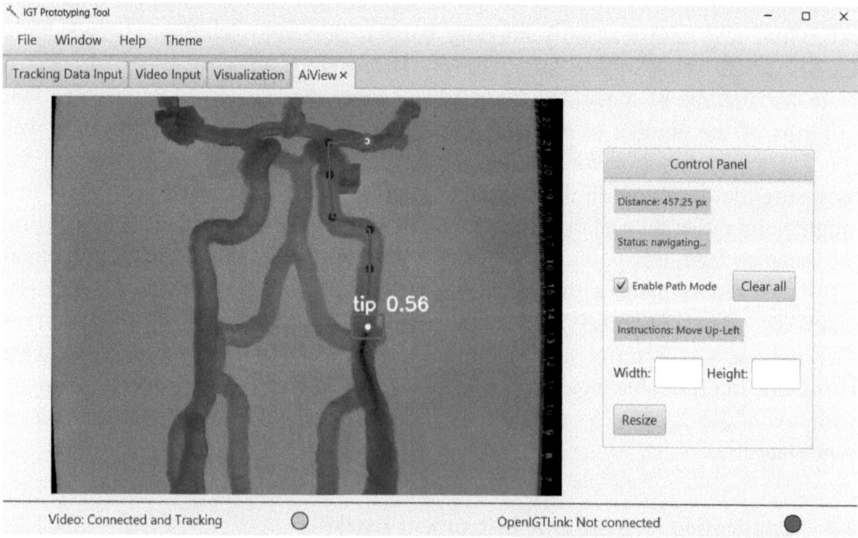

Fig. 2. Screenshot of the AI-based tracking view in the software prototype. The view shows a webcam stream of a 3D-printed vessel tree with a catheter inserted. The detected catheter tip is indicated with a bounding box, and a user-defined navigation path is visualized along with additional guidance information displayed on the side.

3 Results

Our software is available on GitHub (github.com/NAMI-THU/IGTPrototypingTool). The Git tag *2026-03-BVM-basic-version* refers to a basic version that is intended as a starting point for new projects. The tag *2026-03-BVM-instrument-tracking-demonstrator* refers to our sample application for instrument tracking.

Assessing our model fine-tuned with the fluoroscopy dataset, we find both variants, 8n and 8l, are capable of localizing 87.0% of the tips within a radius of 7.8 mm (20 pixels). Decreasing this distance to 3.9 mm (10 pixels) still results in 71.0% of correctly localized tips for 8l, and the 8n variant in 65.9%. Intriguingly, both variants perform similarly, although the 8n variant being slightly less accurate in terms of positioning. As expected for YOLO models, detection works in real time with low latency. Even when testing the execution on a weak GPU such as the Nvidia GTX 1650, the inference on the 8n variant took on average 0.02 s ± 0.07 s per image, and 0.09 s ± 0.14 s with the 8l model (both on $n = 821$ test images). Testing our demonstrator based on the webcam dataset over 15 minutes ($n = 9000$ frames) on a laptop without a dedicated GPU, we found a smooth display of the image with overlay (Fig. 2) and also a stable inference of 0.05 s ± 0.01 s.

4 Discussion

We presented an easily accessible software prototype for IGT research implemented in Java. Using OpenIGTLink, it is possible to access various hardware devices. We tested our prototype on AI-based tracking of instruments in fluoroscopic imaging. Our YOLO models achieved a performance of 87.0% correctly detected tips (max. 7.8 mm offset). Although the 8n model seems to be slightly less accurate, it consists of only 7% the number of parameters of the 8l model, and thus is considerably faster. Our demonstrator shows that a trained model can be used within the Java prototype.

Of course, catheter detection or segmentation tasks were also in focus of related studies. Gherardini et al., for example, could segment catheters with up to 0.97 accuracy in a dice overlap metric in X-ray fluoroscopic images using a U-net architecture [8]. Even though the results are difficult to compare to ours due to synthetic data and different metrics, we can confirm that the well-contrasted instruments in X-ray images of a real angiography device can be detected well with machine learning models.

The vessel phantom made from glued tubes is highly simplified. Nevertheless, we see good chances of achieving good results on real clinical data, as the instruments are usually well contrasted there too. For our automatic annotation approach in this work, we acquired new data; however public data sets such as the WEISS catheter data set [9] also exist and can be considered in future research. While our current model only detects any instrument tips, future work might focus on distinguishing different instruments by adapting the training process to different classes and collecting more data for each instrument category. Besides the use case of researching instrument tracking for stroke treatment, the software prototype already showed benefits in several other projects. Students of THU were, e.g., able to implement: (a) 3D visualization for planning needle insertions, (b) a tool for manual image annotation of fluoroscopic image sequences, and (c) a connection to the open-source tracker Anser EMT [10].

In conclusion, we showed an exemplary application of Java software for IGT prototyping and demonstrated how it can be used to train a neural network for real-time detection of instruments in fluoroscopic images and how to apply such trained networks on image streams in real-time.

Acknowledgement. We are grateful for the many students who contributed to the development of the software prototype. In addition to the authors of this manuscript this includes Veronika Seidel, Raphael Steinborn, Florian Hauptmann, Andrew Sadler and many more. Find a complete list of contributors in the git repository.

References

1. Cleary K, Peters TM. Image-guided interventions: technology review and clinical applications. Annu Rev Biomed Eng. 2010;12(1):119–42.
2. Sindram D, Swan RZ, Lau KN, McKillop IH, Iannitti DA, Martinie JB. Real-time three-dimensional guided ultrasound targeting system for microwave ablation of liver tumours: a human pilot study. HPB. 2011;13(3):185–91.
3. Stevanovic L, Bodanowitz R, Mittmann BJ, Greiner-Perth AK, Marschall E, Kannberg T et al. Localizable instruments for navigated treatment of ischemic stroke. Proc BVM. 2023:279–84.
4. Fichtl A, Sheikhani A, Wagner M, Kleger A, Müller M, Sturm N et al. Implementing an electromagnetic tracking navigation system improves the precision of endoscopic transgastric necrosectomy in an ex vivo model. Sci Rep. 2024;14(1).
5. Tokuda J, Fischer GS, Papademetris X, Yaniv Z, Ibanez L, Cheng P et al. OpenIGTLink: an open network protocol for image-guided therapy environment. Int J Med Robot. 2009;5(4):423–34.
6. Jocher G, Chaurasia A, Qiu J. Ultralytics YOLOv8. Version 8.0.0. 2023. URL: `https://github.com/ultralytics/ultralytics` (visited on 01/02/2026).
7. Ramadani A, Bui M, Wendler T, Schunkert H, Ewert P, Navab N. A survey of catheter tracking concepts and methodologies. Med Image Anal. 2022;82:102584.
8. Gherardini M, Mazomenos E, Menciassi A, Stoyanov D. Catheter segmentation in X-ray fluoroscopy using synthetic data and transfer learning with light U-nets. Comput Meth Prog Biomed. 2020;192:105420.
9. Mazomenos E, Stoyanov D, Gherardini M. WEISS catheter segmentation in fluoroscopy dataset. University College London, 2023.
10. Jaeger HA, Franz AM, O'Donoghue K, Seitel A, Trauzettel F, Maier-Hein L et al. Anser EMT: the first open-source electromagnetic tracking platform for image-guided interventions. Int J Comput Assist Radiol Surg. 2017;12(6):1059–67.

Deep Radiomics with DINOV3 for MRI-based Differentiation of Peripheral Nerve Sheath Tumors in Neurofibromatosis Type 1

Georgii Kolokolnikov [1], Marie-Lena Schmalhofer [2], Lennart Well[2], Inka Ristow [2], René Werner [1]

[1]Institute for Applied Medical Informatics, Institute of Computational Neuroscience, Center for Biomedical Artificial Intelligence (bAIome), University Medical Center Hamburg-Eppendorf

[2]Department of Diagnostic and Interventional Radiology and Nuclear Medicine, University Medical Center Hamburg-Eppendorf

g.kolokolnikov@uke.de

Abstract. This study investigates the potential of DINOv3 as a deep radiomics feature extractor for MRI-based differentiation of peripheral nerve sheath tumors (PNSTs) in neurofibromatosis type 1. We analyzed 3D T2-weighted fat-suppressed MRI scans from two patient cohorts (122 and 36 patients) and compared four feature extraction approaches: classical radiomics, the foundation model for cancer imaging biomarkers (FMCIB), Radio DINO, and DINOv3. In the first experiment, we assessed feature generalizability using k-nearest neighbor classifiers in leave-one-patient-out cross-validation to quantify how well features selected for one tumor differentiation task transfer to another. In the second experiment, we reproduced the prior PNST differentiation benchmark using random forest classifiers to evaluate the clinical relevance of deep radiomics features. DINOv3 demonstrated robust feature generalization and achieved AUC of 0.76–0.96 across tasks in the PNST differentiation benchmark. It consistently outperformed classical radiomics (AUC 0.60–0.94) and FMCIB (AUC 0.60–0.84), and performed on par with Radio DINO (AUC 0.82–0.94). These findings indicate that DINOv3 embeddings provide generalizable and clinically discriminative deep radiomics features for PNST differentiation in NF1.

1 Introduction

Neurofibromatosis type 1 (NF1) is a genetic disorder affecting 1 in 3000 individuals [1]. A hallmark of NF1 is the predisposition to develop peripheral nerve sheath tumors (PNSTs), among which plexiform neurofibromas (PNFs) are clinically most relevant due to the potential for malignization. Pathology describes a spectrum of PNSTs from benign PNFs to atypical neurofibromas (ANFs) and malignant PNSTs (MPNSTs) [1]. The latter often arise from distinct nodular lesions (DNLs) within PNFs [2]. ANFs, as precursors to MPNSTs, show neither local recurrence after

© Der/die Autor(en), exklusiv lizenziert an
Springer Fachmedien Wiesbaden GmbH, ein Teil von Springer Nature 2026
H. Handels et al. (Hrsg.), *Bildverarbeitung für die Medizin 2026*,
Informatik aktuell, https://doi.org/10.1007/978-3-658-51100-5_48

resection nor the ability to metastisize. Therefore, early noninvasive diagnosis of PNSTs is essential for the clinical management of NF1 patients.

MRI is the modality of choice for NF1 surveillance [3]. Benign PNSTs (BPNSTs) typically appear as well-defined, hyperintense masses on T2-weighted (T2w) fat-suppressed MRI sequences (Fig. 1.a and b). ANFs often manifest as DNLs with growth pattern distinct from surrounding PNFs (Fig. 1.a and c). MPNSTs may resemble ANFs (Fig. 1.d), making noninvasive differentiation challenging.

Classical radiomics offers a quantitative approach for tumor characterization by extracting hand-crafted imaging features that describe morphology and texture [3]. When combined with machine learning, these features can be used for tumor classification. Prior studies achieved area under the receiver operating characteristic curve (AUC) values of 0.71–0.94 for benign vs. malignant PNSTs classification [3, 4], though performance declined when ANFs were included in the analysis.

Recently, deep radiomics approaches, that extract image representations using deep neural networks, have outperformed classical radiomics [5], but have not yet been applied to NF1 [3]. Their reliance on large annotated datasets limits use in NF1, where data are scarce. Foundation models pre-trained on large datasets can mitigate this by providing robust, transferable feature embeddings. Examples include the convolutional foundation model for cancer imaging biomarkers (FMCIB) [6] and the transformer-based Radio DINO model [7]. The latest advancement, DINOv3, further improves representation stability and predictive performance [8], achieving competitive results in medical imaging despite being trained on natural images [9]. However, the potential of DINOv3 as a foundation model for deep radiomics and the generalizability of deep radiomics in NF1 have not yet been investigated.

In this study, we hypothesize that DINOv3 can be used as a deep radiomics feature extractor that provides generalizable feature signatures for PNST differentiation, addressing the limitations of classical radiomics. Our contributions are:

- Application of DINOv3 embeddings as a deep radiomics feature space for PNST differentiation in NF1 patients.
- Analysis of feature generalizability across classical and deep radiomics.
- Clinically relevant benchmarking of DINOv3 against classical radiomics for differentiation of BPNSTs, ANFs, and MPNSTs.

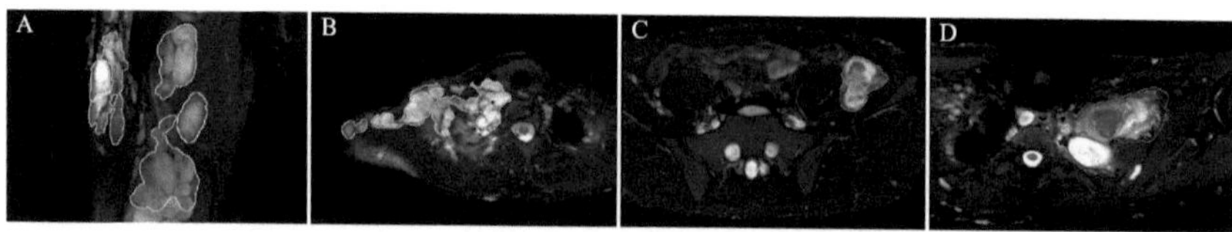

Fig. 1. MRI of peripheral nerve sheath tumors (PNSTs). (A) Plexiform neurofibromas (blue) and distinct nodular lesions (yellow) in a coronal T2w fat-suppressed MRI (Siemens Magnetom 3T scanner). (B) Benign PNSTs (green), (C) atypical neurofibroma (orange), and (D) malignant PNST (red) in axial T2w fat-suppressed MRI (Philips Ingenia 3T scanner).

2 Materials and methods

2.1 Data description

This study was conducted on two cohorts of NF1 patients examined between 2006 and 2024 at the University Medical Center Hamburg-Eppendorf. The first dataset comprised coronal 3D T2w fat-suppressed MRI scans from 122 patients (64 male, age range 8–75 years) acquired on a Siemens Magnetom 3T scanner (voxel spacing $0.6 \times 0.6 \times 7.8$ mm; 20–51 slices). It included 414 DNLs (mean tumor volume of $25.9 \pm 46.4\,\text{cm}^3$) and 1463 PNFs ($11.2 \pm 50.1\,\text{cm}^3$), located in proximity to DNLs (Fig. 1.a). The second dataset consisted of axial 3D T2w fat-suppressed MRI scans from 36 patients (20 male; age range 12–54 years) acquired on a Philips Ingenia 3T scanner (voxel spacing of $0.7 \times 0.7 \times 3.0$ mm; 27–40 slices). It included 117 BPNSTs ($29.0 \pm 70.9\,\text{cm}^3$), 8 ANFs ($60.6 \pm 40.9\,\text{cm}^3$), and 17 MPNSTs ($269.2 \pm 268.8\,\text{cm}^3$) (Figs. 1.b–d). All tumors were manually segmented by two radiologists.

2.2 Feature generalizability analysis

To investigate the generalizability of classical and deep radiomics features, we designed a two-task framework assessing how well features selected for one tumor differentiation task transfer to another: (A) DNL-vs-PNF, and (B) BPNST-vs-ANF/MPNST differentiation. We compared four feature extraction approaches: classical radiomics, feature extraction using FMCIB [6], Radio DINO [7], and DINOv3 [8]. For classical radiomics, 819 hand-crafted features were extracted from masked tumor regions using the default PyRadiomics configuration in 3D, including first-order and texture descriptors. FMCIB processed 3D image patches to produce 4096D embeddings. For Radio DINO and DINOv3, 384D feature vectors were extracted in 2D and averaged across slices to obtain a single tumor-level representation, following the aggregation strategy used by Liu et al. [9]. More advanced 3D aggregation methods, such as the Medical Slice Transformer, offer only moderate performance gains over simple averaging at higher computational cost [10].

To ensure feature robustness to annotation variability, six perturbed variants of each tumor mask (one-voxel morphological dilation, erosion, and in-plane translations by ± 1 pixel along the X and Y axes) were generated. Features were extracted from tumor images using all mask variants, and the features with intra-class correlation coefficient ≥ 0.75 were retained. We further removed near-zero variance features (< 0.1) and redundant features using pairwise Spearman correlation ($|\rho| \geq 0.9$), keeping the more stable feature of each pair. For each feature extractor, four feature signatures were formed: (i) a full signature (all features after redundancy reduction), (ii) a task-specific signature A (top 5 features selected on task A via recursive feature elimination in leave-one-patient-out cross-validation), (iii) a task-specific signature B, and (iv) a random 5-feature subset from the full signature (control). Each signature was evaluated on both classification tasks. We used a k-nearest neighbor classifier with the default scikit-learn configuration ($k = 5$), since it is a simple non-parametric method that reflects the structure of the feature space, enabling an assessment of feature separability rather than classifier capacity.

Tab. 1. Performance comparison of feature signatures across feature extraction methods and classification tasks. Values represent AUC ± standard deviation, obtained using a k-nearest neighbor classifier in leave-one-patient-out cross-validation.

	Classical radiomics	FMCIB	Radio DINO	DINOv3
Task A: DNL-vs-PNF				
Full signature	**0.96 ± 0.08**	0.94 ± 0.09	**0.96 ± 0.07**	**0.96 ± 0.08**
Defined on task A	0.93 ± 0.09	0.92 ± 0.10	**0.95 ± 0.09**	0.93 ± 0.10
Defined on task B	**0.90 ± 0.13**	0.88 ± 0.14	**0.90 ± 0.12**	**0.90 ± 0.13**
Random signature	0.90 ± 0.15	0.86 ± 0.14	**0.91 ± 0.14**	0.88 ± 0.15
Task B: BPNST-vs-ANF/MPNST				
Full signature	**0.85 ± 0.06**	0.70 ± 0.05	0.84 ± 0.04	**0.85 ± 0.04**
Defined on task A	0.77 ± 0.15	0.57 ± 0.13	**0.83 ± 0.11**	0.82 ± 0.12
Defined on task B	0.81 ± 0.11	0.73 ± 0.09	0.87 ± 0.09	**0.93 ± 0.07**
Random signature	0.74 ± 0.16	0.74 ± 0.15	0.76 ± 0.14	**0.80 ± 0.14**

2.3 Peripheral nerve sheath tumor differentiation benchmark

To assess the clinical relevance of DINOv3 features, we reproduced the PNST differentiation benchmark of Ristow et al. [4] on the same NF1 cohort. Following the reference study, the baseline model was a random forest (RF) classifier trained on five texture radiomics features computed from the gray-level co-occurrence matrix. We performed feature selection on the BPNST-vs-MPNST task to identify top five most informative features for FMCIB, Radio DINO, and DINOv3, analogous to the radiomics signature defined by Ristow et al. [4]. The selected features were used for RF training and evaluation using leave-one-patient-out cross-validation across four binary classification tasks: (1) BPNST-vs-MPNST, (2) BPNST-vs-ANF, (3) ANF-vs-MPNST, and (4) BPNST-vs-ANF/MPNST. To account for the RF stochasticity, the entire cross-validation procedure was repeated 10 times with different random seeds, and results were averaged. RF classifiers consisted of 100 trees, following recommendations from Oshiro et al. [11], without further hyperparameter tuning to maintain comparability with the prior study. The optimal operating point on the receiver operating characteristic curve was determined using Youden's index, and performance was reported as AUC.

3 Results

3.1 Feature generalizability analysis

In task A (DNL-vs-PNF), all methods showed moderate AUC declines when using reduced feature subsets instead of the full signatures (Tab. 1). Task-specific signatures (features selected for the same task A) outperformed cross-task (features selected on the other task B) and random signatures, indicating that features optimized for a given task were more informative. Radio DINO showed the highest stability with minimal declines from the full signature. In task B (BPNST-vs-ANF/MPNST), overall AUCs were lower due to greater lesion heterogeneity and smaller cohort size. DINOv3

Tab. 2. Performance comparison of feature extraction methods across PNST differentiation tasks following the setup of Ristow et al. [4]. Values represent the mean AUC ± standard deviation, obtained using a random forest classifier in leave-one-patient-out cross-validation.

	Classical radiomics	FMCIB	Radio DINO	DINOv3
BPNST-vs-MPNST	0.94 ± 0.01	0.84 ± 0.01	0.94 ± 0.01	**0.96 ± 0.01**
BPNST-vs-ANF	0.91 ± 0.01	0.60 ± 0.02	0.91 ± 0.01	**0.94 ± 0.01**
ANF-vs-MPNST	0.60 ± 0.02	0.75 ± 0.03	**0.82 ± 0.02**	0.76 ± 0.02
BPNST-vs-ANF/MPNST	0.94 ± 0.01	0.74 ± 0.02	0.94 ± 0.01	**0.95 ± 0.01**

achieved the best overall performance and strongest cross-task generalization. Radio DINO also remained robust, while classical radiomics showed larger declines and FMCIB yielded the lowest absolute performance. These observations highlight that DINOv3, despite not being fine-tuned on medical images, achieved high tumor classification performance and strong cross-task generalization.

3.2 Peripheral nerve sheath tumor differentiation benchmark

Tab. 2 summarizes the PNST differentiation results, comparing FMCIB- and DINO-based deep radiomics with the prior classical radiomics baseline [4]. Across the BPNST-vs-MPNST, BPNST-vs-ANF, and BPNST-vs-ANF/MPNST tasks, DINOv3 achieved the highest AUC (0.96 ± 0.01, 0.94 ± 0.01, 0.95 ± 0.01), outperforming classical radiomics, Radio DINO, and FMCIB. In contrast, the ANF-vs-MPNST task was most challenging, with substantially lower AUC (0.60 ± 0.02, 0.75 ± 0.03, 0.82 ± 0.02, 0.76 ± 0.02 for classical radiomics, FMCIB, Radio DINO, and DINOv3). Due to the strong class imbalance (8 ANFs, 17 MPNSTs), we additionally examined sensitivity and specificity to better characterize model behavior. Radio DINO achieved the most balanced performance (sensitivity 0.75 ± 0.02, specificity 0.88 ± 0.03), whereas classical radiomics (0.88 ± 0.09, 0.48 ± 0.13) and FMCIB (0.88 ± 0.09, 0.53 ± 0.08) favored sensitivity at the expense of specificity. DINOv3 showed a more balanced trade-off (0.88 ± 0.09, 0.65 ± 0.03) but did not surpass Radio DINO on this task. Overall, both DINO-based methods matched or exceeded the performance of classical radiomics and FMCIB.

4 Discussion

This study demonstrates that deep foundation models such as Radio DINO and DINOv3 can generate generalizable image representations for MRI-based PNST differentiation. Feature signatures from these models maintained strong discriminative power in the cross-task generalizability analysis. In the clinical benchmark replicating Ristow et al. [4], DINOv3 achieved performance comparable to Radio DINO, which was trained on radiological images, and outperformed the classical radiomics baseline despite lacking medical-domain fine-tuning. These findings suggest that DINOv3 embeddings can serve as generalizable deep radiomics features for PNST differentiation.

Several limitations of this study should be acknowledged. The second dataset showed class imbalance and small sample size, preventing the use of a separate hold-out test set. Consequently, we used leave-one-patient-out cross-validation in line with prior NF1 radiomics work [4]. Because testing many radiomics features on small cohorts can inflate type I error [12], we treated the 384D DINO embedding as a feature space and derived compact signatures. Random signatures consistently underperformed task-specific ones, confirming that performance was driven by meaningful rather than arbitrary features. Future work will validate DINOv3 as a deep radiomics feature extractor across additional PNST cohorts, explore medical fine-tuning, and incorporate feature interpretability to advance deep radiomics toward clinically meaningful NF1 biomarkers.

Acknowledgement. This work was supported by the Deutsche Forschungsgemeinschaft (DFG SPP 2177, project number 515277218) and the German lay organization "Bundesverband Neurofibromatose e.V." (grant/project no. n/a).

References

1. Hirbe AC, Dehner CA, Dombi E et al. Contemporary approach to neurofibromatosis type 1 – associated malignant peripheral nerve sheath tumors. Am Soc Clin Oncol Educ Book. 2024;44(3):e432242.
2. Salamon J, Widemann BC, Gross AM et al. Malignant peripheral nerve sheath tumors in neurofibromatosis type 1 arise from distinct nodular lesions: a retrospective imaging analysis. Neurooncol Adv. 2025:vdaf201.
3. Wang Z et al. Radiomics and machine learning in PNST. Peripheral Nerve Sheath Tumors. Ed. by Vetrano IG, Nazzi V. Cham: Springer Nature Switzerland, 2024:211–7.
4. Ristow I, Madesta F, Well L et al. Evaluation of magnetic resonance imaging-based radiomics characteristics for differentiation of benign and malignant peripheral nerve sheath tumors in neurofibromatosis type 1. Neuro Oncol. 2022;24(10):1790–8.
5. Demircioğlu A. Are deep models in radiomics performing better than generic models? a systematic review. Eur Radiol Exp. 2023;7(1):11.
6. Pai S, Bontempi D, Hadzic I et al. Foundation model for cancer imaging biomarkers. Nat Mach Intell. 2024;6(3):354–67.
7. Zedda L, Loddo A, Di Ruberto C. Radio DINO: a foundation model for advanced radiomics and AI-driven medical imaging analysis. Comput Biol Med. 2025;195:110583.
8. Siméoni O, Vo HV, Seitzer M et al. DINOv3. arXiv: 2508.10104. 2025.
9. Liu C, Chen Y, Shi H et al. Does DINOv3 set a new medical vision standard? arXiv: 2509.06467. 2025.
10. Müller-Franzes G, Khader F, Siepmann R et al. Medical slice transformer for improved diagnosis and explainability on 3D medical images with DINOv2. Sci Rep. 2025;15(1):23979.
11. Oshiro TM, Perez PS, Baranauskas JA. How many trees in a random forest? Machine Learning Data Mining Pattern Recognition. Ed. by Hutchison D, Kanade T, Kittler J et al. Vol. 7376. Springer Berlin Heidelberg, 2012:154–68.
12. Chalkidou A, O'Doherty MJ, Marsden PK. False discovery rates in PET and CT studies with texture features: A systematic review. PLoS One. 2015;10(5):e0124165.

Is DINOv3 Ready for Caries Detection on Panoramic Dental X-ray Images?

Christopher J. Hansen [1], Paula Kloehn[2], Anna-Louisa Kollster[2], Toni Gehrmann [2], Jonas Conrad [2], Christian Graetz [2], Christof Dörfer[2], Claus-C. Glüer[1], Jan-Bernd Hövener [1], Coenraad Mouton [1]

[1]Section Biomedical Imaging, Dept. of Radiology and Neuroradiology, University Medical Center Schleswig-Holstein (UKSH), Kiel, Germany
[2]Clinic of Conservative Dentistry and Periodontology, University of Kiel, Kiel, Germany
christopher.hansen@rad.uni-kiel.de

Abstract. Accurate segmentation of dental caries on panoramic radiographs is challenging due to subtle lesion appearance, overlapping anatomy, and domain variability across imaging sites. While task-specific models such as CariesNet and U-Net3+ have been proposed, their generalization to unseen data is rarely examined. We present a controlled, multi-site benchmark for caries segmentation on single-tooth images from panoramic radiographs and compare specialized networks to DINOv3, a vision foundation model. Using an expert-annotated dataset of single-tooth images from the University Medical Center Schleswig-Holstein (UKSH), we evaluate model generalization on an out-of-distribution (OOD) test set from the Federal University of Bahia (UFBA). All models were trained under identical conditions with standardized preprocessing, loss functions, and hyperparameter optimization. Two DINOv3 variants, one with a linear head and one with a U-Net head, were compared to CariesNet and U-Net3+. While CariesNet reached the highest in-distribution (ID) Dice score on carious images (0.4503), it dropped notably OOD (0.2656). DINOv3 with a U-Net head showed more stable performance (0.3724 ID vs. 0.3505 OOD), suggesting stronger robustness to domain shifts. Overall, pretrained foundation models demonstrated competitive and more consistent results without dental specific pretraining. The proposed benchmark provides a reproducible framework for future evaluation of segmentation models in dental radiography.

1 Introduction

Dental caries represents one of the most widespread diseases worldwide, affecting billions of individuals across all age groups and constituting a major cause of tooth loss and treatment demand [1]. Early and accurate detection is therefore critical for preventive dentistry and effective treatment planning. While bitewing radiographs are often considered the standard modality for detecting proximal and secondary caries, panoramic radiographs (orthopantomograms, OPGs) are commonly used in clinical

© Der/die Autor(en), exklusiv lizenziert an
Springer Fachmedien Wiesbaden GmbH, ein Teil von Springer Nature 2026
H. Handels et al. (Hrsg.), *Bildverarbeitung für die Medizin 2026*,
Informatik aktuell, https://doi.org/10.1007/978-3-658-51100-5_49

practice. The task of detecting carious lesions on OPGs is inherently challenging, even for experienced clinicians. Lesions often appear subtle, with low contrast relative to surrounding structures, and may be obscured by overlapping anatomy or imaging artifacts. To automate this process, various caries segmentation neural networks have been proposed, ranging from modified U-Net variants [2] to specialized networks such as CariesNet [3]. Conversely, many other computer vision tasks are increasingly being tackled by fine-tuning generalist networks, such as pretrained foundation models (e.g. CLIP and DINO), which provide powerful, general purpose features obtained from large scale self-supervised learning. In this work, we determine whether finetuning a state-of-the-art vision foundation model, DINOV3, can exceed or match the performance of specialized architectures for caries segmentation on panoramic dental radiographs. Furthermore, we also compare DINOV3-based architectures to specialized models when considering generalization on an out-of-distribution dataset. This is an important consideration, given the known sensitivity of deep learning models to domain shifts, patient populations, and X-ray devices. However, there are two fundamental hurdles. First, there is currently no benchmark dataset for caries segmentation on panoramic radiographs. Existing public datasets are scarce and typically limited to image-level or bounding-box annotations, lacking segmentation labels [4]. As a result, most published models are trained and evaluated on private institutional datasets, which makes fair comparison between methods difficult. Second, there is no established framework or dataset to evaluate the generalization of these models to out-of-distribution (OOD) data. To address these gaps, we assemble a high-difficulty, expert-annotated dataset of panoramic radiographs from the University Medical Center Schleswig-Holstein (UKSH), Kiel, with pixel-level caries masks. In this dataset, positive lesions are sparse relative to the field of view, often subtle and low-contrast, and frequently obscured by overlapping anatomy. These properties make the task non-trivial even for clinicians. We use this dataset to establish a rigorous in-distribution (ID) benchmark and, to explicitly probe robustness, we evaluate the trained models on an OOD test set from the Federal University of Bahia (UFBA), Brazil [5]. On this two-site evaluation, we fine-tune DINOv3 [6] with two segmentation heads and compare it against strong task-specific baselines: CariesNet (a model based on PraNet) and U-Net 3+. This is performed under identical training and evaluation conditions, i.e. identical preprocessing, postprocessing, losses, data splits, and hyperparameter budgets. To our knowledge, this is the first multi-institutional assessment of DINOv3 for caries segmentation on OPGs.

2 Methods

2.1 Data

Our ID dataset from UKSH comprises 1,455 single-tooth images, including 658 carious and 797 healthy teeth, split into 70% training, 20% validation, and 10% test sets. The OOD test set from UFBA consists of 460 images, with 226 carious and 234 healthy teeth. All single-tooth images were extracted from full panoramic radiographs using the automated cropping and preprocessing pipeline described by Hansen et al. [7].

2.2 Training protocol

As a baseline to compare DINOv3 against, we implemented CariesNet and U-Net3+. To ensure a fair comparison across models, we standardized the training protocol for all architectures, using the same loss formulation, training time, and hyperparameter optimization budget. We employed a combined binary cross-entropy and Dice loss, computing the Dice term only on images with carious lesions. This is essential, as without it the healthy images would dominate the objective and bias models toward trivial background predictions. All models were trained with the Adam optimizer and a mile-stone based learning rate decay. Hyperparameters were tuned with Optuna over 100 trials using Bayesian optimization via a tree-structured parzen estimator (TPE) and a successive halving pruning strategy. The search space included learning rate, weight decay, batch size, number of epochs, learning rate decay, and optional data augmentation, among others.

2.3 Models

2.3.1 DINOv3. We employed DINOv3, a state-of-the-art self-supervised vision transformer trained on approximately 17 billion images using a mean-teacher framework. In this setup, a student network learns to match the representations produced by a teacher network, enabling the extraction of rich visual features from unlabeled data [6]. For evaluating the transferability of pretrained representations, we freeze the DINO backbone and train two different segmentation heads on the feature representations. Specifically, we train 1) a linear convolutional layer on the features of the final layer, and 2) a large U-Net architecture using multi-scale features from all layers. The linear head allows us to determine how powerful the DINO features are with minimal supervised finetuning, while the U-Net head serves as a more realistic (and more expensive) indication of the performance attainable. For the linear head, we use the ViT-L/16 transformer DINO backbone (~ 300 M parameters), while for the U-Net head we use the ConvNeXt Large backbone (~ 198 M parameters), so as to be compatible with the U-Net architecture. We employ the same training strategy as used for the other models (Sec. 2.2), with two key exceptions: Learning rate decay - we use a step decay for the baseline models, but opt for a one-cycle cosine decay here as initial experimentation showed this to be more effective. Image size - given that DINO is pretrained using multi-resolution images, we also consider various image sizes during the hyperparameter search (512^2, 392^2, 224^2).

2.3.2 CariesNet. We employed CariesNet, a deep learning architecture specifically designed for dental caries segmentation. It builds upon the PraNet architecture by introducing a Res2Net backbone and a partial decoder. More specifically, the reverse attention module used in PraNet is replaced with a full-scale axial attention module. For our implementation, no official repository was available. We therefore reimplemented the architecture based on the publicly available PraNet code and the modifications described in the CariesNet paper, with ImageNet pretrained weights, to serve as a more standard fine-tuning baseline [3]. We employ the same training

Tab. 1. Dice and IoU scores for all tooth images and only for tooth images with caries on both the ID UKSH test set and the OOD UFBA test set.

	Dice All		Dice Caries Only		IoU Caries Only	
Model	UKSH	UFBA	UKSH	UFBA	UKSH	UFBA
DINOv3 U-Net	0.4432	0.2568	0.3724	**0.3505**	0.2651	**0.2420**
DINOv3 Linear	0.3661	0.2112	0.3515	0.1871	0.2367	0.1238
CariesNet	0.2420	0.3067	**0.4503**	0.2656	**0.3390**	0.1934
U-Net 3+	**0.4690**	**0.4329**	0.0117	0.0029	0.0065	0.0070

strategy as used for the other models (Sec. 2.2). Furthermore, the images are resized to 512×512 pixels.

2.3.3 U-Net3+. We implemented the U-Net 3+ architecture for caries segmentation following the study of Alharbi et al. [2]. We employ the same training strategy as used for the other models (Sec. 2.2), with the exception, that we based our implementation on the original GitHub repository provided by the authors of U-Net 3+ [8] and introduced the same modifications as reported in Alharbi et al., namely the addition of Gaussian noise regularization and Gaussian error linear unit (GeLU) activations in the encoder. In line with the original work, we used input images resized to 256×256 pixels. The original model was trained on a substantially larger dataset than ours and, in the absence of pretrained weights, serves here as a "train-from-scratch" baseline.

2.4 Evaluation

We report segmentation performance using the Dice coefficient and intersection-over-union (IoU). Both metrics are computed at the image level. Dice is defined as Dice $= \frac{2|P\cap G|}{|P|+|G|}$ and measures the overlap between predicted (P) and ground truth (G) lesion regions. For positive images (with caries), Dice is calculated only on lesion pixels to avoid the background from dominating the score. For negative images (without caries), Dice is set to 1.0 if no lesion is predicted ($|P| = 0$) and to 0.0 if any lesion is predicted despite being healthy.

IoU is defined as IoU $= \frac{|P\cap G|}{|P\cup G|}$ and is computed on lesion regions for positive images, following the same rules.

3 Results

In this section, we present the quantitative results of all models on the ID (UKSH) and OOD (UFBA) test sets. For each configuration, we report the Dice coefficient for all images as well as Dice and IoU scores for carious images only (Sec. 2.4).

When evaluating all images (Tab. 1 Dice All), including true negatives, U-Net 3+ achieves the highest Dice scores with 0.4690 ID and 0.4329 OOD. CariesNet shows lower overall scores (0.2420 and 0.3067, respectively), while DINOv3 U-Net reaches 0.4432 ID and 0.2568 OOD. DINOv3 Linear reaches a score of 0.3661

ID and 0.2112 OOD. However, recall that since TN images contribute a Dice of 1.0 to this metrics, these values can potentially mask poor lesion segmentation performance.

For carious images (Tab. 1 Dice Caries Only), CariesNet achieves the highest Dice score on the ID test set (0.4503), while U-Net 3+ shows very low performance (0.0117), indicating limited ability to learn caries-related features. Both models experience a substantial performance drop on the OOD test set, with Dice scores of 0.2656 for CariesNet and 0.0029 for U-Net 3+. DINOv3 Linear shows a similar decline like CariesNet from 0.3515 to 0.1871 Dice score. DINOv3 U-Net reaches a moderate Dice score ID (0.3724) and remains relatively stable OOD (0.3505), suggesting more robust generalization across domains.

IoU follows a similar pattern. CariesNet achieves the highest IoU ID (0.3390) but declines OOD (0.1934), like DINOv3 Linear with IoU 0.2367 and 0.1238 respectively. DINOv3 U-Net remains comparatively stable (0.2651 / 0.2420), while U-Net 3+ and the linear head perform poorly (Tab. 1 IoU Caries Only). Visual inspection (Fig. 1) shows similar segmentations for CariesNet and DINOv3, while U-Net 3+ produces mostly random predictions.

4 Discussion

This study presents a structured, multi-site benchmark for dental caries segmentation on panoramic radiographs, enabling consistent and reproducible evaluation of both specialized and foundation models. By standardizing preprocessing, loss functions, training protocols, and hyperparameter optimization across all architectures, we reduce confounding factors and allow for a more balanced comparison between classical task-specific networks and modern foundation models. Our results show that generalist vision foundation models can perform competitively without dental-specific pretraining. DINOv3 with a U-Net head reached similar ID Dice scores to CariesNet while demonstrating stronger OOD generalization. This finding is particularly relevant for medical domains with heterogeneous imaging conditions, where task-specific networks often overfit to site-specific characteristics [9]. The linear DINOv3 head achieved solid in-distribution performance but showed a noticeable drop

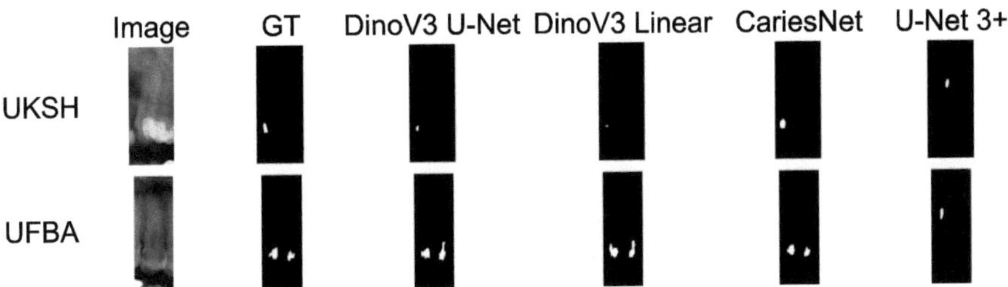

Fig. 1. This figure shows the original image, the ground truth (GT) segmentation mask and the prediction masks of all different models for an example image from the UKSH ID and UFBA OOD testset.

on the OOD dataset, indicating that while the pretrained features capture relevant dental structures, minimal finetuning alone is not sufficient for robust domain transfer. U-Net 3+ obtained the highest Dice when all images were considered, largely due to true negatives, but performed poorly on carious lesions. This underscores the importance of reporting separate results for positive and negative images to avoid misleading metrics in imbalanced datasets. Importantly, the current DINOv3 backbone was pretrained on a broad, non-medical image corpus. Pretraining on large collections of unlabeled OPG images could further enhance feature alignment with the dental domain, likely improving both ID accuracy and robustness to domain shifts. We believe that this is a promising avenue for future work. Overall, DINOv3 exhibited more robust generalization than task-specific baselines, suggesting that foundation models can help overcome data scarcity and domain variability in dental imaging. Nonetheless, absolute performance remains moderate, indicating that additional techniques, such as domain adaptation or semi-supervised finetuning may be required for clinical deployment. Our standardized, multi-site benchmark provides a foundation for further evaluation of those approaches.

References

1. Li Z, Yu C, Chen H. Global, regional, and national caries of permanent teeth incidence, prevalence, and disability-adjusted life years, 1990–2021: analysis for the Global Burden of Disease Study. BMC Oral Health. 2025;25(1):715.
2. Alharbi SS, Al Rugaibah AA, Alhasson HF, Khan RU. Detection of cavities from dental panoramic X-ray images using nested U-net models. Appl Sci. 2023;13(7):4502.
3. Zhu H, Cao Z, Lian L, Guanchen Y, Gao H. CariesNet: a deep learning approach for segmentation of multi-stage caries lesion from oral panoramic X-ray image. Neural Comput Appl. 2023;35:16051–9.
4. Hamamci IE et al. DENTEX: abnormal tooth detection with dental enumeration and diagnosis benchmark. `https://dentex.grand-challenge.org/`. Accessed: 2025-10-21. 2023.
5. IvisionLab. dns-panoramic-images-v2. `https://github.com/IvisionLab/dns-panoramic-images-v2`. Accessed: 2025-07-23. 2021.
6. Siméoni O, Vo HV, Seitzer M, Baldassarre F, Oquab M, Jose C et al. DINOv3. arXiv: 2508.10104. 2025.
7. Hansen CJ, Conrad J, Seidel R, Krekiehn NR, Yilmaz E, Koser N et al. Automated tooth instance segmentation and pathology annotation pipeline for panoramic radiographs. Proc BVM. 2024:310–5.
8. Huang H et al. UNet-Version: official PyTorch implementation of U-net and its variants (U-net++, U-net 3+, etc.) `https://github.com/ZJUGiveLab/UNet-Version`. Accessed: 2025-09-24. 2020.
9. Liu C, Chen Y, Shi H, Lu J, Jian B, Pan J et al. Does DINOv3 set a new medical vision standard? arXiv: 2509.06467. 2025.

Visual Acuity Assessment from Uni- and Multimodal Retinal Image Data using the Foundation Model MIRAGE

Caroline v. Dresky[1], Claus von der Burchard[2], Monty Santarossa[2], Julia Andresen[1], Marc S. Seibel[1], Timo Kepp[3], Johann Roider[2], Heinz Handels[1,3]

[1]Institute of Medical Informatics, University of Luebeck
[2]University Hospital Schleswig-Holstein, Kiel
[3]German Research Center for Artificial Intelligence, Luebeck
caroline.vondresky@uni-luebeck.de

Abstract. This study investigates image-based prediction of visual acuity, the most important measure of eye function, using the ophthalmic foundation model MIRAGE based on uni- and multimodal retinal image input. The three imaging modalities optical coherence tomography (OCT), infrared reflectance scanning laser ophthalmoscopy and fundus autofluorescence as well as multimodal combinations thereof turn out to be suitable for image-based prediction of no/mild, moderate, or severe visual impairment for patients suffering from central serous chorioretinopathy (CSCR). Among these, OCT-based inputs achieve the best performance across evaluation metrics. Multimodal combinations, however, provide no additional benefit over the best unimodal approach, which suggests that OCT captures the most relevant information for estimating visual function in the presence of CSCR.

1 Introduction

Visual acuity (VA) is the key metric for evaluating eye function, providing a concise measure of overall vision quality [1]. It quantifies the minimum angle of resolution (MAR) the eye can distinguish at the fixation point, corresponding to the macular region. Although VA does not capture all aspects of visual impairment, it remains the primary indicator of visual status, particularly in macular diseases such as central serous chorioretinopathy (CSCR). As a psychometric measure, VA can fluctuate in repeated testing [2] but generally offers a robust and clinically meaningful distinction between eyes with no/mild, moderate, or severe visual impairment.

Recent studies have shown that VA can be estimated directly from medical eye images as an alternative to standard chart-based tests [3–5]. This procedure offers several advantages, as it allows for retrospective VA determination and might support a deeper understanding of the structure-function correlations associated with each biomarker influencing VA. While most published image-based approaches to assess VA using deep learning methods rely on large annotated datasets, [5] could show that

© Der/die Autor(en), exklusiv lizenziert an
Springer Fachmedien Wiesbaden GmbH, ein Teil von Springer Nature 2026
H. Handels et al. (Hrsg.), *Bildverarbeitung für die Medizin 2026*,
Informatik aktuell, https://doi.org/10.1007/978-3-658-51100-5_50

the use of a foundation model that requires comparatively little labeled data yields a clinically satisfying classification into three impairment classes. This approach was based on retinal images acquired by optical coherence tomography (OCT), a non-invasive, high-resolution technique capable of visualizing the ultrastructure of the macula within seconds [6]. It is well known that retinal OCT images reveal many structural alterations that affect VA [7]. However, VA might also be impaired by alterations that are only poorly visible in OCT, such as opacities in the optical media (e.g. cataract), intraretinal hemorrhages, or chronic retinal pigment epithelium (RPE) alterations [8, 9].

To better understand how other imaging modalities or a combination may contribute to predicting VA, we compare VA classification for CSCR patients using a foundation model fine-tuned on images of three different modalities. Besides OCT, we employ infrared reflectance scanning laser ophthalmoscopy (IR-SLO, hereafter IR), fundus autofluorescence (FAF) as well as the bimodal combinations OCT+IR and OCT+FAF. IR provides an en-face imaging of the retina and can highlight RPE abnormalities, which might help to predict potential reductions in visual acuity in patients with CSCR. FAF is even more sensitive in detecting RPE abnormalities, since it selectively depicts natural fluorescence from fluorophores, primarily lipofuscin, within the RPE. Lipofuscin, a byproduct of photoreceptor degradation, accumulates under RPE dysfunction and oxidative stress in CSCR, appearing as increased autofluorescence.

2 Materials and methods

2.1 Model architecture

The recently published multimodal retinal foundation model MIRAGE used in this approach has been pretrained on 261,184 triplets of paired OCT and SLO images and automatically generated pseudo-labels of retinal layers [10]. In more detail, a multimodal masked autoencoder [11], based on modality-specific linear projection layers, a vision transformer (ViT) encoder (ViT-Base or ViT-Large), and transformer decoders, has been trained by reconstructing the input images from a masked version, which resulted in a checkpoint set of model weights. For fine-tuning, we used the pretrained projection layers and ViT-Base encoder (12 transformer blocks, 768-dimensional embeddings, 12 attention heads). The decoders were replaced by a fully connected layer with three output neurons representing the probabilities of the three visual acuity categories *no/mild*, *moderate*, and *severe visual impairment*, and the highest probability yields the final classification. The fine-tuning model can handle any subset of the aforementioned input modalities. While previous work [10] focused on single-modality input, this paper explores fine-tuning with multiple modalities for the first time. We compared model performance using unimodal inputs (OCT, IR, FAF and OCT images containing embedded fluorescence markings) and bimodal inputs (OCT+IR and OCT+FAF), with the feasible combinations constrained by the model architecture, allowing up to two specific acquired modalities to be processed simultaneously.

2.2 Dataset and preprocessing

We used a dataset of 1,075 triplets of central OCT slices ("B-scans"), IR images, and FAF images taken from the left and/or right eyes of 117 patients suffering from CSCR in successive visits to the University Hospital Schleswig-Holstein (Campus Kiel) between 2009 and 2023. All images were acquired with a Spectralis OCT scanner (Heidelberg Engineering, Heidelberg, Germany). At each patient visit, standard clinical VA testing using eye charts was performed. The resulting VA values v (logMAR scale) were grouped into three clinically motivated categories: *no/mild impairment* (class 0, $v < 0.1$), *moderate impairment* (class 1, $0.1 \leq v < 0.4$), and *severe visual impairment* (class 2, $v \geq 0.4$), which were used as labels for the corresponding images. This classification yields an assignment of 456 samples to class 0, 404 to class 1, and 215 to class 2.

The acquired images were resized to 512 × 512 pixels using bicubic interpolation and normalized. To project fluorescence regions from FAF onto OCT images, we utilized the registration pipeline of [9] in reverse. This procedure determines the position and width of the fluorescing regions in the OCT image space, which are then represented as white rectangles at the lower edge of the OCT images. According to the requirements of the MIRAGE model, bimodal inputs (OCT+IR and OCT+FAF) were combined in a 3-channel image with OCT in the first and the second modality in the second channel, while the third channel remained empty. An example for each model input is shown in Fig. 1.

2.3 Model fine-tuning

We fine-tuned all model parameters, roughly 86M for the unimodal and 87M for the bimodal approaches, on the training set comprising approximately 60% of the

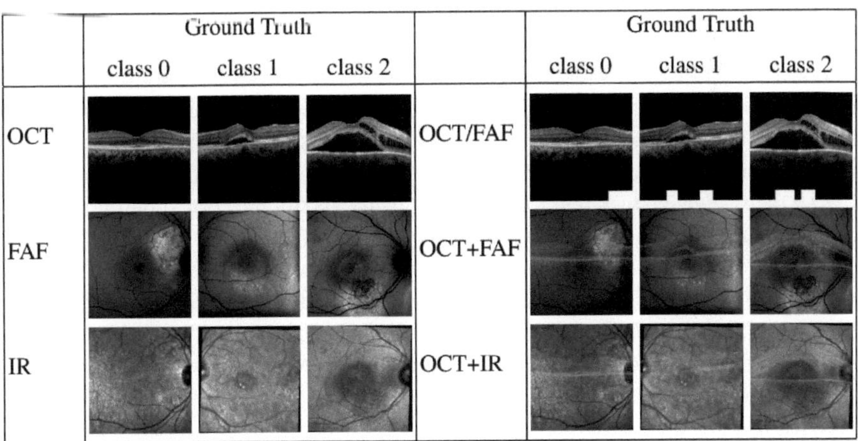

Fig. 1. Example images of all input modalities and their combinations used for fine-tuning MIRAGE, organized by visual impairment level.

Modality	Balanced Accuracy		Macro F1-score	
	Mean	95% CI	Mean	95% CI
OCT	0.56	(0.53, 0.59)	**0.52**	(0.50, 0.55)
FAF	0.43	(0.41, 0.45)	0.39	(0.36, 0.42)
IR	0.45	(0.41, 0.50)	0.42	(0.37, 0.47)
OCT/FAF	0.55	(0.52, 0.59)	0.50	(0.47, 0.54)
OCT+FAF	0.56	(0.53, 0.58)	**0.52**	(0.49, 0.55)
OCT+IR	**0.57**	(0.54, 0.59)	**0.52**	(0.49, 0.56)

Tab. 1. Evaluation metrics of twelve MIRAGE fine-tuning runs.

annotated images. To avoid splitting images of the same patient across different subsets, all images from a single patient were assigned to the same group, which may have resulted in slight deviations from the nominal 60%/20%/20% distribution. We used the AdamW optimizer, a batch size of 16 for unimodal and 8 for bimodal inputs, and trained for a maximum of 300 epochs using early stopping starting from epoch 20 with a patience of 100 epochs. During training, images were augmented using random horizontal flipping, affine transformations, and slight intensity shifts. To mitigate class imbalance, we employed two alternative approaches: a class-balanced focal loss, and a weighted sampling strategy for the training data in combination with a label-smoothing cross-entropy loss. In the following, we focus on the first approach and subsequently complement the analysis with results obtained using the second approach. Each training epoch ended with a validation step on roughly 20% of the annotated images. The model weights achieving the largest balanced accuracy across all validation steps were saved as the checkpoint for testing on the remaining approximately 20% of the labeled data.

3 Results

To evaluate whether visual impairment levels can be inferred from each uni- and bimodal image input, we fine-tuned MIRAGE with four different splits of the dataset into training, validation and test groups. For each split, three training sessions with different shuffles of the training data were performed. As evaluation metrics, we employed balanced accuracy and macro F1-score as meaningful measures in the presence of class imbalance. Tab. 1 and Fig. 2 report the mean values of both metrics across the twelve independent training runs, evaluated on the corresponding test sets for each input modality. The highest mean balanced accuracy values (0.55–0.57) and macro F1-scores (0.50–0.52) were obtained for the OCT-related inputs, namely OCT, OCT/FAF, OCT+FAF, and OCT+IR. Paired t-tests indicated no statistically significant differences among the OCT-related results themselves. In contrast, all OCT-related inputs achieved significantly higher performance with respect to both metrics compared to FAF and IR alone. The same qualitative conclusions were reached using the second approach to mitigate class imbalance, based on weighted sampling during training.

Since MIRAGE achieved its best performance with OCT-related inputs, we provide additional details for the unimodal OCT setting as a representative case. Fig. 3

shows the averaged confusion matrices, including mean, minimum and maximum values across all twelve fine-tuning runs for both class imbalance mitigation strategies. From these, we can particularly deduce the sensitivities (true positive rates) of 0.80 and 0.82 for class 0, 0.35 and 0.42 for class 1 and 0.53 and 0.36 for class 2.

4 Discussion

For all tested image modalities and combinations, the foundation model MIRAGE achieved visual impairment classification results that are better than random guessing (dashed lines in Fig. 2). This confirms the potential of image-based approaches for VA assessment for CSCR patients. Among the tested modalities, OCT-related inputs performed equally well, whereas FAF and IR yielded significantly lower results. As expected from a clinical perspective, this suggests that FAF and IR are less suitable for VA assessment when used as unimodal inputs. Moreover, combining OCT images with information derived from FAF or IR images did not improve classification performance, indicating that OCT alone captures the most relevant structural information for estimating visual function in CSCR. However, as alterations visible in FAF images, such as lipofuscin accumulation, are typically associated with advanced

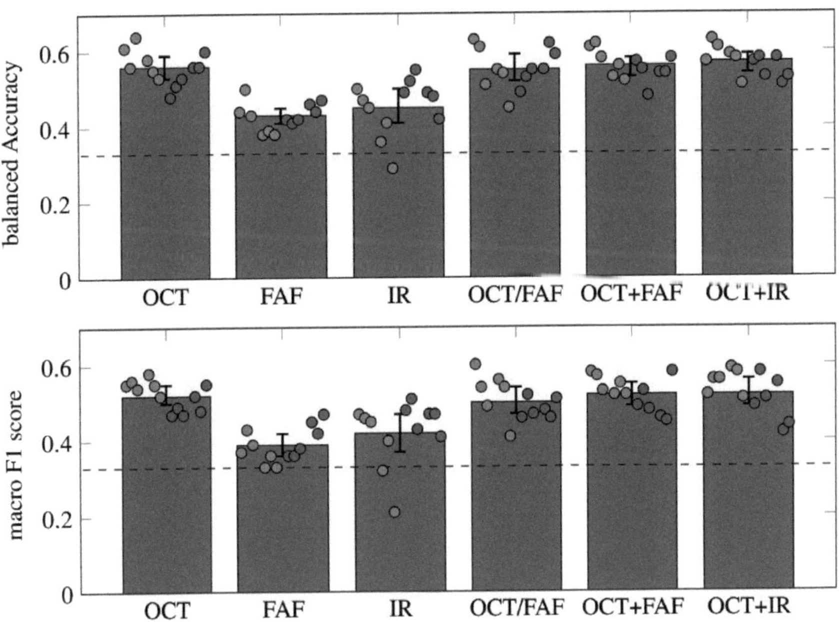

Fig. 2. Balanced accuracy and macro F1-score (dots), mean values (horizontal lines) and 95% confidence intervals (error bars) for twelve training sessions with four different group splittings (color-coded dots) and three different training data shuffles each. The dashed lines represent random guessing.

stages of eye diseases, one could investigate whether a more subtle differentiation within class 2 might benefit from FAF information.

Focusing on the performance of the most efficient approach, i.e., unimodal OCT input, analysis of class sensitivities across both class-imbalance mitigation strategies shows that class 0 (no/mild impairment) is reliably separated from the remaining classes (Fig. 3). In contrast, discrimination between the less represented classes 1 and 2 is substantially more challenging and strongly depends on the imbalance-handling strategy: class-balanced loss enhances sensitivity for the minority class 2, whereas weighted sampling provides better performance for the medium-frequency class 1. However, the off-diagonal elements in both confusion matrices reveal frequent misclassifications between classes 1 and 2. One possible reason for the observed confusion is the limited discriminability of the image data itself, as images from different classes may appear highly similar or class-specific biomarkers may not be visible in the examined imaging modalities. As already discussed in [5], the difficulty of distinguishing adjacent classes is also related to the fact that VA is an imprecise ground truth label. Measured via a subjective test method, it exhibits natural fluctuations, which are particularly problematic near the boundaries between neighboring classes and can adversely affect model training.

To address the above-mentioned problems, we are currently investigating the sources of misclassification in more detail. In particular, we are examining whether incorrectly classified images tend to lie near the boundaries of adjacent VA classes or exhibit specific image characteristics. Furthermore, we are assessing the reliability of the predictions based on the output probability vectors, providing insight into the model's confidence and enabling the development of decision strategies that take prediction uncertainty into account.

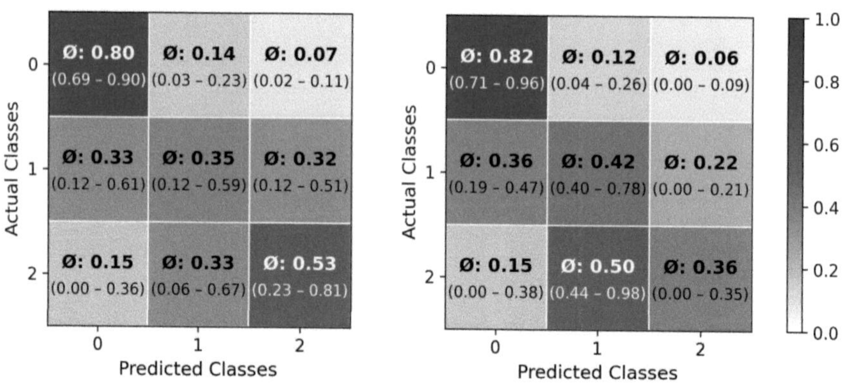

Fig. 3. Results of MIRAGE fine-tuned with OCT images: Averaged confusion matrices presenting the mean values, minima and maxima of the results of twelve fine-tunings. Left: Matrix resulting from class-balanced focal loss approach, right: Matrix resulting from weighted sampling approach.

References

1. Arditi A, Cagenello R. On the statistical reliability of letter-chart visual acuity measurements. Invest Ophthalmol Vis Sci. 1993;34(1):120–9.
2. Lovie-Kitchin JE. Validity and reliability of visual acuity measurements. Ophthalmic Physiol Opt. 1988;8(4):363–70.
3. Lin TY, Chen HR, Huang HY, et al. Deep learning to infer visual acuity from optical coherence tomography in diabetic macular edema. Front Med. 2022;9.
4. Inoda S, Takahashi H, Arai Y, et al. An AI model to estimate visual acuity based solely on cross-sectional OCT imaging of various diseases. Albrecht Von Graefes Arch Klin Exp Ophthalmol. 2023;261(10):2775–85.
5. v. Dresky C, von der Burchard C, Andresen J, et al. Visual acuity assessment from optical coherence tomography images using the foundation model RETFound. Proc SPIE MI CAD. 2025;13407.
6. Bouma BE, de Boer JF, Huang D, et al. Optical coherence tomography. Nat Rev Methods Primers. 2022;2.
7. Scharf A, von der Burchard C, Tatli A, et al. Linking AI-based biomarker analysis to visual acuity changes in central serous chorioretinopathy (CSCR). Invest Ophthalmol Vis Sci. 2024;65.
8. Ouyang Y, Heussen FM, Keane PA, et al. The retinal disease screening study: retrospective comparison of nonmydriatic fundus photography and three-dimensional optical coherence tomography for detection of retinal irregularities. Invest Ophthalmol Vis Sci. 2013;54:5694–700.
9. Santarossa M, Tatli A, Burchard C von der, et al. Chronological registration of OCT and autofluorescence findings in CSCR: two distinct patterns in disease course. Diagnostics. 2022;12(8):1780.
10. Morano J, Fazekas B, Sükei E, et al. Multimodal foundation model and benchmark for comprehensive retinal OCT image analysis. NPJ Digit Med. 2025;8(1).
11. He K, Chen X, Xie S, et al. Masked autoencoders are scalable vision learners. Proc IEEE/CVF CVPR. 2022:15979–88.

Characterization of Foundation Models for Longitudinal Similarity Measurement in Medical Video Data

Luisa Neubig [1], Deirde Larsen [2], Takeshi Ikuma [3], Melda Kunduk [4], Andreas M. Kist [1]

[1]Department Artificial Intelligence in Biomedical Engineering, FAU Erlangen-Nürnberg, Erlangen, Germany
[2]Department of Communication Sciences and Disorders, East Carolina University, Greenville, NC, USA
[3]Department of Otolaryngology – Head and Neck Surgery, Louisiana State University Health Sciences Center, New Orleans, LA, USA
[4]Department of Communication Sciences and Disorders, Louisiana State University, Baton Rouge, LA, USA
luisa.e.neubig@fau.de

Abstract. Foundation models provide general-purpose image representations that promise to capture structural and semantic information. However, their suitability for measuring similarity across image sequences has not been thoroughly examined. Conventional metrics such as the structural similarity index measure (SSIM) are commonly used to assess frame-to-frame consistency but are sensitive to motion, deformation, and intensity changes, which limits their usefulness for dynamic imaging. In this study, we compare embeddings from a variety of pretrained models, including DINOv2, ResNet50, CLIP, SAM, and LPIPS, to evaluate their ability to represent temporal and structural similarity in videos and their ability to assess the quality of image registration. We analyzed sensitivity to global and local motion in two medical imaging datasets. We focused on videofluoroscopic swallowing studies (VFSS) with global and local motion and the BAGLS dataset of vocal fold vibrations with mainly local motion. Our results indicate differences in how models maintain consistent similarity under motion, and suggest that some embedding-based approaches provide a more stable representation than SSIM without additional fine-tuning.

1 Introduction

Foundation models have become widely used for extracting general-purpose visual features from images. These models, trained on large and diverse datasets, provide embeddings that capture structural, semantic, and perceptual aspects of visual information. Although such embeddings have been extensively applied to static image

© Der/die Autor(en), exklusiv lizenziert an
Springer Fachmedien Wiesbaden GmbH, ein Teil von Springer Nature 2026
H. Handels et al. (Hrsg.), *Bildverarbeitung für die Medizin 2026*,
Informatik aktuell, https://doi.org/10.1007/978-3-658-51100-5_51

analysis, their suitability to measure similarity across coherent temporal-variant images in medical imaging remains underexplored. In particular, it remains unclear how well different pretrained models preserve representation consistency over time and whether they can serve as alternatives to conventional similarity metrics. Image similarity in videos is often evaluated using reference-based measures, such as the SSIM, which compares local luminance, contrast, and structure between frames. However, SSIM is sensitive to small spatial shifts and intensity variations and therefore may not accurately reflect perceptual similarity in videos that include motion or deformation, as is often the case in medical imaging. Embedding-based approaches derived from deep neural networks may provide a more robust alternative, as they represent images in high-dimensional feature spaces that can capture higher-level relationships between frames.

In this study, we compare the cosine similarity across image embeddings of five pretrained foundation models with SSIM to assess their ability to reflect temporal and structural similarity in videos, without explicit region analysis. We use models based on different learning paradigms, including the Self-Distillation without labels model (DINO) [1], the supervised ResNet50 [2], the multimodal contrastive language-image pretraining (CLIP) [3] vision encoder, the vision backbone of the segment anything model (SAM) [4], and the learned perceptual image patch similarity model (LPIPS) [5]. We then evaluated their susceptibility to local and global motion using two different medical datasets. By comparing embedding-based similarity with SSIM across these datasets, we aim to identify which representations maintain consistent similarity measures in the presence of different motions. Our results provide insights into the representational stability of foundation models and their potential use for video-based analysis without task-specific finetuning.

2 Methods

2.1 Foundation models

We rely on five pretrained foundation models (see above) to derive image embeddings representing different aspects of visual information. All models were used in their publicly available pretrained form without additional training or task-specific finetuning. DINO and ResNet were trained on ImageNet, SAM on the SA-1B dataset, LPIPS on the BAPPS dataset supplemented with ImageNet and related image sets, and CLIP on the WebImageText (WIT) corpus. The embeddings were extracted and analyzed to study longitudinal representational similarity within images. We access the foundation models in PyTorch and use their embeddings for our quantitative and qualitative analyzes of image-level similarity and representation structure.

2.2 Data

To evaluate image embeddings under conditions of both global and local motion, we analyzed two distinct datasets. The first data set consisted of videofluoroscopic swallowing studies (VFSS) provided by Louisiana State University (LSU), USA. In these recordings, patients must swallow radiopaque contrast material that is visualized in video-rate X-ray examinations of the swallowing process. From this data set, we selected swallow studies that contain only local movement (i.e., no_move_vfss) with changes in the oral cavity and pharynx and swallows with extensive global movement of the patients themselves (i.e., move_vfss). To assess embedding sensitivity to fine-scale motion, we further analyzed sequences from the BAGLS dataset [6], which comprises high-speed endoscopic recordings (>4,000 fps) of vocal fold vibration and primarily captures localized tissue motion. Frame pairs were constructed from consecutive frames (t and $t + 1$) as provided by the dataset. We evaluated shorter and longer clips to characterize how long-term changes in endoscopic footage affect the embedding space. The raw frames were converted to grayscale and encoded with each foundation model to obtain the corresponding embeddings, with dimensionalities of 768 for DINO (ViT-B/14), 2048 for ResNet50, 768 for CLIP, 256 for SAM, and 1472 for LPIPS (VGG).

2.3 Metrics

Image similarity and structural preservation were evaluated using both reference-based and embedding-based metrics. SSIM served as a conventional reference-

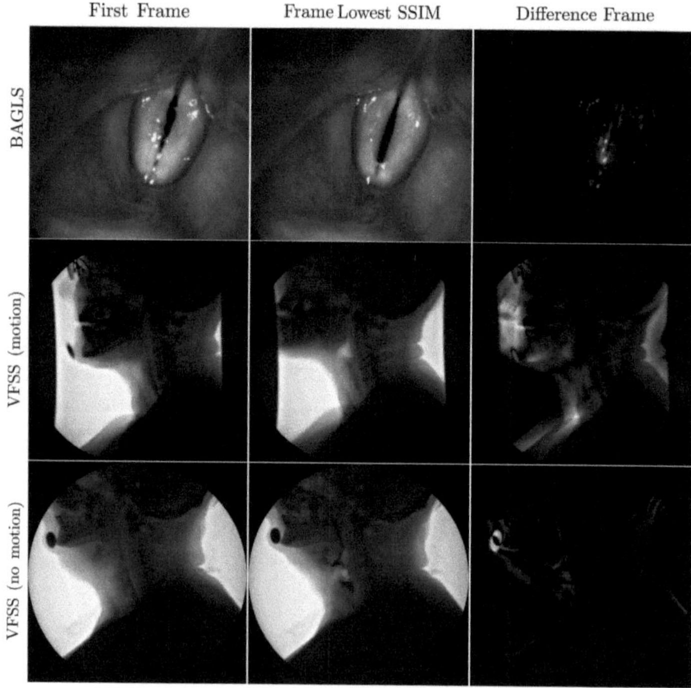

Fig. 1. Visual comparison of the starting frame, the lowest-SSIM frame in a given sequence, and the corresponding difference image across datasets.

based metric that evaluated luminance, contrast, and structural consistency within the video. We used cosine similarity to quantify the similarity between image embeddings. This embedding-based metric measures the alignment of feature vectors in a learned representation space, capturing higher-level semantic and perceptual relationships between images.

3 Results

Motion and deformation are inherent in the imaging of dynamic physiological processes, which can complicate the assessment of structural consistency across frames. A central question is how to obtain a similarity representation that remains stable under such variations. When we investigated SSIM, we observed that SSIM was highly decreased, although adjacent video frames barely changed qualitatively. In Fig. 1, we show the starting frame of a sequence of each dataset, the frame with the lowest SSIM, and the real difference. These images show that local and global motion affect established similarity measures, while the overall global information remains intact. This instability may confound the interpretation of temporal changes by reflecting imaging or motion-related artifacts.

To analyze this in greater detail, we evaluated embeddings from multiple pretrained models to assess their ability to represent global similarity consistently across frames in two medical video datasets. Specifically, we compared the temporal dynamics of cosine similarity between embedding vectors with frame-to-frame SSIM, examining how well each method preserves consistent and smooth similarity throughout a sequence of consecutive frames. Fig. 2 compares SSIM and cosine similarity across both datasets. SSIM exhibits the weakest performance in captur-

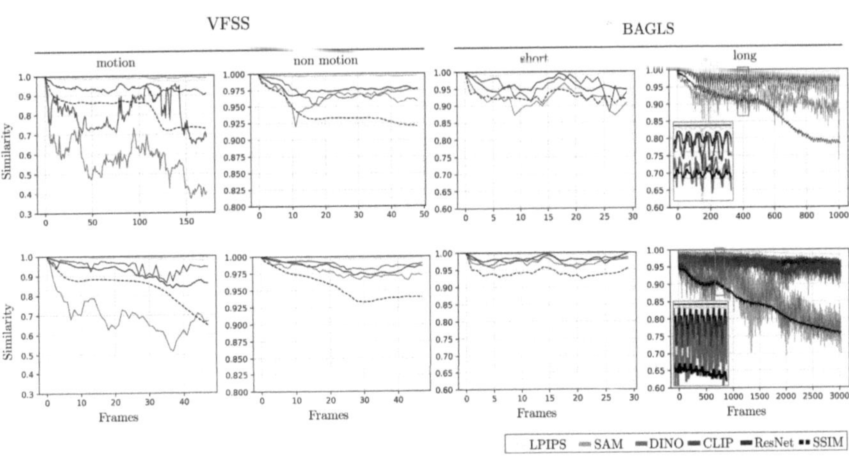

Fig. 2. Exemplary SSIM and cosine similarity across embeddings for VFSS (left local, right local and global motion) and BAGLS (dominating local motion, short snippets and long videos) with representation of oscillating behavior in the enlarged section.

Dataset	SSIM	ResNet	CLIP	DINO	SAM	LPIPS
BAGLS	0.903	0.952	0.982	0.927	1.000	0.992
VFSS (m)	0.784	0.909	0.962	0.909	0.996	0.984
VFSS (nm)	0.922	0.975	0.968	0.933	0.998	0.992

Tab. 1. Summary of quantitative (cosine) similarity values across the datasets BAGLS, VFSS with motion (m) and VFSS with no motion (nm) at the timestamp of the lowest SSIM. Note that SAM has basically identical embeddings for local motion (BAGLS).

ing similarity over entire sequences. DINO and CLIP show substantial fluctuations, while LPIPS, SAM, and ResNet demonstrate more stable behavior. However, SAM appears to be very insensitive by showing minimal variation between frames. In longer videos from the BAGLS dataset, a noticeable oscillatory pattern emerges in the similarity measures, suggesting that the fundamental frequency F_0 could potentially be extracted by FFT analysis of the similarity trajectories.

To quantitatively assess the oscillatory behavior of the vocal folds, we first segmented the glottal area using the publicly available OpenHSV model [7], providing a well-established reference to calculate F_0. We computed the fast Fourier transform (FFT) of the cosine similarity trajectories and extracted the corresponding F_0 for an exemplary longer video of the BAGLS dataset, as shown in Fig. 3a. The region around F_0 is also highlighted in Fig. 3b. The F_0 obtained from the segmented glottal area matches closely that derived from the embedding similarities. In our example video, segmentation yields F_0 = 285.7 Hz, while ResNet and CLIP provide 284 Hz, and DINO and LPIPS yield 288 Hz. This strong agreement suggests that glottal motion can be reliably inferred from the embeddings without additional supervision.

Across all three datasets, LPIPS and SAM embeddings exhibited stable cosine similarity over time. In the case of SAM embeddings, it is saturated for local motion, whereas LPIPS is still able to depict these subtle changes. To further investigate

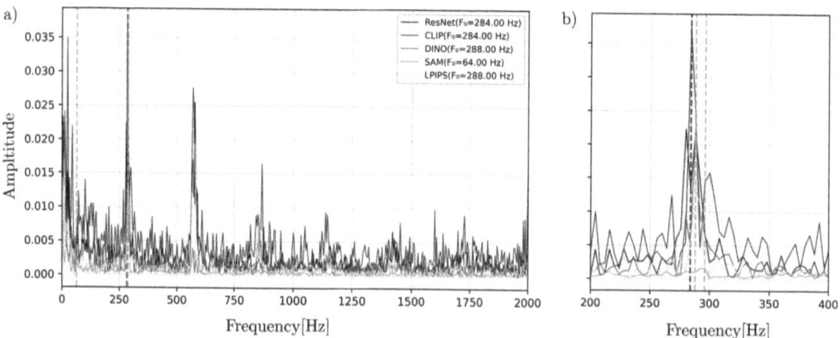

Fig. 3. Power spectrum of the SSIM and cosine similarity trajectories shown in Fig. 2 top right to determine F_0. a) represents the full available spectrum and b) shows an inset around the true F_0.

their relationship with each other, we computed the cross-correlation between the respective embeddings and SSIM, as shown in Fig. 4. The cross-correlation quantifies the temporal alignment between metrics and reflects their robustness to smooth transitions, with higher values indicating similar but differently smoothed responses to image changes. LPIPS showed the strongest correlation with both SSIM and ResNet, while CLIP demonstrated the weakest correlation with all other measures, which is consistent with its rather poor performance and noisy performance in Fig. 2.

To examine whether the embeddings share a similar perception of frame-wise similarity, we selected one representative example from each dataset (Fig. 1) and analyzed the cosine similarity in the frame of the lowest SSIM. The corresponding values are reported in Tab. 1. Across all examples, SAM produced consistently high values, suggesting a limited ability to react to subtle local differences in images. In the BAGLS dataset, where only subtle glottal variations are present, ResNet, CLIP, and LPIPS (0.952, 0.927, and 0.992, respectively) correspond well to visual similarity, while DINO yields considerably lower values despite minimal visual change. A similar pattern was observed in the no-motion VFSS example. In VFSS footage with global motion, the SSIM provides a lower estimation of the similarity of 0.784. ResNet and DINO reflect the increased motion with similarity values around 0.9, whereas CLIP and LPIPS rate the frames as highly similar, likely due to the dominant appearance of the patient's head while overlooking any positional shift.

Since the embeddings appeared to capture perceptual similarity more effectively than SSIM, we further examined whether they can differentiate between local and global motion. Fig. 5 shows the UMAP projections for the BAGLS and VFSS (motion) datasets in all frames. The BAGLS embeddings form relatively compact clusters, consistent with mainly local motion, whereas the VFSS embeddings follow a more continuous trajectory, indicating greater temporal variation.

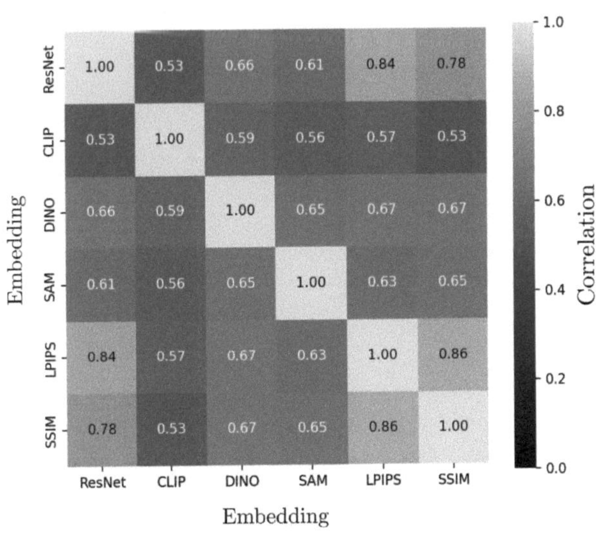

Fig. 4. Heatmap of the correlation of the SSIM and the cosine similarity of the embeddings averaged across videos and datasets.

Fig. 5. UMAP manifolds for BAGLS (left) and VFSS (right) across embedding spaces.

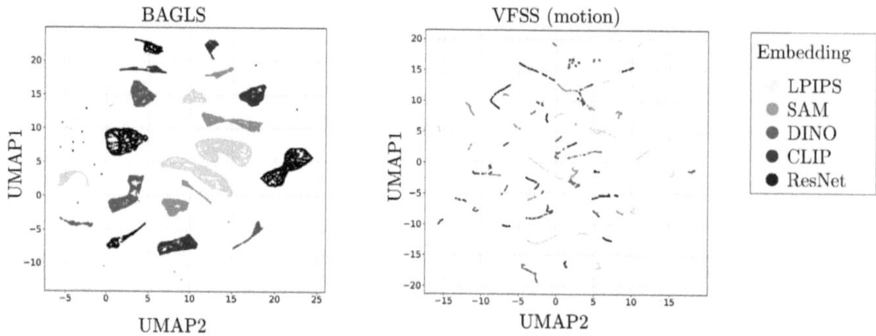

4 Discussion

We showed that SSIM is compared to embeddings not suitable for longitudinal similarity analysis in medical imaging due to its pixel-level sensitivity to spatial shifts, illumination variations, and deformations, resulting in unstable similarity values over time. Among embedding-based approaches, DINO, ResNet50, and CLIP exhibited partial robustness, but remained affected by changes in motion and appearance, and showed easy perturbations even with adjacent frames. In particular, cosine similarity of the embedding spaces enabled us to directly retrieve F_0 of the vibration frequency of the vocal fold. The SAM embeddings were largely insensitive to local and global motion data. In general, embedding-based measures, particularly LPIPS, offer a more stable and informative foundation for longitudinal similarity analysis in dynamic medical image data.

References

1. Caron M, Touvron H, Misra I, Jégou H, Mairal J, Bojanowski P et al. Emerging properties in self-supervised vision transformers. Proc NYSDS. 2021:9650–60.
2. He K, Zhang X, Ren S, Sun J. Deep residual learning for image recognition. Proc NYSDS. 2016:770–8.
3. Radford A, Kim JW, Hallacy C, Ramesh A, Goh G, Agarwal S et al. Learning transferable visual models from natural language supervision. Proc NYSDS. 2021.
4. Kirillov A, Mintun E, Ravi N, Mao H, Rolland C, Gustafson L et al. Segment Anything. Proc NYSDS. 2023:4015–26.
5. Zhang R, Isola P, Efros AA, Shechtman E, Wang O. The unreasonable effectiveness of deep features as a perceptual metric. Proc NYSDS. 2018:586–95.
6. Gómez P, Kist AM, Schlegel P, Berry DA, Chhetri DK, Dürr S et al. BAGLS: a multihospital benchmark for automatic glottis segmentation. Sci Data. 2020;7(1).
7. Kist AM, Dürr S, Schützenberger A, Döllinger M. OpenHSV: an open platform for laryngeal high-speed videoendoscopy. Sci Rep. 2021;11(1).

Adaptive Automatic Prompt Generation Assistant for Segmentation Foundation Models

David Lurz, Luisa Neubig, Andreas Kist

Department Artificial Intelligence in Biomedical Engineering,
Friedrich-Alexander-Universität Erlangen-Nürnberg
david.lurz@fau.de

Abstract. A variety of interactive segmentation foundation models are available, achieving strong performance in various domains of medical image segmentation. Many of these models, such as MedSAM2, require input prompts in the form of point coordinates or boxes. This prompt creation, however, is a time-consuming and error-prone task. To address this, we propose BOB, the Bounding-box Oracle for Biomedicine. By training lightweight 2D object detection models on the bounding boxes of annotated medical segmentation datasets, it can generate box prompts for medical images, videos, and volumes, allowing faster prompt generation while still keeping a human-in-the-loop architecture. We trained YOLOv12n and D-FINE-N with 30 classes on around 50k diverse images across more than 10 modalities. An algorithm to cluster the prompts and filter by object and prompt quality ensures appropriate behavior in multi-dimensional images. By combining the generated prompts with a segmentation foundation model, we are able to quickly perform semantic and instance segmentation with optional human-in-the-loop. Compared to theoretically perfect box prompts generated from the ground truth, we could achieve around 90-110% mIoU performance across scenarios, rivaling state-of-the-art specialized deep neural networks. To allow prompt generation, visualization, interactive refinement, and subsequent segmentation of the prompts, we provide a napari plugin. Our code and full results are openly available at `https://github.com/DavidL-11/BOB`.

1 Introduction

Medical image segmentation plays a crucial role in the field of medical image processing. Recent advancements in deep learning have demonstrated that deep neural networks are particularly effective for image segmentation tasks, although they tend to be specific to certain tasks and are limited to predicting only the classes they were trained on. Consequently, they struggle to generalize to new anatomical structures. Foundation models like the segment anything model (SAM) [1] offer a solution to this issue. These models are trained on extensive datasets and feature zero-shot capabilities, enabling them to potentially segment any user-specified target and adapt to novel tasks. Often, these models require input prompts, such as points

© Der/die Autor(en), exklusiv lizenziert an
Springer Fachmedien Wiesbaden GmbH, ein Teil von Springer Nature 2026
H. Handels et al. (Hrsg.), *Bildverarbeitung für die Medizin 2026*,
Informatik aktuell, https://doi.org/10.1007/978-3-658-51100-5_52

or boxes, to identify areas for segmentation. While this facilitates human-in-the-loop adjustments, it also presents certain drawbacks: on the one hand, prompt creation takes work and needs skilled workers to find and identify objects of interest; on the other hand, low-quality prompts, like boxes that are too large, have a negative impact on segmentation quality.

To address some of these limitations, previous work has already focused on automatically creating prompts for these models. ProxyPrompt [2] automatically generates prompts for SAM in a clinical context by utilizing a pre-annotated mask of similar style, essentially turning the zero-shot segmentation into one-shot segmentation. Wei et al. [3] propose a self-prompting strategy for SAM that generates promising prompts from voxel features. Li et al. [4] create an automatic 3D-based prompt generator for multi-organ CT segmentation. More specifically, Mansoori et al. [5] utilize a YOLOv8 object detection model in combination with SAM for fully automatic polyp segmentation in colonoscopy. MedLSAM [6] combines SAM with MedLAM, a model to localize organs in 3D CT scans. For visualization and interactivity, SAM extensions for napari and 3D Slicer have been created, e.g. napari-sam [7].

While these methods might work in specific cases, the existing solutions are either too task-specific, not of desired quality, don't adapt to multiple dimensions, or do not allow manual refinement of the prompts. Furthermore, a generalized user interface that allows automatic prompt generation, interactive placement of prompts, visualization of data and resulting segmentation, as well as the possibility of easily switching between different segmentation foundation models, is also missing. In this paper, we propose the bounding-box oracle for biomedicine (BOB), that addresses these limitations.

2 Materials and methods

From our previous comparison of current segmentation foundation models [8] we selected SAM2.1 [9] and MedSAM2 [10] for 2D segmentation, as well as MedSAM2, nnInteractive [11] and VISTA3D [12] for 3D segmentation. VISTA3D with label prompts is only used as a comparison baseline, as it does not accept box prompts, to showcase what completely automatic segmentation foundation models are already capable of.

The datasets used for our evaluations include an extension of BAGLS [13] (BAGLS-VF, glottis and vocal fold segmentation), brain electron microscopy [14] (mitochondria segmentation), NeoPolyp [15] (Polyp segmentation), IMed361-M [16] (>50 datasets of varying modalities and segmentation targets, mainly CT/MRI), MedSegBench [17] (35 datasets of more rare segmentation targets), AMOS22 and FLARE22 (grand challenge multi-organ abdomen CT/MRI and CT segmentation), toothfairy3 [18–20] (70 different classes in CBCT head scans) and the medical segmentation decathlon [21] (MSD; 10 different 3D segmentation tasks).

BOB is able to generate box prompts without the ground truth by using 2D object detection models and applying them to 2D and 3D images, as well as videos. This was achieved by training 2D object detection models on more than 50k training images sourced from these datasets. By selecting segmentation targets where foundation models showed promising performance, we obtained the following 30 classes: glottis, left vocal cord, right vocal cord, lung, polyp, tool, organ, liver, right kidney, spleen, mitochondria, aorta, inferior vena cava, pharynx, fetal head, gallbladder, esophagus, stomach, tooth, left kidney, prostate/uterus, skin lesion, glioma, optic disc, optic cup, nucleus, heart myocardium, heart left ventricle, heart right ventricle, heart atrium left. As object detection models, we chose YOLOv12n and D-FINE-N due to their strong real-time performance. We trained them with an AdamW in PyTorch 2.8.0 with CUDA12.8 on an RTX5070TI. After 50 and 70 epochs, the models reached an mAP of 0.92 and 0.93, respectively.

For 3D stacks and videos, prompts are generated for each slice or frame, respectively. After grouping boxes with the same class ID and significant IoU overlap across frames together with a unique object ID, only the `n_prompts_per_object` boxes with the highest confidence score are kept to allow manual human refinement and leave the actual segmentation to the z-propagation of the foundation models.

To use this tool effectively, we created an extension for the multidimensional image viewer, napari. It allows loading and viewing images, applying CT windowing preprocessing, generating prompts, adding prompts manually, segmenting these prompts, and then viewing the resulting segmentation. It supports 2D and 3D images, as well as videos, and includes multiple presets for common segmentation tasks and modalities. Generated prompts can be viewed in 2D, 3D, or across video frames. The usual workflow with this extension consists of importing an image, selecting a preset, running automatic prompt generation, reviewing the prompts, optionally editing them or adding more, running the segmentation, and then removing the prompts (Fig. 1). Currently supported segmentation models include SAM2.1, MedSAM2 and nnInteractive.

To quantify BOB's segmentation performance, we chose the intersection-over-union (IoU) metric, where a value of 1.0 means perfect overlap. We compare the performance of BOB's generated prompts to theoretically perfect prompts generated from the ground truth (point, box) and VISTA3D's label prompts, which support 127 classes.

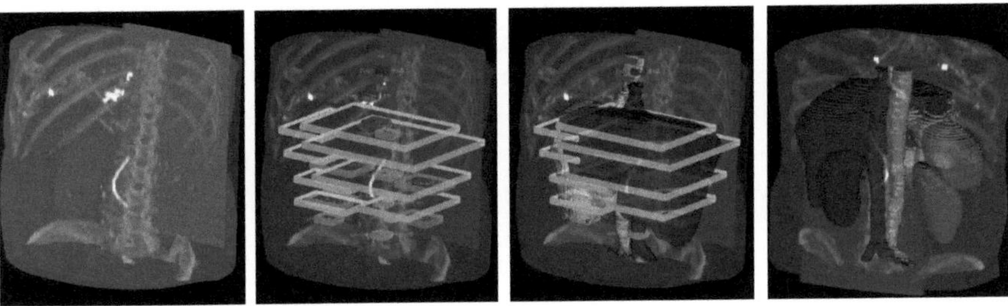

Fig. 1. Multi-organ segmentation steps with BOB-napari (3D view). From left to right: loaded data, BOB-guided bounding-box proposals, after segmentation with MedSAM2 (front view), segmentation result without prompts (back view).

Tab. 1. BOB mIoU performance compared to other prompting strategies and models (evaluated on the test sets; only supported BOB classes included in calculation).

Model	Dataset	Prompting Strategy (mIoU ↑) Box	BOB D-FINE-N	BOB YOLOv12n	Label
SAM2.1 Tiny	BAGLS-VF	0.777	0.771	0.752	–
	BrainEM	0.835	0.828	0.802	–
	NeoPolyp	0.914	0.851	0.740	–
	IMed361	0.774	0.735	0.675	–
	MedSegBench	0.827	0.753	0.690	–
$\text{MedSAM2}_{\text{latest}}$	BAGLS-VF	0.743	0.739	0.724	–
	BrainEM	0.841	0.825	0.801	–
	NeoPolyp	0.940	0.871	0.764	–
	IMed361	0.820	0.782	0.710	–
	MedSegBench	0.876	0.797	0.732	–
	ToothFairy3	0.797	0.771	0.773	–
	MSD	0.844	0.757	0.743	–
	AMOS22	0.728	0.702	0.692	–
	FLARE22	0.879	0.886	0.880	–
nnInteractive	ToothFairy3	0.838	0.774	0.780	–
	AMOS22	0.651	0.692	0.701	–
	FLARE22	0.843	0.887	0.891	–
VISTA3D	AMOS22	–	–	–	0.755
	FLARE22	–	–	–	0.892
	Average	**0.819**	**0.789**	**0.755**	–

3 Results

While BOB is technically only supposed to be a prompt generation assistant with human supervision, we calculated its maximum performance when using all of its generated prompts with no adjustments, but well-selected prompt generation parameters. This allows us to determine the quality of the generated prompts and how much human input is required to refine them. As a reference, we also measured the mIoU of the same model, when using "perfect "box prompts, generated from the ground truth using a bounding box for each object.

The mIoU per model and prompting strategy (Tab. 1). For BAGLS-VF, BOB had to predict left and right vocal folds, as well as the glottis. It was able to do this reliably, in both images and videos, reaching 99% of the average IoU of perfect box prompts, even without any kind of human input and prompt refinement. The challenge with the brain electron microscopy datasets was typically the number (>20) of prompts per image, where BOB also achieved more than 98% of perfect box prompt performance.

The performance on the NeoPolyp dataset was slightly worse, although still yielded commendable results at an mIoU of 0.871 with MedSAM2 and D-FINE-N, resulting in about 92% of perfect box prompt mIoU. For the two large dataset collections, we only evaluated the classes supported by BOB on the official test split, resulting in a box prompt mIoU of 0.82 for IMed361M and 0.876 for MedSegBench.

Once again, BOB delivers around 95% (IMed361M) and 90% (MedSegBench) of these perfect box prompts, almost reaching a very good mIoU of 0.8 in both benchmarks, which indicates strong performance and is often considered clinically usable.

The median values of box, D-FINE-N, and YOLOv12n are relatively close across the many datasets of IMed-361M,Fig. 2, but D-FINE-N handles especially hard cases better and therefore achieves overall superior results. The metrics for ToothFairy3 are computed using a combined volume of all teeth instead of averaging across the individual objects, since BOB doesn't differentiate between the various tooth types. This results in very high metrics, again, more than 98% of box prompt performance. It should be noted that, using manual inspection, YOLOv12n actually produced better results in many cases, leading to fewer unnecessary prompts and fewer false positives.

The MSD included the 3D segmentation tasks for the spleen and a glioma. While spleen segmentation was excellent (mIoU = 0.910), locating the glioma and determining its exact boundaries proved to be quite a challenge (mIoU = 0.626), requiring a possible human-in-the-loop.

For many 3D segmentation tasks, like in FLARE22, the results for BOB are actually higher than the perfect box prompts (Fig. 3). By arguing that the amount of effort required to create one prompt corresponds to reviewing five prompts, we allowed BOB to generate upwards of 5 prompts per object (BOB D-FINE-N) compared to only one (BOB D-FINE-N Single). For nnInteractive we compared both modes and found an average 5% higher mIoU with the additional guidance, especially noticable for large/long organs like the Inferior Vena Cava. This improvement over

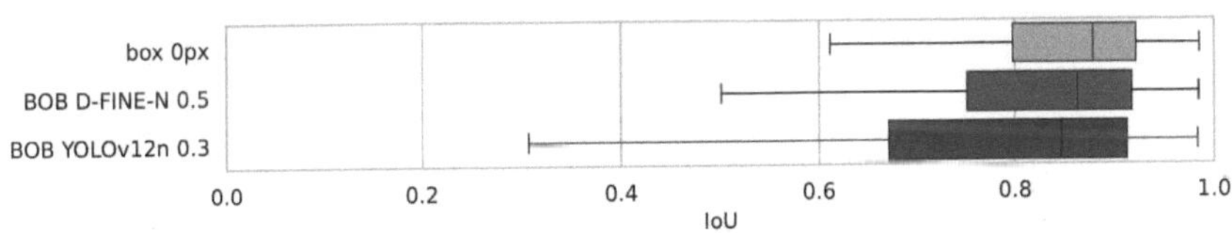

Fig. 2. IMed-361M IoU distribution for supported BOB classes.

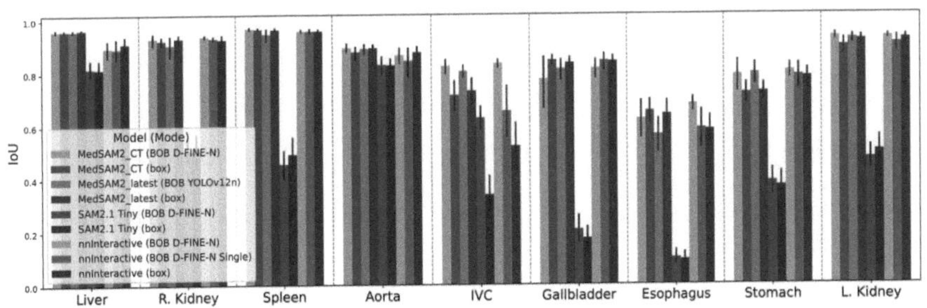

Fig. 3. FLARE22 segmentation results: BOB vs. perfect box prompt.

the perfect box prompt baseline also hints at the fact that this score could be improved even more by manual refinement of the prompts.

The lower mIoU for AMOS22 (Tab. 1) is mainly caused by the gallbladder and prostate, where BOB struggled. The aorta, on the other hand, benefited the most from the additional guidance using multiple prompts, gaining an almost 10% mIoU increase compared to single perfect box prompts.

To qualitatively assess model behavior, Fig. 4 and Fig. 5 visualize predicted bounding boxes for multiple representative object classes, demonstrating BOB's ability to localize objects across diverse targets, modalities and dimensionalities.

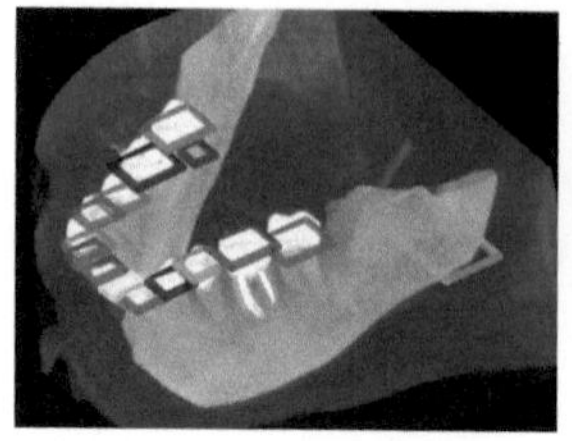
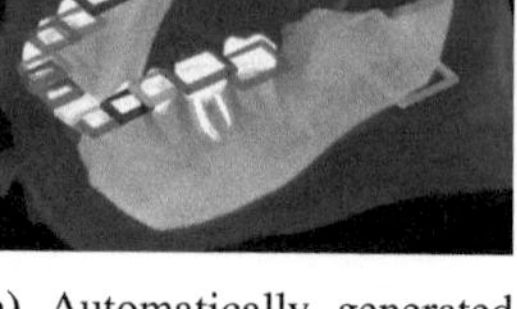
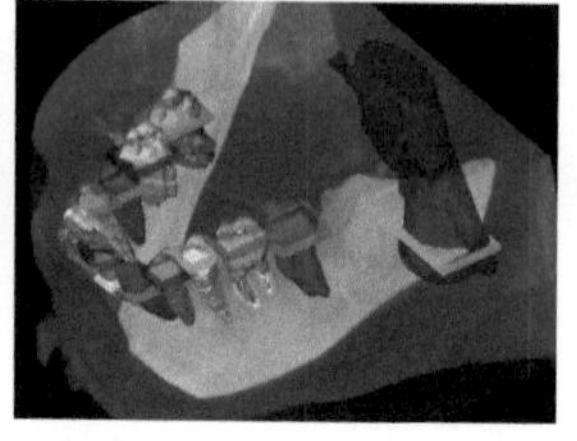
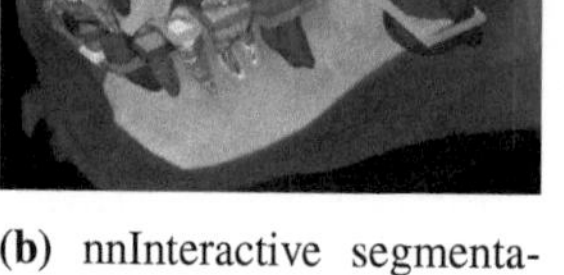
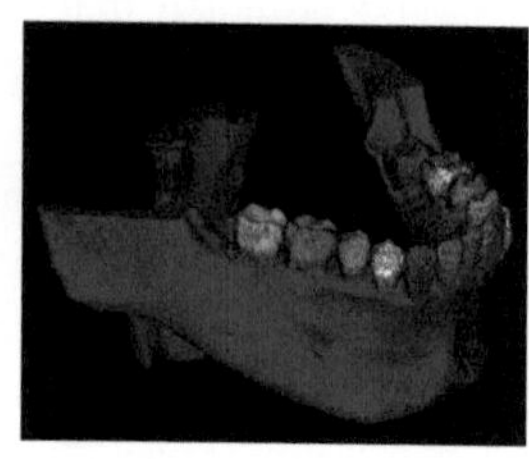

(a) Automatically generated prompts. **(b)** nnInteractive segmentation result. **(c)** Segmentation result + manual prompt for jawbone.

Fig. 4. ToothFairy3 + BOB + nnInteractive workflow.

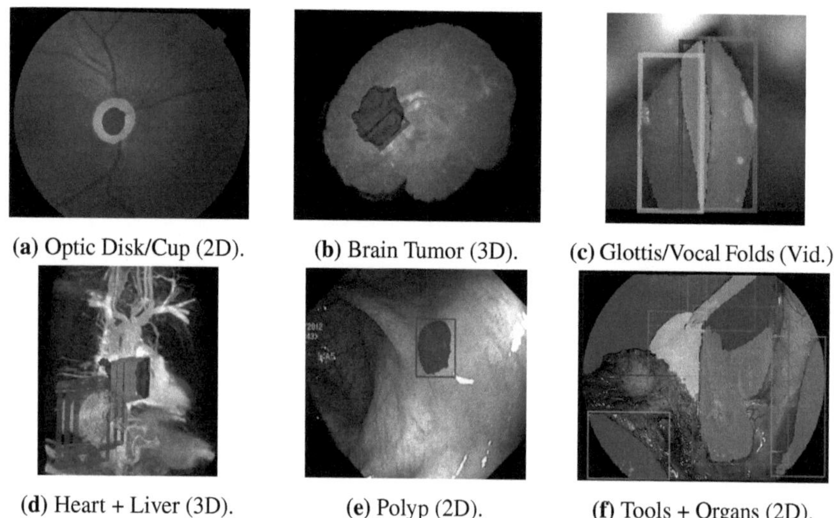

(a) Optic Disk/Cup (2D). **(b)** Brain Tumor (3D). **(c)** Glottis/Vocal Folds (Vid.). **(d)** Heart + Liver (3D). **(e)** Polyp (2D). **(f)** Tools + Organs (2D).

Fig. 5. Examples of supported BOB classes - Predicted bounding boxes + segmentation result with MedSAM2.

4 Discussion

BOB was able to achieve more than 90% of maximum box prompt performance for almost all its supported classes. Even when compared to task-specific models, BOB displays competitive results. A U-Net trained on BAGLS, and its extension BAGLS-RF, reached an mIoU of 0.777 ± 0.003 [22]. In combination with BOB D-FINE-N, we could closely approximate these values with SAM2.1 Tiny at an mIoU of 0.771 ± 0.193, and beat it with SAM2.1-Large at an IoU of 0.794 ± 0.188. The leading model in the Kaggle NeoPolyp competition reached a mean IoU of 0.814 vs. our 0.853. The current FLARE22 leader achieved an mDSC of 0.9373 across the classes supported by BOB, corresponding to an mIoU of 0.8819 vs. our 0.891 (nnInteractive + YOLOv12n). Note that these results are not comparable, since we did not have access to the official competition test split of these datasets, but hint at strong performance across tasks regardless.

For most cases, BOB with the D-FINE-N model produced vastly superior results compared to YOLOv12n (Tab. 1). In the case of 3D prompt generation, though, most notably for the teeth, D-FINE-N produced too many false positives. These quickly add up, as all prompts across the z-slices are accumulated. For these cases, a model with a higher precision and lower recall, like YOLOv12n, or even D-FINE-N with a high confidence threshold, is preferred. For video segmentation of BAGLS, BOB could select the best prompts across the video, and (Med)SAM2 was able to track and segment the object of interest throughout the video, even when it disappeared for a few frames, e.g., the glottis when the vocal folds close. In conclusion, we showed that it is possible to assist the manual prompt generation of segmentation foundation models by chaining them with simple 2D object detection models. Our recommended setup for most tasks consists of BOB D-FINE-N in combination with $\text{MedSAM2}_{\text{latest}}$, as they provide strong performance in most segmentation tasks and use relatively few resources compared to larger models like VISTA3D. nnInteractive is recommended for 3D segmentation tasks where resource constraints are not a problem. Traditional task-bound models, like U-Net, are much more efficient by a noticeable margin, but also require training for each task and typically do not perform instance segmentation. "Foundation models "without box prompts, like VISTA3D, can produce good results for their supported classes, but struggle with unseen objects, whereas the other interactive foundation models showed better zero-shot accuracy [8] and still allow manual box prompt input, even if BOB can't find anything. The combination of BOB and a foundation model also allows semantic segmentation (due to BOB's class prediction) and instance segmentation (due to SAM/MedSAM) at the same time.

Currently, BOB supports 30 classes, which should be extended in the future. A challenge in 3D is that each prompt requires its own propagation, because segmenting multiple prompts at the same time is supported, but has shown insufficient results in our tests. For example, this can cause the segmentation to take very long (>30 prompts for ToothFairy3). Lastly, just like MedSAM2, BOB suffers from the fact that it is also 2D-based and can't utilize all spatial information in multidimensional images, which could be approached in the future by different 2D projections.

References

1. Kirillov A, Mintun E, Ravi N, et al. Segment anything. arXiv: 2304.02643. 2023.
2. Xinyi W, Hongyu K, Peishan W, Li S, Sun Y, Lam SK et al. Proxy Prompt: endowing SAM and SAM 2 with auto-interactive-prompt for medical segmentation. arXiv: 2502.03501. 2025.
3. Wei S, Qiu S, Zhou M, Zhang H, Wang Y, Li Q. Self-prompting driven SAM2 for 3D medical image segmentation. Proc IEEE ICASSP. 2025:1–5.
4. Li C, Khanduri P, Qiang Y, Sultan RI, Chetty I, Zhu D. AutoProSAM: automated prompting SAM for 3D multi-organ segmentation. arXiv: 2308.14936. 2024.
5. Mansoori M, Shahabodini S, Abouei J, Plataniotis KN, Mohammadi A. Self-prompting polyp segmentation in colonoscopy using hybrid Yolo-SAM 2 model. arXiv: 2409.09484. 2024.
6. Lei W, Wei X, Zhang X, Li K, Zhang S. MedLSAM: localize and segment anything model for 3D CT images. arXiv: 2306.14752. 2024.
7. MIC-DKFZ. Napari-sam. https://github.com/MIC-DKFZ/napari-sam. 2025.
8. Lurz D, Neubig L, Kopp M, Kist A. Foundation models in medical image segmentation. Proc BVM. 2026.
9. Ravi N, Gabeur V, Hu YT, Hu R, Ryali C, Ma T et al. SAM 2: segment anything in images and videos. arXiv: 2408.00714. 2024.
10. Ma J, Yang Z, Kim S, Chen B, Baharoon M, Fallahpour A et al. MedSAM2: segment anything in 3D medical images and videos. arXiv preprint: 2504.03600. 2025.
11. Isensee F, Rokuss M, Krämer L, Dinkelacker S, Ravindran A, Stritzke F et al. nnInteractive: redefining 3D promptable segmentation. arXiv: 2503.08373. 2025.
12. He Y, Guo P, Tang Y, Myronenko A, Nath V, Xu Z et al. VISTA3D: a unified segmentation foundation model for 3D medical imaging. arXiv: 2406.05285. 2024.
13. Gómez P, Kist AM, Schlegel P, Berry DA, Chhetri DK, Dürr S et al. BAGLS: a multihospital benchmark for automatic glottis segmentation. Sci Data. 2020;7(1):186.
14. Lucchi A, Li Y, Fua P. Learning for structured prediction using approximate subgradient descent with working sets. Proc IEEE CVPR. 2013:1987–94.
15. An NS, Lan PN, Hang DV, Long DV, Trung TQ, Thuy NT et al. BlazeNeo: blazing fast polyp segmentation and neoplasm detection. IEEE Access. 2022;10:43669–84.
16. Cheng J, Fu B, Ye J, Wang G, Li T, Wang H et al. Interactive medical image segmentation: a benchmark dataset and baseline. arXiv: 2411.12814. 2024.
17. Kuş Z, Aydin M. MedSegBench: a comprehensive benchmark for medical image segmentation in diverse data modalities. Sci Data. 2024;11(1):1283.
18. Bolelli F, Marchesini K, Nistelrooij N van, et al. Segmenting maxillofacial structures in CBCT volume. Proc IEEE/CVF CVPR. 2025:1–10.
19. Bolelli F, Lumetti L, Vinayahalingam S, et al. Segmenting the inferior alveolar canal in CBCTs volumes: the ToothFairy challenge. IEEE Trans Med Imaging. 2024:1–17.
20. Lumetti L, Pipoli V, Bolelli F, et al. Enhancing patch-based learning for the segmentation of the mandibular canal. IEEE Access. 2024:1–12.
21. Antonelli M, Reinke A, Bakas S, et al. The medical segmentation decathlon. Nat Commun. 2022;13(1):4128.
22. Döllinger M, Schraut T, Henrich LA, Chhetri D, Echternach M, Johnson AM et al. Re-training of convolutional neural networks for glottis segmentation in endoscopic high-speed videos. Appl Sci. 2022;12(19):9791.

Abstract: Progressive Growing of Patch Size

Curriculum Learning for Accelerated and Improved Medical Image Segmentation

Stefan M. Fischer[1,2,3,4], Lina Felsner[1,3], Richard Osuala[3,5], Johannes Kiechle[1,2,3,4], Daniel M. Lang[3], Jan C. Peeken[2,6], Julia A. Schnabel[1,3,4,7]

[1]School of Computation, Information and Technology, Technical University Munich
[2]School of Medicine, TUM University Hospital rechts der Isar, Technical University Munich
[3]Institute of Machine Learning in Biomedical Imaging, Helmholtz Munich
[4]Munich Center of Machine Learning (MCML)
[5]Departament de Matemàtiques i Informàtica, Barcelona Artificial Intelligence in Medicine Lab (BCN-AIM), Universitat de Barcelona
[6]Institute of Radiation Medicine, Helmholtz Center Munich
[7]School of Biomedical Engineering and Imaging Sciences, King's College London

stefan.mi.fischer@tum.de

In this work, we extend Progressive Growing of Patch Size, an automatic curriculum learning approach for semantic segmentation, originally introduced at MICCAI2024 [1]. Our approach progressively increases the patch size during model training, resulting in an improved class balance for smaller patch sizes and accelerated convergence of the training process. We evaluate our curriculum approach in two settings: a resource-efficient mode and a performance mode, both regarding Dice score performance and computational costs across 15 diverse and popular 3D medical image segmentation tasks. The resource-efficient mode matches the Dice score performance of the conventional constant patch size sampling baseline with a notable reduction in training time to only 44%. The performance mode improves upon constant patch size segmentation results, achieving a statistically significant relative mean performance gain of 1.28% in Dice Score. Remarkably, across all 15 tasks, our proposed performance mode manages to surpass the constant patch size baseline in Dice Score performance, while simultaneously reducing training time to only 89%. The benefits are particularly pronounced for highly imbalanced tasks such as lesion segmentation tasks. Rigorous experiments demonstrate that our performance mode not only improves mean segmentation performance but also reduces performance variance, yielding more trustworthy model comparison. Furthermore, our findings reveal that the proposed curriculum sampling is not tied to a specific architecture but represents a broadly applicable strategy that consistently boosts performance across diverse segmentation models, including UNet, UNETR, and SwinUNETR. In summary, we show that this simple yet elegant transformation on input data substantially improves both Dice Score performance and training runtime, while being compatible across diverse segmentation backbones.

© Der/die Autor(en), exklusiv lizenziert an
Springer Fachmedien Wiesbaden GmbH, ein Teil von Springer Nature 2026
H. Handels et al. (Hrsg.), *Bildverarbeitung für die Medizin 2026*,
Informatik aktuell, https://doi.org/10.1007/978-3-658-51100-5_53

References

1. Fischer SM, Felsner L, Osuala R, Kiechle J, Lang DM, Peeken JC et al. Progressive growing of patch size: resource-efficient curriculum learning for dense prediction tasks. Proc MICCAI. 2024:510–20.

Abstract: Cross-Modality Supervised Prostate Segmentation on CBCT for Adaptive Radiotherapy

Balint Kovacs [1,2†], Goran Stanic [3,4,5†], Fabian Weykamp[4,6,7,8], Florian Ebert[2], Dimitrios Bounias[1,2], Bouchra Tawk[4,6,7,8], Martin Niklas[3,9], Jakob Liermann[7,8], Oliver Jäkel[3,4,7,8], Klaus H. Maier-Hein[1,8,10], Ralf Floca[1,4‡], Kristina Giske[3,4‡]

[1]German Cancer Research Center (DKFZ) Heidelberg, Division of Medical Image Computing (MIC), Heidelberg, Germany
[2]Medical Faculty Heidelberg, Heidelberg University, Heidelberg, Germany
[3]DKFZ Heidelberg, Division of Medical Physics in Radiation Oncology, Germany
[4]Heidelberg Institute of Radiation Oncology (HIRO), National Center for Radiation Research in Oncology (NCRO), Heidelberg, Germany
[5]Faculty of Physics and Astronomy, University of Heidelberg, Heidelberg, Germany
[6]DKFZ Heidelberg, Clinical Cooperation Unit Radiation Oncology, Germany
[7]Department of Radiation Oncology, Heidelberg Ion-Beam Therapy Center (HIT), Heidelberg University Hospital, Heidelberg, Germany
[8]National Center for Tumor Diseases (NCT), Heidelberg, Germany
[9]DKFZ Heidelberg, Division of Radiology, Germany
[10]Pattern Analysis and Learning Group, Department of Radiation Oncology, Heidelberg University Hospital, Heidelberg, Germany
{balint.kovacs,goran.stanic}@dkfz-heidelberg.de

Accurate organ segmentation is crucial for prostate cancer radiotherapy, but cone-beam computer tomography (CBCT) based models are hindered by low image quality and annotation scarcity. We propose a cross-modality supervision framework where a generative adversarial network translates planning CT (pCT) into synthetic CBCT, enabling segmentation models to train on high-quality pCT-derived annotations while adapting to CBCT characteristics. Additionally, anatomy-aware augmentation enhances robustness to organ deformations. By eliminating the need for manual CBCT annotations, our method enables practical AI-driven segmentation for adaptive radiotherapy, achieving accuracy comparable to pCT-trained models. [1]

References

1. Kovacs B, Stanic G, Weykamp F, Ebert F, Bounias D, Tawk B et al. Cross-modality supervised prostate segmentation on CBCT for adaptive radiotherapy. Proc MICCAI. 2025:121–30.

[†]These authors contributed equally to this work.
[‡]These authors contributed equally to this work.

© Der/die Autor(en), exklusiv lizenziert an Springer Fachmedien Wiesbaden GmbH, ein Teil von Springer Nature 2026
H. Handels et al. (Hrsg.), *Bildverarbeitung für die Medizin 2026*, Informatik aktuell, https://doi.org/10.1007/978-3-658-51100-5_54

Comparative Study of Deep Learning Models for Brain Metastases Autosegmentation

Anqi Wang[1], Florian Putz [2], Yixing Huang [3], Andreas Maier [1]

[1]Pattern Recognition Lab, Friedrich-Alexander-Universität Erlangen-Nürnberg, Germany
[2]Department of Radiation Oncology, University Hospital Erlangen, Germany
[3]Institute of Medical Technology, Peking University Health Science Center, Beijing, China
anqi.wang@fau.de

Abstract. Accurate detection and segmentation of brain metastases (BM) are essential for stereotactic radiosurgery (SRS) planning. This study first systematically compares six loss functions across three representative 3D deep learning models. Results show Dice is a robust baseline, CE improves precision, and Focal has limited effectiveness. While JVSS substantially enhances small-lesion sensitivity, it reduces precision; combined losses achieve the most balanced and robust performance. Furthermore, we propose a novel inference strategy: local overlap fusion for subvolume merging (LOF_SM). By applying axis-wise local weighting in overlapping regions, LOF_SM significantly improves computational efficiency, reducing inference time by approximately 30%, while simultaneously maintaining sensitivity and improving precision over conventional sliding window (SW) methods. These findings underscore the importance of jointly optimizing loss functions and inference strategies to achieve a superior balance between detection performance and computational efficiency, thereby facilitating the clinical application of BM segmentation.

1 Introduction

Brain metastases (BM) are the most common secondary intracranial malignancies in adults [1]. Stereotactic radiosurgery (SRS) has largely replaced whole-brain radiotherapy (WBRT) as the standard treatment, highlighting the need for accurate lesion detection and precise delineation for effective treatment planning [2]. Deep learning has advanced BM segmentation by improving sensitivity and reducing interobserver variability [3]. CNN-based models laid the foundation but remain limited in small-lesion detection and generalization [4]. Transformer-based models have shown improved representational capacity yet still face challenges in detecting tiny lesions and in computational efficiency.

Loss-function design is a key factor. While Dice and cross-entropy (CE) loss are widely used, specialized losses such as Focal [5], and joint volume-level sensitivity-specificity (JVSS) [6] have been proposed to improve small-lesion sensitivity, a systematic, cross-model evaluation of these functions, validated on size-stratified datasets, is notably absent.

© Der/die Autor(en), exklusiv lizenziert an
Springer Fachmedien Wiesbaden GmbH, ein Teil von Springer Nature 2026
H. Handels et al. (Hrsg.), *Bildverarbeitung für die Medizin 2026*,
Informatik aktuell, https://doi.org/10.1007/978-3-658-51100-5_55

Furthermore, the inference stage presents a significant computational bottleneck. Conventional sliding window (SW) inference is computationally expensive and memory-intensive due to global 3D weighting for overlaps. Recent studies, such as end-to-end inference [7], underscore the importance of inference strategies for both accuracy and efficiency.

To address these challenges, we compare six loss functions – Dice, CE, Focal, JVSS, and two combined losses (Dice+CE and Dice+Focal) – across three representative 3D networks (Swin UNETR, DeepMedic, and nnU-Net) on two size-stratified test sets (Test_Tiny and Test_Big). We also propose the local overlap fusion for subvolume merging (LOF_SM) strategy, which replaces the computationally expensive global 3D weighting with an efficient, axis-wise local fusion mechanism. This approach achieves superior efficiency and comparable or better accuracy than conventional SW inference.

2 Materials and methods

2.1 Dataset

We used a clinical BM MRI dataset from the University of California, San Francisco (UCSF) [8], comprising 219 patients and 3,449 annotated lesions. Only the T1-weighted contrast-enhanced (T1CE) sequence was utilized. Ground truth voxel-wise annotations were generated in ITK-SNAP by two board-certified neuroradiologists or fellows, based on consensus and reference to final radiology reports. The dataset was divided by patient into training (102 cases), validation (51 cases), and test (66 cases). To investigate the influence of lesion size on segmentation performance, the test set was further stratified according to the maximum lesion volume per patient: Test_Tiny ($< 2.65\,\text{cm}^3$) and Test_Big ($\geq 2.65\,\text{cm}^3$).

2.2 Networks and loss functions

We employed three representative 3D segmentation networks: the transformer-based encoder-decoder Swin UNETR [9], the dual-pathway multi-scale 3D CNN DeepMedic [10], and the self-configuring U-Net baseline nnU-Net [11]. To examine the impact of loss-function design on BM segmentation, we evaluated six widely used losses: Dice, CE, Focal [5] (emphasizes hard examples for small-lesion detection), JVSS [6] (introduces a lesion-volume-weighted term that penalizes false-negative and false-positive lesions, which is highly relevant for small metastases) and their combinations (Dice+CE, Dice+Focal).

2.3 Local overlap fusion for subvolume merging

Patch-wise inference is widely used to overcome GPU memory limits in 3D medical image segmentation, however conventional SW inference introduces redundant computations and often blends predictions suboptimally in overlapping regions. The recently proposed SM strategy [12] which was originally applied to MRI-to-CT conversion using Swin UNETR, addresses this by performing axis-wise sequential fusion instead of applying a full 3D weight field, thereby improving efficiency and reducing boundary artifacts.

Building on the SM concept, we propose LOF_SM, validated here on the Swin UNETR for BM segmentation. Our refinement minimizes redundant multiply-accumulate operations by restricting weighted computation only to the narrow overlap bands along each fusion axis, while directly concatenating the non-overlapping regions. The fusion is performed using a 1D weighting vector that is broadcast across the remaining two dimensions. This mechanism substantially accelerates inference without compromising segmentation accuracy.

We investigate the effectiveness of three specific weighting schemes within the LOF_SM framework: (i) polynomial (LOF_SM_P), following the original SM formulation; (ii) constant averaging (LOF_SM_C); and (iii) Gaussian weighting (LOF_SM_G) for smooth blending. In our BM segmentation experiments, LOF_SM achieved significantly improved inference efficiency and a crucial balance of reduced false positives with maintained or enhanced sensitivity.

2.4 Experimental setup

Models were implemented using PyTorch, MONAI (for Swin UNETR), and public codebases (for DeepMedic and nnU-Net). Training proceeded for 300 epochs on NVIDIA A100/RTX8000 GPUs, selecting the best validation Dice checkpoint. MRI volumes were skull-stripped, bias-corrected, Z-score normalized, and resampled to $240\times240\times155$ voxels at 1 mm^3 isotropic resolution. Data augmentation included random flips and intensity scaling.

2.4.1 Training.

2.4.1 Training. Swin UNETR used 64^3 patches and Adam (lr 1×10^{-5}, wd 1×10^{-6}). DeepMedic used dual-pathway patches of $25^3/19^3$ voxels, with Adam (lr 1×10^{-3}, wd 1×10^{-4}). nnU-Net was trained on full-resolution volumes with Adam (lr 1×10^{-3}, wd 1×10^{-4}). All models employed cosine annealing for learning rate scheduling.

2.4.2 Inference. Inference comparisons employed Swin UNETR with 128^3 patches and 60% overlap. Baseline SW inference used MONAI's `constant` and `gaussian` modes. The proposed LOF_SM adopted the same patch size and overlap ratio.

2.4.3 Evaluation. Segmentation performance was assessed at the lesion-wise level. A predicted region was counted as a true positive if it overlapped a ground-truth lesion by at least one voxel. Metrics included lesion-wise sensitivity, precision, Dice score, and the mean numbers of false-negative and false-positive lesions per patient.

Tab. 1. Comparative Performance of Loss Functions (Test_Tiny: T, Test_Big: B).

Model	Loss	Sens (T)	Sens (B)	Prec (T)	Prec (B)	Dice (T)	Dice (B)
	Dice	0.68	0.69	0.69	0.61	0.66	0.72
	Dice+CE	0.71	0.70	0.76	0.69	0.63	0.75
Swin UNETR	CE	0.47	0.51	0.80	0.76	0.54	0.77
	Dice+Focal	0.66	0.65	0.75	0.63	0.65	0.76
	Focal	0.50	0.54	0.61	0.38	0.60	0.70
	JVSS_$\alpha = 0.5$	0.48	0.53	0.41	0.18	0.52	0.68
	JVSS_$\alpha = 0.95$	0.69	0.71	0.01	0.01	0.39	0.48
	Dice	0.63	0.81	0.29	0.23	0.58	0.67
	Dice+CE	0.77	0.82	0.43	0.33	0.57	0.65
DeepMedic	CE	0.79	0.84	0.42	0.33	0.55	0.64
	Dice+Focal	0.81	0.85	0.34	0.26	0.56	0.65
	Focal	0.53	0.64	0.58	0.39	0.49	0.56
	JVSS_$\alpha = 0.5$	0.80	0.84	0.59	0.55	0.57	0.66
	JVSS_$\alpha = 0.95$	0.90	0.93	0.16	0.12	0.56	0.66
	Dice	0.86	0.86	0.82	0.90	0.68	0.75
	Dice+CE	0.86	0.85	0.81	0.94	0.68	0.75
nnU-Net	CE	0.56	0.70	0.86	0.89	0.60	0.76
	Dice+Focal	0.87	0.86	0.83	0.91	0.68	0.75
	Focal	0.43	0.66	0.76	0.85	0.57	0.70
	JVSS_$\alpha = 0.5$	0.82	0.80	0.32	0.47	0.61	0.66
	JVSS_$\alpha = 0.95$	0.87	0.86	0.26	0.36	0.60	0.66

3 Results

3.1 Impact of loss functions on segmentation performance

As shown in Tab. 1, the Dice loss provided stable overall performance (Dice: 0.60–0.75), achieving a relatively balanced sensitivity-precision trade-off. In contrast, the CE loss skewed towards higher precision, often at the cost of sensitivity, while the Focal loss performed poorly, likely due to overemphasizing hard examples, which compromised large-lesion detection (e.g., a missed large lesion in Fig. 1e). The JVSS loss was designed to emphasize recall, showing a strong trade-off. With $\alpha = 0.5$, it boosted DeepMedic's sensitivity (0.80 (T), 0.84 (B)), but significantly reduced precision (0.59/0.55). Increasing α to 0.95 further maximized small-lesion sensitivity (e.g., DeepMedic to 0.90 (T)), but caused a drastic drop in precision across all models, often resulting in visible over-segmentation of small lesions (Fig. 2d).

The combined losses generally achieved more balanced performance. Dice+CE prioritized precision, yielding high values for large lesions (e.g., nnU-Net Precision: 0.94 (B)). Conversely, Dice+Focal significantly enhanced the detection of small lesions (e.g., nnU-Net Sensitivity: 0.87 (T); DeepMedic Sensitivity: 0.81 (T)).

Tab. 2. Inference Strategy Metrics: Sens, Prec, Errors, and inference time per patient.

Inference	Datasets	Sens ↑	Prec↑	FP per patient↓	FN per patient↓	Time(s)↓
SW_constant	Test_Tiny	0.52	0.61	2.25	3.27	1.27
	Test_Big	0.59	0.66	1.72	2.29	1.01
SW_gaussian	Test_Tiny	0.52	0.46	4.43	3.42	1.18
	Test_Big	0.60	0.51	3.18	2.16	1.01
LOF_SM_P	Test_Tiny	0.53	0.58	2.78	3.26	**0.89**
	Test_Big	0.61	0.62	2.12	2.05	**0.81**
LOF_SM_C	Test_Tiny	0.52	0.64	**2.08**	3.32	0.92
	Test_Big	0.62	**0.72**	1.61	**2.02**	**0.81**
LOF_SM_G	Test_Tiny	0.52	**0.65**	2.09	3.32	0.95
	Test_Big	0.62	0.68	**1.58**	2.06	**0.81**

3.2 Evaluation of the LOF_SM inference strategy

The LOF_SM family consistently outperformed baseline SW inference across both size-stratified test sets (Test_Tiny and Test_Big) in terms of efficiency and detection accuracy (Tab. 2). On Test_Tiny, LOF_SM_P demonstrated superior efficiency, reducing inference time from 1.27 s to 0.89 s (a nearly 30% gain), while slightly improving lesion-wise sensitivity (0.53 vs. 0.52 for SW). On Test_Big, the LOF_SM variants showed clear advantages in accuracy: both LOF_SM_C and LOF_SM_G increased sensitivity to 0.62. LOF_SM_C achieved the highest precision (0.72), whereas LOF_SM_G delivered the lowest false positives per patient (1.58), indicating superior false positive control.

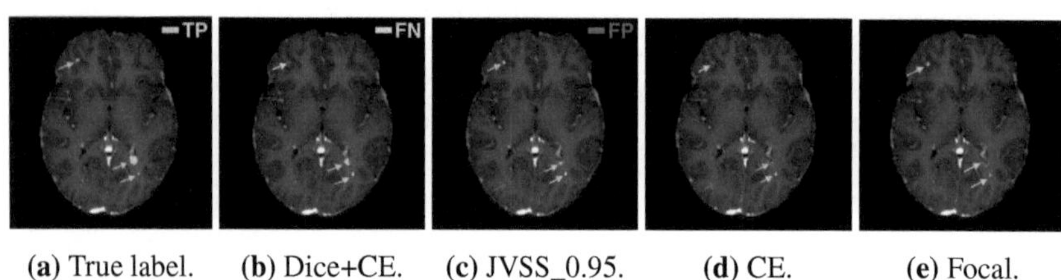

(a) True label. **(b)** Dice+CE. **(c)** JVSS_0.95. **(d)** CE. **(e)** Focal.

Fig. 1. Qualitative comparison of lesion detection performance for different loss functions.

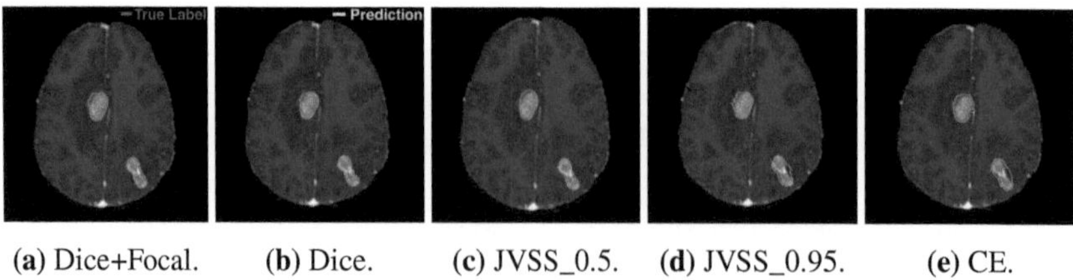

(a) Dice+Focal. **(b)** Dice. **(c)** JVSS_0.5. **(d)** JVSS_0.95. **(e)** CE.

Fig. 2. Qualitative comparison of contouring performance for different loss functions.

4 Discussion

This study identifies loss function design and inference strategy as two key factors for optimizing automated BM segmentation. Among the loss functions, Dice proved to be a robust baseline. CE excelled at precision and false-positive control, while Focal showed limited competitiveness in 3D BM segmentation. Although JVSS notably improved small-lesion sensitivity, the resulting marked drop in precision suggests that prioritizing recall excessively may compromise overall segmentation quality. The combined losses (Dice+CE and Dice+Focal) were more robust overall, but their varied tendencies – prioritizing large-lesion precision vs. small-lesion detection – underscore the need for a choice guided by specific clinical priorities.

Crucially, the inference strategy proved equally critical. The proposed LOF_SM consistently outperformed the conventional SW approach in both efficiency and detection. By employing axis-wise local overlap weighting, LOF_SM reduced redundant computation, achieving an inference time reduction of nearly 30%, while simultaneously improving precision and maintaining sensitivity.

In summary, achieving optimal BM segmentation requires the joint optimization of both training (loss functions) and deployment (inference strategies) to balance detection performance with computational efficiency. Future work will focus on validating LOF_SM on larger multi-center datasets and integrating it into clinical workflows to assess its practical utility.

References

1. Nayak L, Lee EQ, Wen PY. Epidemiology of brain metastases. Curr Oncol Rep. 2012.
2. Gondi V, Bauman G, Bradfield L, Burri SH, Cabrera AR, Cunningham DA et al. Radiation therapy for brain metastases: an ASTRO clinical practice guideline. Pract Radiat Oncol. 2022.
3. Cho SJ, Sunwoo L, Baik SH, Bae YJ, Choi BS, Kim JH. Brain metastasis detection using machine learning: a systematic review and meta-analysis. Neuro Oncol. 2020.
4. Huang Y, Khodabakhshi Z, Gomaa A, Schmidt M, Fietkau R, Guckenberger M et al. Multicenter privacy-preserving model training for deep learning brain metastases autosegmentation. Radiother Oncol. 2024.
5. Lin TY, Goyal P, Girshick R, He K, Dollár P. Focal loss for dense object detection. Proc IEEE ICCV. 2017.
6. Huang Y, Bert C, Sommer P, Frey B, Gaipl U, Distel LV et al. Deep learning for brain metastasis detection and segmentation in longitudinal MRI data. Med Phys. 2022.
7. Jeon YS, Yang H, Fu H, Kway Y, Feng M. No more sliding window: efficient 3D medical image segmentation with differentiable top-k patch sampling. Proc MICCAI. 2025.
8. Rudie JD, Saluja R, Weiss DA, Nedelec P, Calabrese E, Colby JB et al. The University of California San Francisco brain metastases stereotactic radiosurgery (UCSF-BMSR) MRI dataset. Radiol Artif Intell. 2024.
9. Hatamizadeh A, Nath V, Tang Y, Yang D, Roth HR, Xu D. Swin UNETR: swin transformers for semantic segmentation of brain tumors in MRI images. Proc MICCAI. 2022.
10. Kamnitsas K, Ledig C, Newcombe VFJ, Simpson JP, Kane AD, Menon DK et al. Efficient multi-scale 3D CNN with fully connected CRF for accurate brain lesion segmentation. Med Image Anal. 2017.

11. Isensee F, Jaeger PF, Kohl SA, Petersen J, Maier-Hein KH. nnU-net: a self-configuring method for deep learning-based biomedical image segmentation. Nat Methods. 2021;18(2):203–11.
12. Fan F, Qiu J, Huang Y, Maier A. Enhancing cross-modality synthesis: subvolume merging for MRI-to-CT conversion. arXiv: 2409.05982. 2024.

Applying Active Learning to Nipple Segmentation in Breast MRI

Kai Geissler[1], Markus Wenzel[1,2], Susanne Diekmann[1], Robert Grimm[3], Heinrich von Busch[4], Torbjörn Vik[1], Hans Meine[1]

[1]Fraunhofer Institute for Digital Medicine MEVIS
[2]Constructor University, Bremen, Germany
[3]Research and Clinical Translation, Magnetic Resonance, Siemens Healthineers AG, Erlangen, Germany
[4]Digital & Automation, Siemens Healthineers AG, Forchheim, Germany
kai.geissler@mevis.fraunhofer.de

Abstract. Active learning seeks to quickly improve model performance while reducing expert annotation effort, which is especially valuable in medical imaging. We study whether an uncertainty-based active learning scheme scales to a large, heterogeneous data collection and what performance is achievable with a limited annotation budget for nipple segmentation in breast magnetic resonance imaging – a precursor task to report lesion localization that has seen little automation so far. We prospectively evaluated an iterative active learning pipeline on 3,762 examinations from nine institutions / datasets, combining a 3D U-Net with Monte Carlo dropout-based image-wise uncertainty and a simple diversity-aware selection strategy. For almost all institutions, the nipple center-of-gravity error and Dice score improve substantially during the first three iterations, before largely plateauing, indicating diminishing returns. Uncertainty decreases in tandem with performance improvements, making it a practical proxy to guide annotation stopping. Persistent challenges involve absent or ambiguous nipples and institution-specific artifacts. Our results demonstrate that uncertainty-driven active learning can efficiently improve nipple segmentation on multi-center MRI with limited annotations. They highlight the need to detect nipple presence before segmentation and show that even if a model improves on data from most institutions when adding more data to the training, it can still achieve worse results in other institutions.

1 Introduction

Active learning is a machine learning paradigm that aims to reduce the necessary annotation effort by selecting the most informative samples from an unannotated data pool for annotation. This is beneficial in medical imaging, where manual annotations are costly and time-consuming to create because medical experts are required. For instance, segmenting the nipple region in breast magnetic resonance imaging (MRI) is one such challenging task due to the variability in nipple appearance and

© Der/die Autor(en), exklusiv lizenziert an
Springer Fachmedien Wiesbaden GmbH, ein Teil von Springer Nature 2026
H. Handels et al. (Hrsg.), *Bildverarbeitung für die Medizin 2026*,
Informatik aktuell, https://doi.org/10.1007/978-3-658-51100-5_56

occasionally ambiguous anatomy. Nipple localization is relevant because breast lesions are usually described with an o'clock position, using the nipple location as reference. As there is only little previous work on precise and fully automatic nipple detection/segmentation [1–4], we selected this task for our study.

Most active learning studies in the field of medical image analysis use small public datasets with only a few hundred annotated cases from a limited number of clinical institutions [5, 6]. This leaves the question unanswered how well these approaches extend to larger, multi-centric data collections with thousands of cases with varying patient cohorts and image appearance.

In this study, we applied an uncertainty-based active learning scheme to nipple segmentation in breast MRI using a large data collection of 3,762 examinations originating from eight different clinical institutions and one public dataset. Our experiments focused on practical aspects: (i) does an uncertainty-based active learning scheme work well on a large, diverse data collection, (ii) what model performance is achieved with a limited annotation budget, and (iii) how do time required for annotation, model training, and uncertainty estimation influence the annotation process?

2 Materials and methods

We used a multi-centric data collection of T1-weighted MR images of the female breast collected from 3,436 patients in more than nine clinical institutions in Europe, North America, and Asia. The data covers a diverse set of imaging characteristics, such as different fields of view, resolutions, voxel sizes, fat suppression (FS) settings, and MR scanners. The MR scanners include models from Siemens Healthineers, GE HealthCare and Philips. An overview of the most important image characteristics and the number of images and masks for all institutions is shown in Tab. 1. The dataset identified with "ACRIN" is a subset of the ACRIN-6698 dataset [7].

A breast segmentation model from previous work [8] was used to crop images to a region of interest of the breast, reducing the data that needs to be processed by the nipple segmentation model. The cropped images were resampled to $2 \times 2 \times 2\,\mathrm{mm}^3$ and their 0th and 99.5^{th} percentiles are normalized to 0 and 1, respectively.

For nipple segmentation, we used a 3D U-Net with 5 levels and 12 base filters. We used an AdamW optimizer, a batch size of 2 and spatial dropout with a rate of 0.2 on each level – except for the layer acting on input resolution in the encoder and the decoder part of the U-Net. The learning rate was 0.001 with a cosine annealing learning rate scheduler. Batch normalization was employed, and the model was trained for 100,000 iterations. Those hyperparameters settings were manually tuned on the initial data pool to find a proper trade-off between inference time and segmentation quality. For data augmentation, we used the batch generators library.

To compute image-wise uncertainties, Monte Carlo dropout [9] was employed and mean pairwise Dice [10] was used to calculate uncertainty scores for each image from 10 Monte Carlo dropout samples. In Monte Carlo dropout, several inference passes of the same trained model are performed, using a different random configuration of dropout layers for each pass with a specified dropout rate. We used the same dropout rate as during training in our experiments. Mean pairwise Dice is

Tab. 1. Data overview (*: Mean (std. dev.), SHS: Siemens Healthineers, PH: Philips).

	ACRIN	Austria I	Germany I	Germany II	India I
Studies (patients)	378 (378)	999 (990)	45 (45)	1586 (1289)	37 (37)
Nipple Masks (patients)	30 (30)	50 (50)	44 (44)	53 (53)	30 (30)
Age* [years]	n/a	52.0 (13.1)	47.7 (14.1)	55.8 (10.6)	44.8 (13.2)
Fat Suppression	Yes	No	No	No	Yes
Voxel Size (in-plane)* [mm]	0.67 (0.07)	0.44 (0.0)	0.87 (0.08)	0.75 (0.03)	0.75 (0.06)
Slice Thickness* [mm]	1.79 (0.48)	1.8 (0.02)	1.5 (0.0)	2.38 (0.24)	1.45 (0.13)
Resolution (in-plane)*	506 (41)	896 (0)	430 (28)	512 (10)	436 (31)
Number of Slices*	115 (34)	112 (3)	116 (4)	46 (0)	116 (11)
Field Strength [T]	1.5,3	3	1.5,3	1.5	1.5,3
Manufacturer	GE,PH,SHS	SHS	SHS	GE,SHS	SHS
	Japan I	Japan II	Poland I	Switzerland I	
Studies (patients)	306 (304)	199 (199)	60 (60)	161 (134)	
Nipple Masks (patients)	49 (49)	30 (30)	50 (50)	30 (29)	
Age* [years]	53.9 (12.6)	59.0 (13.6)	49.3 (10.8)	46.7 (11.2)	
Fat Suppression	Yes	Yes	Yes	Yes / No	
Voxel Size (in-plane)* [mm]	0.8 (0.12)	0.89 (0.07)	1.02 (0.01)	0.88 (0.06)	
Slice Thickness* [mm]	1.05 (0.38)	1.0 (0.03)	1.2 (0.0)	1.08 (0.26)	
Resolution (in-plane)*	408 (127)	373 (23)	352 (0)	414 (28)	
Number of Slices*	188 (31)	147 (7)	160 (3)	164 (43)	
Field Strength [T]	1.5,3	1.5,3	1.5	1.5,3	
Manufacturer	GE,PH,SHS	SHS	SHS	SHS	

used to derive an uncertainty score from those samples by computing the pairwise Dice coefficients between all the samples and taking the mean of those coefficients.

For training an initial model, 20 cases each from Austria I, Germany I, Germany II, Japan I, and Poland I were annotated by a radiological technologist. Within every active learning iteration, uncertainties and segmentation proposals were computed for all unannotated cases based on the current model. From these, further cases were selected for annotation, and their segmentation masks were corrected by a research scientist and added to the training data used for subsequent iterations.

For the first active learning iteration, the 5 most uncertain cases for each institution were selected. As these were mostly extreme outliers, the strategy was switched for the following iterations. Therefore, from iteration 2 on, 5 cases from each available institution were selected based on model uncertainty using the stochastic batches strategy [5]. This strategy balances model uncertainty and data diversity by sampling random batches of images and selecting the batch where the summed uncertainty is highest. We set the number of batches to sample equal to the cases per institution.

The data split was performed as follows. To grow all of training, validation, and test sets, after each annotation round the newly selected and annotated cases are split 60-20-20 into the three groups. The evaluations shown in the results are done using the final, complete test set, to ensure comparability between active learning rounds.

The model training and inference was performed on a GPU cluster using either NVIDIA RTX A5000 or 2080 Ti graphics cards, depending on the cluster node.

3 Results

The error of predicting the nipple center of gravity from the segmentation masks is shown in Fig. 1. For most institutions, the error reduces until iteration 3 and then saturates. For Austria I, the error tends to increase over time. Upon inspection of the data from this institution, it appeared that it has many breast images after mastectomy or reconstructive surgery, where the nipples are barely visible or missing completely. For Germany I, India I, Japan I, Japan II, Poland I and Switzerland I the final centerpoint error is on the order of 1–3 mm, while for ACRIN, Austria I and Germany II the medians are all above 5 mm. These contain several cases where atypical breast anatomy, bias fields, or the deformation from the breast coil make it difficult to properly delineate the nipple position.

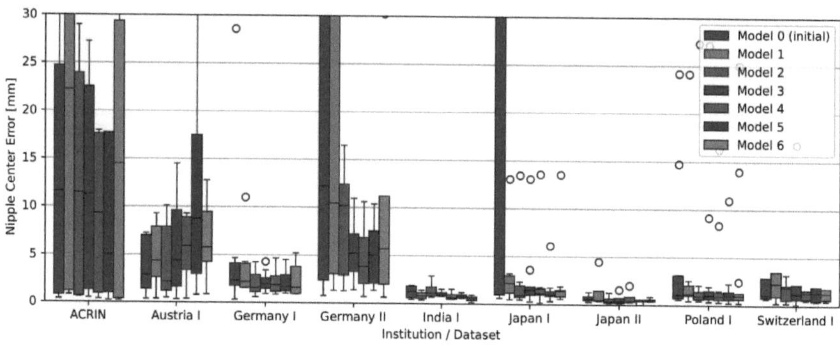

Fig. 1. Nipple center of gravity error on test data per institution / dataset over several annotation rounds. The center of gravity is computed for each breast side separately.

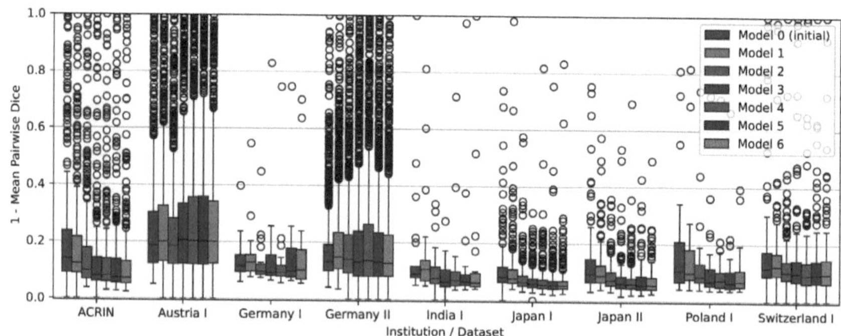

Fig. 2. Uncertainty distribution per institution / dataset over several annotation rounds. Shown are only test, validation and unannotated cases (i.e. cases used for any model training are excluded). For most institutions the uncertainty reduces until model 4 and then saturates, while for Austria I and Germany II there is no trend visible.

The results for the image-wise Dice score per institution provide essentially the same picture as the centerpoint error and are thus omitted here. The mean (stdandard deviation) Dice score of the final model (model 6) over the whole test set is 0.60 (0.27).

Fig. 2 displays the development of uncertainty for validation, test, and unannotated cases over active learning rounds. The uncertainty appears to be negatively correlated with the segmentation performance, being lower for well-performing institutions and higher for institutions which perform badly. It also reduces over time for institutions on which the model improves (Germany I, India I, Japan I and II, Poland I, Switzerland I) and stays roughly constant for the institutions where we do not observe proper model improvement, like Austria I. This indicates that the model uncertainty can serve as surrogate to judge how well the model already performs and if it still improves – without needing explicit test data. The Pearson correlation coefficient between the Dice score (performance) and mean pairwise Dice (uncertainty) on the test data is 0.76 when using data from all seven trained models (508 observations in total). Fig. 3 shows the correlation plot.

Model training took 7–12 hours, depending on the hardware on which the training was performed. The uncertainty and segmentation mask proposal computation of the unannotated data took 7–24 hours per active learning iteration, being executed on 3 GPUs in parallel. The annotation of data in each iteration took about 8–10 hours.

4 Discussion

Our results suggest that uncertainty-based active learning can be used to efficiently annotate data for nipple segmentation on a large, heterogeneous, multi-center breast

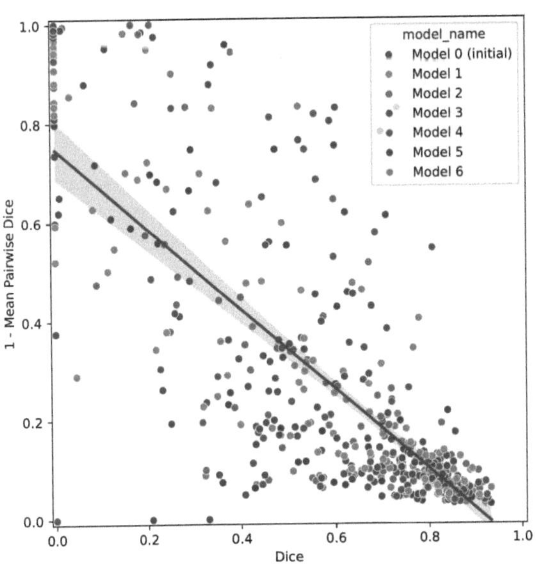

Fig. 3. Correlation between nipple segmentation Dice (segmentation quality) and 1 − mean pairwise Dice (uncertainty). The gray line is the linear regression line between the two variables. The gray, shaded area shows the 95% confidence interval of the regression line (computed via bootstrapping). It is visible that segmentation quality and uncertainty are inversely correlated.

MRI collection, but with clear signs of diminishing returns. Across most institutions, both the nipple center-of-gravity error and the Dice score improved in the first two to three iterations and then largely saturated, indicating that the model quickly benefits from a modest number of targeted annotations and that subsequent rounds yield smaller gains relative to the added effort. The switch from selecting the most uncertain cases per institution to the stochastic batches strategy was important: initial rounds over-emphasized extreme outliers, while later rounds balanced uncertainty and diversity, leading to more stable learning and broader generalization across cohorts. Importantly, the observed negative correlation between uncertainty and performance and the reduction of uncertainty on improving institutions support the practical use of uncertainty as a proxy for progress, potentially guiding when to stop annotating without relying on extensive, fixed test sets.

At the same time, several limitations temper these findings and point to avenues for improvement. First, data heterogeneity contributed to institution-specific performance variability, with Austria I and parts of ACRIN and Germany II showing persistently higher errors, often due to missing nipples, atypical anatomy, or coil-related deformation. This underscores the need for explicit handling of absent nipples (e.g., a pre-classifier for nipple presence) and for domain adaptation and artifact mitigation (bias-field correction, harmonization). Second, Monte Carlo dropout is computationally demanding, and its uncertainty calibration can be imperfect. En-

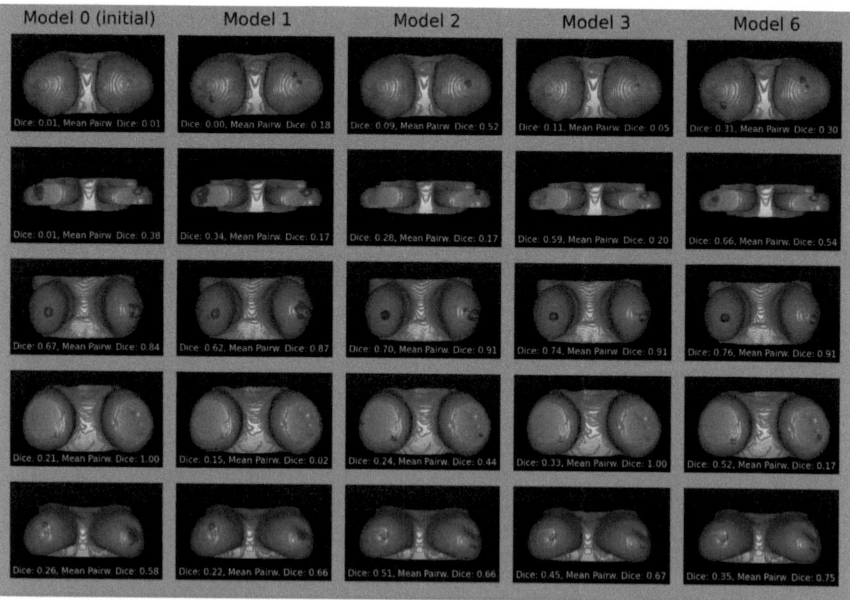

Fig. 4. 3D rendering of breast mask together with manual nipple mask (green) and automatically segmented nipple mask (blue) for the first four and the last active learning iteration(s). Shown is the case for each of five institutions / dataset that had the highest improvement in segmentation quality with respect to their Dice scores.

sembles, heteroscedastic losses, or evidential approaches could yield more reliable and efficient uncertainty estimates. Finally, annotation quality and consistency can vary between annotators, and evaluation metrics (Dice and center error) do not capture clinical acceptability or workflow impact; incorporating point-based annotations, uncertainty-aware correction interfaces, and task-relevant clinical endpoints would provide a more comprehensive assessment of utility and cost.

In summary, this study demonstrates the feasibility and practical benefit of uncertainty-based active learning for nipple segmentation in multi-centric breast MRI, achieving center-of-gravity errors on the order of 1–3 mm for most cohorts with a limited annotation budget and offering an uncertainty signal that can guide annotation stopping. The performance plateau after a few rounds highlights a pragmatic balance between annotation effort and achievable accuracy, while persistent

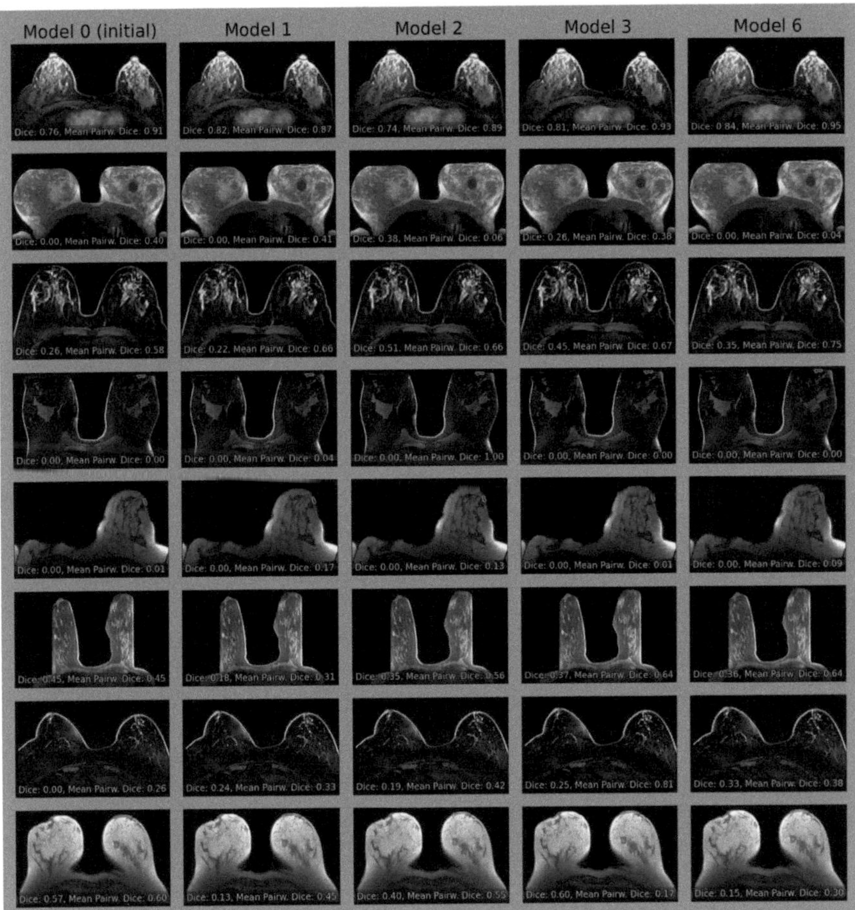

Fig. 5. Slices of worst performing cases for eight different institutions / datasets, showing manual segmentation contours (green) and automatic segmentation contours (blue).

challenges on certain institutions emphasize the importance of handling absent nipples, mitigating artifacts, and adapting to domain shifts. Addressing these points might strengthen generalization, further reduce annotation burden, and support robust deployment of active learning-driven segmentation in clinical practice.

Acknowledgement. We thank our clinical partners that provided data for the study: Dieter Szolar (Diagnostikum Graz, Austria), Sabine Ohlmeyer (Universitätsklinikum Erlangen, Germany), Edyta Szurowska (Medical University of Gdansk, Poland), Uwe Fischer (Diagnostic Breast Center Göttingen, Germany), Nachiko Uchiyama (Nippon Medical School Hospital, Tokyo, Japan), Kazuki Oyama (Shinshu University School of Medicine, Matsumoto, Japan), Noemi Schmidt (University Hospital Basel, Switzerland) and Pratiksha Yadav (Dr. D. Y. Patil Hospital, Pune, India).

References

1. Zhang J, Saha A, Zhu Z, Mazurowski MA. Hierarchical convolutional neural networks for segmentation of breast tumors in MRI with application to radiogenomics. IEEE Trans Med Imaging. 2018;38(2):435–47.
2. Giannini V, Bianchi V, Carabalona S, Mazzetti S, Maggiorotto F, Kubatzki F et al. MRI to predict nipple-areola complex (NAC) involvement: an automatic method to compute the 3D distance between the NAC and tumor. J Surg Oncol. 2017;116(8):1069–78.
3. D'Alonzo M, Martincich L, Fenoglio A, Giannini V, Cellini L, Liberale V et al. Nipple-sparing mastectomy: external validation of a three-dimensional automated method to predict nipple occult tumour involvement on preoperative breast MRI. Eur Radiol Exp. 2019;3(1):31.
4. Gwo CY, Gwo A, Wei CH, Huang PJ. Identification of breast contour for nipple segmentation in breast magnetic resonance images. Med Phys Mex Symp Med Phys. 2014;41(2):022304.
5. Gaillochet M, Desrosiers C, Lombaert H. Active learning for medical image segmentation with stochastic batches. Med Image Anal. 2023;90:102958.
6. Nath V, Yang D, Landman BA, Xu D, Roth HR. Diminishing uncertainty within the training pool: active learning for medical image segmentation. IEEE Trans Med Imaging. 2020;40(10):2534–47.
7. Newitt DC, Partridge S, Zhang Z, Gibbs J, Chenevert T, Rosen M et al. ACRIN 6698/I-SPY2 breast DWI. Cancer Imaging Arch. 2021.
8. Geißler K, Wenzel M, Grimm R, von Busch H, Szolar D, Ohlmeyer S et al. Multi-site segmentation of breast and fibroglandular tissue in MRI with a focus on clinical practicality. Proc SPIE MI IP. 2025;13406:134061R.
9. Gal Y, Ghahramani Z. Dropout as a bayesian approximation: representing model uncertainty in deep learning. Proc ICML. 2016:1050–9.
10. Roy AG, Conjeti S, Navab N, Wachinger C. Inherent brain segmentation quality control from fully convnet Monte Carlo sampling. Proc MICCAI. 2018:664–72.

Hybrid Vessel Wall Segmentation for Assisted Annotation in CT Angiography

Jacopo Bracci [1,2], Alexander Katzmann [2], Leonhard Rist [2], Linda Vorberg [1,2], Michael Sühling[2], Andreas Maier [1]

[1]Pattern Recognition Lab, Friedrich-Alexander-Universität, Erlangen-Nürnberg, Germany
[2]Computed Tomography, Siemens Healthineers AG, Forchheim, Germany
jacopo.bracci@fau.de

Abstract. Cardiovascular diseases are the leading cause of death worldwide, responsible for over 19.8 million deaths annually. Accurate delineation of the vessel lumen and wall is essential for quantifying vascular health, diagnosing disease, and guiding treatment. However, manual annotation, the clinical gold standard, remains time consuming, inconsistent, and prone to human bias, limiting reproducibility and comparability across studies. To address this, we present a fully automatic pipeline designed to assist and standardize vessel annotation. A multi-purpose segmentation network first provides an estimate of the outer vessel boundary, which is then refined through a gradient based algorithm that delineates the inner lumen contour. On a clinically annotated test set of $n = 46$ slices, the method achieved a Mean Absolute Error of 0.197 ± 0.109 mm for the inner lumen and 0.284 ± 0.237 mm for the outer wall. Only 12.16 % of the inner and 19.97 % of the outer contour lines required manual adjustment. This demonstrates the potential of the proposed approach to substantially reduce annotation effort and improve standardization for quantitative vascular analysis.

1 Introduction

Cardiovascular diseases (CVDs) are the leading mortality cause worldwide, responsible for about 32 % of all deaths ($\approx$ 19.8 million annually) [1]. Accurate vessel assessment is crucial for diagnosis, treatment, and prevention. Computed tomography angiography (CTA) allows visualization of the vessel lumen and wall for quantitative measures such as diameter, wall thickness, and plaque burden.

Manual annotation is the clinical standard but remains slow, subjective, and inconsistent, limiting reproducibility and reliable reference generation. Automatic approaches, including unsupervised vesselness or gradient based algorithms [2, 3] and deep learning models [4, 5], have been explored.

In this work, we combine the strengths of both paradigms: a pretrained deep learning network provides an estimate of the outer vessel contour, and an analytical gradient based algorithm estimates the inner lumen boundary. This hybrid design

© Der/die Autor(en), exklusiv lizenziert an
Springer Fachmedien Wiesbaden GmbH, ein Teil von Springer Nature 2026
H. Handels et al. (Hrsg.), *Bildverarbeitung für die Medizin 2026*,
Informatik aktuell, https://doi.org/10.1007/978-3-658-51100-5_57

leverages learned shape priors from deep learning and edge detection to produce consistent and anatomically meaningful vessel annotations with minimal manual correction.

2 Materials and methods

The proposed pipeline consists of two steps: first, a pretrained segmentation network proposes a segmentation mask for the outer contour (*Deep Learning Module*, Fig. 1), second a gradient based method searches through a Region of Interest (ROI) within the proposed outer contour to yield the inner contour (*Analytical Module*, Fig. 2).

2.1 Dataset

A dataset of 3D CT scans acquired at a single site with a NAEOTOM Alpha Photon Counting scanner (Siemens Healthineers AG, Forchheim, Germany) was available for this study. Using manually annotated vessel centerlines, we sampled axial cross-sectional slices (Fig. 1a) along each centerline every 0.5 mm. No noticeable step artifact was introduced in the used slices. Each slice spans $60 \times 60\,\text{mm}^2$ at $128 \times 128\,\text{px}^2$ (isotropic spacing of ≈ 0.47 mm).

For this initial study, an evaluation set of $n = 46$ randomly selected slices was used. Slices were pre-windowed following [6], using the centerline lumen value as intraluminal intensity L. Accordingly, we set the width value as $W_{\text{pre}} = 2.07 \cdot L$ and the center value as $C_{\text{pre}} = 0.72 \cdot L$. All values are expressed in Hounsfield units (HU). The annotator could still adjust the windowing if needed.

For a consistent definition of a calcification we followed [7]. Accordingly, the calcification border value B_{calc} was derived from the maximum calcification intensity value M_{calc} as

$$B_{\text{calc}} = 0.58 \cdot M_{\text{calc}} + 201\,\text{HU} \tag{1}$$

Annotations were created with an in-house tool by correcting model proposals. Images were presented in Cartesian and polar views, with polar used for primary editing [4]. We show an example of this transformation from Cartesian (Fig. 2b) to polar (Fig. 2d).

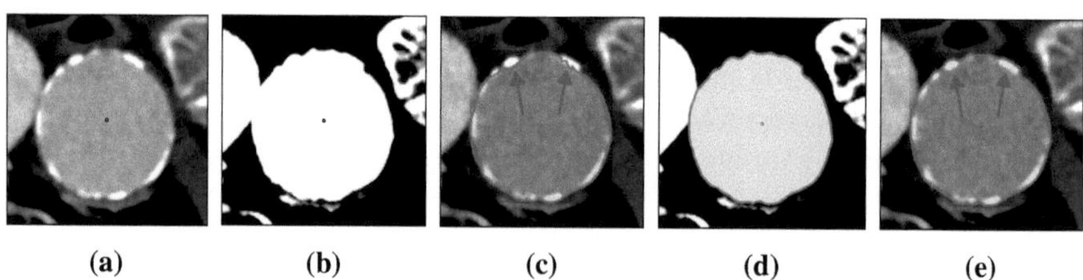

Fig. 1. Inputs, intermediate steps and outputs of the Deep Learning module: (a) Original slice, (b) "Bright" slice, (c) Segmentation for the original slice and missed calcifications, (d) Segmentation for the "bright" slice, and (e) Proposed outer contour.

2.2 Deep learning module

As a first step in our annotation pipeline, we employed the SAM2 segmentation model [8], showing strong performance across diverse domains, including medical applications. For each slice, SAM2 was prompted to segment a single object at the centerline point as shown in (Fig 1a). The output of the model was a binary mask converted to a smooth, continuous contour, as shown in (Fig. 1c). Specifically, only the connected region containing the image center was retained, the mask was smoothed with a Gaussian filter to reduce pixel-level irregularities, and the boundary was extracted and refined into a smooth closed curve that was uniformly resampled to a fixed number of points. We observed that occasionally SAM2 was not consistent in including calcifications within the vessel segmentation, as emphasized by the arrows in (Fig. 1c). To mitigate this, we re-prompted SAM2 with a second "bright" view of the slice by purposely setting relatively low values for the window center and width (Fig. 1b). This view effectively makes the calcifications and the inner lumen visually appear similar, while preserving a difference between the vessel and the background.

One drawback of this approach is that the pre-windowed predicted mask is not guaranteed to be fully contained within the "bright" mask. Therefore, we defined the outer contour as the union of the predicted "bright" mask (Fig. 1d) and the predicted pre-windowed mask (Fig. 1c), resulting in the proposed outer contour (Fig. 1e).

2.3 Analytical module

Next, we derive the inner contour within the provided vessel segmentation. We used a gradient based approach, as gradients are effective for edge detection. The algorithm comprises multiple steps as follows:

2.3.1 Location of calcifications. We first detected calcifications inside the proposed outer contour by finding local maxima. Starting from these maxima, region growing was performed until the calcification border value B_{calc} (Eq. 1) was reached, resulting in a calcification mask (Fig. 2a).

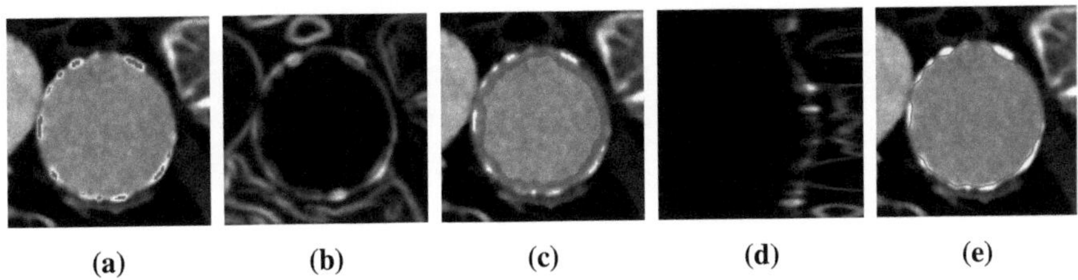

Fig. 2. Inputs, intermediate steps and outputs of the Analytical Module: (a) Detected calcifications, (b) Gradient magnitude image, (c) Ring-shaped Region of Interest (ROI), (d) Gradient magnitude image and ROI in polar coordinates, and (e) Proposed inner contour.

2.3.2 Gradient computation. To capture intensity changes, we computed the image gradient-magnitude on the Cartesian slice without windowing. We worked with discrete 2D images and gradients were approximated with a Sobel filter and smoothed using a Gaussian filter to reduce noise. An example is shown in (Fig. 2b).

2.3.3 Region of interest generation. We formed a ring-shaped ROI by first subtracting the calcification mask from the outer mask, followed by a morphological erosion and a subsequent subtraction (Fig. 2c). These steps guaranteed the ROI to be wide enough to capture vessel-wall edges while being small enough to exclude noise from inside and outside the vessel.

2.3.4 Inner contour proposal. To ensure calcifications were included in the vessel wall, we masked out pixels lying between the outermost edge of each calcification and the outer wall. To maintain plausible wall thickness, we enforced a minimum thickness of 1 px ($\approx$ 0.47 mm), comparable to 0.55 mm in [9]. We therefore clipped the ROI by 1 px on the outer side only. The results of these steps are shown in (Fig. 2d). Finally, to estimate the inner contour, we selected the maximal-gradient points within the final ROI. The resulting contour was smoothed using a mild Gaussian filter (σ = 1.0) and mapped back to Cartesian coordinates (Fig. 2e).

2.4 Evaluation

Our evaluation is twofold. First, to assess the annotation performance, we report the mean, standard deviation, and median of the mean absolute error (MAE, mm), root mean squared error (RMSE, mm), and relative mean absolute error (RMAE, %).

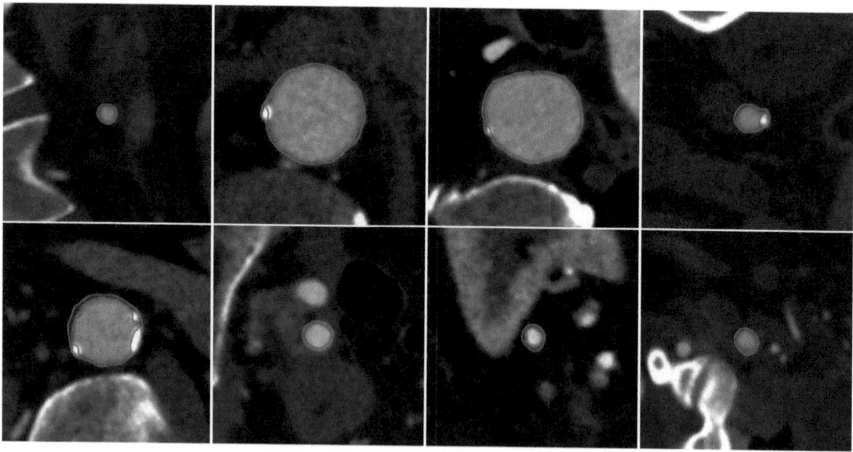

Fig. 3. Qualitative results of the proposed pipeline. Randomly selected axial cross-sections are shown with the automatically generated contours overlaid: inner contour (teal) and outer contour (orange).

Metrics were computed per slice and then aggregated over the dataset of $n = 46$ slices. Second, we quantified annotator intervention. As a metric, we used the proportion of all the contour lines for which the annotator made a change of at least one pixel (≈ 0.47 mm, Sec. 2.1). This captures how often non-visually-trivial edits were required or, in other words, the amount of manual effort needed for clinically accurate segmentation.

3 Results

In Fig. 4 we report quantitative results. For the inner contours, the average MAE was 0.197 ± 0.109 mm (median 0.194 mm) and the average RMAE was 7.1 ± 7.6 % (median 4.53 %). For the outer contours, the average MAE was $0.284 \pm .237$ mm (median 0.240 mm) and the average RMAE was 9.5 ± 4.3 % (median 4.88 %). Across all annotated contours, 4 inner contours and 1 outer contour required no manual modification at all, corresponding to an error of 0. The proportion of the contour line that required a noticeable change of at least 0.47 mm was 12.16 % for inner contours and 19.97 % for outer contours. In Fig. 3 we present qualitative results from randomly selected outputs of our method.

4 Discussion

The proposed pipeline produced accurate and consistent vessel contours. Both the inner and outer contours achieved low errors, with MAE below 1 mm and median

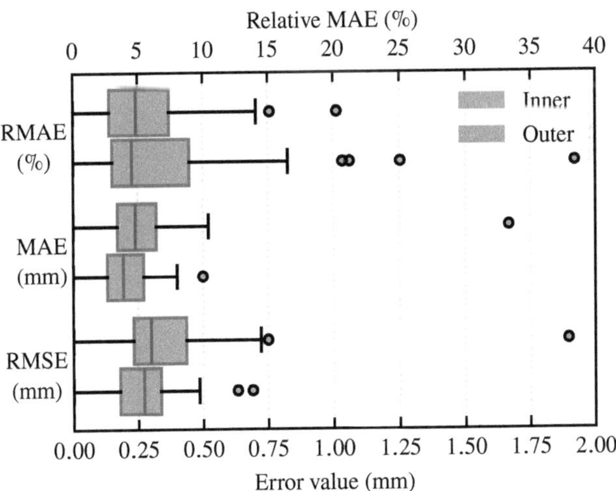

Fig. 4. Comparison of inner and outer contour errors across evaluation metrics. Boxplots show the distribution of RMAE (%), MAE (mm), and RMSE (mm) for inner (teal) and outer (orange) contours.

RMAE below 5 %. The small edit fraction and the presence of zero edits indicate that the automatic proposals were close to the corrected annotations, and that manual effort was limited to local refinements rather than global redraws. Although we did not formally time the process, the annotator reported a noticeable speedup compared with manual contouring, which aligns with the small proportion of edited contour length.

While the results are promising, several limitations should be considered. This initial evaluation was conducted on a small dataset of $n = 46$ slices, which limits the generalizability of the findings. The pipeline depends on the quality of the initial segmentation and on an accurate vessel centerline. Failures of SAM2, for example near bone or in regions affected by strong artifacts, can propagate to later stages. While the "bright" window improves inclusion of calcified regions, it can also overextend toward adjacent high-intensity structures if not properly constrained. Similarly, the gradient based refinement applies a simple maximum-gradient rule, which may become unreliable in low-contrast or noisy regions. Finally, the evaluation relied on a single annotator, which prevents assessment of inter-annotator variability and separation of algorithmic from human error.

Future research will focus on improving robustness, scalability, and evaluation depth. We plan to conduct a timing study and an inter-annotator experiment to quantify efficiency gains and reproducibility. Automatic adaptive windowing strategies could further enhance calcification handling and contour segmentation in general. To conclude, this study shows that the proposed pipeline can produce accurate contour proposals with limited manual correction, and it offers a practical path toward more efficient and reproducible vessel segmentation.

References

1. World Health Organization. Cardiovascular diseases (CVDs). https://www.who.int/news-room/fact-sheets/detail/cardiovascular-diseases-(cvds). Accessed: October 10, 2025. 2025.
2. Lesage D, Angelini ED, Bloch I, Funka-Lea G. A review of 3D vessel lumen segmentation techniques: models, features and extraction schemes. Med Image Anal. 2009;13(6):819–45.
3. Ghanem AM, Hamimi AH, Matta JR, Carass A, Elgarf RM, Gharib AM et al. Automatic coronary wall and atherosclerotic plaque segmentation from 3D coronary CT angiography. Sci Rep. 2019;9(1):47.
4. Chen L, Sun J, Canton G, Balu N, Hippe DS, Zhao X et al. Automated artery localization and vessel wall segmentation using tracklet refinement and polar conversion. IEEE Access. 2020;8:217603–14.
5. Alblas D, Brune C, Wolterink J. Deep-learning-based carotid artery vessel wall segmentation in black-blood MRI using anatomical priors. Proc SPIE MI IP. 2022.
6. Saba L, Mallarin G. Window settings for the study of calcified carotid plaques with multidetector CT angiography. AJNR Am J Neuroradiol. 2009;30(7):1445–50.
7. Okutsu M, Mitomo S, Onishi H, Nakajima A, Yabushita H, Matsuoka S et al. Estimation of coronary artery calcium thickness by computed tomography angiography based on optical coherence tomography measurements. Heart Vessels. 2023;38(11):1305–17.

8. Ravi N, Gabeur V, Hu YT, Hu R, Ryali C, Ma T et al. SAM 2: segment anything in images and videos. arXiv: 2408.00714. 2024.
9. Fayad ZA, Fuster V, Fallon JT, Jayasundera T, Worthley SG, Helft G et al. Noninvasive in vivo human coronary artery lumen and wall imaging using black-blood magnetic resonance imaging. Circulation. 2000;102(5):506–10.

Automatic Deep Learning-Based Segmentation of Abdominal Vessels in CT Scans

Michal Nohel [1,2], Katerina Krejci [2], Constantin Ulrich [3,4], Maximilian Rokuss [3,5,6], Yannick Kirchhoff [3,5,6], Jiri Chmelik [2], Stefan Reguli [7], Jan Hrubovcak [8], Lubomir Martinek [8], Lukas Knybel [9]

[1]Department of Deputy Director for Science and Research, University Hospital & Faculty of Medicine, Ostrava, Czech Republic
[2]Department of Biomedical Engineering, Faculty of Electrical Engineering and Communication, Brno University of Technology, Brno, Czech Republic
[3]German Cancer Research Center (DKFZ) Heidelberg, Division of Medical Image Computing, Heidelberg, Germany
[4]Medical Faculty Heidelberg, University of Heidelberg, Heidelberg, Germany
[5]HIDSS4Health – Helmholtz Information and Data Science School for Health, Karlsruhe/Heidelberg, Germany
[6]Faculty of Mathematics and Computer Science, Heidelberg University, Heidelberg, Germany
[7]Department of Neurosurgery, University Hospital & Faculty of Medicine, Ostrava, Czech Republic
[8]Department of Surgery, University Hospital & Faculty of Medicine, Ostrava, Czech Republic
[9]Department of Oncology, University Hospital & Faculty of Medicine, Ostrava, Czech Republic

michal.nohel@fno.cz

Abstract. Accurate preoperative mapping of abdominal vasculature is essential in colorectal surgery to reduce intraoperative bleeding and postoperative ischemia. We developed deep learning models for automated 3D segmentation of arteries and veins from dual-phase contrast-enhanced CT scans. Our dataset included 55 patients with arterial and venous phase scans, where major vessels down to third-order branching were manually annotated. Three nnU-Net variants (standard 3D U-Net, residual encoder U-Net, and SkeletonRecall) were trained independently for arteries and veins using five-fold cross-validation. Segmentation performance was evaluated using Dice score, centerline Dice score, sensitivity, and precision. All models achieved comparable Dice and centerline Dice scores, with slightly better results for veins segmentation. SkeletonRecall showed the highest sensitivity and superior vessel continuity, despite lower precision. On the independent test set, Dice scores were lower due to incomplete ground truth, yet SkeletonRecall correctly captured vessels up to third-order branching. The trained models are publicly available at `https://github.com/LERCO-FNO/Abdominal-Vessels-Segmentation`.

© Der/die Autor(en), exklusiv lizenziert an
Springer Fachmedien Wiesbaden GmbH, ein Teil von Springer Nature 2026
H. Handels et al. (Hrsg.), *Bildverarbeitung für die Medizin 2026*,
Informatik aktuell, https://doi.org/10.1007/978-3-658-51100-5_58

1 Introduction

Colorectal cancer is one of the most common oncological diagnoses in all developed countries. Each year, malignant tumors of the colon or rectum are diagnosed in approximately 7,200 individuals in the Czech Republic, and nearly 3,300 patients die from this disease annually [1]. Surgical resection represents a crucial component in the treatment, as it remains the only potentially curative modality for removing the primary tumor. Colorectal resections demand a precise understanding of mesenteric angio architecture, where inter individual variation in arterial inflow and venous drainage can precipitate blood loss or compromise perfusion; border zone territories at the splenic flexure and the rectosigmoid junction are particularly exposed. Although arterial and portal venous phase contrast-enhanced CT (CECT) depict these pathways, assembling an actionable, patient-specific vessel map from multiphase data is labor-intensive and prone to omission of small-caliber branches. Preoperative knowledge of the vascular system and large vessels also supports the oncologically correct surgical procedures in malignant tumors, which have a fundamental impact on the patient's prognosis.

To address this, we developed a deep learning-based framework for automatic 3D segmentation of abdominal arteries and veins. Our dataset comprises 55 patients, each with arterial and venous phase CECT scans, where major vessels and their branches (down to the third-order branching) were manually annotated by experienced surgeons. Using the nnUNet segmentation framework [2], we trained models to capture complex anatomical variations, including small and distal vessels that are often difficult to see and segment.

The purpose of this study is to accelerate and improve surgical procedures by providing intuitive, patient-specific vascular maps. Segmented vessels are integrated into a virtual reality (VR) environment, allowing surgeons to explore 3D anatomy prior to surgery. The preoperative familiarization reduces intraoperative uncertainty, improves surgical efficiency, and enhances patient safety. By training and validating these segmentation models, we provide the foundation for a VR-assisted planning pipeline that can make colorectal resections faster, safer, and more precise.

2 Materials and methods

For this study, we used a subset of 55 CECT scans of adult patients, acquired at the University Hospital Ostrava. The dataset will be published and is currently under review in SciData [3]. It consists of CECT scans covering both arterial and venous phases. Only scans acquired for preoperative planning purposes, excluding polytrauma protocols, were included. When chest CT scans were present, only the abdominal region, from the diaphragm to pelvis, was used.

All scans were performed on a Siemens Somatom Force dual-energy CT scanner (2 × 192 detector rows) with a majority slice thickness of 0.75 mm. Arterial phases were captured 25–30 seconds after contrast injection, and venous phases 55–60 seconds post-injection, using either Visipaque 320 or Omnipaque 325 administered intravenously. Each study contained approximately 700–900 axial slices. For each patient, major arteries and veins were manually annotated down to third-order branching, including smaller distal vessels. These annotations served as ground truth for training and evaluating our deep learning models for 3D vascular segmentation.

In this work, we introduced three different nnU-Net-based models for vessel segmentation: the classical nnU-Net [2], the residual encoder U-Net (ResEnc) [4], and the nnU-Net with Skeleton Recall [5]. Although there are several approaches for thin tubular structures segmentation in 3D medical images, such as cl-Dice [6] loss or persistent homology-based losses [7], the Skeleton Recall method has proven particularly effective for vessel segmentation. It works by introducing an additional loss term that emphasizes the skeleton of the structure, specifically applying a recall term to the "*tubed skeleton*". This encourages the network to focus on the centerline connectivity of vessels, regardless of the diameter of individual branches, thereby improving the continuity and topological correctness of the segmented vascular network.

Each of these three model configurations was trained independently for arterial and venous segmentation tasks using the same preprocessing pipeline and data splitting strategy. In total, 50 scans were used for training and validation with five-fold cross-validation, while the remaining 5 scans were used as an independent test set. Training followed the standard nnU-Net framework, including the default data augmentation techniques, spatial transformations, intensity normalization, and patch-based sampling. Optimization followed the standard nnU-Net training schedule, allowing direct comparison of model performance across architectures.

To assess the performance of the segmentation models, we evaluated several complementary metrics. The primary measure was the classical Dice score, quantifying the volumetric overlap between the predicted and reference segmentations. In addition, the centerline Dice score (clDice) [6] was used to evaluate the accuracy of the segmented vessel centerlines, providing a topology-aware assessment of vascular continuity.

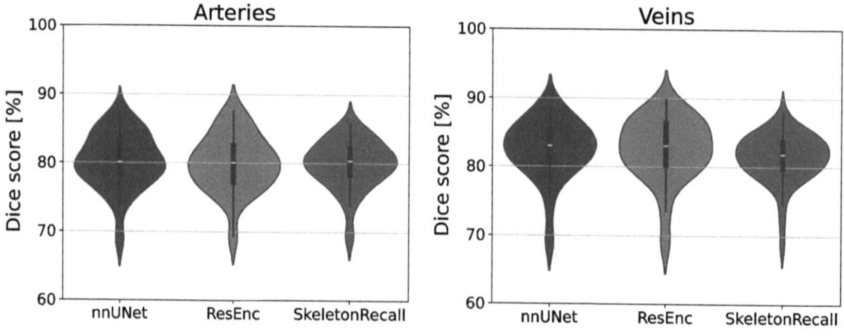

Fig. 1. Comparison of Dice scores for arterial (left) and venous (right) segmentations across three nnU-Net model variants. Violin plots illustrate the distribution of Dice scores obtained from five-fold cross-validation, showing the variability in segmentation performance for each network.

Tab. 1. Mean and standard deviation of Dice score, centerline Dice score, sensitivity, and precision for arterial (A) and venous (V) segmentation using three nnU-Net model variants. Results are reported for five-fold cross-validation and the independent test set.

Models	Dice [%]	clDice [%]	Sensitivity [%]	Precision [%]
A-nnU-Net	80.13 ± 4.06	79.41 ± 3.80	76.28 ± 6.43	84.90 ± 4.97
A-ResEnc	79.99 ± 4.12	79.94 ± 3.60	75.05 ± 6.43	86.18 ± 5.17
A-SkeletonRecall	79.92 ± 3.52	79.63 ± 3.30	82.29 ± 5.59	78.05 ± 5.03
A-SkeletonRecall Test	68.84 ± 6.85	68.66 ± 5.81	88.72 ± 4.95	56.51 ± 7.62
V-nnU-Net	82.43 ± 4.37	77.75 ± 6.65	79.87 ± 7.11	85.68 ± 4.43
V-ResEnc	82.58 ± 4.63	78.63 ± 7.27	78.97 ± 7.26	87.07 ± 4.56
V-SkeletonRecall	81.47 ± 3.53	75.03 ± 5.19	84.54 ± 6.37	79.05 ± 4.61
V-SkeletonRecall Test	73.03 ± 4.63	58.84 ± 11.34	85.05 ± 4.68	64.66 ± 8.02

To further evaluate model performance, sensitivity and precision were calculated, reflecting the proportion of correctly identified vessel voxels and the rate of false-positive predictions. These metrics provided a comprehensive evaluation of both volumetric accuracy and structural fidelity of the vascular segmentation.

3 Results

For the segmentation of abdominal vessels, the nnU-Net framework was employed in its 3D full-resolution configuration. To explore the impact of different architectures and training strategies, three different variants of the nnU-Net trainer were used: standard 3D U-Net, a residual encoder U-Net designed to improve feature propagation in deeper layers, and a topology-aware variant, SkeletonRecall, that incorporates a skeleton-based loss function to better preserve vessel continuity.

The comparison of Dice scores achieved by the three variants of the model for the arteries and veins is presented in Fig. 1, while Tab. 1 summarises the complete set of

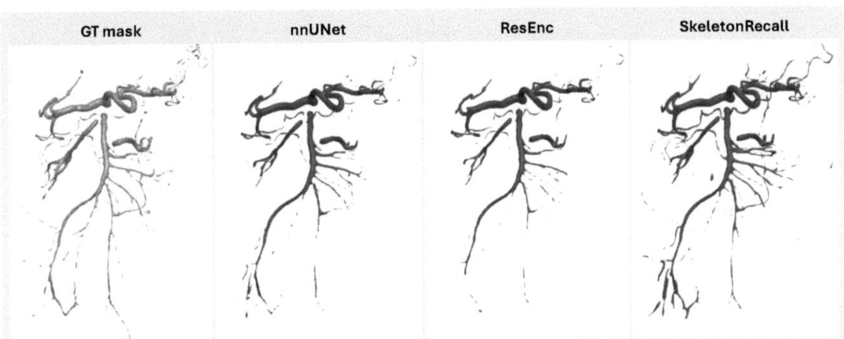

Fig. 2. Example of arterial vessel segmentations from the validation dataset. The ground truth mask is shown in green (left), followed by the predictions from the nnU-Net, ResEnc U-Net, and SkeletonRecall models. The corresponding Dice scores were 80.53, 79.69, and 78.57.

quantitative metrics, including the Dice score, the centerline Dice score, sensitivity and precision, along with their mean values and standard deviations across all folds.

Representative examples of arterial segmentations from the validation dataset are shown in Fig. 2, illustrating the comparison between the three nnU-Net model variants. The visual results correspond well with the quantitative evaluation, with the SkeletonRecall model producing the most coherent and topologically continuous vessel structures. Although its overall Dice score was slightly lower compared to the baseline nnU-Net, manual assessment of the segmentations revealed that SkeletonRecall achieved more anatomically complete and connected results, particularly in distal vessel branches. The model frequently predicted small vascular structures that were not consistently annotated in the ground truth, which likely led to a lower Dice score despite superior visual accuracy and anatomical plausibility.

Based on these findings, the SkeletonRecall model was selected for final testing. Predictions on the independent test set demonstrated good generalization performance (Fig. 3), which shows two representative cases with ground truth (green) and model predictions (red).

4 Discussion

In this study, three different settings for nnU-Net model training were explored and evaluated for the segmentation of abdominal arteries and veins. The quantitative results indicate that, the models performed comparably in terms of Dice and centerline Dice scores, with only minor differences. Slightly higher scores were achieved for venous segmentation, likely due to the fact that veins are generally larger and less affected by labeling inaccuracies.

SkeletonRecall model achieved the highest sensitivity, confirming its ability to capture a greater proportion of the vessel structures present in the ground truth. However, the improvement came at the cost of lower precision, indicating a higher

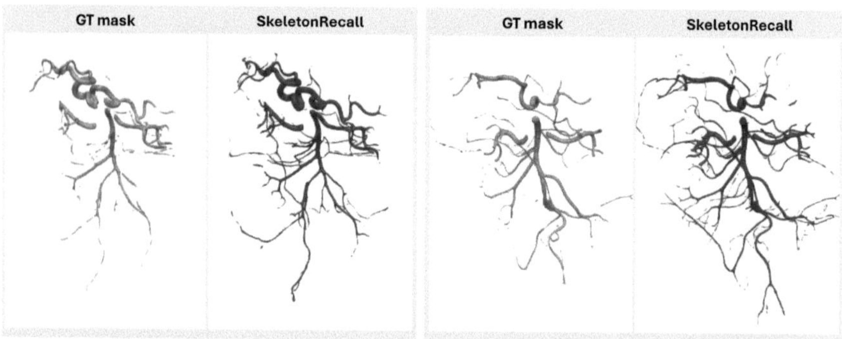

Fig. 3. Examples of arterial vessel segmentations from the independent test dataset. Two representative cases from different patients are shown. The ground truth masks are displayed in green, and the predictions of the SkeletonRecall model are shown in red. The corresponding Dice scores were 77.50 and 75.66.

number of false-positive voxels. Qualitative evaluation further revealed that the SkeletonRecall model maintained better vascular continuity, preserving even fine branches and distal connections that were occasionally missing in the predictions of the standard U-Net and ResEnc U-Net models.

On the independent test dataset, the overall performance metrics were lower; however, this is likely attributable to the incomplete ground truth segmentations(Fig. 3) . In several test cases, the SkeletonRecall model successfully segmented vessels up to the third-order branching, which were not fully annotated in the test ground truth masks.

In conclusion, the SkeletonRecall model provided the most anatomically consistent and clinically relevant results. Despite slightly lower global metrics, its superior representation of vessel continuity and small branches makes it the most suitable for clinical applications, particularly in the context of VR-based preoperative planning and vascular mapping.

Acknowledgement. This article has been produced with the financial support of the European Union under the LERCO project number CZ.10.03.01/00/22_003/0000003 via the Operational Programme Just Transition.

References

1. Majek O, Suchanek S, Zavoral M, Dusek L, Ngo O, Chloupkova R et al. Kolorektum.cz: colorectal cancer screening programme in the Czech Republic. Version 3.0. 2025. URL: `https://www.kolorektum.cz/cs/o-programu/kolorektalni-karcinom/`.
2. Isensee F, Jaeger PF, Kohl SA, Petersen J, Maier-Hein KH. nnU-net: a self-configuring method for deep learning-based biomedical image segmentation. Nat Methods. 2021;18(2):203–11.
3. Strakos P, Hrubovcak J, Kubicek J, Sethia K, Kaushik S, Jaros M et al. A dataset of abdominal CT with artery and vein segmentations for colorectal cancer surgical planning. Nat Methods. 2025. Dataset under review at Scientific Data.
4. Isensee F, Wald T, Ulrich C, Baumgartner M, Roy S, Maier-Hein K et al. nnU-net revisited: a call for rigorous validation in 3D medical image segmentation. Proc MICCAI. 2024:488–98.
5. Kirchhoff Y, Rokuss MR, Roy S, Kovacs B, Ulrich C, Wald T et al. Skeleton recall loss for connectivity conserving and resource efficient segmentation of thin tubular structures. Proc ECCV. 2024:218–34.
6. Shit S, Paetzold JC, Sekuboyina A, Ezhov I, Unger A, Zhylka A et al. clDice: a novel topology-preserving loss function for tubular structure segmentation. Proc IEEE/CVF CVPR. 2021:16555–64.
7. Clough JR, Byrne N, Oksuz I, Zimmer VA, Schnabel JA, King AP. A topological loss function for deep-learning based image segmentation using persistent homology. IEEE Trans Pattern Anal Mach Intell. 2020;44(12):8766–78.

Abstract: Sex-based Bias Inherent in the Dice Similarity Coefficient

A Model Independent Analysis for Multiple Anatomical Structures

Hartmut Häntze [1,2,3], Myrthe Buser [2], Alessa Hering [2], Lisa C. Adams [3], Keno K. Bressem [3]

[1]Charité - Universitätsmedizin Berlin
[2]Radboudumc, Netherlands
[3]Klinikum rechts der Isar, Technical University of Munich
hartmut.haentze@charite.de

Overlap-based metrics such as the Dice similarity coefficient (DSC) penalize segmentation errors more heavily in smaller structures. As organ size differs by sex, this implies that a segmentation error of equal magnitude may result in lower DSCs in women due to their smaller average organ volumes. While previous work has examined sex-based differences in models or datasets, no study has yet investigated the potential bias introduced by the DSC itself. In this work [1], we quantified sex-based differences of the DSC in an idealized setting independent of specific models. The reference was a whole-body MRI dataset of 50 participants (25 male, 25 female) with manual annotations for 40 classes, grouped by volume. Uniform over- and under-segmentation were simulated by adding or removing fixed voxel margins along structure boundaries. Even minimal errors (i.e., a 1 mm boundary shift) produced systematic DSC differences between sexes. Average DSC differences were around 0.03 for small structures, 0.01 for medium-sized structures; only large structures were mostly unaffected. These findings show that fairness studies using the DSC should not expect identical scores between the sexes. This does not indicate a flaw in the metric: the DSC correctly assigns greater relative penalty to the same absolute error when the target structure is smaller. However, interpreting such score differences as evidence of model unfairness can be misleading. Even a sex-neutral model can yield different DSC values simply because male and female anatomy differs in volume.

References

1. Häntze H, Buser M, Hering A, et al. Sex-based bias inherent in the dice similarity coefficient: a model independent analysis for multiple anatomical structures. Proc MICCAI. 2025:125–34.

© Der/die Autor(en), exklusiv lizenziert an
Springer Fachmedien Wiesbaden GmbH, ein Teil von Springer Nature 2026
H. Handels et al. (Hrsg.), *Bildverarbeitung für die Medizin 2026*,
Informatik aktuell, https://doi.org/10.1007/978-3-658-51100-5_59

Medical Image Annotations for AI-based Wound Segmentation

The Rocky Road to High-quality Training Data

Georg Wimmer[1], Christof Kauba[1], Christian Puttinger[2], Pamina Schlager[2], Roland Zauner[2], Carolin Gemeier[2], Tobias Welponer[2], Christine Prodinger[2], Anja Diem[2], Katharina Ude-Schoder[2], Martin Laimer[2], Johann W. Bauer[2], Andreas Uhl[1]

[1]Paris Lodron University Salzburg , Department of Artificial Intelligence and Human Interfaces,Jakob-Haringer-Strasse 2, 5020 Salzburg, Austria
[2]University Hospital of the Paracelsus Medical University, Department of Dermatology and Allergology, Müllner Hauptstr. 48,5020 Salzburg, Austria
gwimmer@cs.sbg.ac.at

Abstract. Image annotations are indispensable to the development of new image-based AI software applications in medicine. The quality of these annotations, which serve as training data for AI methods, significantly impacts the effectiveness of AI-based methods. As a paradigm of the annotation process, we present wound annotation in epidermolysis bullosa (EB). EB is a group of rare genetic skin conditions that result in fragile skin and chronic wounds. Accurate wound segmentation is crucial for monitoring and treatment planning. The wound image annotations are made to train deep learning models for the automated segmentation of skin wounds caused by EB. The initial image annotations were widely different between experts with an average inter-annotator agreement of only 32%, as measured using the Dice similarity coefficient. By countermeasures such as annotation workshops to unify the annotation strategy, more precise annotation guidelines, and revised wound class definitions, we were able to distinctly increase the inter-annotator agreement to 59.3%. By sharing the encountered issues in the annotation process, we aim to help others anticipate and mitigate similar risks in medical image annotation tasks.

1 Introduction

Deep learning (DL)-based segmentation models require high-quality, consistently annotated datasets. For epidermolysis bullosa (EB) patients, the diversity of wound appearances demands a carefully structured annotation strategy. The medical experts in our team (physicians with years of experience treating EB) defined a set of wound classes. Together with the AI developers, a data annotation workflow was initiated. The images to be annotated are recorded from different cameras of

© Der/die Autor(en), exklusiv lizenziert an
Springer Fachmedien Wiesbaden GmbH, ein Teil von Springer Nature 2026
H. Handels et al. (Hrsg.), *Bildverarbeitung für die Medizin 2026*,
Informatik aktuell, https://doi.org/10.1007/978-3-658-51100-5_60

the VECTRA WB360 3D imaging system (https://www.canfieldsci.com/imaging-systems/vectra-wb360-imaging-system/). The aim of the project is to detect and segment the wounds in the 2D images using AI-based segmentation methods, project the segmented images to a 3D whole-body skin image, and then measure the wound sizes in the 3D image. The plan for the next stage of the project is to develop an app where EB patients can record and upload images of their wounds captured by smartphones, which will be classified, segmented and measured and the progression of the wounds will be recorded.

Previous studies have shown the high impact of annotation quality on the development of AI-based methods [1] and the importance of clearly defined labeling instructions [2] and iterative quality control strategies in medical image labeling [3].

This paper describes the specific challenges we faced during the annotation of wound images from EB patients and the practical steps taken to resolve them. By sharing our experiences we aim to offer actionable guidance for similar efforts in other complex clinical domains.

2 Materials and methods

Images were recorded using the VECTRA WB360 3D imaging system. The images have a high resolution of 4016 x 6020 pixels and show the patients from different perspectives covering their entire bodies. At the start of the project, we had 68 images of four patients. Throughout the project, we continuously added new images and now have 272 images from 19 patients.

Our team of medical experts defined the 8 wound classes to categorize EB wounds (wound classes are listed in Tab. 1). An image processing expert first pre-segmented all skin areas and anonymized the images (head area is set to black). Then, the wound segmentations were carried out by six medical experts from our team. Since the annotators are highly qualified medical experts having extensive experience with EB-related skin wounds, we initially did not deem it necessary to provide clear labeling instructions beyond defining the wound classes.

The most significant challenge we encountered was the inconsistency among medical experts in the segmentation of the wounds. We employ the Dice similarity coefficient (DSC) [4] to quantify the agreement between two annotations of the same image from different annotators. The DSC, also known as the Sørensen-Dice index, is defined as

$$\mathrm{DSC}(A, B) = \frac{2|A \cap B|}{|A| + |B|} \tag{1}$$

where A and B represent the sets of pixels labeled as positive (belonging to a particular class) in two segmentation masks. The DSC ranges from 0 (no overlap) to 1 (perfect overlap). The DSC is especially well-suited for segmentation tasks involving class imbalance, which is typical in medical imaging scenarios such as EB wound analysis. Many wound classes, such as blisters or cancerous areas, occupy relatively small portions of the image. The DSC metric emphasizes the overlap between these smaller regions while being less influenced by the large background area, unlike simple accuracy metrics. In our case, using DSC allowed us to sensitively detect annotation disagreements for each wound class and later to validate improvements in consistency following our revised annotation strategy. We report the average DSC for each class.

We also consider one multi-class case, where we compare images annotated from different experts across all classes at once. In this case, the two annotations A and B of an image contain up to 9 different classes (the 8 wound classes indexed with values between 1 and 8 and healthy regions or background indexed with value 0). In this case we employ an adapted multi-class version of the DSC to quantify the agreement between annotators, which is defined as follows

$$\text{MC-DSC}(A, B) = \frac{2|A == B \wedge A \geq 1|}{|A \geq 1| + |B \geq 1|} \tag{2}$$

The MC-DSC compares the area that was identically labeled by both segmentation masks (excluding the background) to the total area of both masks not labeled as background. Like the DSC, the MC-DSC ranges from 0 (no overlap) to 1 (perfect overlap). We use the MC-DSC as a summary metric for evaluating the similarity between annotations from different annotators, rather than simply calculating the mean value of the average DSCs per class as is customary. The reason for that is the huge class imbalance in our dataset. Some wound classes are rare in our dataset, like Blister and Cancer. Others are common, like Scaling-Erythema and Crust-Scaling Crust. In addition, some classes cover large areas of the skin (Unspecifely Altered - Hyperpigmented and Scaling - Erythema), while others cover only very small areas (Blister). The mean value of the average DSCs per class therefore does not correspond to the similarity that the annotations exhibit to the human eye. However, the MC-DSC is perfectly suited for this purpose.

2.1 CVAT annotation tool – deployment and technical and organizational challenges

We selected CVAT (Computer Vision Annotation Tool) for its usability, local server support, and privacy controls. It allowed image-specific permissions and easy export of class-wise binary masks for deep learning (DL) model training.

The initial plan was to host the CVAT server at the Paris Lodron University Salzburg (PLUS). However, a number of unexpected problems emerged:

- Server setup failure: due to unresolved technical issues, specifically the inability to implement two-factor authentication, the CVAT server at PLUS could not be used securely for medical data annotation.
- Delayed server deployment: setting up an alternative CVAT server at the Salzburg University Hospital was delayed by approximately three months due to bureaucratic constraints.
- Temporary laptop-based annotation: to avoid halting progress, a Windows laptop was used temporarily. However, CVAT performed poorly on this device,

Tab. 1. Per-class annotation statistics and inter-annotator agreement measured using the DSC.

Initial Wound Classes	Imgs	Pairs	Mean DSC (Std)
Unspecified altered - hyperpigmented	155	58	0.199 (0.270)
Scaling - Erythema	181	69	0.273 (0.328)
Erosion/Ulcer - Hypergranulating	62	21	0.000 (0.000)
Erosion/Ulcer with Coating	58	36	0.127 (0.225)
Erosion/Ulcer without other features	98	41	0.244 (0.352)
Crust - Scaling Crust	160	67	0.242 (0.280)
Blister	27	15	0.161 (0.288)
Cancer, suspected or confined	8	8	0.000 (0.000)
Affected vs healthy	239	74	0.592 (0.283)
All labels	239	74	**0.320** (0.302)

annotations could only be made at the office and only one person could work at a time. This resulted in slow progress with the image annotations.

- Insufficient amounts of permitted storage space: after successful server launch, Docker-based storage issues emerged. Since storage expansion wasn't feasible, Docker and CVAT were reinstalled monthly to reclaim space, allowing annotation to proceed.

3 Results

3.1 Comparison of annotations from different experts using the initial annotation strategy

In Tab. 1, we show the mean DSC value (along with the standard deviations) between the annotations of images by different annotators for each wound class separately, for the differentiation between affected skin and healthy skin/background ("Affected vs non-affected") and for the differentiation across all classes of an image ("All labels" using the MC-DSC). The column 'Imgs' shows the number of images that include labels from a specific category (wound classes and the two special categories Affected vs healthy and All labels), 'Pairs' denotes the number of comparisons pairs, each between two annotations from different experts of the same image and class. Note that we always compared all possible pairs , but the numbers widely vary depending on how many of the annotated images including a specific class were annotated by more than one expert. We had up to 4 annotations from different experts per image, but about 56% of the images were annotated by only one expert and comparisons for images with only one annotation are not possible. Altogether, 239 annotations were produced from 173 images.

When comparing annotations of the same image produced by different annotators, we observed a low average agreement of only 32% (All labels), measured using the MC-DSC. Looking at the average DSC values per class in Tab. 1, results between 0% and 27.3% were achieved. Clearly, this is insufficient to train DL-based segmentation methods. Each annotator interpreted and applied the wound class definitions slightly differently, leading to substantial variability in the segmentation masks.

In addition to the different interpretations of wound definitions, two other factors contributed to the inconsistencies in the annotations. At the outset of the annotation process, the AI developers did not properly specify that all areas of an image must be annotated in order to obtain suitable training data for the AI-based methods envisioned. Consequently, some annotators only labeled areas where they were certain of the correct classification, leaving ambiguous or unclear areas unlabeled. Second, some clearly visible wounds were missed in the initial annotations, either caused by start-up difficulties with the annotation software or due to distractions in the annotation. Both factors introduced systematic under-annotation, which potentially undermines model performance and generalizability. To visually demonstrate the extent of inter-annotator variability, we show example segmentations from different annotators for four images in Fig. 1. Similar inconsistencies were observed across the dataset, motivating the need for revised definitions and coordinated training.

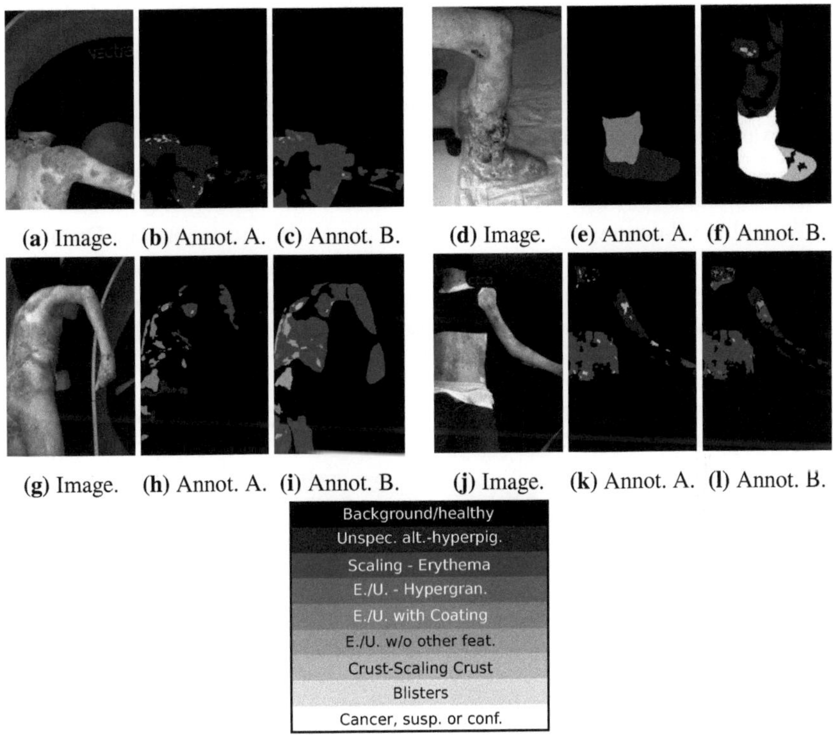

(a) Image. **(b)** Annot. A. **(c)** Annot. B. **(d)** Image. **(e)** Annot. A. **(f)** Annot. B.

(g) Image. **(h)** Annot. A. **(i)** Annot. B. **(j)** Image. **(k)** Annot. A. **(l)** Annot. B.

(m) Class-color mapping.

Fig. 1. Exemplar segmentations with a high inter-annotator variability. The classes in the segmentations are represented in different gray scales as depicted in (m).

3.2 Revised annotation strategy

To address the initially low inter-annotator agreement, the annotation guidelines were revised in collaboration with the medical team. Revisions included merging the wound classes 'Scaling-Erythema' and 'Unspecified Altered-Hyperpigmented' into a new, consolidated class: 'Lesional (Re-)Epithelialized'. The remaining wound classes were renamed (Tab. 2), but otherwise remained the same. The updated guidelines also included more precise class definitions and sessions to discuss how images should be annotated and when each of the classes should be used.

To validate the improvements, the six annotators independently segmented the images on a small validation set consisting of four images using the new schema. We measure the inter-annotator agreement on the resulting 24 segmentation masks. The results showed a substantial improvement in consistency: the average DSC across all annotated wound classes ("All labels" using the MC-DSC) rose from 0.320 to 0.809, and agreement on the overall affected skin area ('Affected vs healthy') increased from 0.592 to 0.885. These results underscore the effectiveness of coordinated guideline refinement. They also demonstrate the importance of early consensus-building and collaborative quality control in the development of clinically useful medical datasets.

To visually demonstrate the improvements in the inter-annotator variability, we show example segmentations from each of the 4 images of the validation dataset in Fig. 2. We can clearly observe that the annotations of different experts using the revised annotation strategy are clearly more consistent than before (Fig. 1).

After this validation, we held a project meeting with the annotators. During this meeting, we reviewed all images and classes in the validation set with low inter-annotator agreement and built a consensus on how to best annotate these images. Then, using the revised annotation strategy, the annotations on the full set of images

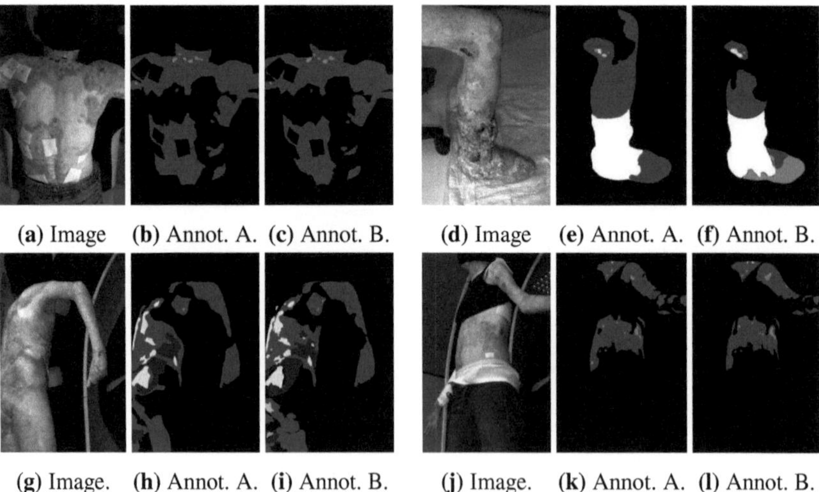

(a) Image **(b)** Annot. A. **(c)** Annot. B. **(d)** Image **(e)** Annot. A. **(f)** Annot. B.

(g) Image. **(h)** Annot. A. **(i)** Annot. B. **(j)** Image. **(k)** Annot. A. **(l)** Annot. B.

Fig. 2. Exemplar segmentations of the validation dataset with the revised annotation strategy.

Tab. 2. Per-class annotation statistics and inter-annotator agreement of the new annotations after the validation.

Revised Wound Classes	Initial Wound Classes	Imgs	Pairs	Mean DSC (Std)
Lesional, (Re-)Epithelialized	Unspec. alt.-hyperpig. Scaling - Erythema	281	64	0.604 (0.245)
Hypergranulating (Les., Dehisc.)	E./U. - Hypergran.	1	0	n/a
Coating (Lesional, Dehiscent)	E./U. with Coating	101	35	0.002 (0.009)
Erosion (Lesional, Dehiscent)	E./U. w/o other feat.	83	25	0.048 (0.167)
Crust (Lesional, Dehiscent)	Crust-Scaling Crust	142	38	0.273 (0.339)
Blister (Lesional, Dehiscent)	Blister	53	8	0.135 (0.220)
Lesional, Suspected Tumor	Cancer, susp. or conf.	18	7	0.812 (0.116)
Affected vs healthy		293	65	0.663 (0.221)
All labels		293	65	**0.593** (0.222)

could be started. Currently, 293 new annotations were produced from 228 images within one month by four annotators. Tab. 2 presents the detailed class-wise inter-annotator agreements of the new annotations. Tab. 2 also shows how the classes were renamed and merged, respectively.

As we can observe, the average DSC across all annotated wound classes decreased from 0.809 (validation set) to 0.593, but is still clearly higher than for the initial annotations (0.32). One remaining problem are the poor results for the three erosion classes (Hypergranulating (Lesional, Dehiscent), Coating (Lesional, Dehiscent), and Erosion (Lesional, Dehiscent)) and blisters. A project meeting is already planned at which the differences in the annotations will be discussed so that a consensus can be reached on how such wounds with differing annotations should be annotated in future and so that the existing annotations can be revised.

For the remainder of the project, we plan to continuously measure the inter-annotator agreement and hold project meetings whenever there are significant discrepancies in the annotations, in order to reach a consensus on how the images should be annotated.

4 Discussion

Our experience yielded several key insights:

- Provide clear annotation guidelines.
- Organize annotation workshops with practical examples to align the understanding of classes and unify the annotation strategy.
- Revised class definitions and class merging can improve annotation consistency.
- Continuously monitor the annotations so that different annotation approaches of the annotators can be recognized and addressed early on and a consensus can be reached on how to standardize the annotations.
- A stable IT infrastructure should be ensured at an early stage to avoid delays in the annotation process.

Future work will focus on completing the annotation task using the refined protocol and finally training and evaluating DL-based segmentation models on the annotated dataset.

Acknowledgement. This work has been partially supported by the Salzburg State Government WISS2025 project "servEB: Global Data and Patient Management for Rare Genetic Skin Diseases". The data and samples for this project have been provided by the EB Biobank of the EB Research Institute GmbH, Salzburg, Austria

References

1. Sambasivan N, Kapania S, Highfill H, Akrong D, Paritosh P, Aroyo LM. "Everyone wants to do the model work, not the data work": data cascades in high-stakes AI. Proc CHI. 2021.
2. Rädsch T, Reinke A, Weru V, Tizabi MD, Schreck N, Kavur A et al. Labelling instructions matter in biomedical image analysis. Nat Mach Intell. 2023;5:1–11.
3. Freeman B, Hammel N, Phene S, Huang A, Ackermann R, Kanzheleva O et al. Iterative quality control strategies for expert medical image labeling. Proc AIII HCOMP. 2021;9(1):60–71.
4. Dice LR. Measures of the amount of ecologic association between species. Ecology. 1945;26:297–302.

Label, Refine, Repeat

Extending nnInteractive with Dataset Traversal and nnU-Net Proposals

Nico Schmutzenhofer[1,2†], Lukas Förner[1,2,3†], Sina Wendrich[1,2], Kartikay Tehlan[1,2,3], Thomas Wendler[1,2,3,4,5]

[1]Department of Diagnostic and Interventional Radiology and Neuroradiology, Augsburg, Germany
[2]Digital Medicine, University Hospital Augsburg, Augsburg, Germany
[3]Computer-Aided Medical Procedures and Augmented Reality, Technical University of Munich, Garching bei München, Germany
[4]Center of Advanced Analytics and Predictive Sciences, University of Augsburg, Germany
[5]Bavarian Cancer Research Center (BZKF) Augsburg, Germany
lukas.foerner@uk-augsburg.de

Abstract. Interactive segmentation tools accelerate annotation but often operate on a single image at a time and lack robust initialization. We extend nnInteractive with (i) dataset-aware traversal that supports sequential/on-the-fly loading of images and volumes, similar to MONAI Label's iteration approach, and (ii) model-assisted pre-segmentation via nnU-Net to warm-start the interaction. Our traversal module adds persistent progress tracking and resume-from-last functionality, enabling efficient, dataset-scale labeling sessions. The nnU-Net integration generates class-wise candidate masks (2D/3D) that are overlaid in the UI for immediate acceptance, editing, or rejection. Users can toggle structures, adjust thresholds, and refine them with standard nnInteractive tools. The system supports batch precomputation or on-the-fly inference, and logs edits to facilitate auditability and reproducibility. We illustrate end-to-end workflows on the pediatric BraTS dataset of 2024 and outline evaluation protocols (clicks, correction time, Dice-Sørensen score after refinement) to quantify annotation efficiency. Together, these additions turn nnInteractive into a scalable, dataset-centric labeling environment that leverages state-of-the-art segmentation priors while preserving expert control. The code is available at: https://github.com/Clinical-Computational-Medical-Imaging/label-refiner

1 Introduction

Accurate and efficient tumor segmentation plays a central role in medical image analysis, forming the foundation for reliable diagnosis, personalized treatment plan-

[†]These authors contributed equally to this work.

© Der/die Autor(en), exklusiv lizenziert an
Springer Fachmedien Wiesbaden GmbH, ein Teil von Springer Nature 2026
H. Handels et al. (Hrsg.), *Bildverarbeitung für die Medizin 2026*,
Informatik aktuell, https://doi.org/10.1007/978-3-658-51100-5_61

ning, and effective disease monitoring. Despite its importance, this process is often challenging, as manual delineation of organ and anomaly boundaries is both time-consuming and highly dependent on the operator's expertise, especially when structures exhibit complex shapes or heterogeneous tissue characteristics. Among the available software solutions, *3D Slicer* [1, 2] stands out as a widely used open-source platform that offers a flexible and extensible environment for medical image visualization, processing, and quantitative analysis. To accelerate the segmentation process for clinical staff, new tools have been developed that leverage pretrained models to automatically identify and segment entire connected structures, whether benign or malignant. Approaches such as *nnInteractive* [3] exemplify this trend, offering flexible frameworks that adapt to various imaging modalities and anatomical regions while reducing the need for extensive manual input. However, most of these methods assume single-image workflows and start from scratch per case without leveraging strong priors [4, 5]. We address these challenges by combining dataset-aware traversal, model-assisted segmentation, and scalable logging with standardized evaluation protocols, resulting in an interactive segmentation tool that preserves expert control over the output. The proposed tool is implemented as an open source extension within 3D Slicer, enabling seamless integration into existing clinical and research workflows. By integrating manual segmentation with predictions from a pretrained *nnU-Net* [6], and offering interactive refinement through nnInteractive prompts, we aim to reduce the time required for accurate expert segmentation. Users can substitute any task-specific nnU-Net model by specifying the model path in the configuration; nnU-Net requires training a new model for each segmentation task. Our primary objective is to reduce annotation time and interaction effort while maintaining segmentation quality comparable to purely manual annotation. We hypothesize that, in cases where models are available, nnU-Net proposals provide a useful initialization that reduces corrective interactions, particularly for challenging cases.

2 Materials and methods

The advancements to the nnInteractive plugin [7] comprise three components: volume loading, automatic segmentation, and assisted refinement.

2.1 Volume Loading

To enable rapid loading of subsequent imaging volumes, we implemented a *Next Volume* action that automatically loads the next volume from a specified input directory, supporting both NIfTI and DICOM formats.

For NIfTI, the user selects a root directory and all `.nii` and `.nii.gz` files are indexed recursively and grouped by patient ID, with each group shown as a separate case. For DICOM, we traverse the standard Patient-Study-Series levels and group the series of one patient into a selectable case.

This design ensures efficient and reproducible loading of imaging data for both single- and multi-volume analyses.

2.2 Automatic Segmentation

We integrate nnU-Net to provide an initial proposal that warm-starts the interactive session (Fig. 1, left). Two execution modes are supported: *on-the-fly* inference at load time, and *batch precomputation* prior to labeling sessions.

2.2.1 Pre-processing. Each input modality is resampled to the model's target spacing and intensity-normalized according to nnU-Net conventions. Missing modalities can be set to *None*; dummy channels are inserted to match the expected channel count without aborting the workflow.

2.2.2 Inference. Given an image volume $I \in \mathbb{R}^{X \times Y \times Z \times C}$, the model predicts per-voxel class probabilities

$$\mathbf{p}(\mathbf{x}) = \left(p_c(\mathbf{x})\right)_{c=1}^{K}, \quad \sum_{c=1}^{K} p_c(\mathbf{x}) = 1$$

and an initial hard labelmap

$$\hat{y}(\mathbf{x}) = \arg \max_{c \in \{1,\ldots,K\}} p_c(\mathbf{x})$$

where $\mathbf{x} \in \mathbb{R}^3$ denotes voxel coordinates, $p_c(\mathbf{x})$ is the predicted probability for class c, and K is the total number of classes (including background).

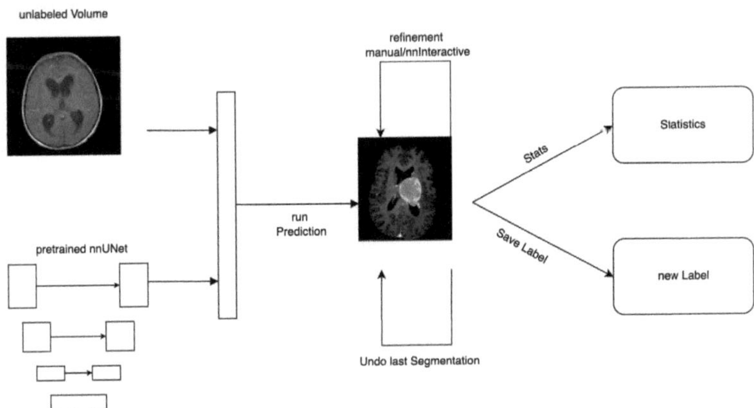

Fig. 1. Overview of the interactive segmentation pipeline. The workflow consists of two main components: (1) a computer-aided segmentation stage, where a pretrained model automatically generates an initial structure segmentation (here: tumor), and (2) a user refinement stage, where experts can iteratively refine the segmentation using either manual editing tools or nnInteractive functionalities. The refined segmentation can then either be saved for downstream use or used to compute quantitative statistics, such as the volume of the segmented structures in mm^3.

We display task-specific label classes as defined in the model's `dataset.json` file. For BraTS, these correspond to enhancing tumor (ET), tumor core (TC), and whole tumor (WT); for other tasks, class names are read directly from the model configuration. Softmax probabilities can optionally be saved to disk for uncertainty-aware inspection.

2.2.3 Post-processing and import. The predicted labelmap is mapped to a Slicer label entity with class-specific color/opacity tables. Optional small-component removal and morphological smoothing are available as a toggle to suppress spurious fragments. If precomputed results exist in a parallel `pred/` directory, they are loaded instantly; otherwise, on-the-fly inference is triggered on user request.

2.3 Assisted Correction

Experts refine $\hat{y}$ using nnInteractive prompts and, when desired, Slicer's native editing tools (Fig. 1, right). We also add an undo function for reverting the most recent label change without requiring a full restart, as well as a save function for persisting the result. We model the refinement loop as a sequence of prompt-conditioned updates

$$S_t = \mathcal{F}_\theta(I, S_{t-1}, e_t), \quad t = 1, 2, \ldots$$

where $S_0 = \hat{y}$ is the nnU-Net proposal, e_t is the user prompt at step t, and $\mathcal{F}_\theta$ is the nnInteractive update operator.

Prompt types. Positive/negative points ($+1/-1$), 2D bounding boxes, scribbles, and lasso selections. Each prompt is encoded with tool type, polarity, and 3D coordinates in scanner space.

Update cycle. On each event e_t, the client sends a compact message to the nnInteractive backend and receives an updated mask S_t which is immediately overlaid.

Class handling. Users may toggle class visibility (e.g. for BraTS, ET/TC/WT) or collapse to a single foreground for coarse editing; class-specific corrections are propagated consistently across slices.

Undo. Each accepted state S_t is pushed onto a bounded history stack $\mathcal{H}$. *Undo* pops and restores S_{t-1}. To limit memory consumption, the history stack retains at most ten states, and the oldest entry is discarded once this limit is exceeded.

Traversal integration. When a case is accepted, *Export* writes the final labelmap. *Next Volume* then advances to the next case, with resume-from-last-session supported via a lightweight manifest.

Stopping rule. The process ends when the expert accepts the segmentation.

3 Results

We evaluated the proposed workflow on 6 brain MRI cases from the BraTS-PED dataset (T1, T1ce, T2, FLAIR, per case). The unblinded segmentation approach began with the generated segmentation from the pretrained nnU-Net (BraTS-PED 2024 training dataset) and subsequently underwent iterative refinements with nnInteractive prompts. Each case was loaded using the *Next Volume* action and processed using two segmentation methods:

1. a blinded segmentation without a generated segmentation by nnU-Net. The segmentation was done using only nnInteractive prompts (positive/negative points, 2D bounding boxes, scribbles, lasso).
2. an unblinded segmentation that started from the generated segmentation by the pretrained nnU-Net and later iterative refinements with nnInteractive prompts.

We recorded per-case time (s), number of lesions, prompt count (P + N) (clicks) and difficulty (Tab. 1).

In the blinded runs, the annotator needed about 3–4 min per case (median $\approx$ 3.7 min) to obtain an acceptable tumor mask, with around 7 prompts in the typical case. This confirms that the baseline nnInteractive setup is already fast for small, well-contrasted lesions. When starting from the nnU-Net proposal, the effort shifted: for the easier cases (C03, C04, C09), annotation time dropped to about 1.5–2.5 min, and the number of corrective prompts was reduced to a few clicks, because the user mainly had to tighten boundaries or recover small missed foci. However, not every case benefited equally: for C05, C06, and C08, the unblinded runs were longer and required more corrections, indicating that a suboptimal proposal can also introduce extra work.

Segmentation accuracy remained nearly unchanged between the two modes. Blinded annotation achieved a median DSC of 0.850 (IQR 0.784–0.891), while unblinded annotation reached 0.888 (IQR 0.822–0.911), i.e., the median difference ΔDSC was close to zero. This is consistent with human-in-the-loop segmentation: once a trained rater is allowed to correct the mask, DSC saturates, and the main benefit of a proposal is reduced interaction, not higher final overlap. The per-case results nevertheless show that interactive refinement rescued difficult cases where the initial nnU-Net proposal was poor: for C05, the initial DSC of 0.159 was corrected to 0.911 (unblinded) and 0.913 (blinded) through user interaction. In contrast, cases that were already easy to segment manually saw little to no gain, or even a reduction (e.g., C04).

Finally, the dataset-aware traversal contributed to overall efficiency by removing non-annotation overhead: loading the next volume and, if desired, its proposal could be done from within 3D Slicer without reconfiguring paths or models. For labeling sessions that process multiple consecutive studies, this reduces friction and helps keep the annotator in a continuous workflow.

Tab. 1. Per-case results for blinded and unblinded segmented studies (6 cases: C03, C04, C05, C06, C08, C09). Initial: raw nnU-Net prediction without refinement, where Time, Prompts, and Difficulty do not apply. Difficulty: subjective rating by the annotator when using the plugin based on tumor boundary clarity and contrast of the images (–: hard, 0: moderate, +: easy). Prompts (P+N): positive clicks + negative clicks. Blinded: median time 220 s [215–280], mean time 242.5 s; median prompts 4 [4–6] + 3 [1–3], mean prompts 4.33 + 2.17. Unblinded: median time 215 s [150–285], mean time 228 s; median prompts 2 [1–3] + 5 [0–8], mean prompts 3.33 + 5.67. Dice: blinded median DSC 0.850 [0.784–0.891], mean 0.776; unblinded median DSC 0.888 [0.822–0.911], mean 0.787; ΔDSC (unblinded – blinded) median –0.002 [–0.002–0.035], mean 0.011. Volume of ground truth, V_{GT}, and segmentation, V_{Seg}, is given in cm^3. Difficulty is a qualitative measure of how easy/hard it was to differentiate between the tumor and the background.

Case	Setting	Time (s)	Prompts (P+N)	Difficulty	V_{GT}	V_{Seg}	DSC
	Initial	–	–	–	16.60	19.45	0.825
C03	Blinded	215	6 + 1	+	16.60	15.53	**0.876**
	Unblinded	150	1 + 4	+	16.60	16.24	0.874
	Initial	–	–	–	138.66	133.02	**0.930**
C04	Blinded	225	7 + 3	+	138.66	115.91	0.784
	Unblinded	110	3 + 0	+	138.66	135.48	0.902
	Initial	–	–	–	17.24	180.51	0.159
C05	Blinded	160	1 + 0	0	17.24	16.58	**0.913**
	Unblinded	285	0 + 8	+	17.24	16.20	0.911
	Initial	–	–	–	4.95	14.82	0.170
C06	Blinded	280	4 + 3	–	4.95	21.13	**0.367**
	Unblinded	393	13 + 6	–	4.95	29.33	0.285
	Initial	–	–	–	84.23	78.92	0.817
C08	Blinded	360	4 + 3	–	84.23	87.23	**0.824**
	Unblinded	270	1 + 16	0	84.23	96.52	0.822
	Initial	–	–	–	101.67	102.10	0.892
C09	Blinded	215	4 + 3	0	101.67	106.40	0.891
	Unblinded	160	2 + 0	0	101.67	110.46	**0.926**

4 Discussion

Our goal was not to train a better segmentation network, but rather to utilize already trained networks (here, nnU-Net) in combination with nnInteractive to create a toolchain for faster annotation by experts. The experiments demonstrate that this is feasible through the integration of dataset-aware traversal, nnU-Net proposals, and nnInteractive.

Initializing the workflow with an nnU-Net proposal slightly improved the median DSC (0.850 vs. 0.888), but it achieved the intended effect of reducing annotation effort, showing a trend toward time reduction (p=0.011 in Wilcoxon signed-rank test with n=6) and corrective interactions. Given that human-in-the-loop refinement tends to saturate segmentation overlap rapidly, this shift from "better accuracy" to "less work" is expected. The benefit was most pronounced in the more challenging cases (C04, C09), where the proposal provided a spatial prior that could be efficiently adjusted; in straightforward cases, purely interactive segmentation was already near-optimal. The dataset-aware traversal further decreased non-annotation overhead by enabling case-to-case progression within 3D Slicer, thereby maintaining workflow continuity for annotators.

Our evaluation has several constraints: (1) a single annotator limits assessment of inter-rater variability; (2) six cases are insufficient for robust statistical conclusions; (3) we evaluated only brain tumor segmentation, and generalization to other anatomies remains untested; (4) cognitive load and usability were not formally measured. Future work should address these gaps through studies with diverse annotators and segmentation tasks.

The natural next step is to close the loop by fine-tuning the base model using accepted expert corrections. This involves developing an intelligent acquisition layer that prioritizes which cases experts should label next. The system would combine multiple complementary strategies: identifying regions where the model is uncertain or ambiguous, selecting diverse batches of cases that provide non-redundant information when experts label multiple examples at once, and maintaining broad coverage across different types of cases in the dataset. Additionally, practical signals such as the effort required to correct previous cases (editing time and number of corrections needed) and the model's confidence scores can be leveraged to identify high-value cases that would most improve the model, focusing expert effort where it matters most.

Acknowledgement. This research was partially funded by the German Childhood Cancer Foundation under grant number A 2024/05 / DKS 2025.01, the Intramural Research Funding "Precision Medicine for pHGG" of the Faculty of Medicine, University of Augsburg, the Bavarian Center for Cancer Research as part of the Lighthouse "Local Therapies", as well as by the Bavarian Ministry of Economic Affairs, Regional Development and Energy (StMWi) under grant number DIK-2310-0004// DIK0556/02.

References

1. Fedorov A, Beichel R, Kalpathy-Cramer J, Finet J, Fillion-Robin JC, Pujol S et al. 3D Slicer as an image computing platform for the Quantitative Imaging Network. Magn Reson Imaging. 2012;30(9):1323–41.
2. 3D Slicer. 3D slicer image computing platform. `https://www.slicer.org`. Accessed: 2025-10-27. 2025.
3. Isensee F, Rokuss M, Krämer L, Dinkelacker S, Ravindran A, Stritzke F et al. nnInteractive: redefining 3D promptable segmentation. arXiv: 2503.08373. 2025.
4. Diaz-Pinto A, Alle S, Ihsani A, Asad M, Nath V, Pérez-García F et al. MONAI label: a framework for AI-assisted interactive labeling of 3D medical images. Med Image Anal. 2022;95:103207.
5. Diaz-Pinto A, Mehta P, Alle S, Asad M, Brown R, Nath V et al. DeepEdit: deep editable learning for interactive segmentation of 3D medical images. Proc MICCAI. 2022:11–21.

6. Isensee F, Jaeger PF, Kohl SA, Petersen J, Maier-Hein KH. nnU-net: a self-configuring method for deep learning-based biomedical image segmentation. Nat Methods. 2021;18(2):203–11.
7. de Vente C, Venkadesh KV, van Ginneken B, Sánchez CI. SlicerNNInteractive: a 3D slicer extension for nnInteractive. arXiv: 2504.07991. 2025.

This chapter is published under the Creative Commons Attribution 4.0 International License (http://creativecommons.org/licenses/by/4.0/deed.en).

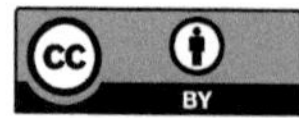

Bridging Radiology and Pathology

A DICOM-based Framework for Multimodal Mapping and Integrated Visualization

Nilesh P. Rijhwani [1,2], Titus J. Brinker [1], Neher Peter [2], Nolden Marco [2], Klaus Maier-Hein [2,3,4,5,6], Christoph Wies [1,3‡], Maximilian Fischer [2,3,4,5‡]

[1]Division of Digital Prevention, Diagnostics and Therapy Guidance, German Cancer Research Center (DKFZ), Heidelberg, Germany
[2]Division of Medical Image Computing , German Cancer Research Center (DKFZ), Heidelberg, Germany
[3]Medical Faculty, University Heidelberg, Heidelberg, Germany
[4]Research Campus M^{2}OLIE, Mannheim, Germany
[5]German Cancer Consortium, DKFZ Core Center Heidelberg, Heidelberg, Germany
[6]Pattern Analysis and Learning Group, Department of Radiation Oncology, Heidelberg University Hospital, Heidelberg, Germany

maximilian.fischer@dkfz-heidelberg.de

Abstract. Accurate disease diagnosis depends on effective collaboration between medical specialties, yet departments often use distinct data systems and proprietary formats. This heterogeneity hinders joint analysis and integration of complementary diagnostic information. The use of separate viewers for each modality further restricts cross-specialty collaboration. Although multimodal integration, particularly between radiology and pathology, has demonstrated potential for identifying novel biomarkers, it still relies heavily on manual, time-consuming data pairing. This project introduces an interdisciplinary toolbox that can operate within the Kaapana framework or as a standalone tool to bridge radiology and pathology. By linking modality-specific viewers and extending them with automated image registration and alignment, the platform enables efficient, scalable multimodal analysis. The integrated environment promotes reproducible workflows, accelerates cross-disciplinary research, and facilitates deeper insights into disease mechanisms and patient care. The method will be integrated in the Kaapana toolkit and as standalone package `https://github.com/MIC-DKFZ/combinedmodalityviewer`.

1 Introduction

The increasing availability of multimodal medical data, particularly the combination of radiological and pathological data, offers great potential for comprehensive disease characterization. However, integrating and visualizing these data streams is

[‡]These authors contributed equally to this work.

© Der/die Autor(en), exklusiv lizenziert an
Springer Fachmedien Wiesbaden GmbH, ein Teil von Springer Nature 2026
H. Handels et al. (Hrsg.), *Bildverarbeitung für die Medizin 2026*,
Informatik aktuell, https://doi.org/10.1007/978-3-658-51100-5_62

technically challenging due to fundamental differences in their scale and acquisition. Currently, few systems support the spatially registered and interactive inspection of these distinct modalities within a unified environment. Radiology has undergone extensive digitization, supported by standardized DICOM-based infrastructures and well-established analytical tools [1]. In contrast, digital pathology is still transitioning toward routine digital adoption, and specialized microscopy viewers often operate in isolation from radiological systems [2]. This data fragmentation limits consistent multimodal exploration and hinders the interpretability of complex algorithmic pipelines. In response, we developed a lightweight, modular viewer for the synchronized visualization of spatially registered radiological and histopathological data. This system integrates established open-source components into a single, coherent web interface, demonstrating a practical and extensible solution for multimodal data exploration. The proposed viewer serves as a bridge between radiological and pathological workflows and establishes a foundation for future research.

2 Methods

For improving multimodal image evaluation, two requirements must be fullfilled: the modalities must be mapped onto each other, and the linked dataset must be visualized appropriately. Both branches are tackled with our proposed framework. This section presents the methods that are used to link radiology and pathology images onto each other, as well as the visualization tools to visualize the linked datasets.

2.1 Data preprocessing

The integration of both modalities requires preprocessing, including DICOM conversion of whole slide images (WSIs) and definition of their anatomical origin.

2.1.1 Dicom conversion. A unified data format is essential for integrating multiple imaging modalities. In radiology, DICOM is the established standard, and with the DICOM-WSI extension it now also supports pathology [3]. Our pipeline therefore requires both modalities in DICOM format and linked through the corresponding DICOM tags[2]. To achieve this, we employ the wsi-dicomizer[3], which is also natively integrated into other multimodal imaging platforms such as Kaapana [4]. The tool can be used within Kaapana or independently, supported by the comprehensive documentation.

2.1.2 Localization of WSI in radiology. Once both modalities are available in the picture archiving and communication system (PACS), the mapping pipeline can be initiated after verifying data completeness. A key step is aligning WSIs with their corresponding radiological images by resolving the anatomical region. The routine

[2]`https://dicom.nema.org/medical/dicom/current/output/html/part18.html`

[3]`https://github.com/imi-bigpicture/wsidicomizer`

evaluates multiple DICOM tags: *BodyPartExamined, Anatomic Region Sequence, Admitting Diagnoses Code Sequence* and parses textual fields (*StudyDescription, SeriesDescription, ProtocolName, ...*) if codes are missing. Free-text entries are normalized to canonical organ labels (heart, prostate, ...) using master JSON derived from controlled DICOM concept lists. The resolver prioritizes exact matches, then broader anatomy groups, and supports substring matching for common label variants.

2.2 Segmentation pipeline

After identifying the anatomical site from the WSI file, the corresponding region in the radiological image is determined. The radiological volume is converted to Neuroimaging Informatics Technology Initiative (NIfTI)-format format using dcm2niix [5] and, together with the identified body part, passed to TotalSegmentator[6] for segmentation. The resulting mask is then converted via itkimage2segimage[4] into a single DICOM-SEG object referencing the original MR images, using dcmqi tooling and a generated meta.json [7]. The resulting multimodal dataset includes (i) the original radiological DICOM volume, (ii) the DICOM-WSI file, (iii) the anatomical site, and (iv) a dicom segmentation (DICOM SEG) object delineating the organ or biopsy subregion. This step creates a standardized, spatially coherent link between the radiological image, its anatomical context, and the corresponding histopathology. For organs such as kidneys or lungs, a post-processing step merges left and right masks into a single binary mask by voxelwise union, ensuring consistent downstream handling with one segment per anatomical target.

2.3 Combined viewer

Navigation across radiological and pathological image viewers typically requires two separate systems, each optimized for its modality. Radiology viewers like Open Health Imaging Foundation (OHIF)-viewer [1] offer advanced tools for volumetric DICOM studies, while pathology viewers such as SLIde microscopy (SLIM)-viewer provide interfaces for exploring high-resolution WSIs [2]. However, cross-modality assessments in separate environments hinder efficient correlation between findings, requiring manual synchronization of spatial context and metadata. To address this, we developed a unified viewer that integrates both modalities within a coordinated web interface. The system embeds the OHIF radiology viewer and SLIM microscopy viewer in a synchronized split-screen layout, enabling interactive, side-by-side exploration of linked regions of interest while preserving full functionality of both viewers. Radiology data such as magnetic resonance imaging (MRI) are stored as DICOM series, and microscopy images (WSI, TIFF, or proprietary formats) are standardized to DICOM via an optional conversion step. All subsequent operations use standard DICOM services and objects. The overall architecture comprises three main components:

[4]https://qiicr.gitbook.io/dcmqi-guide/opening/cmd_tools/seg/itkimage2segimage

- *PACS and services*: A dcm4chee-arc[5] instance can be queried via DICOM web[6] protocols.
- *Backend API*: A java script service with endpoints for (i) study retrieval and packaging, (ii) body-part recognition and concept mapping, and (iii) segmentation pipelines producing DICOM SEG objects [7].
- *Web application*: A React-based client lists PACS studies, launches segmentation tasks, and opens the split viewer. OHIF displays radiology data, and SLIM renders microscopy data [1, 2]. The interface is served by NGINX, which also proxies API and archive traffic.

On the client, the study table lists PACS studies. The user selects a radiological study and as default setting, the OHIF viewer opens as entry point to examination for the selected subject.

2.4 Human interaction

Interactive linking between radiological and pathological data is implemented entirely within the web client. The interface captures user selections on radiological images and dynamically loads the corresponding pathology view, enabling synchronized cross-modal navigation. The clickable segmentation overlay is generated directly in the browser by sampling the Cornerstone canvas RGBA buffer after each OHIF rendering event and identifying segmentation pixels using a predefined red-dominant color criterion. A stack-based flood-fill algorithm groups adjacent pixels

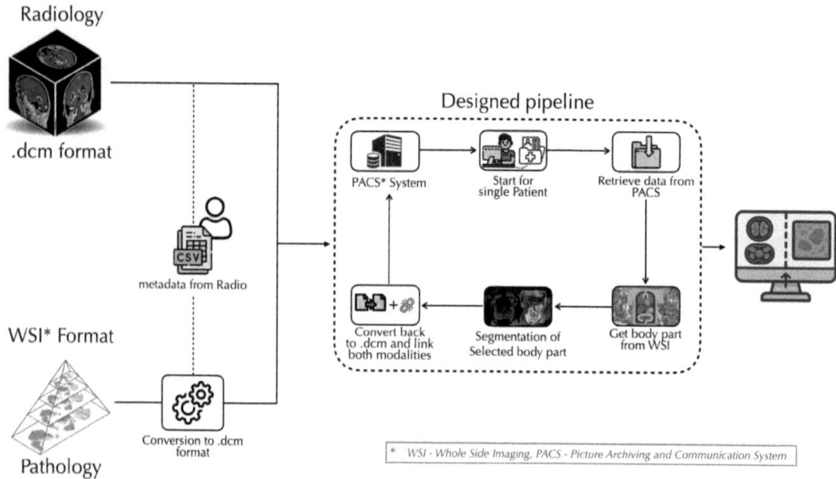

Fig. 1. End-to-end pipeline. The flow runs from the user action in the web UI to a DICOM SEG created by dcmqi, with SM-driven body-part inference and master JSON mapping in the middle.

[5] `https://github.com/dcm4che/dcm4chee-arc-light`
[6] `https://www.dicomstandard.org/using/dicomweb`

into contiguous regions, records their bounds, and converts them to screen coordinates based on the current canvas scale. For each region, a semi-transparent, dashed rectangle with a numeric label is rendered as an interactive target without obscuring the underlying image or interfering with OHIF tools [1]. When selected, the client queries the PACS to locate the corresponding WSI study, retrieves the appropriate images, and displays it in the SLIM viewer on the left while maintaining the OHIF view on the right [2]. This interaction model enables direct navigation from localized radiological findings to corresponding histopathological data, supporting efficient and spatially consistent multimodal exploration.

2.5 Implementation

The Java script backend service calls an PACS endpoint (here we use the dcm4chee-arc PACS) using DICOM web. The anatomic master JSON is mounted into the container and loaded at startup. External tools are invoked with child processes. The service runs inside a container that installs dcm2niix from the system repository [5], *TotalSegmentator* and *SimpleITK* inside a Python virtual environment [6], and dcmqi from a release archive so that itkimage2segimage is available within the pipeline [7].

3 Results

We verified that MRI studies can be discovered and downloaded through the API, that WSI metadata correctly identifies the intended organ in typical cases, and that the systematized nomenclature of medicine – clinical terms (SNOMED CT) resolver returns consistent codes for common targets. The pipeline produces a DICOM SEG for the selected organ and uploads it to the archive. The user interface reflects the outcome and provides clear prompts that indicate what was generated. The archive is always addressed through the internal hostname inside the compose network, which avoids connection errors. The master JSON is mounted with an absolute bind path

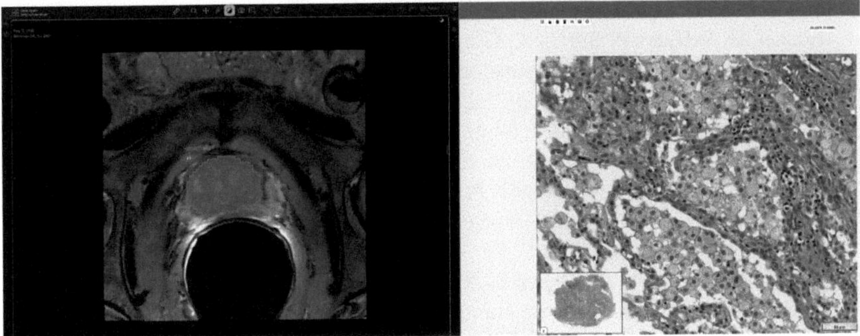

Fig. 2. The screenshot of the combined split-viewer which demonstrates simultaneous viewing of images with auto-segmented "Prostate" along with clickable overlay box.

to prevent inadvertent directory mounts. Python packages are isolated in a virtual environment to honor Debian's external management policy.

4 Discussion

We developed a modular and extensible pipeline that integrates radiological and pathological imaging within a unified, DICOM-based framework. Using DICOM as the sole input format enables seamless integration with existing PACS infrastructures and clinical data environments. All components are containerized with Docker, ensuring reproducibility and flexible extension of the processing chain. Beyond organ-level mapping, users can incorporate advanced registration methods for fine-grained spatial alignment. The visualization layer follows the same modular design, allowing interchangeable viewer components such as SLIM, OHIF, or other viewers like QuPath[7] depending on the use case or institutional preference. This architecture ensures interoperability and adaptability across research and clinical settings. In summary, it provides a robust foundation for collaborative diagnostics and multimodal imaging research.

Acknowledgement. This work was funded by the German Cancer Research Center CORE-funding program (grant-number: 1010001158/1010001159).

References

1. Ziegler E, Urban T, Brown D, Petts J, Pieper SD, Lewis R et al. Open Health Imaging Foundation viewer: an extensible open-source framework for building web-based imaging applications to support cancer research. JCO Clin Cancer Inform. 2020;4:336–45.
2. Gorman C, Punzo D, Octaviano I, Pieper S, Longabaugh WJ, Clunie DA et al. Interoperable slide microscopy viewer and annotation tool for imaging data science and computational pathology. Nat Commun. 2023;14(1):1572.
3. Herrmann MD, Clunie DA, Fedorov A, Doyle SW, Pieper S, Klepeis V et al. Implementing the DICOM standard for digital pathology. J Pathol Inform. 2018;9(1):37.
4. Fischer M, Schader P, Braren R, Götz M, Muckenhuber A, Weichert W et al. DICOM whole slide imaging for computational pathology research in Kaapana and the joint imaging platform. Proc BVM. 2022:273–8.
5. Li X, Morgan PS, Ashburner J, Smith J, Rorden C. The first step for neuroimaging data analysis: DICOM to NIfTI conversion. J Neurosci Methods. 2016;264:47–56.
6. Wasserthal J, Breit HC, Meyer MT, Pradella M, Hinck D, Sauter AW et al. TotalSegmentator: robust segmentation of 104 anatomic structures in CT images. Radiol Artif Intell. 2023.
7. Herz C, Fillion-Robin JC, Onken M, Riesmeier J, Lasso A, Pinter C et al. dcmqi: an open source library for standardized communication of quantitative image analysis results using DICOM. Cancer Res. 2017;77(21):e87–e90.

[7] https://qupath.github.io/

Flexible Multiplanar Viewer with Easy Adaptability for Expert Studies, Questionnaires, and Investigational Imaging Biomarker Assessment

Maja Schlereth [1,2], Filippo Fagni[2], Moritz Schillinger [1], Katharina Breininger [3]

[1]Department Artificial Intelligence in Biomedical Engineering, Friedrich-Alexander-Universität Erlangen-Nürnberg, Erlangen, Germany
[2]Department of Internal Medicine 3, Friedrich-Alexander Universität Erlangen-Nürnberg and Universitätsklinikum Erlangen, Erlangen, Germany
[3]Center for AI and Data Science (CAIDAS), Julius-Maximilians-Universität Würzburg, Würzburg, Germany
maja.schlereth@fau.de

Abstract. Assessing volumetric image data, both for investigational imaging biomarker assessment and for technical research, is a frequent task. Often, the focus is on comparing methods, e.g., for image quality improvement or examining image artifacts in a series of images. However, easily adaptable tools to assess several 3-D images in an organized sequence are limited. To address this gap, we developed a web-based, interactive multiplanar viewer with a focus on streamlined, guided image quality assessment through expert studies and questionnaires, as well as easy adaptability to study-specific requirements. The viewer has a modular structure, and users can add or remove different predefined modules as needed. In this work, we showcase the viewer for hand magnetic resonance imaging (MRI) assessment. To evaluate the usability of our presented graphical user interface (GUI), we performed a small user study across medical imaging and clinical experts. They rated the system as very intuitive and flexible, and highlighted its generalizability to different settings and images. We release our code and application on github.com/MajaSchle/dash_multiplanar.

1 Introduction

In medical image computing, we frequently encounter the need to efficiently review or assess 3-D medical image data. However, current multiplanar viewers are often cumbersome to adapt to specific applications such as expert studies or questionnaires. Furthermore, these expert studies require strict guidance to minimize potential errors and to ensure users follow well-defined steps, such as specific image orders. To address these challenges, we present a lightweight, modular multiplanar viewer that focuses on simple adaptation to specific applications, reproducibility in expert

© Der/die Autor(en), exklusiv lizenziert an Springer Fachmedien Wiesbaden GmbH, ein Teil von Springer Nature 2026
H. Handels et al. (Hrsg.), *Bildverarbeitung für die Medizin 2026*, Informatik aktuell, https://doi.org/10.1007/978-3-658-51100-5_63

studies, and integration of downstream analyses. The tool enables guided viewing protocols and standardized user interactions by defining a rigid, step-by-step process. Its modular design allows easy adaptation to diverse study setups and supports downstream tasks such as 3-D annotations, interactive scoring, or automated model evaluation. Our tool aims to bridge the gap between research prototypes and robust, study-ready visualization environments, supporting efficient data inspection and reproducible user interaction in medical imaging research. While many tools for multiplanar visualization are available, they target different use cases. For instance, 3-D Slicer [1] and MITK [2], both built on VTK, are highly flexible visualization tools that include multiplanar viewing. However, these tools are built in C++ using Python bindings, which requires profound background knowledge of the tool and makes fast customization to specific setups and integration of an expert study protocol and user guidance difficult. While PyVista [3] integrates VTK as a Pythonic interface and enables easy visualization of volumetric data, it lacks a suitable GUI and modules for guided or constrained user interactions. Several web-based multiplanar viewers exist [4]; for example OHIF [5], and NiiVue [6] provide a plugin framework to create task-based workflows. However, these tools are not designed for guided expert studies and are difficult to adapt to highly specific experimental tasks. Compared to the existing multiplanar viewers that lack interactive, study-oriented layouts, our work presents an easily adaptable, modular architecture. We emphasize a study-based design that supports reproducible, fully guided interactions, allowing for strict control of the study progress. We demonstrate the viewer for quality assessment on hand MRI data, and describe how its modularized architecture allows seamless integration of different imaging modalities and for different study setups, such as expert studies with interaction tracking, 3-D landmark annotation, backend model integration, and volumetric representation.

2 Materials and methods

2.1 User interface

We present a web-based tool for interactive volume visualization and assessment. An overview of the core module and several additional modules can be seen in Fig. 1. The core module features a multiplanar viewer that displays volumetric medical images along the three standard anatomical planes: axial, coronal, and sagittal. Users can interactively navigate using a crosshair synced across all three views, allowing selection of a specific anatomical point in all three views by clicking in one view. Additionally, the user can navigate through each view by using the scroll wheel while hovering over a view, a slider, or left and right arrows for a more fine-grained navigation. During the development of the multiplanar viewer, we incorporated feedback from experienced clinicians familiar with various multiplanar viewer tools. To complement the core module, we provide several additional modules that extend the usability of the GUI for various applications:

- An interactive volumetric rendering of the 3-D image using VTK can be added to provide a better spatial understanding of anatomical structures.

- Automatic and manual windowing of the image volume can be included in the GUI to highlight regions of interest and enhance specific image features.
- A module for interactive landmark annotations allows easy landmark placement in the volume by clicking in one of the views. The landmark can be labeled and saved to a CSV file. Incorrect landmarks can be removed again, as well as all landmarks at once. Previously saved landmarks can be loaded and re-annotated.
- A guided expert study module enables the capture of structured expert input. The two main parts of the GUI can be seen in Fig. 2. The user is guided through a predefined sequence of images, ensuring consistency. The expert study starts with a questionnaire, while the slice viewer is faded out. Subsequently, the user can explore the 2-D slices and answer a collapsible hypothesis-specific quality assessment. The system provides feedback on missing answers and controls proceeding to the next step.
- A module for downstream analysis on the example of rheumatoid arthritis allows landmark detection and ROI scoring. The module allows to select different MRI contrasts and to generate disease-specific landmarks and scores. One can choose to display either all landmarks or a specific landmark. When a particular landmark is selected, the disease-specific score for this region can be calculated. To allow for expert feedback, one can adapt or confirm the estimated score.
- A module to assess and track user interactions via mouse movements, scrolls, and clicks within the three slice views can help to assess the thought process of a study participant or clinical expert while evaluating and analyzing volumetric data.

These modules are intended as examples and can be adapted or exchanged by custom implementations.

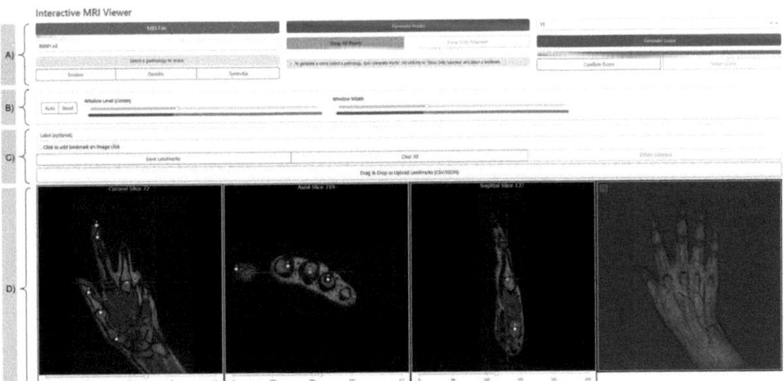

Fig. 1. Overview of the user interface setup. The interactive 3-D viewer includes several optional modules: A) automated landmark detection in hand MRI and automated scoring of pathologies, B) windowing for contrast enhancement, C) manual landmark annotation, D) volumetric rendering of the image, and the core module for multiplanar viewing.

2.2 Implementation

Our tool is implemented as a web-based application. It builds upon Dash, a Python-based framework for interactive data apps, using Plotly to generate interactive charts. The connection between the individual modules, callbacks, and functions is shown in Fig. 3. The backend uses Python with Flask handling the web server (WSGI). Dash callbacks coordinate the loading of NIfTI/DICOM files, adjust image brightness and contrast, create 2-D and 3-D views (via Plotly and dash_vtk), and update the interface. During an expert study setup, we employ an in-memory cache with asynchronous prefetch to minimize latency when loading a new image. All study outputs, such as questionnaire answers, mouse/scroll activity, and annotations, are saved to CSV/JSONL files.

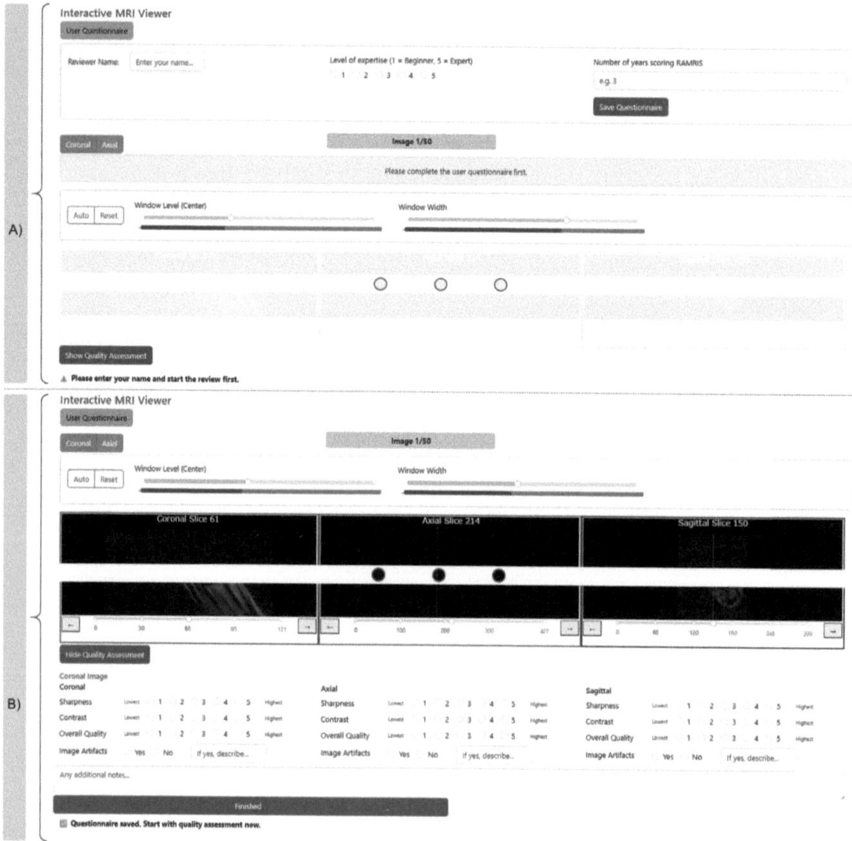

Fig. 2. Depiction of an exemplary expert questionnaire routine. A) First screen for a guided expert study, including a collapsible expert questionnaire and a masked out slice viewer. B) Second part of the expert study with collapsible quality assessment and expert feedback at the bottom.

2.2.1 Module-specific details.

Landmarks and annotations. The user can choose to display either all available landmarks or a single selected landmark. When selecting one landmark, all three views display it, and a rectangular bounding box is shown around the landmark.

Image loading. Different settings can be chosen for image loading. Either a predefined list of image paths can be loaded during a session, or an image can be loaded via drag and drop or via file selection in the explorer. Accordingly, different image formats like .nii, .nii.gz, .dcm, and zipped DICOM folders can be handled.

2-D slice views. The crosshair and landmarks are synced across 2-D views (Fig. 1). Clicking on a view updates the crosshair and the slices in the other views. Each 2-D view is framed in red, green, or blue, corresponding to the respective crosshairs across views. This enables precise localization of features across views.

Expert studies and questionnaires. This interactive viewer is designed to capture structured feedback from experts for a specific task. We emphasize the dynamic GUI progression for viewing and assessing images in a structured manner. A gated logic reduces user errors, such as unintended interactions or erroneously loaded images, and enables a uniform representation across multiple repetitions.

3 Results

To assess the usability of our proposed user interface, we performed a user study across four technical medical imaging experts and one clinical expert specialized in rheumatic disease. We introduced the viewer and the different modules to the users and gave them time to familiarize themselves with the system. They were asked to complete the first section of a predefined MR expert study for the evaluation of hand image quality and the assessment of inflammation in finger joints. They used the multiplanar viewer, interacted with the volume rendering, and used the other modules. After the participants explored the viewer, we asked them to fill out a user questionnaire based on the system usability scale (SUS) [7]. The SUS is a Likert scale

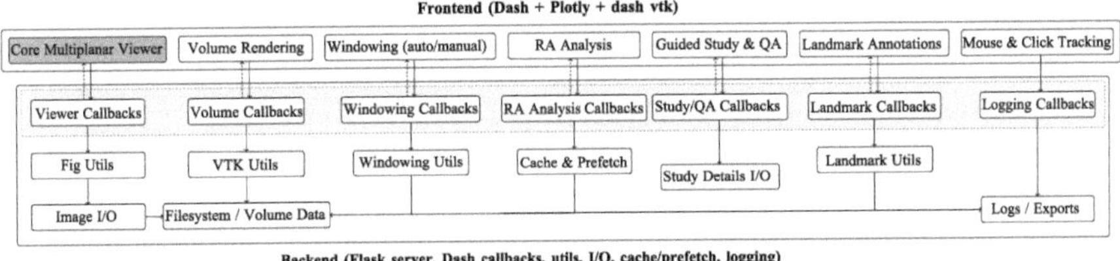

Fig. 3. Overview of backend and frontend, including main modules, callbacks, and functions. The multiplanar viewer module is highlighted in grey. All callbacks in light grey. Solid arrows: data/control flow; dashed arrows: GUI feedback.

that includes 10 predefined questions on a range of 1–5, alternating between positive and negative connotation to prevent user bias. The system usability is calculated by a predefined formula with a maximum value of 100 and an average value of 68. The SUS is not diagnostic, but it helps to indicate the general usability. Scores above 68 indicate acceptable usability, while scores above 80.8 correspond to an "A" grade on a standardized scale. In our assessment across all participants, we reached a mean SUS score of 90, corresponding to an A+ usability rating. In addition to the SUS, we asked the participants for general feedback on the GUI and possible improvements or additional modules. Participants suggested adding a progress indicator in each view during image loading and automatically resetting the zoom when changing the selected landmark. These improvements were subsequently implemented in the GUI. Additional ideas for future functionalities included maximum intensity projection visualization, a time module for 4-D visualization, faster response times, larger buttons in the questionnaire, and automated orientation correction to new settings. Users particularly appreciated the flexibility of our GUI, noting that it generalizes well to new images and is highly intuitive to use.

4 Discussion

We present the first web-based multiplanar viewer specifically designed for easy adaptation to a wide range of applications. The framework provides several modules that can be used out of the box or customized efficiently to meet specific requirements. The tool can be used for fast data exploration, landmark annotation, expert studies, including interaction tracking for better understanding of the participants' behavior, or interactive visualization of downstream tasks such as integration with trained models. In the future, the viewer can be extended for multi-user support, faster rendering speed, and support for time series data. The tool is released as open-source and runs directly in a web browser.

Acknowledgement. We acknowledge support by d.hip campus - Bavarian aim (Ma.S.) and HPC resources provided by the Erlangen National High Performance Computing Center (NHR@FAU) of FAU Erlangen-Nürnberg.

References

1. Slicer 3. 3D slicer image computing platform. 2025.
2. Wolf I, Vetter M, Wegner I, Nolden M, Bottger T, Hastenteufel M et al. The medical imaging interaction toolkit (MITK): a toolkit facilitating the creation of interactive software by extending VTK and ITK. Proc SPIE MI VIGPD. 2004:16.
3. Sullivan C, Kaszynski A. Pyvista: 3D plotting and mesh analysis through a streamlined interface for the visualization toolkit (VTK). J Open Source Softw. 2019;4(37):1450.
4. Pereira H, Romero L, Miguel Faria P. Web-based DICOM viewers: a survey and a performance classification. J Imaging Inform Med. 2025;38(3):1304–22.

5. Ziegler E, Urban T, Brown D, Petts J, Pieper SD, Lewis R et al. Open health imaging foundation viewer: an extensible open-source framework for building web-based imaging applications to support cancer research. JCO Clin Cancer Inform. 2020;4:336–45.
6. Hanayik T, Rorden C, Drake C, Ochsenmeier J, Zhang J, Taylor P et al. NiiVue: a WebGL2 based medical image viewer. J Open Source Softw. 2021.
7. Brooke J. SUS: a quick and dirty usability scale. Usability Evaluation In Industry. CRC Press, 1996:207–12.

Differentiable Approximate Truncation Robust CBCT Reconstruction via Known Operator Learning

Chengze Ye, Linda-Sophie Schneider, Yipeng Sun, Siyuan Mei, Siming Bayer, Paula A. Pérez-Toro, Andreas Maier

Pattern Recognition Lab, FAU Erlangen-Nürnberg
chengze.ye@fau.de

Abstract. The proposed algorithm is a differentiable approximate truncation robust computed tomography (ATRACT) reconstruction algorithm for end-to-end trainable cone-beam CT reconstruction, offering enhanced robustness to truncated geometries and a significant reduction of truncation artifacts. The proposed method utilizes known operator learning to map the analytical reconstruction into a neural network. This approach preserves physical consistency while enabling data-driven optimization of redundancy weights under the 180° limited-angle condition. The experimental results demonstrate that the proposed frame work surpasses the Parker-weighted analytical reconstruction, achieving a 1.5% higher SSIM and a 1.1% lower MSE. This outcome validates the accuracy and efficacy of the analytical-to-neural mapping procedure. The differentiable formulation integrates the interpretability of analytical reconstruction with the adaptability of learning-based methods, thereby providing a robust and extensible foundation for imaging applications under truncated geometries.

1 Introduction

In computed tomography (CT), analytical reconstruction algorithms such as filtered backprojection (FBP) and the Feldkamp-Davis-Kress (FDK) algorithm have been widely adopted due to their computational efficiency and closed-form solutions. However, these methods require complete projection data for accurate reconstruction and are highly sensitive to data truncation. The underlying one-dimensional ramp (or Ram-Lak) kernel employed in FBP represents a global filter. When convolved with truncated projection data, this kernel can severely degrade reconstruction quality. This limitation is particularly pronounced in cone-beam C-arm systems utilized for interventional and low-dose imaging, where acquiring a full set of projections is often infeasible due to mechanical or radiation constraints. These challenges have motivated the development of reconstruction methods that are more robust to truncated data.

To address this issue, Dennerlein and Maier [1] introduced the approximate truncation robust computed tomography (ATRACT), which enables region-of-interest

© Der/die Autor(en), exklusiv lizenziert an
Springer Fachmedien Wiesbaden GmbH, ein Teil von Springer Nature 2026
H. Handels et al. (Hrsg.), *Bildverarbeitung für die Medizin 2026*,
Informatik aktuell, https://doi.org/10.1007/978-3-658-51100-5_64

(ROI) reconstruction from truncated cone-beam data without relying on prior object information.

In recent years, deep learning has seen a surge in applications in CT reconstruction and artifact reduction, signifying its considerable potential in enhancing image quality. However, for complex inverse problems such as cone-beam CT, directly mapping raw projection data to volumetric images typically requires a substantial number of trainable parameters and extensive training datasets, which can result in decreased interpretability. To address these challenges, Maier et al. [2] proposed the concept of known operator learning, which incorporates physically interpretable operators into neural networks. This approach has been shown to significantly reduce the number of learnable parameters, accelerate convergence, and provide theoretical guarantees on maximum error bounds.

In this study, we present a differentiable ATRACT reconstruction framework that connects analytical modeling with data-driven optimization. The known operator learning method is used to map the analytical ATRACT reconstruction to a neural network representation. This approach preserves robustness under truncated geometries while enabling adaptive learning of redundancy weights. This work provides a foundation for interpretable and trainable CT reconstruction frameworks suitable for practical clinical imaging scenarios.

2 Materials and methods

2.1 ATRACT

Building upon the conventional Feldkamp-Davis-Kress (FDK) algorithm, Dennerlein and Maier [1] reformulated the reconstruction process to achieve improved robustness against laterally truncated projection data. Their method introduces a 2D filtering scheme derived from a reformulation of the classical 1D ramp filter. The reconstruction pipeline can be summarized as follows.

First, the projection data are pre-weighted to compensate for the divergent beam geometry

$$g_1(\lambda, u, v) = \frac{D\, m(\lambda, u)}{\sqrt{D^2 + u^2 + v^2}}\, g(\lambda, u, v) \tag{1}$$

where $g(\lambda, u, v)$ denotes the measured projection data at projection angle λ, (u, v) correspond to the detector coordinates, D is the source-to-detector distance, and the weighting term $m(\lambda, u)$ is replaced by a Parker-like function for short-scan to compensate for redundancy.

Next, a 2D Laplacian operator is applied to enhance high-frequency components

$$g_2(\lambda, u, v) = \left(\frac{\partial^2}{\partial u^2} + \frac{\partial^2}{\partial v^2}\right) g_1(\lambda, u, v) \tag{2}$$

The filtered projection is then obtained by performing a 2D Radon-based filtering operation, which can be efficiently implemented as a 2D convolution with a shift-invariant kernel $h_{2d}(u, v)$

$$g_F^{2D}(\lambda, u, v) = \int_{u_1}^{u_2} \int_{v_1}^{v_2} g_2(\lambda, u', v') h_{2D}(u - u', v - v')\, du'\, dv' \quad (3)$$

In practice, this convolution is computed using fast Fourier transform-based circular convolution, which substantially reduces computational effort compared to direct spatial-domain filtering. Finally, the reconstructed voxel intensity is obtained by backprojection of the filtered projections.

2.2 Differentiable ATRACT

Building on the analytical ATRACT reconstruction algorithm (Section 2.1), this section extends ATRACT into a differentiable framework using known operator learning [2]. This enables an end-to-end trainable reconstruction network that preserves physical-model constraints while leveraging data-driven optimization to adaptively learn redundancy weights from the actual projection-data redundancy.

As Eq. 1 demonstrates, the initial phase of the analytical algorithm involves cosine and redundancy weighting. We express these operations as two differentiable weighting layers, denoted as W_{cos} and W_{red}, respectively. In the differentiable implementation, W_{cos} corresponds to the fixed cosine weighting, while W_{red} is defined as a trainable layer that adaptively learns redundancy weights from data to compensate for the incomplete angular coverage in short-scan acquisitions.

The second and third components of the analytical pipeline, corresponding to Eq. 2 and 3 in Section 2.1, map to 2D Laplace filtering L and 2D residual filtering layers C, respectively. We formulate both operations as differentiable convolution layers with Laplacian and residual kernels.

Finally, a differentiable 3D backprojection layer $A_{3\text{d}}^{\text{T}}$ maps the filtered projections back into the volumetric domain. To ensure physically meaningful reconstructions, we apply a non-negativity constraint in the final layer of the network.

The reconstruction pipeline forms a neural network representation by assembling the above differentiable operators in the same order as the analytical algorithm, resulting in

$$f(x) = W_{\text{cos}} W_{\text{red}} L C A_{3\text{d}}^{\text{Tg}}(\lambda, u, v) \quad (4)$$

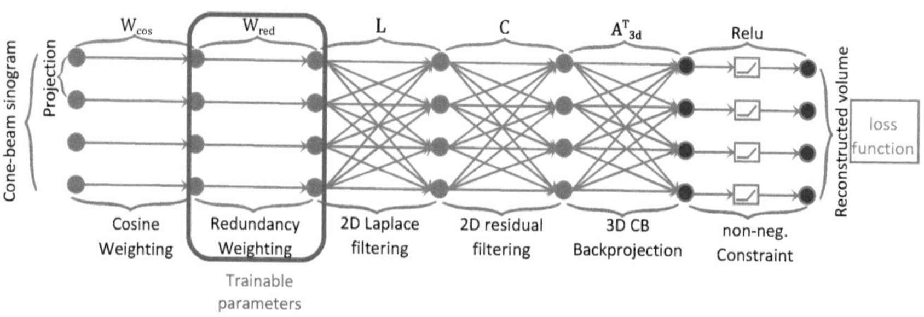

Fig. 1. Differentiable ATRACT framework architecture.

where f(x) denotes the reconstructed volume. This representation, illustrated schematically in Fig. 1, preserves the physics-based structure of the original analytical model and introduces trainable components optimized through backpropagation.

2.3 Experiments

2.3.1 Geometry configuration. To evaluate the stability and robustness of the differentiable ATRACT framework, we used a clinical C-arm system (Artis zeego, Siemens Healthineers AG, Forchheim, Germany). The flat-panel detector runs in 4×4 binning, yielding 620×480 pixels with 0.616 mm isotropic pixel size. The source-detector distance is 1200 mm, and the source-isocentre distance is 750 mm. The reconstructed volume contains $128 \times 512 \times 512$ voxels with 0.25 mm isotropic spacing.

2.3.2 Data preparation. We train the proposed model on a simulated dataset and subsequently evaluate it on real clinical data. Adopting the procedure of [5], this study generates 30 simulated samples and allocates 24 for training and 6 for validation. During training, the network input comprises 180° limited-angle sinograms with a total of 360 projections, whereas the corresponding ground-truth volumes are reconstructed from 360° full-scan acquisitions with 720 projections. For quantitative evaluation on real data, we select five patient cases from the Pancreatic-CT-CBCT-SEG dataset [6]. Using the Pyro-NN framework [7] and the same system geometry as in the simulation stage, we generate the respective cone-beam forward projections. We fed the resulting forward-projection sinograms as input to the pretrained network for evaluation. The network reconstructs the volumes, and we compare these volumes with the corresponding clinical ground-truth volumes.

2.3.3 Implementation details. We implement the proposed method in PyTorch 2.1.1 and train it on an NVIDIA A40 GPU. The 3D cone-beam backprojection relies on differentiable operators from the PyroNN framework [7]. To enforce spatial smoothness of the learned redundancy weights, we add a Gaussian smoothing layer

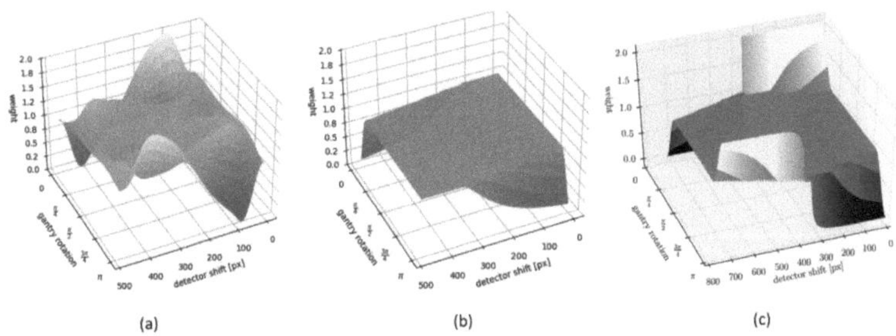

Fig. 2. Presentation of redundancy weights: (a) Learned weights by our proposed method (b) Parker weights. (c) Weights as proposed by Riess et al. [3, 4].

(σ = 20, kernel size = 121) after the redundancy-weight layer. All weights are initialized to one before training. Training uses mean squared error (MSE) loss, and we optimize the parameters with the Adam optimizer following a one-cycle learning-rate schedule ranging from 0.001 to 0.01 over 50 epochs.

3 Results

After 110 epochs, the network reached convergence. Fig. 2 presents the learned redundancy weights obtained from the proposed differentiable ATRACT model. For reference, we also show the Parker weights and the weights proposed by Riess et al. [3, 4]. The similarity to the weights of Riess et al. suggests that the network effectively learned a redundancy weighting pattern consistent with the underlying imaging geometry.

The corresponding reconstruction results are presented in Fig. 3. Reconstruction with learned redundancy weights yields noticeably more homogeneous images than the Parker-weighted result. Furthermore, compared to the FDK reconstruction shown in Fig. 2 (a), the differentiable ATRACT method effectively reduces truncation artifacts.

Complementing the visual results, Table 1 summarizes quantitative observations, including MSE, peak signal-to-noise ratio (PSNR), and structural similarity index measure (SSIM). The proposed method achieves lower MSE and higher PSNR and SSIM values than the Parker weighted model, indicating an improvement in overall reconstruction quality.

4 Discussion

The experimental results confirm the ability of the proposed differentiable ATRACT model to learn meaningful redundancy weighting patterns, thereby verifying the correctness of gradient backpropagation through the pipeline. This demonstrates that

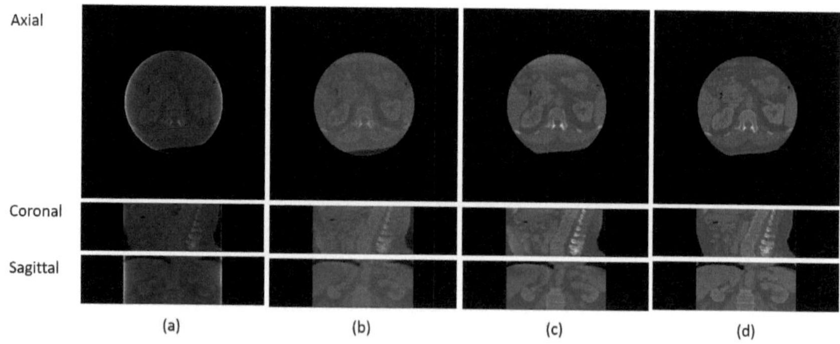

Fig. 3. Reconstructed results. (a) FDK reconstruction. (b) ATRACT using Parker weights. (c) ATRACT using the learned weights. (d) Ground truth.

Tab. 1. Comparison of Image Quality Metrics with Mean ± Standard Deviation.

	MSE↓	PSNR (dB)↑	SSIM↑
Learned	0.4369 ± 0.1089	23.74 ± 1.62	0.8773 ± 0.0127
Parker weight	0.4424 ± 0.1163	23.67 ± 1.64	0.8642 ± 0.0130

the analytical-to-neural mapping preserves differentiability across all reconstruction stages and ensures stable end-to-end optimization. In addition, the proposed framework preserves the fundamental physical principles and geometric constraints of analytical reconstruction, thereby ensuring interpretability. Furthermore, in comparison with the differentiable FDK framework, our model demonstrates enhanced robustness to truncated geometries. The proposed approach offers a flexible foundation for dual-domain optimization under truncated geometric conditions and can be seamlessly integrated with upstream tasks (e.g., calibration) and downstream tasks (e.g., segmentation). Subsequent research will focus on exploring the potential applications of this framework to more specialized imaging tasks.

Acknowledgement. The authors gratefully acknowledge the scientific support and HPC resources provided by the Erlangen National High Performance Computing Center (NHR@FAU) of the FAU Erlangen-Nürnberg.

References

1. Dennerlein F, Maier A. Approximate truncation robust computed tomography-ATRACT. Phys Med Biol. 2013;58(17):6133.
2. Maier AK, Syben C, Stimpel B, Würfl T, Hoffmann M, Schebesch F et al. Learning with known operators reduces maximum error bounds. Nat Mach Intell. 2019;1(8):373–80.
3. Riess C, Berger M, Wu H, Manhart M, Fahrig R, Maier A. TV or not TV? That is the question. Proc NYSDS. 2013:341–4.
4. Würfl T, Hoffmann M, Christlein V, Breininger K, Huang Y, Unberath M et al. Deep learning computed tomography: learning projection-domain weights from image domain in limited angle problems. IEEE Trans Med Imaging. 2018;37(6):1454–63.
5. Ye C, Schneider LS, Sun Y, Thies M, Mei S, Maier A. DRACO: differentiable reconstruction for arbitrary CBCT orbits. Phys Med Biol. 2025;70(7):075005.
6. Hong J, Reyngold M, Crane C, Cuaron J, Hajj C, Mann J et al. Breath-hold CT and cone-beam CT images with expert manual organ-at-risk segmentations from radiation treatments of locally advanced pancreatic cancer [Data set]. Cancer Imaging Arch. 2021.
7. Syben C, Michen M, Stimpel B, Seitz S, Ploner S, Maier AK. PYRO-NN: Python reconstruction operators in neural networks. Med Phys Mex Symp Med Phys. 2019;46(11):5110–5.

Abstract: DRACO
Differentiable Reconstruction for Arbitrary CBCT Orbits

Chengze Ye, Linda-Sophie Schneider, Yipeng Sun, Mareike Thies, Siyuan Mei, Andreas Maier

Pattern Recognition Lab, FAU Erlangen-Nürnberg
chengze.ye@fau.de

Objective: this study introduces a novel method for reconstructing cone beam computed tomography (CBCT) images for arbitrary orbits [1], addressing the computational and memory challenges associated with traditional iterative reconstruction algorithms. Approach: the proposed method employs a differentiable shift-variant filtered backprojection neural network, optimized for arbitrary trajectories. By integrating known operators into the learning model, the approach minimizes the number of trainable parameters while enhancing model interpretability. This framework adapts seamlessly to specific orbit geometries, including non-continuous trajectories such as circular-plus-arc or sinusoidal paths, enabling faster and more accurate CBCT reconstructions. Main results: experimental validation demonstrates that the method significantly accelerates reconstruction, reducing computation time by over 97% compared to conventional iterative algorithms. It achieves superior or comparable image quality with reduced noise, as evidenced by a 38.6% reduction in mean squared error, a 7.7% increase in peak signal-to-noise ratio, and a 5.0% improvement in the structural similarity index measure. The flexibility and robustness of the approach are confirmed through its ability to handle data from diverse scan geometries. Significance: this method represents a significant advancement in interventional medical imaging, particularly for robotic C-arm CT systems, enabling real-time, high-quality CBCT reconstructions for customized orbits. It offers a transformative solution for clinical applications requiring computational efficiency and precision in imaging. Code availability: code is available at `https://github.com/ChengzeYe/Defrise-and-Clack-reconstruction`.

References

1. Ye C, Schneider LS, Sun Y, Thies M, Mei S, Maier A. DRACO: differentiable reconstruction for arbitrary CBCT orbits. Phys Med Biol. 2025;70(7):075005.

© Der/die Autor(en), exklusiv lizenziert an
Springer Fachmedien Wiesbaden GmbH, ein Teil von Springer Nature 2026
H. Handels et al. (Hrsg.), *Bildverarbeitung für die Medizin 2026*,
Informatik aktuell, https://doi.org/10.1007/978-3-658-51100-5_65

Abstract: Bake Your Phantom

Low-cost Recipes for Dough-based, Tissue-mimicking CT Phantoms

Sonja Wichelmann[1], Florian Weiler[1], Thomas Friedrich[2], Joerg Barkhausen[3], Roman Kloeckner[4], Franz Wegner[2,4], Malte M. Sieren[3,4]

[1]Fraunhofer Institute for Digital Medicine MEVIS, Lübeck / Bremen
[2]Fraunhofer Research Institution for Individualized and Cell-Based Medical Engineering IMTE, Lübeck
[3]Institute of Radiology and Nuclear Medicine, UKSH, Lübeck, Germany
[4]Institute of Interventional Radiology, UKSH, Lübeck, Germany
sonja.wichelmann@mevis.fraunhofer.de

Phantoms are an essential tool for conducting research experiments, quality control and teaching with radiation based imaging devices. While many phantoms are commercially available, their widespread use is limited by manufacturing complexity, high costs and lack of modification options. Also, 3D printing techniques exist for creating CT phantoms, but they require expensive equipment and the printing can be time-consuming. In [1], a study was performed to demonstrate a dough-based method to create customizable, realistic CT phantoms using affordable, readily available ingredients. For this study, various doughs composed of flour, salt, water, and oil were created, scanned, and evaluated with CT scans. The effects of storage conditions, preservation, and temperature were analyzed. As an example, a liver was segmented from a 3D CT scan, scaled to 1:2, a negative mold was printed and it was filled with the most suitable dough. The evaluation of the scanned ingredients and doughs show that Hounsfield unit (HU) values ranging from below −200 HU to above 1200 HU can be achieved. Based on the analysis, simple recipes are proposed to replicate radiodensities of different anatomical structures. The results from the liver phantom confirm the feasibility of mimicking liver tissue and morphology. CT phantoms imitating human tissues can be created using simple recipes, as demonstrated with our liver CT phantom. Refrigeration or freezing extends the usability, but temperature effects must be considered to ensure accurate HU values in CT scans. This approach holds substantial promise for expanding access to affordable, customizable CT phantoms and has various potential applications such as experimental research, test data generation for evaluating image processing algorithms and training.

© Der/die Autor(en), exklusiv lizenziert an
Springer Fachmedien Wiesbaden GmbH, ein Teil von Springer Nature 2026
H. Handels et al. (Hrsg.), *Bildverarbeitung für die Medizin 2026*,
Informatik aktuell, https://doi.org/10.1007/978-3-658-51100-5_66

References

1. Wichelmann S, Weiler F, Friedrich T, Barkhausen J, Kloeckner R, Wegner F et al. Bake your phantom: low-cost recipes for dough-based, tissue-mimicking CT phantoms. Eur Radiol. 2025:1–11.

AI-based Dual-domain Framework for Gridline Suppression in Digital Radiography

Shadi Khamseh [1,2], Florian Wolz [2], Joshua Scheuplein [1], Thorsten Ergler[2], Andreas Maier [1]

[1]Pattern Recognition Lab, Department of Computer Science, Friedrich-Alexander-Universität Erlangen-Nürnberg, Erlangen, Germany
[2]Diagnostic Imaging, Siemens Healthineers AG, Forchheim, Germany
`shadi.khamseh@fau.de`

Abstract. Anti-scatter grids enhance image contrast in digital radiography but can introduce gridline artifacts when grid and detector sampling frequencies misalign. We propose a dual-domain AI framework that integrates a frozen DINO Vision Transformer with a FiLM-conditioned U-Net, combining global semantic encoding with frequency-aware reconstruction. The DINO embeddings modulate U-Net activations via Feature-wise Linear Modulation, enabling anatomically consistent correction through the joint prediction of a spatial residual and a frequency-domain attenuation mask, which are adaptively fused to suppress gridline artifacts while preserving tone and structural detail. A physics-based synthetic dataset comprising 1,475 clean and 4,425 grid-contaminated radiographs was generated from real detector captures. On 555 test images with available clean references, the model achieved a mean PSNR of 36.9 dB and an SSIM of 0.98, demonstrating high-fidelity and structurally consistent reconstruction across varying grid frequencies and exposure conditions.

1 Introduction

Anti-scatter grids are widely used in digital radiography to reduce scattered radiation and enhance image contrast at clinically acceptable dose levels [1]. When the spatial frequency of the grid approaches the detector sampling frequency, aliasing effects may arise, producing visible gridline interference patterns in reconstructed images [2]. Such artifacts result from partial spectral overlap between grid and detector lattices and may be exacerbated by grid tilt or rotational misalignment [3]. Because grid-related frequencies can overlap with anatomical structures, conventional filtering methods often fail to remove these artifacts without degrading diagnostic detail.

Deep learning has emerged as an effective tool for artifact reduction and image restoration in medical imaging [4, 5]. Convolutional architectures such as U-Net [6] perform well in many reconstruction tasks but primarily operate in the spatial domain, limiting their ability to address structured periodic artifacts [7, 8]. Hybrid

© Der/die Autor(en), exklusiv lizenziert an
Springer Fachmedien Wiesbaden GmbH, ein Teil von Springer Nature 2026
H. Handels et al. (Hrsg.), *Bildverarbeitung für die Medizin 2026*,
Informatik aktuell, https://doi.org/10.1007/978-3-658-51100-5_67

spatial–frequency approaches improve robustness by explicitly modeling spectral components [5, 7, 8]; however, most existing methods rely on local receptive fields and lack global semantic awareness, which is essential for distinguishing grid artifacts from anatomically meaningful patterns across varying acquisition conditions.

Vision transformers (ViTs) pretrained with the self-supervised DINO framework [9] learn globally coherent representations that capture long-range dependencies and semantic structure. Feature-wise linear modulation (FiLM) [10] enables efficient conditioning of convolutional networks using such global context by modulating intermediate activations through learned scaling and shifting parameters.

Building on these insights, we propose a dual-domain gridline suppression framework that integrates global semantic representations from a frozen DINO encoder with the local reconstruction capability of a FiLM-conditioned U-Net. The model jointly predicts a spatial residual and a frequency-domain attenuation mask, which are adaptively fused to suppress grid-induced artifacts while preserving anatomical structure, tone, and contrast.

We (i) introduce a dual-domain gridline suppression framework combining global semantic encoding with FiLM-based modulation, (ii) design an adaptive fusion of spatial and frequency components conditioned by semantic context for tone-preserving correction, and (iii) construct a physically realistic dataset with quantitative evaluation demonstrating robust gridline suppression across varying frequencies and exposure conditions.

2 Materials and methods

2.1 Dataset

A dataset of 1,475 clean clinical radiographs and 4,425 corresponding gridline-contaminated images was prepared for model training and evaluation. The clean radiographs were acquired using a single digital radiography detector under consistent clinical acquisition protocols and anonymized in compliance with institutional data protection guidelines. To enable controlled training and quantitative evaluation with reliable clean references, gridline artifacts were synthesized using a physically motivated grid extraction and application procedure rather than relying on paired acquisitions alone. This approach allows precise control over grid characteristics while preserving anatomical realism (Fig. 1).

2.1.1 Stage 1: Extraction of grid masks. Grid patterns were derived from detector captures acquired with and without an anti-scatter grid under identical exposure settings. A logarithmic ratio formulation was employed to isolate the multiplicative periodic grid modulation while suppressing low-frequency illumination trends such as the heel effect. This process preserves the original spatial frequency, phase, and orientation of the stationary grid while separating it from anatomical content. The resulting grid masks were normalized to unit mean within a central detector region to ensure consistent overall brightness across synthesized images.

2.1.2 Stage 2: Synthesis of gridline images. Each clean radiograph was multiplied by a randomly selected grid mask, reflecting the multiplicative nature of grid formation in digital radiography. To avoid boundary artifacts during training and inference, the grid-modulated images were smoothly blended using a Tukey window. Grid contrast was subsequently adjusted to maintain clinically realistic brightness and highlight levels, yielding tone-stable gridline images across multiple grid frequencies and acquisition conditions.

The dataset was deterministically split into training, validation, and test subsets, with 555 test images reserved exclusively for quantitative evaluation using available clean reference images. The dataset is not publicly released due to clinical data protection and institutional restrictions.

2.2 Model architecture and training

The proposed framework performs gridline removal through a dual-domain design that combines semantic understanding with frequency-aware reconstruction. It integrates a frozen DINO encoder with a FiLM-conditioned U-Net to jointly exploit global contextual information and localized feature restoration. This design bridges semantic perception and spectral filtering, enabling the model to address both periodic grid artifacts and non-periodic anatomical structures within a unified formulation.

2.2.1 Architecture. A vision transformer small (ViT-S/16) pretrained using the self-supervised DINOv1 framework [9] is used as a frozen feature extractor to encode global radiographic structure, illumination context, and coarse anatomical composition. Its latent representation is injected into the U-Net through Feature-wise linear modulation (FiLM), where layer-dependent scaling and shifting parameters condition intermediate convolutional activations.

This modulation allows the U-Net to adapt its feature processing dynamically based on global semantic context, without introducing additional spatial mixing.

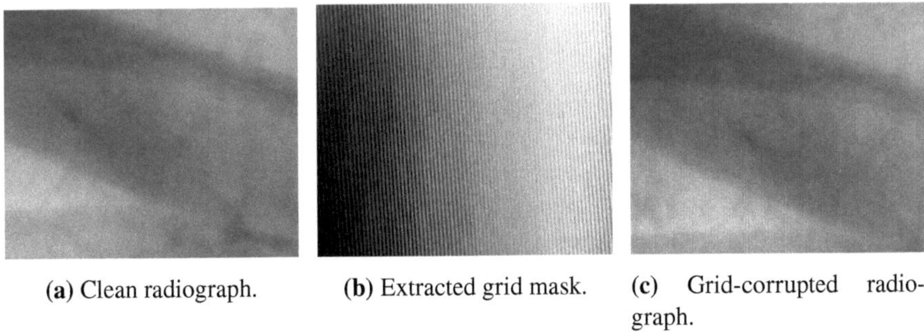

(a) Clean radiograph. **(b)** Extracted grid mask. **(c)** Grid-corrupted radiograph.

Fig. 1. Dataset generation: (a) clean radiograph, (b) extracted grid mask, and (c) resulting gridline-corrupted image.

The network produces two complementary outputs: a frequency-domain attenuation mask, designed to selectively suppress periodic grid components, and a spatial residual responsible for fine-detail recovery. An adaptive fusion of both domains, followed by tone normalization, ensures anatomically faithful and contrast-consistent reconstruction.

2.2.2 Training strategy. Model optimization is performed end-to-end using paired grid-contaminated and clean radiographs (Fig. 2). To encourage frequency-selective suppression, training includes FFT-derived regularization that emphasizes gridline frequency bands. The ViT-S/16 encoder pretrained with the self-supervised DINO v1 framework remains frozen, while the FiLM-conditioned U-Net is optimized. A composite objective combining ℓ_1 reconstruction, gradient consistency, high-frequency FFT loss, and spectral wedge regularization enforces accurate, tone-stable reconstruction. This formulation yields robust gridline suppression across varying grid frequencies and exposure conditions.

3 Results

The proposed framework was evaluated on a held-out test set of 555 radiographs with available clean reference images. Quantitative results are summarized in Tab. 1. The input grid-contaminated images exhibit pronounced periodic interference patterns and reduced structural similarity, motivating targeted gridline suppression while preserving anatomical content.

High-fidelity reconstruction was achieved, with mean/median PSNR values of 36.91/36.54 dB and MS-SSIM values of 0.989/0.993 on the held-out test set. These results indicate strong pixel-wise agreement and excellent tone preservation with respect to the clean reference images. For context, Pavitha et al. [5] reported learning-based gridline artifact suppression using a CNN operating primarily in the spatial domain. Because datasets, acquisition settings, and evaluation protocols differ, a direct quantitative comparison is not possible; nevertheless, the consistently high PSNR and MS-SSIM values observed here support robust reconstruction fidelity under grid-contaminated conditions.

Spectral analysis further demonstrates the selective nature of the proposed method. A mean grid-band attenuation of −0.138 dB indicates targeted suppression of periodic grid-frequency components, while the off-band spectral shift remains limited to +0.419 dB. This behavior confirms that the model attenuates grid-induced frequencies without introducing excessive distortion into non-periodic anatomical structures, consistent with the intended frequency-aware design.

Edge-based metrics characterize the balance between artifact removal and detail preservation. The low Sobel-MAE value of 0.0123 reflects strong gradient consistency with the clean reference images, while an edge-F1-score of 0.441 indicates controlled smoothing that avoids excessive edge degradation. No checkerboard or tiling artifacts were observed, as confirmed by a checkerboard index of 0.999, validating the stability of the tiled inference procedure.

The proposed framework effectively suppresses gridline artifacts while maintaining anatomical sharpness and contrast (Fig. 3). Fine structures such as bone edges and soft-tissue gradients remain visually consistent with the clean references, indicating minimal loss of diagnostic information. Overall, the results demonstrate robust performance across varying grid frequencies and exposure conditions within the evaluated dataset.

4 Discussion

The results demonstrate that the proposed dual-domain framework effectively suppresses gridline artifacts while maintaining diagnostic image quality (Tab. 1). The consistently high PSNR (36.91 dB) and MS-SSIM (0.989) values indicate strong

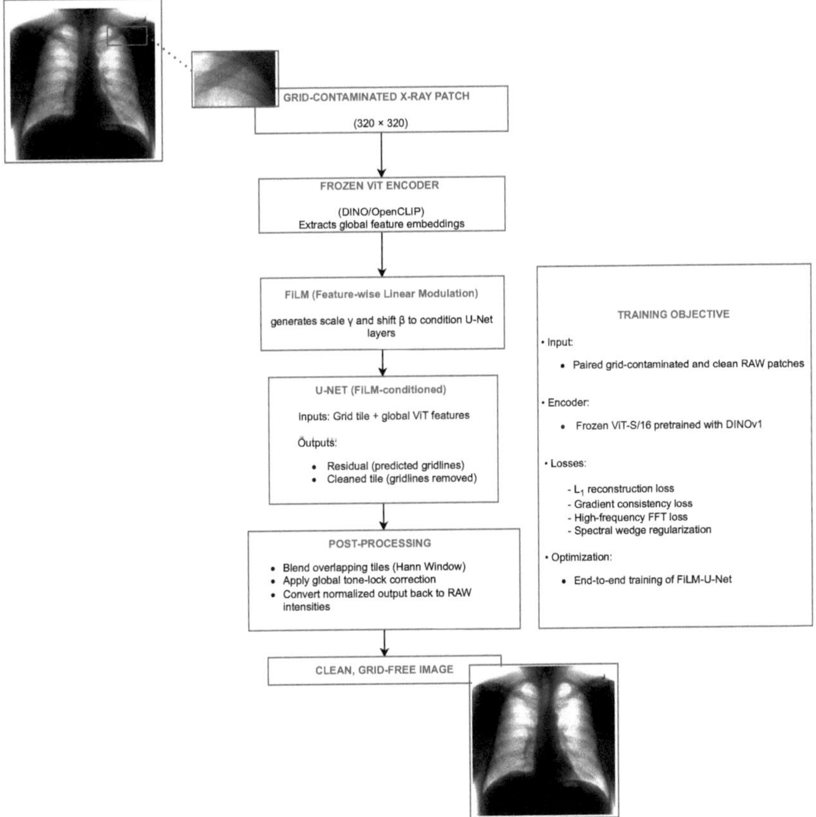

Fig. 2. Overview of the proposed DINO-conditioned FiLM-U-Net framework. Left: inference pipeline combining semantic conditioning and dual-domain reconstruction. Right: training objective and loss formulation used for end-to-end optimization.

Tab. 1. Quantitative evaluation of the proposed gridline-removal model on 555 test radiographs. Mean and median values demonstrate high image fidelity, selective spectral attenuation, and minimal artifact presence.

Metric	Mean	Median	Interpretation
Image fidelity			
PSNR [dB]	36.91	36.54	High reconstruction fidelity
SSIM	0.961	0.981	Strong structural similarity
MS-SSIM	0.989	0.993	Excellent tone preservation
Spectral behavior			
Grid-band Δ dB	-0.138	-0.107	Grid suppression strength
Off-band Δ dB	+0.419	+0.238	Minimal anatomical distortion
Gradients and edges			
Sobel-MAE	0.0123	–	Edge consistency (lower is better)
Edge-F1	0.441	0.392	Sharpness and contour recovery
Artifacts			
Checkerboard index	0.999	0.999	No tiling artifacts

reconstruction fidelity and excellent tone preservation across varying grid frequencies and exposure conditions. These results are consistent with, and in some cases exceed, the performance reported by recent learning-based approaches for gridline artifact suppression, such as the hybrid spatial–frequency CNN proposed by Pavitha et al. [5], while additionally incorporating explicit frequency-aware modeling and global semantic conditioning.

Frequency-domain analysis shows that the proposed method selectively attenuates grid-related spectral components, as reflected by the negative grid-band shift, while introducing only minimal changes in non-grid frequency regions. In contrast, classical notch or band-stop filtering approaches are known to apply indiscriminate frequency suppression, which can lead to loss of anatomical detail when grid frequencies overlap with structural content [2, 3]. The limited off-band spectral shift

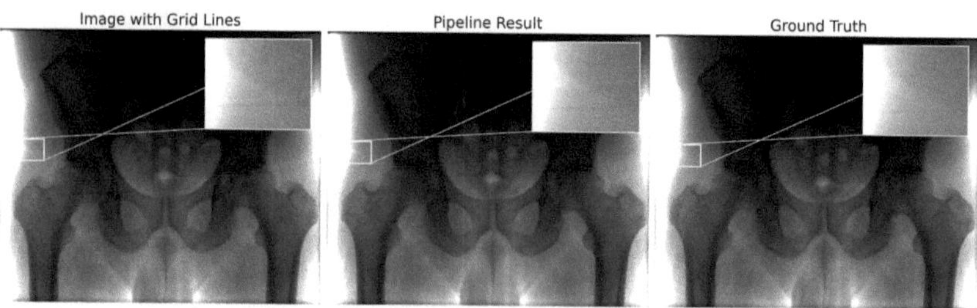

Fig. 3. Visual comparison of gridline removal results. From left to right: (a) input image with visible gridline artifacts, (b) reconstructed output produced by the proposed framework, and (c) clean reference radiograph. Insets highlight effective suppression of gridline patterns while preserving anatomical detail and tone consistency.

observed for the proposed method suggests improved preservation of diagnostically relevant frequencies.

Edge-based evaluations further highlight the balanced behavior of the proposed framework. The low Sobel-MAE indicates stable gradient reconstruction, while the edge-F1-score reflects a conservative trade-off between artifact removal and edge sharpness. Visual inspection confirms that the DINO-guided FiLM conditioning effectively integrates global semantic context into the reconstruction process, reducing residual grid patterns without introducing blurring or texture loss commonly observed in baseline methods.

Compared to purely spatial or hybrid spatial–frequency CNNs, the explicit incorporation of global semantic conditioning enables the model to better distinguish structured grid artifacts from anatomical features across varying acquisition conditions. These findings support the effectiveness of combining global context with frequency-aware local reconstruction for robust gridline suppression.

Future work will focus on enhancing edge sharpness through adaptive spatial–spectral weighting and extending the evaluation to additional detector types and grid geometries to further assess clinical generalization.

Disclaimer. The clinical radiographs used in this study were provided by Siemens Healthineers AG within an internal research collaboration. The dataset is proprietary and not publicly available due to corporate policies and patient data protection regulations. The views and conclusions expressed in this work are those of the authors and do not necessarily reflect the views of Siemens Healthineers.

References

1. Tanaka N, Yoon Y. Effect of anti-scatter grids on the image improvement factor in digital radiography for various phantom thicknesses and irradiation fields. Phys Eng Sci Med. 2023;46(3):1187–92.
2. Lin CY, Lee WJ, Chen SJ, Tsai CH, Lee JH, Chang CH et al. A study of grid artifacts formation and elimination in computed radiographic images. J Digit Imaging. 2006;19(4):351–61.
3. Kim DS, Lee S. Grid artifact reduction for direct digital radiography detectors based on rotated stationary grids with homomorphic filtering. Med Phys Mex Symp Med Phys. 2013;40(6):061905.
4. Litjens G, Kooi T, Bejnordi BE, Setio AAA, Ciompi F, Ghafoorian M et al. A survey on deep learning in medical image analysis. Int J Comput Exp Sci Eng. 2017;42:60–88.
5. Pavitha US, Nikhila S, Mohan M. Hybrid deep learning based model for removing grid-line artifacts from radiographical images. Proc IJCESEN. 2024;10(4):763–74.
6. Ronneberger O, Fischer P, Brox T. U-net: convolutional networks for biomedical image segmentation. Proc MICCAI. 2015;9351:234–41.
7. Sheng Z, Liu X, Cao SY, Shen HL, Zhang H. Frequency-domain deep guided image denoising. IEEE Trans Multimedia. 2023;25:6767–81.
8. Zhang Q, Hu Z, Jiang C, Zheng H, Ge Y, Liang D. Artifact removal using a hybrid-domain convolutional neural network for limited-angle computed tomography imaging. Phys Med Biol. 2020;65(15):155010.

9. Caron M, Touvron H, Misra I, Jégou H, Mairal J, Bojanowski P et al. Emerging properties in self-supervised vision transformers. Proc IEEE/CVF ICCV. 2021:9650–60.
10. Perez E, Strub F, de Vries H, Dumoulin V, Courville A. FiLM: visual reasoning with a general conditioning layer. Proc AAAI CAI. 2018;32(1).

Evaluation of Time-of-flight Camera Positioning for AI-based Patient Pose Assessment in Radiography

Manuel Laufer[1], Julius Haas[1], Dominik Mairhöfer[1], Malte Sieren[2], Hauke Gerdes[2], Fabio Leal dos Reis[2], Arpad Bischof[2,3], Thomas Käster[4], Erhardt Barth[1], Jörg Barkhausen[2], Thomas Martinetz[1]

[1]Institute for Neuro- and Bioinformatics, University of Lübeck
[2]Institute of Radiology and Nuclear Medicine, University Medical Center Schleswig-Holstein
[3]IMAGE Information Systems Europe GmbH, Rostock
[4]Pattern Recognition Company GmbH, Lübeck
m.laufer@uni-luebeck.de

Abstract. In recent years, medical technology companies have increasingly been integrating time-of-flight cameras into their X-ray devices to support optimal collimation and the patient positioning process. However, for many hospitals, it is not financially viable to acquire a new X-ray device with such a camera for those features. In order to still have support for e.g. patient positioning, without having to buy a new X-ray device and be dependent on proprietary algorithms, it is possible to only acquire a time-of-flight camera, attach it to the X-ray device, and use custom algorithms. In this work, we evaluated the ideal camera position for AI-supported patient pose assessment based on depth images for such a setup and assessed the usefulness of a setup with multiple cameras. For this, we generated a total of 461,550 synthetic depth images from CT scans from 50 different camera positions and synthetic radiographs in order to investigate in 1,500 experiments how accurately patients' poses can be assessed with different camera positions. We found that a camera position perpendicular to the target anatomy being radiographed is particularly well suited, and that adding a second camera does not significantly improve performance.

1 Introduction

Incorrect positioning of the patient during the X-ray examination is one of the main reasons for the need of a retake due to the inadequate diagnostic quality of the resulting radiograph [1]. Retaking a radiograph implies avoidable additional exposure of the patient to radiation and costs the hospital time and money. Since furthermore the positioning process is not standardized and depends heavily on the patient and the experience of the radiographer, a system that automatically assesses the patient's pose before the radiograph is taken could help reduce or prevent retakes and ensure quality standards. In order to be able to potentially support the

© Der/die Autor(en), exklusiv lizenziert an Springer Fachmedien Wiesbaden GmbH, ein Teil von Springer Nature 2026
H. Handels et al. (Hrsg.), *Bildverarbeitung für die Medizin 2026*, Informatik aktuell, https://doi.org/10.1007/978-3-658-51100-5_68

positioning process, medical technology companies have been integrating time-of-flight (ToF) cameras into their X-ray devices in recent years. However, many hospitals cannot afford to acquire a new X-ray device or carry out expensive upgrades for these features, and potentially pay for proprietary algorithms. A more cost-effective alternative, that still enables positioning support, is to purchase a standalone ToF camera and integrate it into the positioning process along with custom algorithms for pose assessment. Furthermore, our recent research showed that it is possible to attach ToF cameras to X-ray devices in order to improve the X-ray process, including, in particular, assessing patients' poses using depth images [2–4]. In our work we have only chosen few camera positions that are easy to implement in practice, but for these systems it is necessary to determine which position of the camera relative to the target anatomy to be radiographed is actually ideal for assessing the pose. Since installing cameras in various positions in clinical practice would have been costly, we used our recently published framework that can generate synthetic depth images and corresponding radiographs from CT scans [5]. Using this framework, we were able to generate a dataset of 461,550 synthetic depth images from 50 different camera positions and two zoom levels of upper ankle joints, and evaluated the camera positions in 1,500 experiments to assess their suitability for pose assessment. We have also investigated the extent to which the use of multiple cameras can improve performance. Our experiments were conducted exclusively on upper ankle joints as the target anatomy, as they are difficult to position and, due to their anisotropic shape, are likely to have a greater impact on different camera positions than, for example, a knee. To the best of our knowledge, this is the first empirical evaluation of different camera positions for pose assessment.

2 Materials and methods

In order to assess a patient's pose based on depth images, radiographs taken together with corresponding depth images are mandatory, as only these radiographs allow for an assessment of the diagnostic quality of the pose. Therefore, we applied our

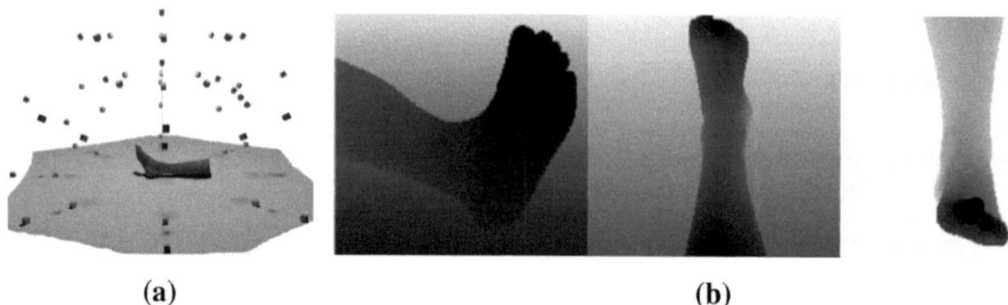

Fig. 1. In 1a the different virtual camera positions are shown. The cameras marked in red indicate the camera positions at ($z = 0°, x = 0°$) and thus perpendicular to the target anatomy. In 1b, three examples of synthetic depth images are shown from the following camera positions, left to right: ($z = 315°, x = 60°, \text{zoom} = 0$), ($z = 180°, x = 30°, \text{zoom} = 0$), ($z = 0°, x = 0°, \text{zoom} = 0$).

framework [5], as it enables generating synthetic depth images and the corresponding radiographs from CT scans. The synthetic depth image is generated by projecting a point cloud of the surface of the target anatomy, which is extracted from the CT scan and then placed onto a previously recorded point cloud of an X-ray room including an X-ray table, into 2D. In order to increase the diversity of the data and the dataset size, and to generate poses other than those taken in the CT scan, we used the two augmentations presented in [5] and also rotated the target anatomy around the longitudinal axis to create 181 different realistic poses. A synthetic radiograph can then be generated for each of those poses from the CT scan using a monte carlo simulation [6]. To evaluate the influence of camera positions on pose assessment, we expanded our framework to generate depth images of upper ankle joints from 50 different camera positions and two zoom levels for each pose and augmentation. We chose the camera positions as spherical coordinates centered around the upper ankle joint, with a rotation around the global vertical z-axis in 45° increments (azimuth), where for a left foot 0° = distal, 90° = lateral, 180° = proximal, and 270° = medial, and a rotation around the x-axis (elevation) in 30° increments; see Fig. 1a and 2 for visualization. Note that for an azimuth angle of 180°, no 30° elevation angle increment was applied, and the elevation angles only go up to 50°, as larger angles would lead to anatomically impossible depth images. We have also distinguished between two zoom levels, whereby zoom level 1 is 30 cm closer to the target anatomy than zoom level 0. This generation process enabled us to use CT scans from 10 patients with 17 upper ankle joints and two additional augmentations in 181 poses each from 50 different camera positions to generate a total of 461,550 synthetic depth images. Since the corresponding radiographs depend only on the pose for each upper ankle joint, and not on augmentation and camera position, the 3,077 synthetic radiographs generated in [5] could be used. They were labeled by four radiologists regarding their diagnostic quality with a rating of 1 being the best and 3 being the worst. Radiographs with a rating above 2.5 can furthermore be classified as non-diagnostic and would have to be retaken in clinical practice. Note that the generation process takes into account the camera-specific intrinsic and extrinsic parameters, so that this dataset can also be generated for a specific ToF camera model. Fig. 1b shows examples of the generated images.

In order to determine the ideal camera position for pose assessment, we conducted experiments for each of the 50 positions. The experiment design followed Laufer et al. [5] for comparability reasons and involved training an EfficientNet-B0 [7] with the depth images from one camera position as a regression with regard to the diagnostic quality of the corresponding radiographs to predict the quality of the pose. In order to be robust against outliers, three different testsets on patient level were defined for each camera position and each of them trained with ten different seeds, resulting in 30 experiments per position, which amounts to a total of 1,500 experiments. The results of the testsets and seeds were averaged for each individual camera position.

In order to further evaluate the extent to which the addition of another camera can improve pose assessment performance, we also evaluated combinations of two camera positions. For this, we averaged the predictions of identical images from the testset of two models trained with depth images from two different camera positions and evaluated them regarding the corresponding quality label. All experiments were evaluated with regard to the mean absolute error (MAE), the accuracy, which counts a deviation of the prediction from the label of less than 0.5 as correct (Eq. 1), and the diagnostic accuracy, which indicates how many images were correctly predicted as diagnostic or non-diagnostic (Eq. 2)

$$\text{Accuracy} = \frac{1}{N}\sum_{j=1}^{N} \mathbf{1}(|y_j - x_j| < 0.5) \tag{1}$$

$$\text{Diag. Accuracy} = \frac{1}{N}\sum_{j=1}^{N} \mathbf{1}((y_j < 2.5 \wedge x_j < 2.5) \vee (y_j \geq 2.5 \wedge x_j \geq 2.5)) \tag{2}$$

where y_j is the (average) networks prediction of the diagnostic quality of the pose based on the depth image, x_j is the label of the pose, based on the corresponding radiograph, N is the number of samples, and $\mathbf{1}$ is the indicator function. For the sake of clarity, not all metrics are specified in all cases, but only the diagnostic accuracy, as it has the highest clinical relevance.

3 Results

Fig. 2 shows the results of the experiments and provides the average diagnostic accuracy for each of the 50 camera positions and both zoom levels. The results show that there are indeed camera positions such as ($z = 45°, x = 60°$, zoom = 1) that should be avoided for pose assessment due to their significantly poorer diagnostic accuracy.

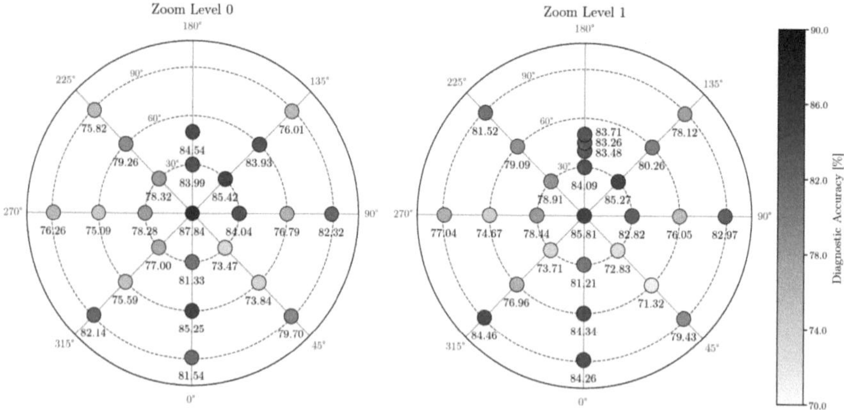

Fig. 2. Visualization of the diagnostic accuracy for pose assessment of the different camera positions and two zoom levels. The best camera position is the one perpendicular to the target anatomy.

At both zoom levels, the best of all 50 camera positions is at ($z = 0°, x = 0°$), i.e., directly vertical above the target anatomy. At zoom level 0, this position achieves a diagnostic accuracy of 87.84%, creating a discrepancy of up to 17 percentage points (p.p.) between the best and worst camera position. There is no significant difference between the two zoom levels across camera positions (Fig. 2 and 3a). Therefore, the subsequent results no longer differentiate between the two zoom levels. To determine whether specific elevation or azimuth angles are more advantageous for pose assessment, Fig. 3b and 4 show the diagnostic accuracies averaged over the corresponding angles. Fig. 3b shows a decline in diagnostic accuracy as the elevation angle increases, until diagnostic accuracy rises slightly at 89°. An improvement of more than 7 p.p. of elevation angle 0° compared to the other angles, underscores that a view directly perpendicular to the target anatomy is particularly advantageous. Regarding the azimuth angles, Fig. 4 shows that the camera positions on the longitudinal axis at $z = 0°$ and $z = 180°$ perform best on average. The azimuth angle of 45° stands out as one that yields results that are almost 7 p.p. worse than its neighboring angles of 0° and 90°. Note that the small standard deviation at an angle of 180° is due to the fact that only the elevation angles 30°, 60°, and 89° were used for averaging for one azimuth angle in this evaluation, and that at 180° this results in averaging only two camera positions.

Tab. 1 shows the results of the 10 best camera position pair combinations by averaging the predictions of the individual camera positions, split by MAE, accuracy, and diagnostic accuracy. The best diagnostic accuracy is achieved at position ($z = 0°, x = 0°, \text{zoom} = 0$) and ($z = 135°, x = 60°, \text{zoom} = 0$) with a value of 87.61% which is slightly worse than the best diagnostic accuracy of one camera. The MAE and accuracy metrics show only marginal improvements over the performance of only

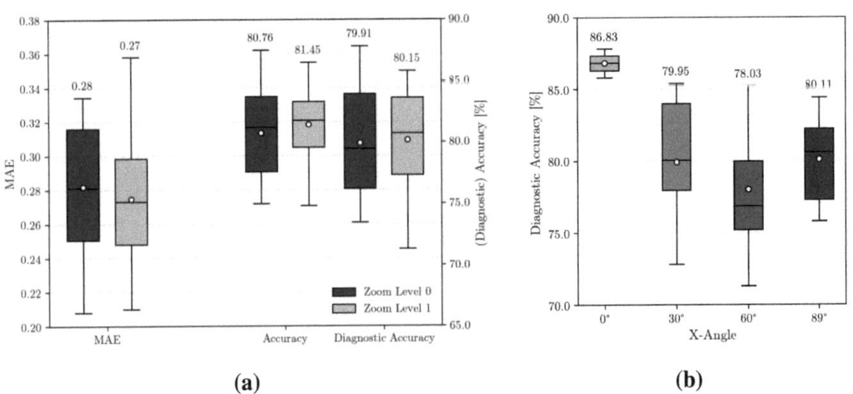

(a) **(b)**

Fig. 3. In 3a, boxplots of the mean MAE (left), accuracy, and diagnostic accuracy (right) are shown across all azimuth and elevation angles, split by zoom level. Note that there is no significant difference between the zoom levels. Fig. 3b shows boxplots of the averaged diagnostic accuracy of the azimuth angles split by elevation angle. An elevation angle of 0° performs better than the other angles. The respective mean values are shown above the boxes.

Tab. 1. Results of the best 10 camera position pair combinations per metric. Only the MAE and accuracy metrics show little improvements compared to the performance of one camera.

	Camera 1			Camera 2					
Rank	z	x	zoom	z	x	zoom	MAE	Accuracy	Diag. Accuracy
1	0 °	0 °	1	0 °	0 °	0	0.20 ± 0.01	88.43% ± 1.22%	87.61% ± 1.60%
2	0 °	0 °	0	0 °	60 °	1	0.21 ± 0.02	88.02% ± 1.88%	87.59% ± 1.30%
3	0 °	0 °	0	315 °	89 °	1	0.21 ± 0.01	87.89% ± 2.27%	87.51% ± 1.49%
4	0 °	0 °	0	0 °	60 °	0	0.21 ± 0.01	87.87% ± 2.39%	87.50% ± 1.36%
5	0 °	0 °	1	315 °	89 °	1	0.21 ± 0.01	87.82% ± 2.01%	87.49% ± 1.37%
6	0 °	0 °	1	0 °	60 °	0	0.21 ± 0.01	87.59% ± 1.20%	87.41% ± 1.36%
7	0 °	0 °	1	135 °	60 °	0	0.21 ± 0.01	87.47% ± 1.30%	87.40% ± 1.48%
8	0 °	0 °	1	0 °	60 °	1	0.21 ± 0.01	87.46% ± 2.30%	87.35% ± 1.68%
9	0 °	0 °	0	135 °	60 °	0	0.21 ± 0.01	87.42% ± 1.48%	87.30% ± 1.55%
10	0 °	0 °	1	135 °	30 °	1	0.21 ± 0.02	87.35% ± 2.39%	87.29% ± 1.30%

one camera. Tab. 2, which shows the 5 most frequent individual camera positions in Tab. 1, illustrates that positions ($z = 0°, x = 0°$, zoom $= 0$) and ($z = 0°, x = 0°$, zoom $= 1$) occur most often within the best camera position pair combinations and that, of the 50 camera positions, only a few contribute most frequently to the best pairs.

4 Discussion

The significant discrepancy of up to 17 p.p. in the results obtained from the different camera positions underscore the necessity of the experiments conducted in this

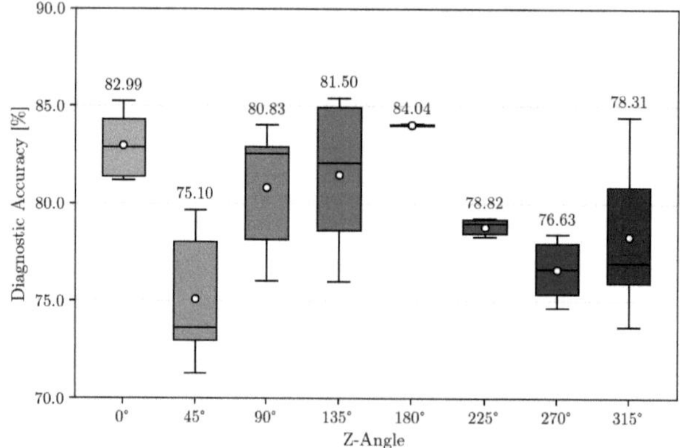

Fig. 4. Boxplots of the averaged diagnostic accuracy of the elevation angles 30°, 60°, and 89° split by azimuth angle. Azimuth angles on the longitudinal axis at $z = 0°$ and $z = 180°$ perform best on average.

Tab. 2. The 5 most frequent individual camera positions appearing in Tab. 1, split by metric and overall. Camera positions that perform well individually are also more likely to be part of the best camera position pair combinations.

Rank	Camera Position	n_{MAE}	n_{Accuracy}	$n_{\text{Diagnostic Accuracy}}$	n_{Total}
1	$(z = 0°, x = 0°, \text{zoom} = 0)$	5	5	9	19
2	$(z = 0°, x = 0°, \text{zoom} = 1)$	6	3	2	11
3	$(z = 315°, x = 89°, \text{zoom} = 1)$	2	3	1	6
4	$(z = 135°, x = 60°, \text{zoom} = 0)$	2	2	1	5
5	$(z = 135°, x = 30°, \text{zoom} = 1)$	1	3	1	5

work. These differences can be partly attributed to the anisotropic shape of the foot, which can lead to the occlusion of features that are potentially important for pose assessment from certain positions. A target anatomy with a more isotropic shape, such as that of the knee joint, could be expected to produce a more uniform distribution of accuracies across the various positions, which should be verified in future experiments. However, a change of the best camera position for isotropic shapes is not to be expected due to its position directly perpendicular to the target anatomy. The lack of difference between the two zoom levels is expected, as the different zoom levels essentially change the resolution of the images, which does not vary greatly over a distance of 30 cm. The results of the analyses regarding the different azimuth and elevation angles show that camera positions on the longitudinal axis, especially directly perpendicular to the target anatomy, are particularly advantageous for pose assessment. The latter position in particular indicates that both ankles are important features for pose assessment and is also suitable for attaching a ToF camera directly to the X-ray device. Furthermore, due to the lack of great performance improvements when combining two cameras, an additional camera is not needed. However, it is possible that fusion strategies that use images from both camera positions already during training will result in a greater performance improvements. Further experiments are required to verify this. Tab. 2 confirms the intuitive expectation that camera positions that perform well individually are more likely to be part of the best combined camera position pairs, so further experiments should focus on these positions. Even though we did not use the same camera positions in our previous experiments with real depth images, a diagnostic accuracy of 89.08% [5] for camera positions between $(z = 180°, x = 30°, \text{zoom} = 0)$ and $(z = 0°, x = 30°, \text{zoom} = 0)$ are in a comparable range, which indicates that our results should generalize well to real data.

The results of this work suggest that hospitals could benefit from their own vendor-agnostic solutions for patient positioning assistance. By purchasing a standalone ToF camera using positioning algorithms independent of the device manufacturer, they could improve patient care and avoid expensive device replacements. This also ensures that older devices that are still functional can be used for longer, as new features can be upgraded inexpensively with custom solutions.

References

1. Little KJ, Reiser I, Liu L, Kinsey T, Sánchez AA, Haas K et al. Unified database for rejected image analysis across multiple vendors in radiography. J Am Coll Radiol. 2017;14(2):208–16.
2. Mairhöfer D, Laufer M, Berkel L, Bischof A, Barth E, Barkhausen J et al. AI-based collimation optimization for X-ray imaging using time-of-flight cameras. Proc ESANN. 2024:703–8.
3. Mairhöfer D, Laufer M, Berkel L, Sieren M, Bischof A, Barth E et al. AI-based collimation optimization for X-ray imaging using depth cameras. Neurocomputing. 2026;661:131881.
4. Laufer M, Mairhöfer D, Sieren M, Gerdes H, Reis FL dos, Bischof A et al. Patient pose assessment in radiography using time-of-flight cameras. Proc SPIE MI IP. 2024;12926:129261J.
5. Laufer M, Mairhöfer D, Sieren M, Gerdes H, Reis FL dos, Bischof A et al. Synthetic data generated from CT scans for patient pose assessment. Proc MIDL. 2025. Accepted but not yet published.
6. Badal A, Badano A. Accelerating Monte Carlo simulations of photon transport in a voxelized geometry using a massively parallel graphics processing unit. Med Phys. 2009;36(11):4878–80.
7. Tan M, Le Q. EfficientNet: rethinking model scaling for convolutional neural networks. Proc ICML. 2019:6105–14.

Abstract: Physiological Neural Representations in Dynamic Imaging

Kartikay Tehlan [1,2], Thomas Wendler [1,2]

[1]Department of Diagnostic and Interventional Radiology and Neuroradiology, University Hospital Augsburg, Augsburg, Germany
[2]Computer-Aided Medical Procedures and Augmented Reality, Technical University of Munich, Garching bei München, Germany
kartikay.tehlan@med.uni-augsburg.de

Dynamic positron emission tomography (PET) with [^{18}F]FDG enables quantitative analysis of tissue metabolism through kinetic modelling. Conventional voxel-wise estimation methods based on non-linear curve fitting are computationally intensive, while data-driven deep neural networks require large training datasets and memory resources. To counter these, we present a physiological neural representation that employs implicit neural representations (INRs) for continuous, patient-specific tracer kinetic parameter estimation in dynamic PET [1]. We predict the parameters K_1, K_2, K_3 , and V_b [2] of an irreversible two-compartment model minimising the mean-squared error between modelled and measured time-activity curves. The dataset included dynamic [^{18}F]FDG PET/CT studies of 24 oncological patients, the INRs were trained per patient, including models augmented with voxel-wise CT Hounsfield units or feature embeddings from a 3D CT foundation model [3]. These anatomical descriptors acted as implicit regularisers, helping robustness. Across the patients, we observed statistically significant reductions in modelling errors as well as computation time. Kinetic maps of K_1, K_2, K_3, and V_b were consistent across liver, spleen, lungs, and kidneys when compared with organ-specific ranges from Sari et al. [4]. The method provides a continuous, data-efficient approach for tracer kinetics estimation, adaptable to anatomy and multi-modal physiological modelling.

References

1. Tehlan K, Wendler T. Physiological neural representation for personalised tracer kinetic parameter estimation from dynamic PET. Proc MICCAI. 2025:491–500.
2. Dimitrakopoulou-Strauss A et al. Kinetic modeling and parametric imaging with dynamic PET for oncological applications: general considerations, current clinical applications, and future perspectives. Eur J Nucl Med Mol Imaging. 2021;48:21–39.
3. Pai S et al. Foundation model for cancer imaging biomarkers. Nat Mach Intell. 2024;6(3).
4. Sari H et al. First results on kinetic modelling and parametric imaging of dynamic 18F-FDG datasets from a long axial FOV PET scanner in oncological patients. Eur J Nucl Med Mol Imaging. 2022:1–13.

© Der/die Autor(en), exklusiv lizenziert an
Springer Fachmedien Wiesbaden GmbH, ein Teil von Springer Nature 2026
H. Handels et al. (Hrsg.), *Bildverarbeitung für die Medizin 2026*,
Informatik aktuell, https://doi.org/10.1007/978-3-658-51100-5_69

Einsatz Künstlicher Intelligenz zur Zellsegmentierung und Klassifikation in histologischen Bildern von Pankreaskarzinomen

Sorel T. Djoumsi[1], Laura Lemberger-Viehmann[2], Tatyana Ivanovska[1], Christian Bergler[1], Thiha Aung[2], Silke Härteis[3]

[1]Ostbayerische Technische Hochschule Amberg-Weiden
[2]Technische Hochschule Deggendorf
[3]Universität Regensburg
s.tahata-djoumsi@oth-aw.de

Zusammenfassung. In dieser Studie wurde eine modulare KI-Pipeline zur Analyse histopathologischer Whole-Slide-Images (WSI) von Pankreaskarzinomen implementiert. Die Pipeline umfasst sämtliche Verarbeitungsschritte von der Vorverarbeitung und Gewebedetektion über die WSI- und Ausschnitt-Extraktion bis hin zur Region-of-Interest (ROI)-Klassifikation, Zellkernsegmentierung und Markerquantifizierung. Ziel ist eine vollständig automatisierte, reproduzierbare und objektive Auswertung histopathologischer Bilddaten. Zum Einsatz kommen moderne Deep-Learning-Ansätze, darunter Basismodelle wie UNI, nnU-Net und EfficientNet, in Kombination mit der Open-Source-Software QuPath. Erste Ergebnisse zeigen, dass Transfer Learning und domänenspezifisches Feintuning auch bei begrenzter Datenmenge zu robusten Klassifikations- und Segmentierungsergebnissen führen. Ein systematischer Vergleich mit bestehenden Ansätzen ordnet die Leistungsfähigkeit der entwickelten Pipeline im aktuellen Forschungsumfeld ein.

1 Einleitung

Pankreaskarzinome [1] zählen zu den aggressivsten malignen Tumoren und weisen mit einer 5-Jahres-Überlebensrate von unter 10% eine der ungünstigsten Prognosen überhaupt auf. Eine präzise histopathologische Beurteilung ist daher von zentraler Bedeutung für die Therapieentscheidung und Prognoseabschätzung.

Die Beurteilung erfolgt häufig anhand sogenannter Markerindizes, beispielsweise des Ki-67-Index [2]. Ki-67 ist ein Proliferations- bzw. Zellwachstumsmarker, der in Krebsgewebe teilungsaktive Tumorzellen rot und nicht proliferierende Zellen blau anfärbt. Der Ki-67-Index beschreibt somit die Zellteilungs- bzw. Wachstumsrate des Tumors; ein hoher Ki-67-Index ist in der Regel mit einer ungünstigeren Prognose assoziiert.

Fortschritte in der digitalen Pathologie [3, 4] und im Deep Learning ermöglichen mittlerweile die automatisierte Quantifizierung histologischer Merkmale aus

© Der/die Autor(en), exklusiv lizenziert an
Springer Fachmedien Wiesbaden GmbH, ein Teil von Springer Nature 2026
H. Handels et al. (Hrsg.), *Bildverarbeitung für die Medizin 2026*,
Informatik aktuell, https://doi.org/10.1007/978-3-658-51100-5_70

Whole-Slide-Images (WSI). Diese Verfahren erfordern jedoch komplexe Schritte der Vorverarbeitung, Detektion und Segmentierung, um verlässliche und reproduzierbare Ergebnisse zu erzielen. Zudem sind Pankreaskarzinome stark heterogen, und bislang steht kein ausreichend präzises KI-Modell zur histopathologischen Evaluierung zur Verfügung. In verwandten Arbeiten wurden hierzu verschiedene Ansätze verfolgt. Saednia et al. stellen ein kaskadiertes Deep-Learning-Framework zur Kernsegmentierung vor, das mehrere Modellstufen sequenziell kombiniert, um die Segmentierungsgenauigkeit in digitalen Histologiebildern zu verbessern [5]. HoverNet nutzt eine kombinierte Architektur, um Zellkerne und deren Subtypen gleichzeitig zu extrahieren und zu klassifizieren [6]. CellPose, ein generalistischer Zellsegmentierungsalgorithmus auf Basis eines deep learning-basierten Vektorfeldmodells, erzielt robuste Segmentierungen über unterschiedliche Zelltypen und Färbungen hinweg und eignet sich insbesondere für heterogene Datensätze [7].

In dieser Arbeit entwickeln wir eine vollständig modulare Pipeline, die den gesamten Prozess von der digitalen Bildaufnahme bis zur Markerquantifizierung abbildet und moderne Deep-Learning-Modelle in einen reproduzierbaren, skalierbaren Workflow integriert. Dabei kombinieren wir erstmals mehrere existierende State-of-the-Art-Komponenten – BiRefNet, UNI und nnU-Net – zu einer spezifischen Pipeline für die Analyse von Pankreaskarzinomen im CAM-Modell [8] und evaluieren diese Integration systematisch, anstatt neue Einzelarchitekturen vorzuschlagen. Durch die Automatisierung zentraler Schritte ermöglicht der entwickelte Ansatz eine erhebliche Zeitersparnis, etwa beim bisher manuellen Auszählen proliferierender Tumorzellen, und führt zu einer präziseren sowie objektiveren histopathologischen Beurteilung, die über die bisher häufig subjektive Expertenanalyse hinausgeht. Insgesamt stellt die vorgestellte Lösung ein praxisnahes Werkzeug dar, das insbesondere für Pathologinnen und Pathologen eine spürbare Entlastung im diagnostischen und quantifizierenden Arbeitsalltag bieten kann.

2 Material und Methoden

2.1 Datensatz

Die Studie basiert auf zehn Whole-Slide-Images (WSI) von Pankreaskarzinomen. Sie wurde gemäß den ethischen Richtlinien der Deklaration von Helsinki durchgeführt (positives Ethikvotum mit der Nr. 20-1989-101 der Ethikkommission der Universität Regensburg liegt vor). Die zehn WSI wurden mit dem PreciPoint-Scanner M8 bei 40-facher Vergrößerung (0,75 – 0,95 NA) und einer Scan-Auflösung von 0,28 µm/Pixel digitalisiert.

Die Daten wurden im TIF-Format gespeichert und in QuPath [9] manuell mit Tumor-, Normal- und Artefaktregionen annotiert (Abb. 1). Die WSIs besitzen unterschiedliche Pixelabmessungen, da sich die Scanbereiche und Zuschnitte zwischen den Präparaten unterscheiden. Im Mittel weisen die Bilder eine Auflösung von 14 070 × 16 035 Pixeln auf. Diese Variabilität der Auflösung spiegelt die heterogenen Gewebeflächen der Präparate wider und ist für die Beurteilung der Generalisierbarkeit der entwickelten Pipeline von Bedeutung.

2.2 Vorverarbeitung, Gewebedetektion und Erzeugung von Bildausschnitten

Für die automatisierte Gewebeextraktion wird auf einer stark herunterskalierten WSI-Vorschau BiRefNet [10] angewendet, um eine binäre Gewebemaske zu erzeugen. Das vortrainierte Modell erwies sich dabei als deutlich robuster gegenüber Artefakten (z. B. Rissen, Glasrändern, variierender Färbung) als klassische Verfahren wie Otsu. Die Maske wird postprozessiert, auf die Originalauflösung rückprojiziert, in Polygone überführt und für eine gewebebereinigte Darstellung genutzt, die als Grundlage aller weiteren Schritte dient. Auf Basis dieser Maske werden zusammenhängende Gewebebereiche über Begrenzungsrahmen identifiziert und als Sub-WSIs gespeichert (Abb. 2); zugehörige Metadaten wie Slide-ID, Auflösung, Pixelgröße und Gewebefläche werden automatisch protokolliert.

Die Sub-WSIs werden anschließend in überlappende Bildausschnitte von 224 × 224 Pixeln zerlegt, wobei die Schrittweite kleiner gewählt wird, um Randeffekte zu minimieren und eine implizite Datenaugmentation zu erzielen. Die Ausschnittgröße entspricht der etablierten Standard-Eingabe vieler Deep-Learning-Modelle und erlaubt eine effiziente Verarbeitung bei ausreichender Detailauflösung. In von Expert:innen markierten Regionen erfolgt ein gezieltes Oversampling durch zusätzliche Ausschnitte im erweiterten Umfeld der Annotationen. Die Klassenzuweisung basiert auf der Flächenüberlappung mit den Klassen *Tumor*, *Normalgewebe* und *Artefakte*; ein Ausschnitt erhält ein Label ab einer Überdeckung von mindestens 90%, Ausschnitte mit Mehrfachüberlappung werden verworfen.

Insgesamt wurden 5070 Bildausschnitte extrahiert (Tab. 1).

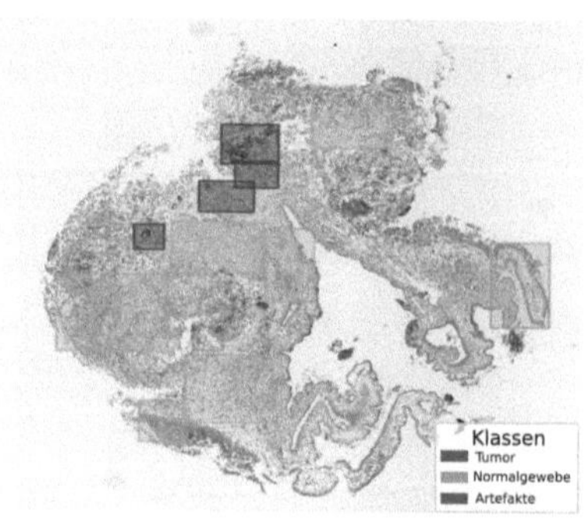

Abb. 1. Schematische Darstellung eines WSI: Rote (Tumor), graue (Artefakte) und orange (Normalgewebe) Quadrate repräsentieren die manuell von Experten definierte Ground Truth. Die überlappenden Bildausschnitte (224 × 224) werden aus diesen Regionen erzeugt.

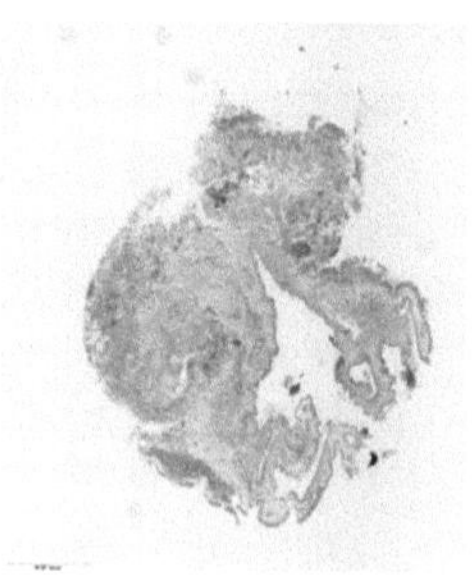

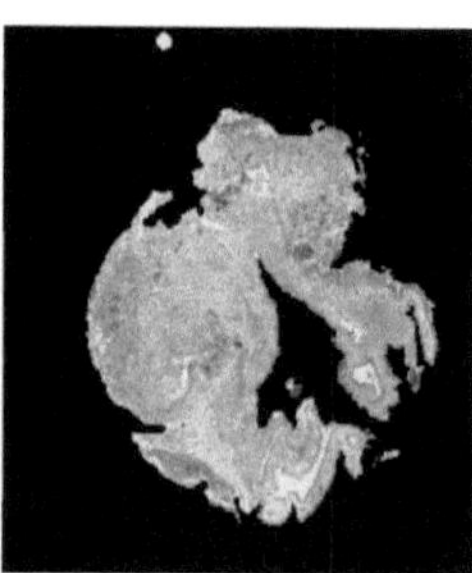

Abb. 2. BiRefNet-gestützte Gewebedetektion: links herunterskalierte WSI-Vorschau, rechts binäre Gewebemaske nach Postprocessing und Rückprojektion.

Klasse	Anzahl	Anteil [%]	Beschreibung
Normalgewebe	2943	58	Gesunde Stromaanteile
Tumorgewebe	1190	23,5	Tumor-Regionen
Artefakte	937	18,5	Leere/überfärbte Bereiche
Gesamt	5070	100	10 WSI

Tab. 1. Verteilung der extrahierten Bildausschnitte.

2.3 Klassifikation der Regionen von Interesse (ROI)

Die ROI-Klassifikation basiert auf dem Basismodell *UNI* (Vision Transformer) [11]. Das vortrainierte Backbone wurde für die dreiklassige Unterscheidung *Tumor*, *Normalgewebe* und *Artefakte* um einen Softmax-Head erweitert. Eingaben waren gewebebereinigte, überlappend extrahierte Bildausschnitte (224 × 224 Pixel) nach Reinhard-Farbnormalisierung [12] und Standardaugmentierungen (Rotation, Spiegelung, leichte Helligkeitsvariation).

2.3.1 Training/Validierung. Zweistufiges Fine-Tuning mit Warm-up des Klassifikationskopfs (Backbone teilweise eingefroren), anschließend end-to-end; Optimierung mit Adam ($\eta = 10^{-4}$), Batchgröße 32, bis zu 100 Epochen mit Early Stopping auf den Validierungsverlust. Validierung per 4-fache Kreuzvalidierung auf einem stratifizierten Datensatz mit slideweisen Splits: Bildausschnitte eines Slides bleiben innerhalb eines Folds zusammen; pro Fold dienen exakt zwei Slides der Validierung.

2.4 Zellkernsegmentierung

Für die Segmentierung wurde nnU-Net (2D) eingesetzt, ein selbstkonfigurierendes Framework, das Auflösung, Ausschnittgröße, Batchgröße, Datenaugmentation und Architektur automatisch an die Bildcharakteristika anpasst [13]. Als Eingabe dienten gewebebereinigte ROI-Ausschnitte der Klassen *Normalgewebe* und *Tumorgewebe*; insgesamt wurden 4 000 Ausschnitte ausgewählt. Die Zellkerne in diesen Ausschnitten wurden in QuPath semi-automatisch segmentiert und als Masken exportiert, die als Ground Truth für das Training dienten. Der Datensatz wurde im Verhältnis 70 %, 15 %, 15 % in Trainings-, Validierungs- und Testmenge aufgeteilt. Als Verlustfunktion kam die Kombination aus Dice- und Cross-Entropy-Loss zum Einsatz, ergänzt durch Standardaugmentierungen (Rotation, Spiegelung, Farb- und Helligkeitsjitter).

2.5 Markerquantifizierung mit EfficientNet-B0

Aus insgesamt 4 000 semi-automatisch segmentierten Bildausschnitten (224 × 224 Pixel) wurden durch Expertinnen und Experten in 547 Fällen einzelne Zellen manuell annotiert; daraus wurden einzelne Zellkerne als 100 × 100-Pixel-Ausschnitte unter Einbezug des lokalen Kontexts extrahiert. Eine Auswahl dieser Zellen wurde von einer Expertin manuell in drei Klassen annotiert (Tab. 2): *Ki-67-positiv*, *Ki-67-negativ* und *Other* (Zelltrümmer bzw. Artefakte).

Zur Markerklassifikation wurde ein EfficientNet-B0-Modell eingesetzt. Das Modell wurde per Transfer Learning trainiert: zunächst mit eingefrorenem Backbone

Klasse	Anzahl	Anteil [%]	Beschreibung
Ki-67-positiv	406	12,9	Proliferierende Tumorzellen
Ki-67-negativ	333	10,5	Nicht-proliferierende Tumorzellen
Other	2 422	76,6	Artefakte/debris
Gesamt	3 161	100,0	Manuell markierte Zellen

Tab. 2. Verteilung der extrahierten und manuell klassifizierten Zellkerne für die Markerquantifizierung.

(Warm-up), anschließend end-to-end mit Adam (Lernrate 10^{-3}) und Early Stopping. Die dreiklassige Softmax-Ausgabe unterschied *Ki-67-positiv*, *Ki-67-negativ* und *Other*. Zur Robustheitssteigerung wurden Standardaugmentierungen genutzt (Rotation, Spiegelung, Farb-/Helligkeitsjitter). Der Datensatz wurde im Verhältnis 70 %, 15 %, 15 % in Trainings-, Validierungs- und Testmenge aufgeteilt. Dabei wurde strikt darauf geachtet, dass die Aufteilung WSI-bezogen erfolgte, sodass Bildausschnitte desselben Whole-Slide-Images ausschließlich einer der drei Teilmengen zugeordnet wurden, um Datenleckagen zu vermeiden und eine realistische Generalisierbarkeit der Modelle sicherzustellen.

3 Ergebnisse

3.1 Klassifikation der ROI

Das Basismodell UNI erzielte in der dreiklassigen ROI-Klassifikation (*Tumor*, *Normalgewebe*, *Artefakte*) einen mittleren F1-Score von 0,86 über alle Folds. Die Präzision für *Tumor* lag bei 0,89 und für *Normalgewebe* bei 0,84, während der Recall für *Tumor* 0,83 erreichte. Fehlzuordnungen traten vor allem an Grenzbereichen zwischen Tumor und Stroma auf, wo Mischstrukturen und Färbungsvariationen die Unterscheidung erschweren. Die Klasse *Artefakte* blieb klar abgegrenzt, was die resultierende Konfusionsmatrix auf Ausschnitt-Ebene (Abb. 3a) zeigt. Die diagonale Dominanz belegt eine konsistente Zuordnung der Klassen, mit geringen Verwechslungen zwischen Tumor- und Normalgewebe. Qualitativ entspricht die Klassifikation den manuell erstellten Expertenannotationen: großflächige Tumorregionen werden zuverlässig erkannt, während in Übergangsbereichen vereinzelt fehlerhafte Bildausschnitte auftreten, die jedoch auf Slide-Ebene kaum Einfluss auf die Gesamtbewertung haben.

3.2 Zellkernsegmentierung

nnU-Net erzielte einen mittleren Dice Koeffizienten von 0,80. Qualitativ gelingt eine klare Trennung benachbarter Zellkerne; in stark gefärbten Arealen kommt es vereinzelt zu Übersegmentierungen.

3.3 Markerklassifikation

Auf dem Testdatensatz erzielt das eingesetzte EfficientNet B0 eine Gesamtgenauigkeit von 97,7%. Für die Klasse *Ki-67-positiv* beträgt der F1 Score 98%. Fehlzuordnungen treten fast ausschließlich in *other/debris* auf, während *Ki-67-positiv* und *Ki-67-negativ* nahezu perfekt getrennt werden. Der Ki-67-Index pro Slide wurde aus den Einzelvorhersagen aggregiert. Abb. 3b zeigt die Konfusionsmatrix der Zellebene.

4 Diskussion

Zur Einordnung der Pipeline werden ROI-Klassifikation, Zellkernsegmentierung und Ki-67 Klassifikation mit ausgewählten Studien verglichen (Tab. 3). Insgesamt liegt die Leistung unserer Pipeline im erwarteten Bereich aktueller Verfahren: Der ROI F1 von 86% entspricht dem Niveau transformatorbasierter Ansätze, der mittlere Dice von $\sim$ 80% reiht sich in publizierte Kerndetektionen ein, und die Ki-67 Klassifikation erreicht mit 99% F1 auf Zellebene eine sehr hohe Trennschärfe.

Wichtiger Hinweis zur Vergleichbarkeit: Die Metriken sind nur bedingt direkt vergleichbar, da sich die Studien in mehreren Aspekten unterscheiden: Domäne (Pankreas vs. Mamma vs. generische Datensätze), Färbungen und Scanner, Annotationsgranularität (Ausschnitt vs. Slide Ebene), Validierungsprotokolle (z. B. 4×Kreuzvalidierung vs. Leave One Out) sowie Aufgabenformulierung (ROI Klassifikation vs. Fallklassifikation, Kernsegmentation vs. Regionssegmentation). Die hier berichteten Werte sollten daher als *orientierende* Bezugsgrößen verstanden werden, nicht als streng äquivalente Benchmarks.

Um einen direkten Vergleich mit bestehenden Methoden zu ermöglichen, wurden die 547 manuell annotierten Bildausschnitte in Trainings- (328 Bilder), Validierungs- (116 Bilder) und Testmenge (103 Bilder) aufgeteilt und die HoverNet-Pipeline [6] in MONAI (`https://colab.research.google.com/github/Project-MONAI/tutorials/blob/main/pathology/hovernet/hovernet_torch.ipynb`) für 100 Epochen feinjustiert; dabei erzielte das Modell die besten Dice-Koeffizienten von etwa 65% auf dem Validierungsdatensatz und etwa 57% auf dem Testdatensatz.

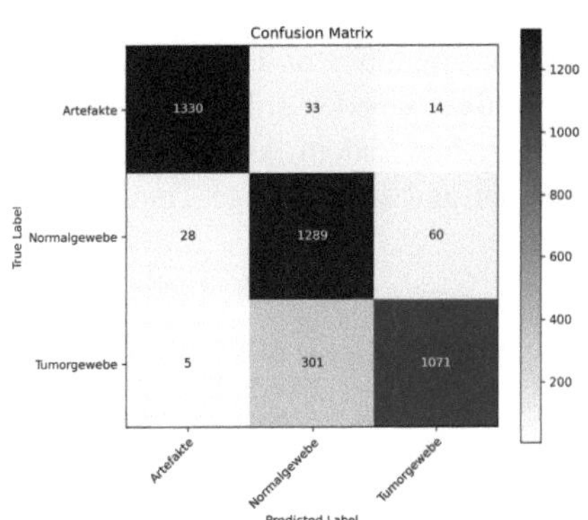

(**a**) ROI-Klassifikation mit dem UNI-Basismodell.

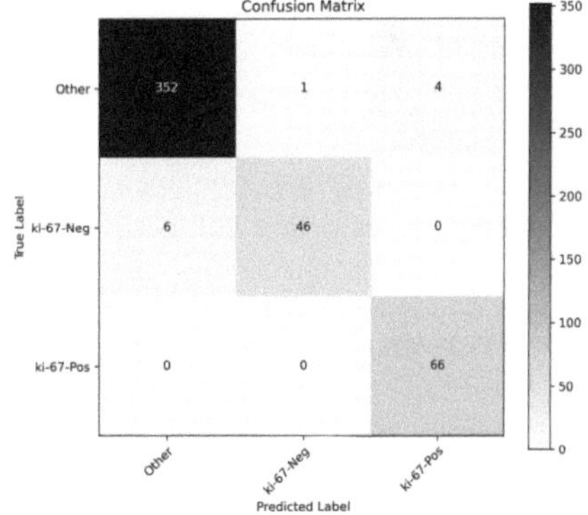

(**b**) Markerklassifikation mit EfficientNet-B0.

Abb. 3. Konfusionsmatrizen für die ROI- (links) und Zellklassifizierung (rechts).

Tab. 3. Vergleich zentraler Teilaufgaben mit publizierten Arbeiten (Domänenunterschiede beachten).

Studie	Aufgabe	Domäne	Daten	ROI F1	Segm. F1	Ki-67 F1
Diese Arbeit	Pipeline	Pankreas	10 WSI	0.86	~0.80	~0.99
Niazi 2018 [14]	Inception V3	PanNET	33 WSI	~0.95	–	–
Matsumoto 2024 [15]	DenseNet/HALO	Mamma	494 WSI	~0.86	–	–
Mola 2025 [16]	CNNs	NET (G1)	10 Fälle	–	–	0.70
Saednia 2022 [5]	U-Net-Ensemble	MoNuSeg	MoNuSeg	–	0.83	–

Unsere Pipeline erzielt zwar höhere Leistungswerte (ca. 80 – 82% Dice-Koeffizient für die Zellklassifizierung auf der 224 × 224-Ausschnittebene in den Validierungs- und Testmengen), besteht jedoch aus mehreren aufeinanderfolgenden Verarbeitungsschritten; wird dabei beispielsweise die ROI-Klassifizierung fehlerhaft durchgeführt, kann dieser Fehler in den nachfolgenden Stufen nicht mehr kompensiert werden, sodass die betroffenen Zellen nicht korrekt klassifiziert werden. Ein wesentlicher Vorteil unseres Modells besteht darin, dass einzelne Komponenten in jedem Verarbeitungsschritt flexibel ausgetauscht oder gezielt erweitert werden können.

Die Kombination eines domänenspezifisch vortrainierten Basismodels (UNI) mit einer selbstkonfigurierenden Segmentierung (nnU-Net) und einem leichten Klassifikator (EfficientNet-B0) ermöglicht einen durchgängigen Workflow für WSIs. Die Architektur adressiert Herausforderungen wie Gigapixel-Auflösung, Färbungsvariabilität und Gewebeheterogenität bei gleichzeitig praktikabler Integration in QuPath. Die implementierte KI-Pipeline bietet eine verlässliche Alternative zur manuellen oder semi-automatisierte Analyse Ki-67-positiver Tumorzellen und erlaubt eine standardisierte, hochdurchsatzfähige Auswertung, die die Reproduzierbarkeit experimenteller und klinischer Studien verbessert.

Diese Arbeit stellt damit einen wichtigen Schritt hin zu KI-gestützten Ansätzen dar, die zelluläre Heterogenität von Pankreaskarzinomen quantitativ erfassen können. Aktuelle Limitationen betreffen den begrenzten Datenumfang und die Datenvielfalt sowie potenzielle Inter-Observer-Effekte. Zukünftige Arbeiten sollten multizentrische, scanner- und stain-diverse Kohorten einbeziehen zudem Aspekte wie Unsicherheitskalibrierung, domänenadaptive Verfahren und slide-skalige Transformer-Modelle stärker in den Fokus rücken.

References

1. Eosewicz S, Wiedenmann B. Pancreatic carcinoma. J Lancet. 1997;349(9050):485–9.
2. Jonat W, Arnold N. Is the Ki-67 labelling index ready for clinical use? Ann Oncol. 2011;22(3):500–2.
3. Deng S et al. Deep learning in digital pathology image analysis: a survey. Front Med. 2020;14(4):470–87.
4. Boor P. Deep learning applications in digital pathology. Nat Rev Nephrol. 2024;20(11):702–3.

5. Saednia K, Tran WT, Sadeghi-Naini A. A cascaded deep learning framework for segmentation of nuclei in digital histology images. Proc IEEE EMBC. 2022:4764–7.
6. Graham S, Vu QD, Raza SEA, Azam A, Tsang YW, Kwak JT et al. Hover-net: simultaneous segmentation and classification of nuclei in multi-tissue histology images. Med Image Anal. 2019;58:101563.
7. Pachitariu M, Rariden M, Stringer C. Cellpose-SAM: superhuman generalization for cellular segmentation. bioRxiv. 2025.
8. Vakilipoor F et al. The CAM model: an in vivo testbed for molecular communication systems. IEEE Trans Mol Biol Multiscale Commun. 2025.
9. Bankhead P et al. QuPath: open source software for digital pathology image analysis. Sci Rep. 2017;7:16878.
10. Zheng P et al. Bilateral reference for high-resolution dichotomous image segmentation. arXiv: 2401.03407. 2024.
11. Chen RJ et al. A universal representation for pathology. Nature. 2024;627:878–86.
12. Reinhard E, Adhikhmin M, Gooch B, Shirley P. Color transfer between images. IEEE Comput Graph Appl. 2002;21(5):34–41.
13. Isensee F et al. nnU-net: a self-configuring method for biomedical image segmentation. Nat Methods. 2021;18:203–11.
14. Niazi MKK et al. Identifying tumor in pancreatic neuroendocrine neoplasms from Ki-67 images using transfer learning. PLoS One. 2018;13(4):e0195621.
15. Matsumoto H et al. Ki-67 evaluation using deep-learning model-assisted digital image analysis in breast cancer. Histopathology. 2024;86(3):460–71.
16. Mola N et al. Comparing non-machine learning vs. machine learning methods for Ki67 scoring in gastrointestinal neuroendocrine tumors. Sci Rep. 2025;15:27700.

Improving Generalization in Mitotic Cell Detection via Domain Transformations

Max Gutbrod[1,2], David Rauber[1], Christoph Palm[1,2]

[1]Regensburg Medical Image Computing (ReMIC), OTH Regensburg, 93053, Germany
[2]Regensburg Center of Health Sciences and Technology (RCHST), OTH Regensburg, 93053, Germany

max.gutbrod@oth-regensburg.de

Abstract. We address domain generalization (DG) in mitotic-cell (MC) detection by combining a β-variational autoencoder (VAE) for domain transformations with feature-space alignment together with an object detector. The β-VAE synthesizes domain-transformed images, and the detector is trained to map originals and their transformed counterparts to equal representations. On the MIDOG++ dataset, this approach improves out-of-domain detection F1 scores by 7 and 3 percentage points compared to the color-variation augmentation and stain-normalization baselines. Results further suggest that morphology shifts hinder generalization more than stain shifts.

1 Introduction

Cancer remains a leading cause of mortality worldwide, and its overall burden continues to grow. A predictor of survival outcomes is the tumor grade, for which the number of cells undergoing division plays a central role. Despite its importance, inter-rater variability in counting dividing cells is high, motivating machine-learning approaches for improved reproducibility and accuracy. In this work, we present a deep-learning-based method to detect mitoses in whole slide images (WSIs) that addresses domain generalization (DG): applying a model trained on one set of domains to unseen domains with different staining, scanners, or tissue morphology.

2 Materials and methods

Our approach comprises two parts. We use the MIDOG++ dataset (Sec. 2.1) to train a domain transformation network (Sec. 2.2) to synthesize domain-transformed images. These images are leveraged during training of a downstream MC detection model to improve generalization to unseen domains (Sec. 2.3).

2.1 Dataset and H&E distance

We use the MIDOG++ dataset [1], comprising ten different Hematoxylin & Eosin (H&E) domains across two species (human and canine) stemming from multiple

© Der/die Autor(en), exklusiv lizenziert an
Springer Fachmedien Wiesbaden GmbH, ein Teil von Springer Nature 2026
H. Handels et al. (Hrsg.), *Bildverarbeitung für die Medizin 2026*,
Informatik aktuell, https://doi.org/10.1007/978-3-658-51100-5_71

scanners and different institutions, introducing stain differences. The dataset also spans diverse tumor types and organs, introducing variation in cell morphologies. Annotations include mitotic cells (MCs) and visually similar lookalikes (imposter cells) as 50 px squares centered on each cell. To quantify stain differences we deconvolve H&E stain vectors from an input x ($\mathrm{s}_h(x)$ and $\mathrm{s}_e(x)$) using Macenko's stain deconvolution [2] and calculate domain-specific centroids $\mathrm{c}_n \in \mathbb{R}^3, n \in \{h, e\}$. The H&E distance (HED) measures the distance between an image and a domain centroid

$$\mathrm{HED_d}(x, \mathrm{c}) = \|\mathrm{c}_n - \mathrm{s}_n(x)\|_2 = \sqrt{\sum [\mathrm{c}_n - \mathrm{s}_n(x)]^2} \tag{1}$$

We split the dataset into seven training ($\mathcal{S}$: $\{1_{\text{a–d}}, 2, 3, 5\}$) and three test domains ($\mathcal{T}$: $\{4, 6, 7\}$). Domain 4 (canine) was chosen as test domain for having the largest HED to all other domains. Domains 6 (canine) and 7 (human) were selected for including spindle cell morphology, a morphology not present in $\mathcal{S}$. Training domain images are split into 80 % training ($\mathcal{S}_{\text{train}}$) and 20 % validation data ($\mathcal{S}_{\text{val}}$).

2.2 Domain transformation network

We adopt the approach from Nguyen et al. [3], which aligns representations of an image and its domain-transformed counterparts, but instantiate the transformation with a β-variational autoencoder (β-VAE) instead of a GAN, avoiding adversarial training instabilities while remaining effective for moderate domain shifts.

Our β-VAE domain transformation network comprises one shared encoder f_ϕ and multiple domain-specific decoders $g_\theta^{d_i}, d_i \in \mathcal{S}$ (Fig. 1). Given an input image x^{d_i}, the encoder produces a representation $z^{d_i} \in \mathbb{R}^{ld}$. The domain-specific decoder

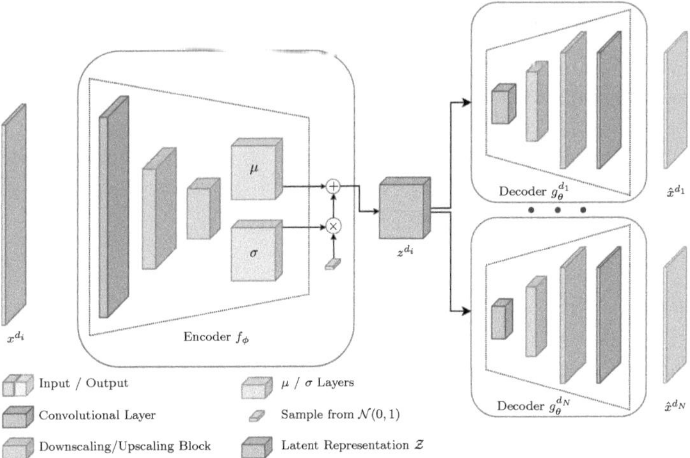

Fig. 1. Architecture of the proposed VAE domain transformation network. For each target domain j, the decoder $g_\theta^{d_j}$ generates a domain-transformed image from an input originating in source domain i.

$g_\theta^{d_i}$ reconstructs x^{d_i}, whereas $g_\theta^{d_j}$ $(d_j \neq d_i)$ generates a domain-transformed image $\hat{x}^{d_j}$. This architecture provides a direct way to synthesize corresponding images for all known source domains without requiring paired cross-domain training images. We train the VAE with L1 reconstruction loss using stochastic gradient descent (momentum 0.9, weight decay 4.5e-5) for 30 epochs with a OneCycle scheduler (maximum learning rate (LR) 0.33), and batch size 14. Each batch comprises 2 patches from each domain. Training patches come from a 512×512 sliding window (50 px overlap), yielding 61 709 patches from $\mathcal{S}_{\text{train}}$.

2.3 Downstream task: FCOS for mitosis detection

The objective of the downstream task is to detect MCs against background and imposter cells in H&E WSIs. We extract 512×512 random crops constrained around each annotation such that the annotated cell is fully contained. Models are trained for 8 epochs with batch size 12, SGD (momentum 0.9, weight decay 1e-5) and a OneCycle scheduler with a maximum LR 0.05.

All downstream experiments use the fully convolutional one-stage object detection (FCOS) [4] architecture, an anchor-free object detector that performs pixel-wise classification and box regression over a feature pyramid network with an auxiliary centerness branch. As downstream encoder h, we use a ResNet-50 model pre-trained on ImageNet. The employed FCOS criterion $\mathcal{L}_{\text{FCOS}}$ consists of a cross entropy loss, intersection-over-union (IoU) regression, and a center-ness term.

We leverage domain-transformed counterparts for each image in $\mathcal{S}_{\text{train}}$ to improve domain generalization (Sec. 2.2). For this, the encoder h of the downstream task encodes the original input image and all domain-transformed counterparts, yielding N feature representations. Finally, the distance between the representation of the original image and the $N-1$ feature representations from domain-transformed images is minimized using the l^2-norm, yielding the full loss criterion for the downstream task

$$\mathbb{E}_{d,d' \in \mathcal{S}}\left[\mathcal{L}_{\text{FCOS}}\left(x^d, y^d\right) + \rho \left\|h\left(x^d\right) - h\left(g^{d'}\left(f\left(x^d\right)\right)\right)\right\|_2^2\right] \tag{2}$$

The scalar ρ balances detection supervision against feature alignment strength. During inference, we first discard predictions with $p<0.5$, then apply class-wise non-maximum suppression with an IoU threshold of 0.3.

3 Results

We evaluate the quality of domain-transformed images by assessing the structure with the structural similarity index measure (SSIM) and HED for stain authenticity. Results for HED are multiplied by 10 for readability. Evaluation follows the MIDOG challenge: the primary metric is F1 for which a detected cell counts as true positive if the predicted box center lies within 25 px of the nearest ground-truth annotation with the same label. Additionally, we report precision and recall.

Tab. 1. Ablation on the depth of the downscaling- and upscaling blocks l and latent dimensions ld (second row). These results were obtained with β=0.1.

Metric	(l=2, ch=32)					(l=3, ch=32)					(l=4, ch=32)				
	64	128	256	512	1024	64	128	256	512	1024	64	128	256	512	1024
SSIM ↑	0.85	0.91	**0.93**	0.94	0.95	0.61	0.77	0.84	0.88	0.91	0.48	0.55	0.62	0.71	0.78
HED ↓	0.63	0.65	**0.64**	0.68	0.73	0.76	0.67	0.63	0.68	0.70	0.99	0.86	0.79	0.69	0.72

3.1 Domain transformation network

The shared encoder has a depth of l downscaling blocks. Each block consists of a strided convolution, batch normalization, ReLU, a skip connection, and a conv+ReLU refinement. The l upscaling blocks from the decoder mirror this design. The initial encoder width is set by ch, which is doubled/halved by subsequent stages. Finally, we denote the latent size as ld.

To avoid a combinatorial search, we first fix ch=32 and β=0.1, and vary l and ld (Tab. 1). Subsequently, we vary $ch \in \{2, 4, 8, 16, 32\}$ and $\beta \in \{0.01, 0.05, 0.1, 0.2, 0.5\}$ (Tab. 2). As the model selection criterion, we choose the model with the lowest HED subject to SSIM ≥ 0.7 on $\mathcal{S}_{\text{val}}$. The results favor l=2 over deeper variants (l=3, 4), and within l=2 recommend ld=256 over ld=512. Finally, with l and ld fixed, ch=8 achieves the lowest HED with competitive SSIM. For this setting, β=0.1 is confirmed as the best SSIM-HED trade-off. Qualitative comparisons for different ld are shown in Fig. 2. Fig. 3 presents domain-transformed examples from our final model, which are later used for feature alignment in the downstream task.

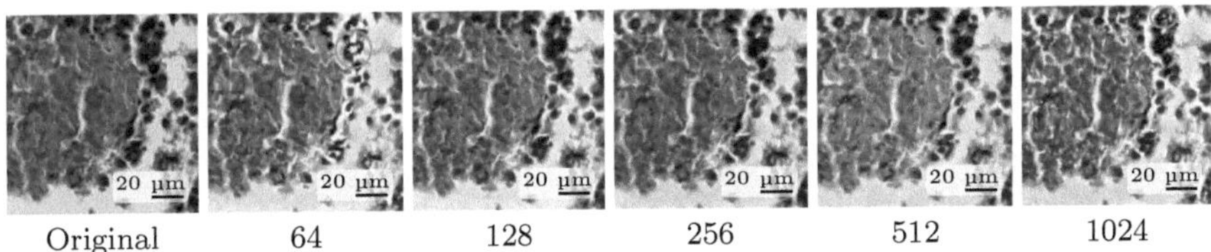

Fig. 2. An original image x^{1_b} and its domain-transformed images $\hat{x}^{1_d}$. Transformations use the models from Tab. 1 with l=2 and ch=32. Models with low (ld=64) or high (ld=1024) show artifacts, highlighted with green circles.

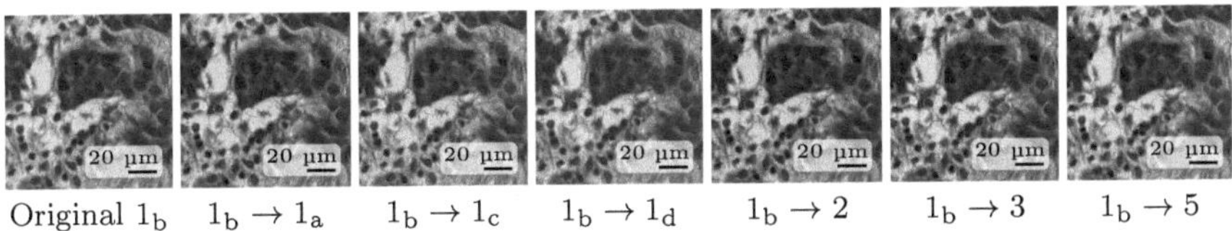

Fig. 3. Domain transformation results from the best-performing VAE.

Tab. 2. Ablations of our β-VAE architecture on width ch and regularization β.

(a) Varying ch (l = 2, ld = 256, β = 0.1).

ch	2	4	**8**	16	32
SSIM ↑	0.87	0.90	**0.92**	0.92	0.93
HED ↓	1.13	0.62	**0.61**	0.67	0.64

(b) Varying β (l = 2, ld = 256, ch = 8).

β	0.01	0.05	**0.1**	0.2	0.5
SSIM ↑	0.94	0.92	**0.92**	0.89	0.84
HED ↓	0.70	0.75	**0.61**	0.63	0.66

Tab. 3. Bootstrapping results averaged across three test domains for all mitosis detection models. Full per-domain results are omitted for space.

		FCOS		VAE FCOS				
		CJ	M	0.75	1.0	1.25	**1.5**	1.75
F1	μ	0.57	0.61	0.60	0.60	0.61	**0.64**	0.60
	$\pm\sigma$	0.11	0.09	0.10	0.10	0.09	0.10	0.09

3.2 Mitotic cell detection

Two baselines are trained: color jitter (CJ) FCOS with color variation augmentations, and Macenko (M) FCOS with a Macenko stain normalization on top. Additionally, we trained domain invariant FCOS models (denoted as VAE FCOS) with loss-balancing values for $\rho \in \{0.75, 1.0, 1.25, 1.5, 1.75\}$.

We bootstrap at the slide level (10 000 resamples), preserving domain balance by resampling slides within each domain and aggregating slide-level precision/recall/F1. Results of each model are presented in Tab. 3 and Fig. 4.

3.3 Discussion

3.3.1 Domain transformation networks. With ch=32 fixed, shallow models worked best. At l=2, increasing ld from 128 to 256 improved SSIM from 0.91 to 0.93 with a slight HED gain (0.65 to 0.64). In contrast, ld=512 brought a marginal SSIM gain (0.94) but a worse HED (0.68). Deeper variants (l=3, 4) reduced SSIM and generally worsened HED. Consequently, we adopt l=2, ld=256 which also reduces parameters by 40% compared to ld=512. Qualitatively, extreme ld values show

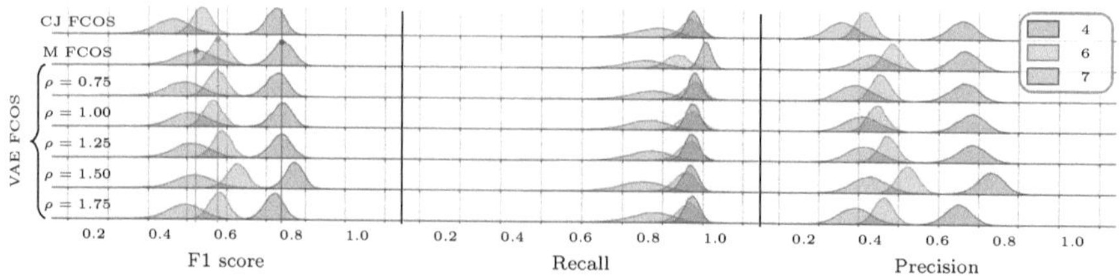

Fig. 4. Bootstrapping results of all FCOS models on our test domains. Bootstrapping was repeated 10 000 times. For better comparison, the green, orange, and blue lines indicate the mean values of the Macenko FCOS baseline.

artifacts (Fig. 2). Further, with ch=2 underfitting (HED 1.13) and widths above 8 yielding no consistent HED gains (Tab. 2a), we choose ch=8. Finally, a β-ablation confirmed β=0.1 as the best SSIM-HED trade-off (Tab. 2b).

3.3.2 Mitotic cell detection. For the downstream MC detection, the feature-alignment weight ρ behaved as anticipated: in-domain validation ($\mathcal{S}_{\text{val}}$) was insensitive to ρ because the detector already saw those domains during training. Thus, out-of-domain testing ($\mathcal{T}$) required evaluating the full set of $\rho \in \{0.75, 1.0, 1.25, 1.5, 1.75\}$.

It was shown that, with a suitable balance between the object detector and feature alignment loss, DG performance can be enhanced (Tab. 3). Experiments employing the VAE FCOS show an average F1 score improvement of +7 percentage points (pp) over the CJ FCOS and of +3 pp over the M FCOS baseline for ρ=1.5. The largest gain from feature alignment appears on domain 6, containing stain and cell morphology shifts (+5 pp over M FCOS). Domain 4 differs primarily in stain while matching source domains in cell morphology, achieving the highest scores. If morphology shifts were adequately addressed, domains 6 and 7 would approach the performance of domain 4. Their lower scores therefore indicate insufficient generalization to morphology changes. This likely reflects a limitation of our domain-transformation network, which successfully transforms stain variation but only weakly alters cell shape. Consequently, most gains arise from improved robustness to stain shifts.

4 Conclusion

This work demonstrates that β-VAE-based domain transformations, paired with a lightweight feature-alignment objective, can improve mitosis detection under domain shifts. A shallow architecture with a mid-sized latent space and modest width provided the best balance between structural fidelity and stain authenticity, and the feature-aligned detector outperformed DG baselines. Observations across test domains suggest that differences in cell morphology pose a greater generalization challenge than staining alone. Future work should benchmark against other state-of-the-art DG approaches and explore alternative alignment losses.

References

1. Aubreville M, Wilm F, Stathonikos N, Breininger K, Donovan TA, Jabari S et al. A comprehensive multi-domain dataset for mitotic figure detection. Sci Data. 2023;10(1):484.
2. Macenko M, Niethammer M, Marron JS, Borland D, Woosley JT, Guan X et al. A method for normalizing histology slides for quantitative analysis. Proc IEEE ISBI. 2009:1107–10.
3. Nguyen AT, Tran T, Gal Y, Baydin AG. Domain invariant representation learning with domain density transformations. Proc NeurIPS. 2021;34:5264–75.
4. Tian Z, Shen C, Chen H, He T. FCOS: fully convolutional one-stage object detection. Proc IEEE/CVF ICCV. 2019:9626–35.

Computer-assisted Detection of Lesions in Cystoscopy

Continuous Improvement by Data Extension and Model Selection

Thomas Eixelberger [1], Philipp Maisch[2], Christian Bolenz[2], Thomas Wittenberg [1,3]

[1]Friedrich-Alexander-Universität Erlangen-Nürnberg, Germany
[2]Department of Urology, University Hospital Ulm, Ulm, Germany
[3]Fraunhofer Institute for Integrated Circuits IIS, Erlangen, Germany
thomas.wittenberg@fau.de

Abstract. Bladder cancer is among the most common malignancies, with early detection being critical for effective treatment. This work investigates AI-based lesion detection in cystoscopic images, leveraging both YOLO and visual transformer (VT) architectures. Multiple datasets, including newly collected and publicly available sources, were systematically combined to train and evaluate detection models. Results show that increasing diversity and volume of training data significantly improves detection performance. Pretraining with colonoscopic images further improved model accuracy, indicating similarities in the appearance of lesions across different organs. While VT initially performed better, advanced YOLO outperformed VT with enriched data. These findings highlight the importance of heterogeneous datasets and model selection to advance automated bladder cancer detection.

1 Introduction

Worldwide, urinary bladder cancer (BCa) is one of the top ten cancer occurrences [1], especially for men it is known as the sixth most common cancer [2]. In 2020, more than 573,000 new cases of bladder cancer have been reported [2]. The primary method to diagnose BCa is cystoscopy, which is a visual examination of the urinary bladder using rigid or flexible endoscopes. More specifically, the gold standard for BCa diagnosis is white light cystoscopy [3]. During cystoscopy, the surface tissue of the urinary bladder wall is systematically examined for suspicious lesions and abnormalities, see examples in Fig. 1. However, early detection and diagnosis of flat, small, or weakly textured tissue lesions (such as carcicnoma in situ) is clinically challenging.

In recent years, many approaches have been investigated with respect to AI-based computer-assisted detection (CEDe) of lesions, such as, e.g., in the fields of mammography or colonoscopy. One key factor for the rapid development and establishment of such methods in the field was the availability of sufficient curated reference data to train and evaluate deep neural network models. However, in the

© Der/die Autor(en), exklusiv lizenziert an
Springer Fachmedien Wiesbaden GmbH, ein Teil von Springer Nature 2026
H. Handels et al. (Hrsg.), *Bildverarbeitung für die Medizin 2026*,
Informatik aktuell, https://doi.org/10.1007/978-3-658-51100-5_72

field of cystoscopy, publicly available datasets have not been widely available. Hence, there exists only some sparse literature in this field so far. E.g., Shkolyar et al. [2] were the first to introduce DNNs for automatic lesion detection in cystoscopy. They trained a DNN using images from 95 patients (417 with, 2,335 without lesions). Evaluation was based on data from 54 patients (23 with tumors, 31 controls) and resulted in a detection rate of F1 = 90%. Lazo et al. [3] used transfer learning with different network architectures (ResNet50, VGG, IncV3) to distinguish conspicuous and inconspicuous regions in urological white and NBI images (bladder, kidney, ureter, urethra) and achieved an AUC value of 0.987. Ikeda et al. [4] conducted a study using cystoscopic white-light images (1671 without, 431 with lesions) from 109 patients. Images were split 80% : 20% for training and testing, the reported precision was 97%, recall was 90%. Ye et al. [5] used an HRNetV2 network to detect and segment bladder tumors. They used >33,000 annotated frames (from a private collection of 102 videos) for training (80% of the data) and testing (20%); and achieved an overall sensitivity and precision of 91.6% and 91.3%, respectively, with a mDice score of 80.3%. [6].

Based on these observations, the objective of our contribution is two-fold: (1) We show that AI-based lesion detection in cystoscopy can be continuously improved by systematically adding heterogeneous learning data collected from various sources. (2) Furthermore, the choice of the network model applied is also a crucial parameter.

2 Methods and materials

2.1 Network models

2.1.1 YOLO-based networks. Deep neural networks using two-stage approaches involve separate steps for detection and prediction, making them slow for real-time object detection tasks. YOLO (You Only Look Once) architectures, on the contrary, are one-stage detector networks that have been specifically designed for efficient real-time object detection applications. Wang et al. [7] have recently introduced the YOLOv7 architecture, building on previous versions and incorporating advancements to improve accuracy and performance. YOLOv7 includes innovative features such as the extended efficient layer aggregation network (E-ELAN) and unique model scaling techniques, allowing for efficient and precise object detection. Compared to YOLOv7, YOLOv11 [8] introduces a more modernized network architecture, improved training and optimization techniques, and enhanced accuracy-efficiency trade-offs while preserving real-time inference performance.

2.1.2 Visual transformer (VT) networks. Detection transformers (DETR) are an object detection framework [9] that use transformer-based architectures. Using an end-to-end approach, DETR simultaneously performs detection and recognition without anchor boxes or proposal networks. Using a VT encoder-decoder architecture and self-attention mechanism, DETR captures global and local contextual information for accurate object predictions. Its training approach treats object detection as a prediction problem, simplifying the architecture and eliminating the need for additional components.

2.1.3 Data collections. For this research a set of different image collections $\mathcal{D}_X$have been gathered from various sources and applied for either training or testing. These collections are denoted as follows:

- $\mathcal{D}_{C.1}$ (>38.000 images) [10] and $\mathcal{D}_{C.2}$ (>340.000 images) [11] relate to our previous work in the field of colonoscopy and were used to pre-train the investigated network models (YOLO, VT).
- $\mathcal{D}_M$ denotes a collection of 12,066 images obtained from 19 cystoscopic videos depicting 112 unique lesions from the Mannheim Urology Department.
- $\mathcal{D}_B$ are 1.533 fiberscopic images with and without lesions from the Bamberg Urology Department, including a large number of PDD (photodynamic detection) images. The honeycomb structures based on the fiberscope were automatically removed using automated image processing [12].
- $\mathcal{D}_{U.3}$ was collected in three batches from the Ulm Urology Department and includes in total 731 images (554 positive, 277 negative) from 130 patients. The first batch included 558 and the second one 730 images.
- $\mathcal{D}_E$ refers to 67 images with lesions and 32 controls of 32 patients collected by the Fraunhofer IIS.
- $\mathcal{D}_R$ is a collection of 671 annotated cystoscopic images recently found on a public image server ('RoboFlow')[1].
- Finally, $\mathcal{D}_S$ refers to a publicly available cystoscopy collection of 1.754 images in four clinical classes – high-grade carcinoma (HGC), low-grade carcinoma (LGC), no tumor lesion (NTL), and non-suspicion tissue (NST) – recently provided by Sharma et al. [6]. Due to its available metadata and for purposes of compatibility, this data was only used for testing.

Where necessary, the depicted lesions were manually annotated by experienced annotators and furthermore verified by urological specialists.

2.2 Experiments

During experiments #1.1 – #1.3 in a first step, a pre-trained YOLO7 network (using the COCO database) was retrained on cystoscopy data $\mathcal{D}_M$ and tested on data sets $\mathcal{D}_E \cup \mathcal{D}_{U.1}$. As expected due to the sparse and non-representative training data, the baseline results were obtained (Tab. 1, line 1) [13]. In the second step, a pre-trained YOLO7 network N_2 was retrained using colon data $\mathcal{D}_{C.1}$, and was tested on data sets $\mathcal{D}_E \cup \mathcal{D}_{U.1}$. Interestingly, a gain was observed (Tab. 1, line 2), although *no* cystoscopic training data was used for training [13]. In step three, a transfer learning approach was employed, as suggested by Ikeda et al. [14]. Hence, the colonoscopy

[1] https://universe.roboflow.com

network was extended using cystoscopy data $\mathcal{D}_{C.1} \cup \mathcal{D}_{M}$, yielding improved results (Tab. 1, line 3) [13].

In the second experiment (#2.1 – #2.2) the YOLO7 model was evaluated against a visual transformer (VT) using the same training data as before, but with an extended test set $\mathcal{D}_{E} \cup \mathcal{D}_{U.2}$. In addition, an 8-fold cross-validation scheme was applied. The YOLO7 yielded results with a slight decrease with respect to the first experiments (Tab. 1, line 4), indicating that the new test data was possibly not adequately represented by the available training data. In contrast, the VT model trained and tested on the same data minimally improved the results (Tab. 1, line 5) [15].

In experiment #3 training data was extended by fiberscopic images $\mathcal{D}_{B}$, also including PDD images. As previously (Exp. #2.2) VT have outperformed the YOLO7 model, only VT was evaluated, giving slightly improved results (Tab. 1, line 6) [12].

As both – new cystoscopy data and new AI models – have recently become available, two more experiments were carried out. As until now, the VT model had slightly outperformed the YOLO7 network, experiments #4.1 – #4.2 were conducted using VT with respect to extended data collections. These new collections relate (a) to network pretraining using an extended colon dataset $\mathcal{D}_{C.2}$ with > 340.000 images, and (b) to two publicly available cystoscopic datasets $\mathcal{D}_{R}$ and $\mathcal{D}_{S}$, where the second even differentiates between four types of lesions [6]. As for the testing, the publicly available and labeled reference data $\mathcal{D}_{S}$ could be applied, for the training almost all available images $\mathcal{D}_{C2,M,N,P,R}$ could be used (#4.1), Furthermore, our previously collected test-data $\mathcal{D}_{U.U3}$ was also used for additional training (#4.2).

3 Results

Examples of cystoscopy images from $\mathcal{D}_{S}$ with detected lesions are displayed in Fig. 1. The 4 × 4 blocks of images relate to the four classes of this data set, namely (from left to right) HGC, LGC, NTL, and NST. The upper row shows detections from YOLO11 network, the lower row depicts detections from VT. Green boxes mark ground truth, red boxes automatic detections.

All results achieved with respect to precision, recall, and F1 score of all performed experiments are collected in Tab. 1 and depicted in Fig. 2. The order of results in the

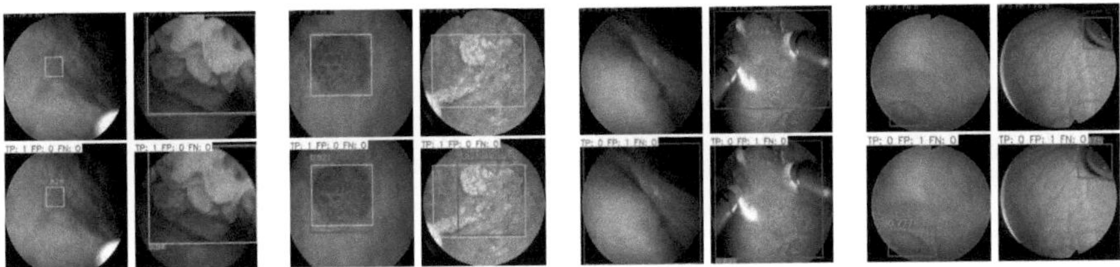

Fig. 1. Examples of cystoscopy images from $\mathcal{D}_{S}$. 4 blocks of 4 images are depicted, from left tor right, these relate to HGC, LGC, NTL, and NST. The top row depicts detections from YOLO11, the bottom from VT. Green boxes indicate ground truth, red ones automatic detections.

Tab. 1. Results of all performed experiments w.r.t precision, recall, and F1 score.

Experiment	Prec.	Rec.	F1	Training Data	Testing Data	Model	
Experiment #1.1	0.48	0.74	0.58	$\mathcal{D}_{M}$	$\mathcal{D}_{E+U.1}$	YOLO7	
Experiment #1.2	0.70	0.74	0.72	$\mathcal{D}_{C.1}$	$\mathcal{D}_{E+U.1}$	YOLO7	
Experiment #1.3	0.58	0.77	0.79	$\mathcal{D}_{C.1,M}$	$\mathcal{D}_{E+U.1}$	YOLO7	
Experiment #2.1	0.82	0.74	0.78	$\mathcal{D}_{C.1,M}$	$\mathcal{D}_{E+U.2}$	YOLO7	8fcv
Experiment #2.2	0.85	0.80	0.82	$\mathcal{D}_{C.1,M}$	$\mathcal{D}_{E+U.2}$	DETR50	8fcv
Experiment #3	0.88	0.76	0.83	$\mathcal{D}_{C.1,M,B}$	$\mathcal{D}_{E+U.2}$	DETR50	
Experiment #4.1	0.80	0.88	0.84	$\mathcal{D}_{C.2+M+B+P+R}$	$\mathcal{D}_{S}$	DETR50	
Experiment #4.2	0.81	0.88	0.85	$\mathcal{D}_{C.2+M+B+P+R+U.3}$	$\mathcal{D}_{S}$	DETR50	
Experiment #5.1	0.91	0.93	0.92	$\mathcal{D}_{C.2+M+B+P+R}$	$\mathcal{D}_{S}$	YOLO11	
Experiment #5.2	0.92	0.94	0.93	$\mathcal{D}_{C.2+M+B+P+R+U.3}$	$\mathcal{D}_{S}$	YOLO11	

table and the graph is provided chronologically and on the other hand, by improving results. In addition, all experiments related to visual transformers have been clustered, as indicated in Fig. 1.

Although the entries in Tab. 1 have been intentionally arranged in order of increasing results along the timeline, it is obvious that an increasing number of learning data with a great variety of depicted content and from different sources can improve the results, regardless of the network model used. Secondly, it can be observed that the improved YOLO11 outperforms the VT approach. Also, the pre-training of all investigated network models with colonoscopic image data seems to have a positive effect on the results, also giving a hint, that the tissues and lesions in the colon and bladder have to some extent a similar appearance.

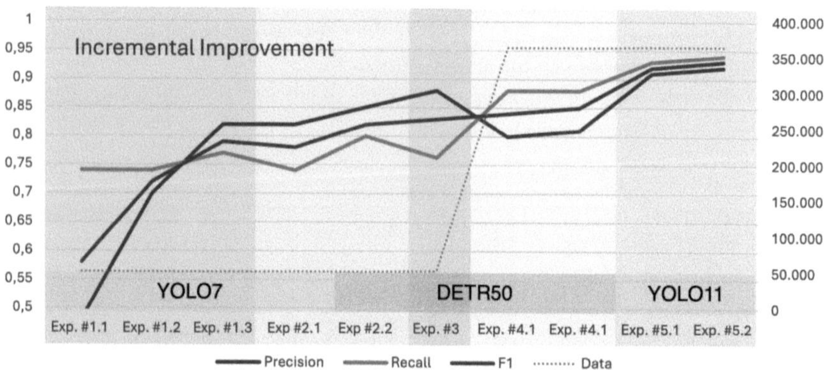

Fig. 2. Overview of experiments with increasing data (left to right), using two network models (YOLO and VT): The values for precision, recall and F1 are increasing with the amount of training data (dotted blue line).

4 Discussion

This contribution demonstrates that AI-based lesion detection in cystoscopy benefits significantly from both the quantity and heterogeneity of the training data. By systematically increasing and diversifying the datasets, the detection performance has consistently improved. Interestingly, pretraining on colonoscopic images also has enhanced the performance, suggesting cross-domain similarities in tissue and lesion appearance between the colon and bladder. Among the network models evaluated, visual transformers (VT) initially outperformed the YOLO7-based architectures, but later YOLO11 versions surpassed VT with further data augmentation and model refinement. This highlights the importance of model selection and continuous adaptation to new data. The inclusion of fiberscopic and PDD images further has enriched the dataset and led to incremental gains. Despite these advancements, challenges remain in generalizing to novel or underrepresented lesion types. Publicly available annotated datasets, like $\mathcal{D}_S$ and $\mathcal{D}_R$ were crucial for robust evaluation. Overall, the study underlines the potential of deep learning in improving early and accurate bladder cancer detection during cystoscopy, but also emphasizes the ongoing need for diverse, high-quality annotated data. Large-scale heterogeneous pretraining, as applied in this work, mirrors the initial supervised training stage employed in recent gastrointestinal and surgical foundation model pipelines [16–19].

Acknowledgement. This work was partially supported by the Richard & Annemarie Wolf-Stiftung.

References

1. Zhang Y, Rumgay H, Li M et al. The global landscape of bladder cancer incidence and mortality in 2020 and projections to 2040. J Glob Health. 2023;(13):04109.
2. Shkolyar E et al. Augmented bladder tumor detection using deep learning. Eur Urol. 2019;76(6):714–8.
3. Lazo J et al. A transfer-learning approach for lesion detection in endoscopic images from the urinary tract. arXiv: 2104.03927v1. 2021.
4. Ikeda A et al. Support system of cystoscopic diagnosis for bladder cancer based on AI. J Endourol. 2020;34(3):352–8.
5. Ye Z et al. Leveraging deep learning in real-time intelligent bladder tumor detection during cystoscopy: a diagnostic study. Ann Surg Oncol. 2025;32(5):3220–6.
6. Sharma P et al. Bladder lesion detection using efficientNet and hybrid attention transformer through attention transformation. Sci Reports. 2025;15(1).
7. Wang C, Bochkovskiy A, Liao H. YOLOv7: trainable bag-of-freebies sets new state-of-the-art for real-time object detectors. Proc IEEE/CVF CVPR. 2023:7464–75.
8. Jocher G, Qiu J, Chaurasia A. Ultralytics YOLO. 2023.
9. Carion N et al. End-to-end object detection with transformers. arXiv: 2005.12872. 2020.
10. Eixelberger T, Wolkenstein G, Hackner R et al. YOLO networks for polyp detection: a human-in-the-loop training approach. Curr Dir Biomed Eng. 2022;8(1):277–80.
11. Biffi C, Antonelli G, Bernhofer S, and others. REAL-Colon: a dataset for developing real-world AI applications in colonoscopy. Sci Data. 2024;(11):539.

12. Eixelberger T et al. Real-time fiberscopic image improvement for automated lesion detection in the urinary bladder. Proc BVM. 2025:25–30.
13. Eixelberger T, Maisch P et al. Deep learning by domain transfer for early tumor detection in the urinary bladder. Curr Dir Biomed Eng. 2023;9(1):53–6.
14. Ikeda A et al. Cystoscopic imaging for bladder cancer detection based on stepwise organic transfer learning with a pretrained CNN. J Endourol. 2021;35(7):1030–5.
15. Eixelberger T, Maisch P, Belle S et al. Comparison of YOLO and transformer based tumor detection in cystoscopy. Curr Dir Biomed Eng. 2024;10(4):228–31.
16. Devkota A, Amireskandari A, Palko Ja. Federated foundation model for GI endoscopy images. arXiv: 2505.24108. 2025.
17. Noh S, Lee BD. A narrative review of foundation models for medical image segmentation: zero-shot performance evaluation on diverse modalities. Quant Imaging Med Surg. 2025;15(6):5825–58.
18. Kerdegari H, Higgins K, Veselkov D et al. Foundational models for pathology and endoscopy images: application for gastric inflammation. Diagnostics. 2024;14(17):1912.
19. Boers TG, Fockens KN, van der Putten JA et al. Foundation models in gastrointestinal endoscopic AI: impact of architecture, pre-training approach and data efficiency. Med Image Anal. 2024;98:103298.

Filtering Scheme for Confocal Laser Endomicroscopy (CLE)-video Sequences for Self-supervised Learning

Nils Porsche [1], Flurin Müller-Diesing [2], Sweta Banerjee [1], Miguel Goncalves[3], Marc Aubreville [1],

[1]Flensburg University of Applied Sciences, Flensburg, Germany
[2]University Hospital RWTH Aachen, Department of Otorhinolaryngology, Aachen, Germany
[3]Department of Oto-Rhino-Laryngology, Head and Neck Surgery, University Hospital Würzburg, Würzburg, Germany
nils.porsche@hs-flensburg.de

Abstract. Confocal laser endomicroscopy (CLE) is a non-invasive, real-time imaging modality that can be used for in-situ, in-vivo imaging and the microstructural analysis of mucous structures. The diagnosis using CLE is, however, complicated by images being hard to interpret for non-experienced physicians. Utilizing machine learning as an augmentative tool would hence be beneficial, but is complicated by the shortage of histopathology-correlated CLE sequences with respect to the plurality of patterns in this domain, leading to overfitting of models. To overcome this, self-supervised learning (SSL) can be employed on larger unlabeled datasets. CLE is a video-based modality with high inter-frame correlation, leading to a non-stratified data distribution for SSL training. In this work, we propose a filter functionality on CLE video sequences to reduce the dataset redundancy in SSL training and improve training convergence and training efficiency. We use four state-of-the-art baseline networks and a SSL teacher-student network for the evaluation. These networks were evaluated on downstream tasks for a sinonasal tumor dataset and a squamous cell carcinoma of the skin dataset. On both datasets, we found the highest test accuracy on the filtered SSL-pretrained model, with 67.48% and 73.52%, both considerably outperforming their non-SSL baselines. Our results show that SSL is effective for CLE pretraining. Further, we show that our proposed video filter can be utilized to improve training efficiency in self-supervised scenarios, resulting in a reduction of 67% in training time.

1 Introduction

In the process of tumor characterization and outline delineation, tissue samples are taken as targeted biopsies from the most suspicious regions under endoscopic and/or image guidance. However, this procedure is limited by potential negative side effects such as hemorrhage and infection and – importantly for margin confirmation – by sampling error, because only a fraction of the circumference can be interrogated.

© Der/die Autor(en), exklusiv lizenziert an
Springer Fachmedien Wiesbaden GmbH, ein Teil von Springer Nature 2026
H. Handels et al. (Hrsg.), *Bildverarbeitung für die Medizin 2026*,
Informatik aktuell, https://doi.org/10.1007/978-3-658-51100-5_73

Margins abutting the skull base (e.g., dura), orbit, brain, the optic nerve, or the internal carotid artery may be inaccessible, where biopsy risks include not only bleeding or infection but also functional loss and/or cerebrospinal fluid leak, which substantially complicates potential reconstruction. The surgical removal is a complex procedure which aims at complete excision with histologically negative margins (R0 resection) while preserving functionally critical tissue whenever feasible. Functional and essential tissue such as muscles, nerves, and blood vessels may be damaged or removed in the process.

One adjunct to the classical biopsy that has been shown in many recent studies to be used non-invasively and in-vivo in the anatomic region of the head and neck is confocal laser endomicroscopy (CLE), an optical biopsy technique [1]. It delivers real-time diagnostic information about tissue structures at a highly magnified scale [1] and supports intraoperative margin assessment and surgical guidance [2]. The challenging aspect of CLE images is in interpreting the data, especially for untrained readers [2], where computer-assisted classification can be valuable in the intraoperative field. At present, CLE is not universally available and is routinely implemented only in a limited number of centers. Moreover, obtaining labeled data is challenging, as reliable correlates are hard to obtain given the margin-sampling constraints described above. For models with a vast amount of parameters, such as current deep learning models, this data shortage easily leads to overfitting, and hence to a severely reduced performance at inference. Few-shot learning methods, recently evaluated for CLE imaging [3], offer a potential solution, though classification with limited patient data remains challenging. Another recent strategy in this field is pretraining using self-supervised learning (SSL) methods, combined with adaptation to downstream tasks using limited datasets. Given the difficulty of obtaining histopathologic labels in CLE, exploiting unlabeled data becomes particularly valuable. This is especially relevant since ImageNet pretraining introduces a major domain shift, with features poorly capturing the distinct texture and contrast of CLE images.

In this work, we show that utilizing SSL schemes in pretraining is viable also for the domain of CLE images, even in the context of limited data cohorts. We also propose a novel data filtering scheme specifically tailored for CLE video sequences (CLE-VSs), allowing us to reduce the computational time in pretraining while at the same time not sacrificing any performance. In addition, we show in two downstream tasks that our model is able to classify CLE images of sinonasal tumors and squamous cell carcinoma of the skin with significantly increased accuracy than multiple ImageNet-pretrained baseline approaches.

2 Materials

We used a total of three datasets from the domain of CLE in this work, all obtained using CellVizio (Mauna Kea Technologies, Paris, France) devices . The ethics approval was granted by the respective IRBs (243 12 B, 60_14 B from Universitätsklinikum Erlangen, EK 370/20 from RWTH Aachen, 154/23_mpz-sc Julius-Maximilians-Universität Würzburg). For one, we used a dataset of sinonasal tumors (SNT-DS), an anatomical region known for its highly complex and diverse structure. The dataset comprised 42 CLE-VSs from six patients; only two included both tumor and healthy sequences, while the others contained only healthy tissue, resulting in a total of 6,669 frames with image resolutions between 336px to 512px. To enhance the validity of the experiments, we utilized another dataset which consisted of squamous cell carcinoma of the skin (SCCS-DS). It included six patients and 23 CLE-VSs, totalling 15,740 frames with resolutions of 572–578 pixels. In this dataset, one patient had only tumor sequences, while the others had both tumor and healthy tissue sequences. The labels for those datasets were retrieved by histopathologic analysis of the resected tissue as part of the clinical routine.

For self-supervised model pretraining, we used an extended and unlabeled dataset of 458 CLE-VSs, which we denote as the head and neck (HAN) dataset. This dataset contains images from various anatomical locations in the field of otorhinolaryngology and oral surgery, including the areas of the vocal folds, squamous cell carcinoma from the oral and sinonasal cavity, as well as from the auricle, nasal cavity, pharynx and larynx. To avoid data bleed in our experiments, both the SCCS and the SNT dataset were not part of the pretraining dataset. The total number of frames in this HAN dataset was 155,025 (95 GB of raw data), considerably exceeding the scale of the downstream task datasets (SCCS-DS and SNT-DS).

3 Methods

3.1 Self supervised learning

Training of models with a self-created supervisory signal, has recently emerged as a valuable tool in few-shot learning scenarios in medical imaging [4]. At its core is the idea to utilize large amounts of unlabeled data to pre-train feature extractors, which are subsequently used in downstream tasks using methods such as linear probing or adaptation. This setup helps to regularize the training process, which is key in few-shot scenarios. Caron et al. proposed self-distillation of vision transformer models by training a teacher and a student on crops of the same image, encouraging the student to mimic the teacher's predictions across views [5]. This yields robust, view-invariant representations that generalize well to downstream few-shot medical tasks, outperforming vanilla pre-training and providing a simple yet powerful regularization that mitigates overfitting [5]. SSL was shown to significantly benefit from data deduplication [6], which can be attributed to eliminating conflicting signals in the loss function.

In this work, we train a vision transformer using the original DINO loss [5]. To avoid overfitting, allow for larger batch sizes, and expedite training, we chose the small configuration (ViT-small). We trained the model with AdamW and default DINO hyperparameters until convergence, as observed by the training loss. We then retrospectively selected the model with the best loss during training.

3.2 CLE video sequence filtering (CLE-ViFi)

A characteristic of CLE video sequences is their high inter-frame correlation, resulting from the relatively steady positioning of the CLE probe during surgical observation. Repeatedly showing nearly identical frames during training is inefficient and, more critically, can introduce conflicting supervisory signals and exacerbate dataset imbalance. As demonstrated by Oquab et al. [6], dataset variability is a key factor for successful SSL. To reduce the redundancy in the dataset, we propose a tailored video filtering scheme for CLE (CLE-ViFi). Our goal is to effectively remove all duplicates or near-duplicates in the pretraining dataset. Our work is based on the assumption that the structural similarity of neighboring frames in a sequence can be utilized as a feature for deduplication. However, due to the high noise level in CLE images (Fig. 1), inter-frame differences in full-resolution data can be strongly influenced by image entropy. Our approach utilizes and combines both of these observations.

Using the SNT dataset, we randomly selected 50 reference frames and identified for each a sufficiently dissimilar (i.e., depicting a different anatomical location) and a similar subsequent frame, yielding a total of 100 pairs. We then determine the structural similarity index measure (SSIM) for all pairs. To support the SSIM kernel and reduce sensor-noise within the CLE images, we compared different image scalings for their discriminatory power and found the optimum scaling factor of 1/32. We found a sensible operating point for our application at a compromise between false negatives rate (0.1) and false positives (0.32) at a classification threshold τ of 0.411. Using this frame-based similarity classifier, we now process the entire HAN dataset. We select a first key frame and compare all subsequent frames until we reach a SSIM $< \tau$. This new frame is then added to the filtered dataset and selected as next key frame. We repeat this until we reach the end of the sequence. This filtering results in the HAN-ViFi dataset, comprising 52,250 non-redundant CLE frames.

3.3 Experiments

3.3.1 Downstream task. We employed SSL-pretrained models using both versions (HAN, HAN-ViFi) of the dataset. We used linear probing, i.e., the training of

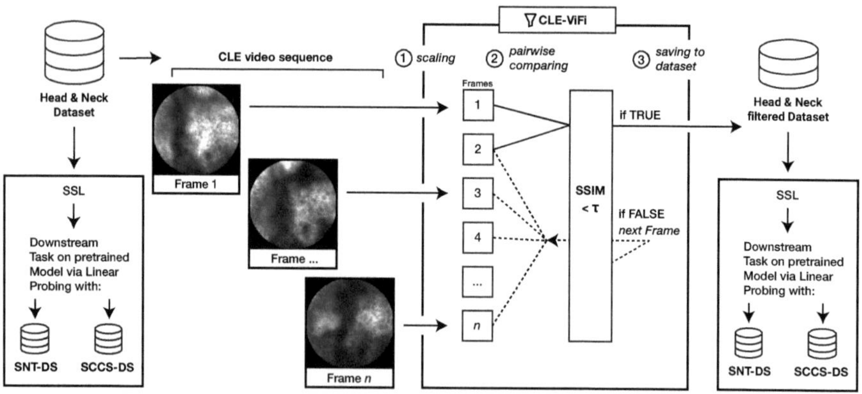

Fig. 1. Overview of the approach: We used self-supervised pre-training on a dataset utilizing our proposed CLE video filter (ViFi) and investigated two downstream tasks (SNT-DS, SCCS-DS).

a final classification layer on top of the SSL-trained feature extractor. We trained the network until convergence, using SGD with a momentum of 0.9 and an initial learning rate of 0.0001 with cosine annealing.

3.3.2 Baselines. We compared the SSL-based pretraining against four state-of-the-art baseline models. For the first two baselines, we used two convolutional neural networks (CNNs), based on the ResNet-18 and ResNet-50 architectures, respectively, which were pretrained on ImageNet and finetuned on the SNT- and SCCS-Dataset. For the third and fourth baseline we used the vision transformer (patch size 16) base and small which were pretrained on ImageNet-21k and also finetuned on the SNT- and SCCS-Dataset. For all model architectures, we evaluated both full fine-tuning and linear probing. We trained the model with early stopping based on validation accuracy, using a learning rate of 0.0001 and the Adam optimizer; the input images were resized to 224×224 pixels.

3.3.3 Cross-Validation. Given the small size of both of our datasets and the expected data shift between patients, we utilized leave-one-patient-out cross-validation to evaluate all of our model trainings. In this, we always determined one patient to be the hold-out (test) patient in each run. We then split the remainder of the dataset randomly into train and validation on sequence level in a ratio of 80/20, with the condition that at least one sequence of each class was to be present in the training and validation split. We performed the validation split on sequence level instead of the patient level, because the model training needs learning signals for both, the tumor- and the non-tumor class in each training and validation run. Given the distribution of tumor- and non-tumor cases across patients, a standard split on patient level would not have provided this. We repeated the cross-validation three times to counter random effects in training (initialization, sampling).

4 Results and discussion

The pretrained models on ImageNet consistently showed lower performance on the test set of the SNT-dataset and the SCCS-dataset (Tab. 1). The SSL models, which were pretrained on CLE data, increased the performance, as measured in the mean accuracy considerably, although not statistically significant (t Test, $p > 0.05$). We furthermore can see a slight advantage in downstream task performance for the feature extractors trained on the filtered (HAN-ViFi) dataset, leading to the conclusion that the video filtering was not detrimental to SSL training. However, by reducing the number of frames in SSL-based pretraining by approximately a factor of three, we significantly reduced the training time, as we found model convergence already after 2:27 RTX4090-GPU hours, compared to 7:23 GPU hours for the unfiltered dataset.

Our investigations support the findings of the current studies in the field of AI research, which predominantly found that SSL-based pretraining can lead to improved results in specialized medical imaging tasks [7]. Specifically, our results show that

Tab. 1. Comparison of the average accuracy +/- standard deviation for various baseline architectures and training strategies.

Model arch.	Pretraining dataset	Pretraining strategy	Finetuning strategy	Datasets SNT-DS	SCCS-DS
ResNet18	ImageNet	supervised	full fine-tuning	58.87% ± 19.11	69.70% ± 9.72
			linear probing	56.98%±22.53	54.42%±12.15
ResNet50			full fine-tuning	48.78%±20.29	69.38%±11.07
			linear probing	66.30%±29.05	61.36%±16.15
ViT-small			full fine-tuning	59.87%±25.99	68.38%±11.04
			linear probing	55.93%±18.39	63.79%±17.42
ViT-base			full fine-tuning	56.48%±26.45	70.06%±10.93
			linear probing	48.43%±16.23	66.57%± 13.92
ViT-small	HAN [ours]	unsupervised	linear probing	67.20%±33.83	72.53%±13.19
	HAN-ViFi [ours]		linear probing	**67.48%**±34.28	**73.52%**±12.52

SSL approaches enable more effective use of unlabeled data, which is a major advantage in a field with limited annotated image material. At the same time, our dataset filtering approach demonstrated a reduction in training time without any decrease in test accuracy across both downstream datasets. Our results show considerable fluctuations, as can be seen in the high standard deviations in Tab. 1. This stems from the substantial heterogeneity of the datasets rather than from training instability: the test set, in particular, includes patients with highly diverse and complex anatomical structures, leading to the observed high standard deviations.

Acknowledgement. This work was partially funded by the Deutsche Forschungsgemeinschaft (DFG, grant number 545049923).

References

1. Sievert M, Auberville M, Oetter N et al. Confocal laser endomicroscopy of head and neck squamous cell carcinoma: a systematic review. Laryngorhinootologie. 2021;100:875–81.
2. Villard A, Breuskin I, Casiraghi O et al. Confocal laser endomicroscopy and confocal microscopy for head and neck cancer imaging: recent updates and future perspectives. Oral Oncol. 2022;127:105826.
3. Aubreville M, Pan Z, Sievert M et al. Few shot learning for the classification of confocal laser endomicroscopy images of head and neck tumors. Proc BVM. 2024:143–8.
4. Ouyang C, Biffi C, Chen C et al. Self-supervised learning for few-shot medical image segmentation. IEEE Trans Med Imaging. 2022;41(7):1837–48.
5. Caron M, Touvron H, Misra I et al. Emerging properties in self-supervised vision transformers. Proc IEEE/CVF ICCV. 2021:9650–60.
6. Oquab M, Darcet T, Moutakanni T et al. Dinov2: learning robust visual features without supervision. arXiv: 2304.07193. 2023.
7. Huang SC, Pareek A, Jensen M et al. Self-supervised learning for medical image classification: a systematic review and implementation guidelines. NPJ Digit Med. 2023;6(1):74.

Tracking Cancer Through Text

Longitudinal Extraction from Radiology Reports using Open-source Large Language Models

Luc Builtjes, Alessa Hering

Department of Radiology and Nuclear Medicine, Radboud University Medical Center
luc.builtjes@radboudumc.nl

Abstract. Radiology reports capture crucial longitudinal information on tumor burden, treatment response, and disease progression, yet their unstructured narrative format complicates automated analysis. While large language models (LLMs) have advanced clinical text processing, most state-of-the-art systems remain proprietary, limiting their applicability in privacy-sensitive healthcare environments. We present a fully open-source, locally deployable pipeline for longitudinal information extraction from radiology reports, implemented using the `llm_extractinator` framework. The system applies the `qwen2.5-72b` model to extract and link target, non-target, and new lesion data across time points in accordance with RECIST criteria. Evaluation on 50 Dutch CT Thorax/Abdomen report pairs yielded high extraction performance, with attribute-level accuracies of 93.7% for target lesions, 94.9% for non-target lesions, and 94.0% for new lesions. The approach demonstrates that open-source LLMs can achieve clinically meaningful performance in multi-timepoint oncology tasks while ensuring data privacy and reproducibility. These results highlight the potential of locally deployable LLMs for scalable extraction of structured longitudinal data from routine clinical text.

1 Introduction

Radiology reports are a central means of documenting and communicating oncologic findings between specialists, particularly between radiologists and oncologists. They describe tumor burden, treatment response, and disease progression according to standardized criteria such as the response evaluation criteria in solid tumors (RECIST) [1]. Beyond their role in clinical decision-making, these reports represent a vast, underutilized source of longitudinal information on cancer progression. If automatically extracted, such information could provide large-scale, high-quality data for clinical research, enable retrospective population analyses, and support the development and evaluation of AI models across diverse patient cohorts. Yet, the narrative nature and heterogeneous structure of radiology reports make this information difficult to access in a systematic and scalable way.

© Der/die Autor(en), exklusiv lizenziert an
Springer Fachmedien Wiesbaden GmbH, ein Teil von Springer Nature 2026
H. Handels et al. (Hrsg.), *Bildverarbeitung für die Medizin 2026*,
Informatik aktuell, https://doi.org/10.1007/978-3-658-51100-5_74

Early information extraction efforts relied on rule-based algorithms [2] or supervised deep learning models [3], but these approaches often lacked generalizability and required substantial data annotation and engineering resources. The emergence of large language models (LLMs) has markedly advanced the ability to process unstructured clinical text without the need for task-specific model training [4]. Nevertheless, many state-of-the-art LLMs are proprietary, raising important privacy, security, and reproducibility concerns in healthcare contexts. Open-source LLMs offer a compelling alternative, as they can be deployed locally to ensure that sensitive patient data remain within institutional boundaries.

Current clinical text extraction efforts largely treat radiology reports as independent documents, even though oncologic interpretation is inherently longitudinal. Changes in lesion size and appearance across timepoints determine treatment response under RECIST, and processing reports at the patient level enables linking of corresponding findings across follow-up studies, capturing disease evolution and ensuring consistent interpretation.

In this work, we present a fully open-source and locally deployable pipeline for longitudinal information extraction from Dutch CT Thorax/Abdomen radiology reports. Using the language-agnostic `llm_extractinator` framework [5] with the `qwen2.5-72b` model, the system extracts and links target lesions (TLs), non-target lesions (NTLs), and new lesions (NLs) across timepoints in accordance with RECIST guidelines. To our knowledge, this is the first demonstration of LLM-based longitudinal extraction from radiology reports. We contribute (i) a reproducible open-source pipeline for clinical text extraction using locally deployable LLMs, (ii) a new task formulation for multi-timepoint lesion linkage under RECIST, and (iii) a quantitative evaluation demonstrating high extraction accuracy (>93% attribute-level) while preserving data privacy and reproducibility. An overview of our study design is shown in Fig.1.

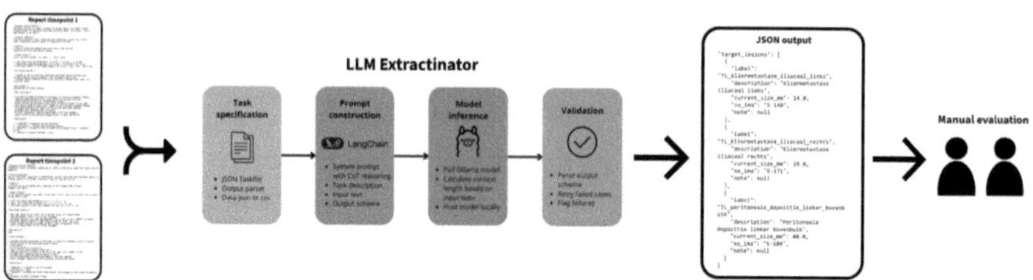

Fig. 1. Overview of the study design. Fifty pairs of Dutch thorax/abdomen radiology reports were analyzed using the `llm_extractinator` package [5], configured with tailored prompts and a customized output parser. The generated structured JSON outputs, representing all lesions extracted from each report pair, were manually assessed for quality by two independent readers.

2 Materials and methods

2.1 Dataset

As a staring point, we retrieved all radiology reports from patients who received a thoracic and/or abdominal CT scan at the [anonymized hospital] between March 2021 and March 2025. To focus on longitudinal data, we first identified patients with more than one report available across distinct timepoints. Within this subset, we performed a text-based search to identify cases in which the term "target" appeared in at least two reports for the same patient, ensuring the inclusion of longitudinal references to target lesions. Following this automated filtering, 60 report pairs were manually reviewed to confirm their suitability for inclusion. The curated dataset was subsequently partitioned into two subsets: 10 pairs allocated as a debug set for prompt engineering and refinement, and 50 pairs reserved as the final test set for evaluation.

2.2 LLM extractinator

We employed the open-source framework `llm_extractinator` [5] to perform structured information extraction. This framework provides a language-agnostic, locally deployable pipeline for clinical text processing using open-source LLMs. It enables users to define extraction tasks through JSON configuration files, specify the model backend, and enforce structured outputs via schema validation (e.g., using Pydantic models).

After identifying the relevant report pairs for each patient, we processed these pairs using the Extractinator pipeline to produce structured outputs suitable for downstream quantitative analyses. We selected `qwen2.5:72b-instruct-q4_K_M` as the underlying large language model (LLM) following a comparative evaluation on a debug dataset, where it achieved the best overall performance among models compatible with our computational constraints. All inferences were conducted on two NVIDIA A100 GPUs (40 GB each) with the temperature parameter set to 0

2.2.1 Prompt engineering. The final prompt was designed to ensure accurate and longitudinally consistent extraction of lesion information. Reports were always processed in concatenated pairs, enabling the model to recognize recurring lesions and maintain temporal continuity. For the LLM, this meant reasoning across both reports to determine whether each lesion persisted, resolved, or appeared newly, while still extracting only the *current timepoint* measurements.

The prompt included an in-context example illustrating the Dutch RECIST table format and its corresponding structured output. This improved both schema adherence and temporal label stability.

Key prompt rules reflecting RECIST conventions were summarized as follows: (i) in tabular data, the *rightmost* numeric value immediately preceding the last valid series–image (`SE-IMA`) reference represents the current measurement; (ii) valid `SE-IMA` identifiers match the pattern `^\d{1,3}-\d{1,4}$` and are never interpreted as sizes; (iii) lesions are categorized as *target*, *non-target*, or *new*, with prose-only findings included using `null` sizes when appropriate; (iv) each lesion receives a stable label (`TL_`, `NTL_`, or `NL_`) derived from its anatomical description to ensure consistent tracking; and (v) outputs must use integer millimetre sizes.

2.2.2 Output parser design. The output parser serves as a blueprint guiding the LLM to produce JSON outputs that strictly adhere to a predefined structure, as specified by a Pydantic v2 schema. It consists of three nested models: *Lesion* containing `label`, `description`, `current_size_mm`, `se_ima`, and `note`, *Report* grouping TLs, NTLs, and NLs under a unique StudyInstanceUID, and *OutputParser* aggregating multiple reports. All fields are optional so the model can opt to return an empty list if no lesions in a given category are present.

2.3 Experiments

To evaluate the LLM's performance in longitudinal lesion extraction, its outputs were compared with manual annotations from two independent readers across 50 patient report pairs. Both readers independently identified all TLs, NTLs, and NLs in each report. The goal was to assess how accurately the LLM detected, linked, and characterized corresponding lesions over time.

Each lesion was evaluated on three attributes per report: (i) *label consistency*: correct lesion identification and naming across timepoints; (ii) *size accuracy*: correct extraction of lesion measurements; and (iii) *series/image (se_ima) accuracy*: correct retrieval of DICOM identifiers for lesion localization.

For TLs and NLs, each attribute received a binary label ("correct"/"incorrect"), yielding six total attributes per lesion pair. For NTLs, 20 cases were evaluated at the attribute level and 30 at the report level for efficiency. Reader annotations were pooled to compute overall accuracy, and inter-reader variability was quantified by lesion-level agreement on identification and correspondence.

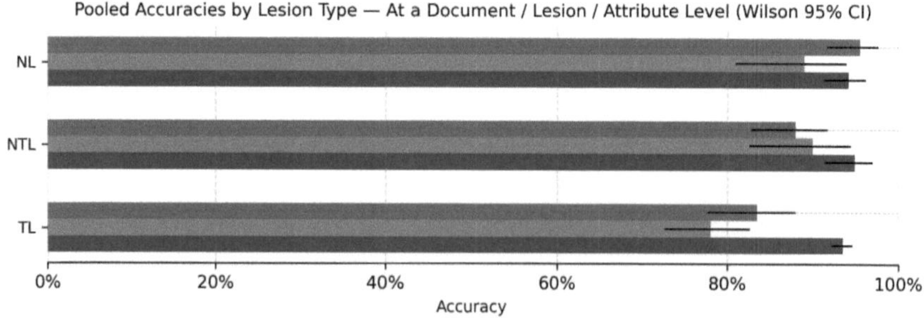

Fig. 2. Comparison of LLM extraction accuracy across lesion types: target lesions (TL), non-target lesions (NTL), and new lesions (NL). Accuracy is shown at three levels: document (green), lesion (orange), and attribute (blue).

3 Results

A total of 50 longitudinal report pairs (100 individual reports) were evaluated. On average, each report pair contained 2.6 TLs, 5.0 NTLs, and 0.91 NLs. A visual overview of the results is shown in Fig. 2.

Across both readers, the pooled accuracy for complete TL extraction was 78.1% (95% CI: 72.5–83.0). At the attribute level, 93.7% (95% CI: 92.2–95.0) of TL attributes were correctly extracted, and 83.5% (95% CI: 77.4–88.2) of reports contained no TL extraction errors.

For NTLs, performance was similarly high, with a pooled accuracy of 90.0% (95% CI: 84.9–93.7) for correct identification. The attribute-level accuracy reached 94.9% (95% CI: 92.5–96.6), and 88.0% (95% CI: 82.1–92.0) of reports showed no NTL extraction errors.

Extraction of NLs demonstrated comparable performance, with 89.1% (95% CI: 80.7–94.2) of lesions identified without error. Attribute-level accuracy was 94.0% (95% CI: 91.1–96.1), and 95.5% (95% CI: 91.2–97.8) of reports were free from NL extraction errors.

Each longitudinal report pair contained on average 30 total attributes; in 62.0% of pairs (95% CI: 52.2–70.9), all attributes were extracted without any errors.

Inter-reader agreement was high overall at a *93.3%* agreement lesion-level agreement rate. Differences between readers were small and not statistically significant for any category (two-proportion z-test, $p > 0.05$).

4 Discussion

This study demonstrates that open-source large language models can achieve high performance in extracting and linking longitudinal lesion data from radiology reports. Using the `llm_extractinator` framework with the `qwen2.5-72b` model, we obtained attribute-level accuracies above 93% across lesion types. These results highlight that open and locally deployable LLMs can reach a level of reliability suitable for clinical research while ensuring data privacy and reproducibility.

The longitudinal setting introduces challenges distinct from single-report extraction, as the model must not only identify findings but also link them coherently across timepoints. Labeling consistency between timepoints was excellent for target lesions (TLs), where all label attributes were correct. This indicates that the stable label design worked effectively for longitudinal tracking. For non-target lesions (NTLs), consistency was somewhat lower, which likely reflects the more variable wording used by radiologists across follow-up reports rather than model limitations. For example, lymph nodes could be described collectively (e.g., "multiple lymph nodes") in one report and individually in another, leading to apparent inconsistencies in label matching despite correct underlying detection. Additionally, the handling of the "Other findings" section was occasionally inconsistent, with the model sometimes classifying them as NTLs and other times omitting them.

The distribution of target lesion errors was balanced, with 45% involving the size attribute and 55% the `se_ima` identifier. This even split is expected, as errors in one attribute often coincide with errors in the other when interpreting tabular data, highlighting that the model's understanding of lesion identity was generally robust. While the model showed resilience to differences in report layout, it occasionally struggled when tabular sections were wrapped across lines or split into multiple parts, sometimes selecting the last value from the first segment instead of continuing correctly. These formatting-related errors are understandable given the loss of visual table cues in plain-text form, and providing more specific in-context examples could further improve consistency in such cases.

Lesions described as difficult to measure posed a specific challenge. They could be indicated in various ways, such as by using an asterisk with a corresponding footnote under the table or by simply noting "nm" (not measurable) without further context. The model sometimes failed to return a `null` value when no measurement was provided, or conversely returned `null` despite an approximate value being available. Nevertheless, it often handled these edge cases correctly, showing that the model can interpret nuanced clinical phrasing with reasonable consistency. Similar variability was observed when lesions were indicated as resolved with a dash ("–"), suggesting that additional examples or explicit rules could further improve stability in these scenarios.

Overall, the presented pipeline performs strongly in a demanding multi-timepoint clinical text task using fully open-source components. Despite minor challenges related to formatting, measurement ambiguity, and heterogeneous report structure, the approach achieves accurate, reproducible, and privacy-preserving longitudinal information extraction. These findings support the feasibility of open LLMs for clinical natural language processing and highlight their potential to enable scalable data extraction in oncology.

References

1. Therasse P, Arbuck SG, Eisenhauer EA, Wanders J, Kaplan RS, Rubinstein L et al. New guidelines to evaluate the response to treatment in solid tumors. J Natl Cancer Inst. 2000;92(3):205–16.
2. Draelos RL, Dov D, Mazurowski MA, Lo JY, Henao R, Rubin GD et al. Machine-learning-based multiple abnormality prediction with large-scale chest computed tomography volumes. Med Image Anal. 2021;67:101857.
3. Tushar FI, D'Anniballe VM, Hou R, Mazurowski MA, Fu W, Samei E et al. Classification of multiple diseases on body CT scans using weakly supervised deep learning. Radiol Artif Intell. 2021;4(1):e210026.
4. Bigolin Lanfredi R, Zhuang Y, Finkelstein M, Thoppey Srinivasan Balamuralikrishna P, Krembs L, Khoury B et al. LEAVS: an LLM-based labeler for abdominal CT supervision. Proc MICCAI. 2025:316–26.
5. Builtjes L, Bosma J, Prokop M, van Ginneken B, Hering A. Leveraging open-source large language models for clinical information extraction in resource-constrained settings. JAMIA Open. 2025;8(5):ooaf109.

Explainable Radiologist-aligned VLM for CT Image Quality Assessment

Jiajun Wang, Yipeng Sun, Siming Bayer, Andreas Maier

Pattern Recognition Lab, Friedrich-Alexander Universität Erlangen-Nürnberg, Germany
jiajun.wang@fau.de

Abstract. The assessment of computed tomography (CT) image quality has traditionally relied on manual evaluation by radiologists, a method that is both subjective and time-consuming. Deep learning-based methods usually only give quantitative scores and are not explainable. Additionally, the application of general-purpose, closed-source vision-language models (VLMs) is constrained by patient privacy regulations and the highly specialized requirements of clinical data. To overcome these limitations, we propose a parameter-efficient supervised fine-tuning (SFT) framework for the medical VLM, MedGemma-4B-IT, designed to automate CT image quality scoring and generate professional textual explanations within the clinical environment. We employed quantized low-rank adaptation (QLoRA) for parameter-efficient fine-tuning, aiming to align the model's visual perception with expert quantitative judgment. Experimental results demonstrate that our fine-tuned model achieves a substantial improvement in correlation with expert scores (SRCC = 0.7950, PLCC = 0.7907), outperforming zero-shot baselines such as Gemini 2.5 Pro and Gemini 2.5 Flash. Furthermore, the model generates explainable text that emulates the reasoning and explanation style of radiologists, thereby advancing the application of eXplainable AI (XAI) in medical image analysis. The project is publicly available at https://github.com/atJessc/VLM-CT-IQA.

1 Introduction

The diagnostic utility of computed tomography (CT) depends critically on image quality, as degradation due to noise, artifacts, or insufficient contrast may lead to misdiagnoses and repeated examinations, thereby increasing patient radiation exposure and healthcare costs [1, 2]. Consequently, objective and consistent assessment of CT image quality is of paramount importance.

Traditionally, the assessment of CT image quality has relied heavily on manual evaluation by expert radiologists. Although this approach provides high accuracy, it is time-consuming, labor-intensive, and prone to inter-observer variability [3, 4]. Most conventional objective methods require predefined regions of interest (ROIs),

© Der/die Autor(en), exklusiv lizenziert an
Springer Fachmedien Wiesbaden GmbH, ein Teil von Springer Nature 2026
H. Handels et al. (Hrsg.), *Bildverarbeitung für die Medizin 2026*,
Informatik aktuell, https://doi.org/10.1007/978-3-658-51100-5_75

making full automation difficult and limiting their applicability to anatomically complex images that lack uniform areas [5].

Deep learning-based methods have been widely applied to CT image quality assessment (CT-IQA). Such methods have achieved remarkable success in no-reference image quality assessment (NR-IQA) tasks [6], with advanced approaches even leveraging cross-modal data, such as breathing signals, to inform quality prediction [7]. However, the decision-making process of deep learning models remains opaque, making it difficult to interpret why specific quality scores are assigned. This lack of transparency poses a challenge in clinical settings where reliability and explainability are critical, thereby restricting their practical adoption.

The rapid advancement of vision-language models (VLMs) has opened new avenues for automating this critical task. Although image quality assessment (IQA) frameworks based on natural images have achieved notable success [8], extending these methods to the medical domain remains challenging due to greater visual complexity, subtler anatomical cues, and the scarcity of large, diverse labeled datasets.

MedGemma-4B-IT [9], an instruction-tuned medical VLM with 4 billion parameters, provides a strong baseline. However, when applied zero-shot to CT-IQA, it fails to produce accurate evaluations. The model lacks an understanding of human scoring nuances, and its predictions deviate substantially from expert ratings.

To bridge this gap, we propose a supervised fine-tuning (SFT) framework for MedGemma-4B-IT that formulates CT-IQA as a multimodal reasoning task within the vision-language instruction-tuning paradigm (Fig. 1). The objective is to enable the model to derive both quantitative quality scores and qualitative explanations directly from the visual features of CT images. We construct a dataset pairing radiologists' scores with textual explanations derived from the best-performing zero-shot

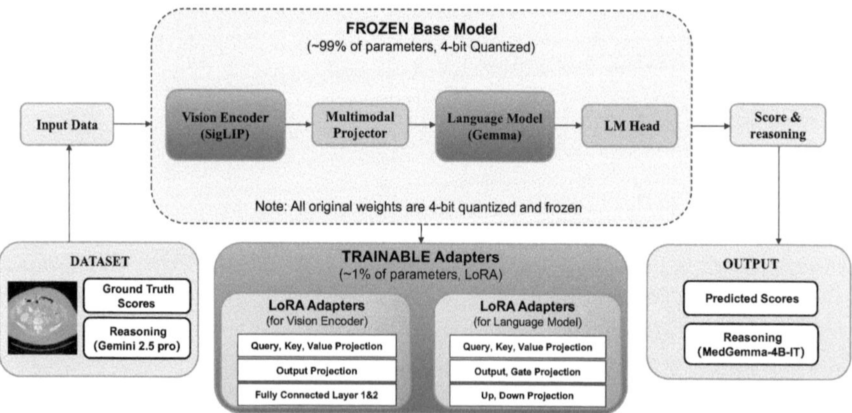

Fig. 1. Overview of the proposed framework. Left: Training data construction. Middle: QLoRA architecture distinguishing frozen 4-bit weights from trainable adapters. Right: Output score and textual explanation.

baseline model and apply quantized low-rank adaptation (QLoRA) for parameter-efficient tuning.

Our results demonstrate that this approach substantially enhances the model's ability to perform nuanced CT-IQA, achieving high correlation with expert scores and outperforming leading VLMs in zero-shot settings. The fine-tuned, locally deployable VLM thus serves as a reliable and explainable solution for automated CT-IQA, offering a privacy-preserving alternative to closed-source, cloud-based systems constrained by patient data regulations.

2 Materials and methods

2.1 Dataset construction

This study is based on the low-dose computed tomography perceptual image quality assessment (LDCTIQA) dataset released for the MICCAI 2023 Challenge, which provides CT images annotated with expert perceptual quality scores [10]. The dataset contains 1,000 CT slices covering various anatomical regions and noise levels. It was randomly split into 800, 100, and 100 samples for training, validation, and testing, respectively.

To obtain rich, human-aligned textual reasoning consistent with expert labels, we employed Gemini 2.5 Pro, which demonstrated the best zero-shot performance to generate explanatory quality assessment texts for each image in the training and validation sets. Numerical quality scores were then paired with these expert-level textual explanations and formatted into structured instruction-response pairs. This process resulted in a novel, explainable CT image quality dataset that integrates expert quantitative ratings with semantically aligned textual reasoning, making it suitable for multimodal supervised fine-tuning.

2.2 Model overview

We selected MedGemma-4B-IT as our base model, leveraging its strong medical priors and multimodal reasoning capabilities. The model's architecture features a Sigmoid-based language-image pre-training (SigLIP) vision encoder, which captures local anatomical and noise patterns from CT images. A multimodal projection layer then aligns these visual representations with the Gemma language space, while the language model, equipped with a language modeling (LM) head, autoregressively generates textual reasoning and the final quality scores.

2.3 Parameter-efficient fine-tuning (PEFT)

We adopt the QLoRA strategy for parameter-efficient fine-tuning applied to all linear projections in both the vision encoder and language model. Specifically, the backbone weights are quantized to 4-bit precision and frozen to significantly reduce memory consumption, while the learnable low-rank adapters are kept in 16-bit precision. This design enables the model to learn task-specific vision-language alignment with minimal trainable parameters and limited computational cost, while preserving the general knowledge encoded in MedGemma.

2.4 Training setup

All experiments were performed using a single NVIDIA RTX 5060Ti GPU with 16GB of VRAM. We trained the model for 3 epochs using AdamW (fused) optimizer with a learning rate of 2×10^{-4}, linear decay, warmup ratio of 0.03, and gradient clipping of 0.3. The per-device batch size was set to 4, and gradient accumulation (×4) was used to achieve an effective batch size of 16. We enabled gradient checkpointing and bfloat16 precision for memory efficiency. Although the loss was computed solely on textual outputs, the cross-modal architecture allowed gradients to propagate through the multimodal projector, effectively tuning both visual and textual alignment. This ensures that visual feature extraction is optimized concurrently with textual reasoning, thereby improving score generation accuracy.

3 Results

All metrics were computed on the held-out LDCTIQA test set (Sec. 2.1). The ground truth quality scores ranged from 0 to 4 and were broadly distributed across the entire range, indicating a balanced representation of low-, medium-, and high-quality CT images. The original MedGemma-4B-IT model, when evaluated in a zero-shot setting on 100 CT images from the test sets, produced 96 predictions clustered around 3.0–3.5. This concentration demonstrates that the unfine-tuned model lacked sensitivity to image quality variations, and its text-based outputs were not diagnostically meaningful.

As shown in Tab. 1, the strong Spearman rank correlation (SRCC = 0.7950) demonstrates that the fine-tuned model learned to preserve the correct ordinal relationships among images, effectively distinguishing "higher-quality" from "lower-quality" CT scans. The Pearson correlation (PLCC = 0.7907) further indicates that the model's predictions not only follow the same trend but also approximate the absolute

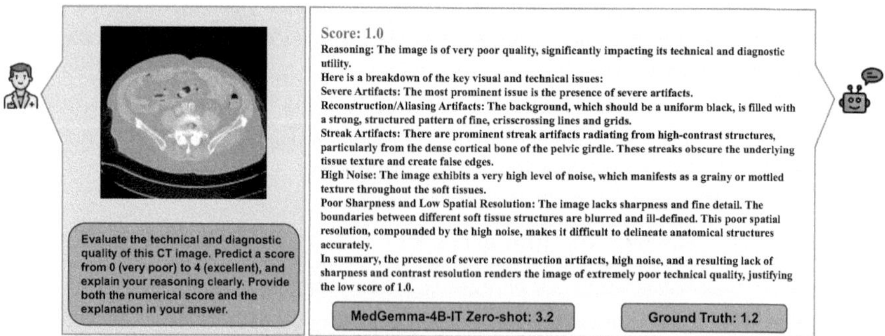

Fig. 2. Sample inference comparing the fine-tuned model against the baseline. The proposed model correctly identifies severe artifacts and noise, predicting a score (1.0) closely aligning with the Ground Truth (1.2). In contrast, the zero-shot MedGemma baseline incorrectly assesses the image as high quality (3.2).

Tab. 1. Comparison of three zero-shot baselines (Gemini 2.5 Flash, Gemini 2.5 Pro, MedGemma-4B-IT) and the fine-tuned MedGemma-4B-IT model.

Model	SRCC	PLCC	MAE	RMSE
Gemini 2.5 Flash (Zero-shot)	0.7170	0.6946	0.7360	0.8800
Gemini 2.5 Pro (Zero-shot)	0.7328	0.7204	0.6540	0.8340
MedGemma-4B-IT (Zero-shot)	-0.2438	-0.2029	1.4790	1.7566
MedGemma-4B-IT (Fine-tuned)	**0.7950**	**0.7907**	**0.5780**	**0.7275**

numerical scale of expert scores. The reduction in mean absolute error (MAE) and root mean squared error (RMSE) confirms that the fine-tuned model provides more precise and stable numerical predictions, aligning closely with radiologist-assigned reference values. Compared with its original weights, the fine-tuned MedGemma-4B-IT improved by over +1.0 SRCC and reduced MAE by 60.92%. The fine-tuned model substantially outperformed all zero-shot baselines.

A paired t-test [11] was conducted to compare absolute prediction errors between the original and the fine-tuned MedGemma-4B-IT models. The MAE decreased from 1.4790 to 0.5780, yielding a t-statistic of 8.03 and a p-value < 0.0001, indicating a statistically significant reduction in prediction error at the 95% confidence level. The computed Cohen's $d = 0.8034$ represents a large effect size, confirming that the improvement is not only statistically significant but also practically meaningful.

As shown in Fig. 2, the model before fine-tuning assigned a misleadingly high score of 3.2/4.0, incorrectly suggesting that the image quality was acceptable. In contrast, the expert-annotated ground truth score for this case was 1.2, indicating the image was almost diagnostically useless. The fine-tuned model not only provided a nearly correct score but also identified multiple specific, critical issues that rendered the image invalid, such as severe reconstruction/aliasing artifacts. Furthermore, the model conducted a comprehensive evaluation across multiple dimensions, demonstrating the soundness of its reasoning logic. It correctly attributed the degradation in sharpness and contrast to the high noise and artifacts as the root cause.

Together, these findings confirm that the fine-tuned MedGemma-4B-IT achieved a marked enhancement in both correlation and accuracy, demonstrating genuine learning of visual quality features beyond text bias.

4 Discussion and conclusion

We have demonstrated the efficacy of transforming a specialized medical VLM, which underperforms in a zero-shot setting, into a powerful tool that accurately emulates the reasoning style of radiologists. This provides a locally deployable, privacy-preserving, and explainable solution for automated CT-IQA.

However, this study has several limitations. First, the textual explanations for fine-tuning were generated by a top-performing zero-shot model (Gemini 2.5 Pro) rather than sourced directly from radiologists' reports. While high in quality, these texts may lack the subtle linguistic nuances of human experts. Second, although the LDCTIQA dataset is representative, the model's generalization capacity must be validated on more diverse data, encompassing a broader spectrum of anatomical regions, scanner models, and artifact types.

Future research could explore reinforcement learning from human feedback (RLHF) to better align the model's generated reasoning with radiologist diagnostic standards. This would advance its development toward an AI assistant capable of delivering consistent, explainable, and clinically reliable IQA across diverse CT protocols, thereby accelerating the adoption of explainable AI (XAI) in medical imaging.

References

1. Xun S, Li Q, Liu X, Huang P, Zhai G, Sun Y et al. Charting the path forward: CT image quality assessment – an in-depth review. J King Saud Univ Sci. 2025;37.
2. Mill L, Bier B, Syben C, Kling L, Klingberg A, Christiansen S et al. Towards in-vivo X-ray nanoscopy. Proc BVM. 2018:115–20.
3. Lorch B, Vaillant G, Baumgartner C, Bai W, Rueckert D, Maier A. Automated detection of motion artefacts in MR imaging using decision forests. J Med Eng. 2017;2017(1):4501647.
4. Preuhs A, Manhart M, Roser P, Stimpel B, Syben C, Psychogios M et al. Image quality assessment for rigid motion compensation. arXiv: 1910.04254. 2019.
5. Patwari M, Gutjahr R, Raupach R, Maier A. Measuring CT reconstruction quality with deep convolutional neural networks. Proc MLMIR. 2019:113–24.
6. Lee W, Wagner F, Galdran A, Shi Y, Xia W, Wang G et al. Low-dose computed tomography perceptual image quality assessment. Med Image Anal. 2025;99:103343.
7. Schwarz A, Dickmann J, Hofmann C, Szkitsak J, Bert C, Maier A et al. Cross-modality image quality prediction for time-resolved CT from breathing signals. Proc MICCAI. 2024:147–56.
8. You Z, Cai X, Gu J, Xue T, Dong C. Teaching large language models to regress accurate image quality scores using score distribution. Proc IEEE/CVF CVPR. 2025:14483–94.
9. Sellergren A, Kazemzadeh S et al. MedGemma technical report. arXiv: 2507.05201. 2025.
10. Lee W, Wagner F, Maier A, Wang A, Baek J, Hsieh SS et al. Low-dose computed tomography perceptual image quality assessment grand challenge dataset (MICCAI 2023). Zenodo, 2023.
11. Hsu H, Lachenbruch PA. Paired t-test. Wiley StatsRef: Stat Ref Online. 2014.

Exploring General-purpose Autonomous Multimodal Agents for Pathology Report Generation

Marc Aubreville [1], Taryn A. Donovan [2], Christof A. Bertram [3]

[1]Flensburg University of Applied Sciences, Flensburg, Germany
[2]Schwarzman Animal Medical Center, New York, USA
[3]University of Veterinary Medicine Vienna, Vienna, Austria
marc.aubreville@hs-flensburg.de

Abstract. Recent advances in agentic artificial intelligence, i.e. systems capable of autonomous perception, reasoning, and tool use, offer new opportunities for digital pathology. In this pilot study, we evaluate whether two agentic multimodal AI systems (OpenAI's ChatGPT 5.0 in agentic mode, and H Company's Surfer) can autonomously navigate, describe, and interpret histopathologic features in digitized tissue slides on a slide viewing platform. A set of 35 veterinary pathology cases, curated for training purposes, was used as the test dataset. The agent was tasked with autonomously exploring whole-slide images using a web-based slide viewer, identifying salient tissue structures, generating descriptive summaries, and proposing provisional diagnoses. We fed different prompts to explore three scenarios: 1) analysis without knowledge of the signalment, 2) analysis with organ and species provided, and 3) diagnosis based on a morphological description provided. All outputs were reviewed and validated by a board-certified pathologist for accuracy and diagnostic consistency. We further tasked another board-certified pathologist with the same task to establish a baseline. We found the systems to yield accurate diagnoses in up to 28.6% of cases with only images, signalment and organ provided (scenario 2), and up to 68.6% when a morphological description was provided (scenario 3). With only the whole slide image (WSI) provided (scenario 1), the models were only correct in up to 5.7% of cases. The human expert, on the other hand, achieved 85.7% diagnostic accuracy with only a single WSI, and 88.6% when also signalment and organ was provided.
The study demonstrates that while the agentic AI system can meaningfully engage with web-based slide viewing software to assess complex visual pathology data and produce contextually aligned feature descriptions, diagnostic precision remains limited compared with a human expert.

1 Introduction

The establishment of digital pathology workflows in labs allows for the use of artificial intelligence (AI) based solutions to be embedded into the diagnostic process. While current research shows that methods based on deep learning models can

© Der/die Autor(en), exklusiv lizenziert an
Springer Fachmedien Wiesbaden GmbH, ein Teil von Springer Nature 2026
H. Handels et al. (Hrsg.), *Bildverarbeitung für die Medizin 2026*,
Informatik aktuell, https://doi.org/10.1007/978-3-658-51100-5_76

achieve performance on the same level of or even exceeding pathology experts, the tasks considered are typically narrowly defined tasks, such as mitotic figure identification [1], cell or tissue segmentation [2], or tumor grading [3].

Report generation is the final step in the pathological diagnosis and involves a multitude of pattern recognition steps, in combination with reasoning and navigation on the pathology slide(s) at various magnifications. Given the complexity of this task, it could be assumed that this is an unachievable task for current artificial intelligence systems. Yet, recent models released in the field of agentic artificial intelligence have demonstrated emerging capabilities for autonomous reasoning, multimodal perception, and iterative goal-directed behavior. In particular, the use of large vision and language models, in combination with tool use, has enabled browser-based navigation of websites, supported by planning and reasoning of workflows. Large-language models models have gained remarkable capabilities across a wide range of domains, and while domain-specific training does improve on the results, even general-purpose models can be applied successfully – albeit with limitations – to specialized fields such as medicine [4]. This raises an intriguing question: Can such general-purpose AI agents emulate aspects of the diagnostic workflow, specifically, the exploration, recognition, and verbal synthesis steps performed by pathologists?

In this study, we investigate the feasibility of deploying an agentic AI system within an open source digital slide viewing environment to autonomously perform slide navigation, tissue feature description, and preliminary diagnostic reasoning. To the best of our knowledge, this is the first attempt at testing the capability of commercially available general-purpose AI tools at this highly specialized task. While we do not advocate for the automation of pathology report generation in real-world clinical settings (given the significant ethical and safety concerns involved), we propose that this task offers a valuable benchmark for assessing the emerging capabilities of agentic vision-language models.

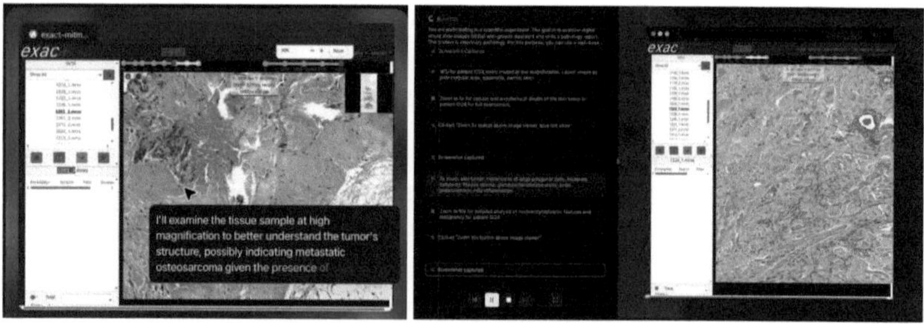

Fig. 1. Screenshots of the experiment, showing ChatGPT 5.0 (OpenAI, left panel) and Surfer (H Company, right panel). Both investigated agentic AI frameworks were able to successfully navigate the slides and complete the tasks.

2 Methods

We prepared an online slide viewing platform [5] with a dataset of 35 cases from veterinary pathology, retrieved from the diagnostic archive of the University of *anonymized*. These cases were part of a panel of educational cases of neoplastic and tumor-like lesions for the training of students and residents in veterinary pathology. Naturally, this means that the cases were selected to be interesting, rather than representative of the general sample distribution, and had an overall good quality. Furthermore, it means that these cases were selected to be diagnostically characteristic, which facilitates the evaluation in this experiment. For each case, we have the following data records:

1. A single whole slide image (WSI) for each case using hematoxylin and eosin stain.
2. The organ the specimen was retrieved from.
3. The signalment, i.e., the animal's species and breed, as well as age and sex.
4. The complete morphologic description by a board-certified pathologist, following a structured catalog, but given in plain text. The morphological description contains all features required to infer the diagnosis.
5. The diagnosis, including information which type of growth disorder (benign or malignant tumor, hyperplasia, ...) was determined by a board-certified veterinary pathologist.

Out of the 35 cases, 28 were from dogs, six from cats, one from a guinea pig, and one from a horse. Regarding organs, the largest organ represented was the skin (13/35), reflecting the high sampling frequency of this organ in domestic animal diagnostic pathology. Furthermore, there were samples from adrenal gland (N=4), spleen (N=4), mammary gland / breast (N=2), eye (N=2), intestine (N=2), joint (N=2), oral mucosa (N=2), uterus (N=2), vulva (N=1), and central nervous system (N=1), covering a wide range of organs. From this, we define three scenarios with progressively more conditioning or context provided to the model:

- Scenario A – WSI only: The model received only the WSI and was tasked with inferring both the organ of origin and the diagnosis solely from the image content.
- Scenario B – WSI + brief case description: The model was provided with the WSI along with a concise case description, including signalment (species, breed, sex, age, and neuter status) and the organ of origin.
- Scenario C – Morphologic description only: The model received only a textual morphologic description. Because the complete morphology was already represented in the description, the WSI was not provided to accelerate inference.

From the dataset, we derived prompts, requiring the model to provide a structured JSON object per case. In this, we requested the model to provide the organ, the diagnosis, as well as multiple morphologic descriptions to provide the model with an incentive to investigate the specimen thoroughly. This list consists of shape (of mass), demarcation (of tumor/surrounding tissue), invasion, cellularity (of mass), growth pattern, stroma and matrix (amount and type), other subgross features (such as hemorrhage or superficial ulceration), tumor cells (size, shape, cell borders, differentiation), tumor cytoplasm (amount, character, content), tumor nuclei (shape, location, chromatin distribution), tumor nucleoli (number and size), malignancy criteria (nuclear pleomorphism and mitotic activity), and other tumor features (necrosis, inflammation, or multinucleation). The detailed prompts and example videos are provided in our github repository[1]. We used batches of three to expedite the experiment, striking a compromise between potentially running into the context limits of the model (as a result of having too many cases) and limiting the time required for the initial setup of the model and the log-in process. In the slide viewing platform, a single dataset was created to be visible for the client. We specifically instructed the model with hints on navigation on the slide and in the software, which we found to be beneficial in early experiments.

We surveyed two agentic multimodal AI solutions that allow for the direct formulation of tasks to be executed on websites: OpenAI's ChatGPT 5.0 in agentic mode, as well as H Company's Surfer [6], which is built on the publicly available Holo1 v1.5 model [7]. Both frameworks were utilized using their respective web user interfaces. If available, caches and memories were turned off for the experiment. After retrieving results from each suite, a board-certified veterinary pathologist evaluated all responses for accuracy. We evaluated the detailed textual morphologic descriptions only for the leading model, as the second-best model yielded notably subpar performance, making an in-depth analysis of its morphologic descriptions less informative. As a benchmark for the AI agents, we asked a second board-certified pathologist to evaluate the WSIs at two time points with the same (limited) information available as the AI agents.

3 Results

Our results indicate that both frameworks had considerable difficulties performing this highly complex task, as opposed to a pathologist who made the correct diagnosis in >85% of the cases (Tab. 1). While we did not observe major obstacles involving the navigation within the slide viewing software, the correctness of the models was generally low. However, we observed that the models did, in many cases, not visually inspect the most relevant parts of the slide, which contributes to a low performance, since slide areas containing potentially important visual features were never inspected. This is reflected by numerous erroneous descriptions of ChatGPT in 336 of 455 features (73.85%, Fig. 2). An important observation was that the models never avoided providing a diagnosis or detailed morphologic descriptions, but delivered an answer that might be probable based upon the information provided (i.e. signalment and organ), listing common tumors for a given species and organ, but not the actual tumor type depicted in the case being examined. This is also reflected by the increased rate of correct diagnoses and descriptions (error rate of ChatGPT:

[1]https://github.com/DeepMicroscopy/AgenticPathologyReports/

Tab. 1. Results of our experiment, evaluated by a board-certified pathologist. Both evaluated frameworks benefit from knowing the organ and signalment, and more so by a morphological description.

Framework	Trial	Organ correct	Diagnosis correct	Wrong dignity	Wrong subtype
ChatGPT 5.0	A: Only WSI available	28.6%	5.7%	5.7%	2.9%
	B: WSI + signalment + organ given	100.0%	28.6%	2.9%	2.9%
	C: Morphological description given	100.0%	68.6%	8.6%	2.9%
Surfer	A: Only WSI available	11.4%	2.9%	0.0%	5.7%
	B: WSI + signalment + organ given	97.1%	8.6%	2.9%	17.1%
	C: Morphological description given	97.1%	68.6%	5.7%	17.1%
Pathologist	A: Only WSI available	91.5%	85.7%	5.7%	0%
	B: WSI + signalment + organ given	N/A	88.6%	5.7%	0%

270 of 455 features, 59.3%) once the signalment and organ were provided to the model.

In the identification of the corresponding organ, we saw a considerable difference between both frameworks, with the ChatGPT framework having a higher performance across all conditions. We also found that this model was better at contextualizing the provided brief case description in scenario B. If a morphological description was provided to the models, the likelihood of a correct diagnosis of both models was much higher (Tab. 1). If the organ was provided; either as part of the brief case description (scenario B) or as part of a verbal morphological description, the models had almost no difficulty in identifying the corresponding organ.

4 Discussion

The observations in our study align with prior observations of model hallucination in large (vision and language) models being more likely in the long tail of the data distribution [8], which this use case is certainly representative of. Given the improved rate of diagnostic success in the third scenario (with morphological description given),

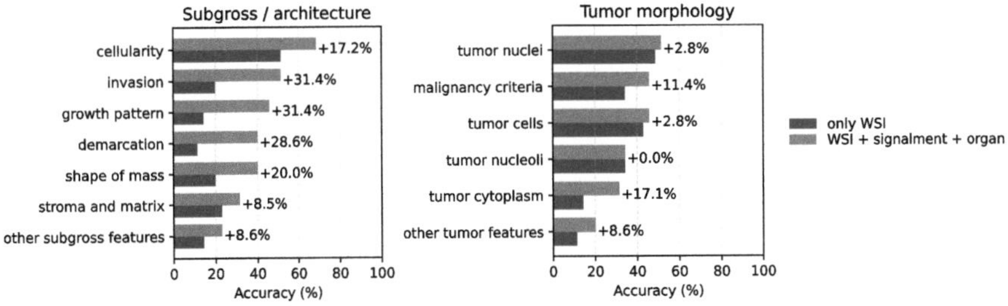

Fig. 2. Accuracy of individual morphologic descriptions given by the leading model (ChatGPT 5.0), as evaluated by a board-certified pathologist.

we can hypothesize that the most challenging part of this task might have been the targeted navigation, in search for diagnostically relevant features, and the extraction and description thereof. This would also correlate with expectations, as the training data for vision-language models (VLMs) is likely to be underrepresented with examples executing diagnostic workflows in pathology, while textual descriptions linking morphological descriptions and diagnoses are likely to be part of the scientific literature that was used in training the models. Although pathology-specific VLMs have recently been introduced [9], this study focused on evaluating general-purpose VLMs due to their broad accessibility and frequent use. In our observation, both students and medical practitioners increasingly rely on these general models as informal knowledge resources for medical inquiries. While the evaluated VLMs demonstrated the ability to employ appropriate medical terminology – potentially conveying an impression of domain competence – our findings reveal a considerable rate of error in diagnostic interpretation and in the description of histopathological images. These results underscore the importance of exercising caution when using VLMs in educational or clinical contexts.

We acknowledge that our study was limited to only two frameworks that provided integration of web-based browsing with agentic models, and that other, and in particular specialized, models and/or pipelines [9] might be more suitable for this task. However, our primary objective was not to benchmark performance across the full spectrum of available models, but rather to explore the feasibility and qualitative behavior of current general-purpose VLM-based agents when applied to a highly domain-specific diagnostic task.

References

1. Aubreville M, Stathonikos N, Donovan TA et al. Domain generalization across tumor types, laboratories, and species: insights from the 2022 edition of the mitosis domain generalization challenge. Med Image Anal. 2024;94:103155.
2. Ma J, Xie R, Ayyadhury S et al. The multimodality cell segmentation challenge: toward universal solutions. Nat Methods. 2024;21(6):1103–13.
3. Bulten W, Kartasalo K, Chen PHC, Ström P, Pinckaers H, Nagpal K et al. Artificial intelligence for diagnosis and Gleason grading of prostate cancer: the PANDA challenge. Nat Med. 2022;28(1):154–63.
4. Saab K, Tu T, Weng WH et al. Capabilities of Gemini models in medicine. arXiv: 2404.18416. 2024.
5. Marzahl C, Aubreville M, Bertram CA et al. EXACT: a collaboration toolset for algorithm-aided annotation of images with annotation version control. Sci Rep. 2021;11(1):4343.
6. Andreux M, Skuk BB, Benchekroun H et al. Surfer-H meets Holo1: cost-efficient web agent powered by open weights. arXiv: 2506.02865. 2025.
7. Hcompany. Holo15. `https://huggingface.co/collections/Hcompany/holo15-68c1a5736e8583a309d23d9b`. Accessed: 2025-12-12. 2025.
8. Huang L, Yu W, Ma W et al. A survey on hallucination in large language models: principles, taxonomy, challenges, and open questions. ACM Trans Inf Syst. 2025;43(2):1–55.

9. Zhang W, Guo J, Zhang H et al. Patho-AgenticRAG: Towards multimodal agentic retrieval-augmented generation for pathology VLMs via reinforcement learning. arXiv: 2508.02258. 2025.

Abstract: BigReg

An Efficient Registration Pipeline for High-resolution X-ray and Light-sheet Fluorescence Microscopy

Siyuan Mei[1], Fuxin Fan[1], Mareike Thies[1], Mingxuan Gu[1], Fabian Wagner[1], Oliver Aust[2], Ina Erceg[3], Zeynab Mirzaei[4], Georgiana Neag[2], Yipeng Sun[1], Yixing Huang[5], Andreas Maier[1]

[1]Pattern Recognition Lab, Friedrich-Alexander University Erlangen-Nuremberg
[2]Department of Internal Medicine 3, University Hospital Erlangen
[3]Fraunhofer Institute for Ceramic Technologies and Systems - IKTS
[4]Institute for Nanotechnology and Correlative Microscopy - INAM GmbH
[5]Institute of Medical Technology, Health Science Center, Peking University
siyuan.mei@fau.de

X-ray microscopy (XRM) and light-sheet fluorescence microscopy (LSFM) have emerged as pivotal tools in preclinical research, particularly for studying bone remodeling diseases such as osteoporosis. To enable micrometer-level structural correspondence and facilitate functional analysis, we introduce BigReg, an automatic, two-stage registration pipeline optimized for high-resolution XRM and LSFM volumes [1]. The first stage involves extracting surface features and applying two successive global-to-local point cloud-based methods for coarse alignment. The subsequent stage refines this alignment in the 3D Fourier domain using a modified cross-correlation technique, achieving precise volumetric registration. Evaluations using expert-annotated landmarks and augmented test data demonstrate that BigReg approaches the accuracy of landmark-based registration with a landmark distance (LMD) of 8.36 µm ± 0.12 µm and a landmark fitness (LM fitness) of 85.71% ± 1.02%. Moreover, BigReg can provide an optimal initialization for mutual information-based methods which otherwise fail independently, further reducing LMD to 7.24 µm ± 0.11 µm and increasing LM fitness to 93.90% ± 0.77%. To the best of our knowledge, BigReg is the first automated method to successfully register XRM and LSFM volumes without requiring manual intervention or prior alignment cues, thus opening up new avenues for multimodal analysis of bone microarchitecture and disease pathology.

References

1. Mei S, Fan F, Thies M, Gu M, Wagner F, Aust O et al. BigReg: an efficient registration pipeline for high-resolution X-ray and light-sheet fluorescence microscopy. J Med Imaging. 2025;12(5):54004–4.

© Der/die Autor(en), exklusiv lizenziert an
Springer Fachmedien Wiesbaden GmbH, ein Teil von Springer Nature 2026
H. Handels et al. (Hrsg.), *Bildverarbeitung für die Medizin 2026*,
Informatik aktuell, https://doi.org/10.1007/978-3-658-51100-5_77

Abstract: Bone-guided Semi-supervised Registration

Lukas Förner [1,2,3], Thomas Wendler [1,2,3,4,5]

[1]Department of Diagnostic and Interventional Radiology and Neuroradiology, University Hospital Augsburg, Augsburg, Germany
[2]Computer-Aided Medical Procedures and Augmented Reality, Technical University of Munich, Garching bei München, Germany
[3]Digital Medicine, University Hospital Augsburg, Augsburg, Germany
[4]Center of Advanced Analytics and Predictive Sciences, University of Augsburg, Germany
[5]Bavarian Cancer Research Center (BZKF) Augsburg, Germany
lukas.foerner@uk-augsburg.de

Learning-based deformable image registration (DIR) achieves accurate correspondences but struggles with intensity changes [1], e.g., COVID-19, where evolving ground-glass opacities, consolidations, and inflation differences alter Hounsfield distributions. We incorporate rigid anatomical guidance [2]: bone masks define rigidly-moving regions, with per-structure pre-alignment and a differentiable rigid-consistency loss constraining the field within masks while allowing flexible soft-tissue deformations. Using TransMorph [3] on Learn2Reg NLST thoracic CT [4] (209 volumes; 1.5 mm isotropic; 224×192×224), we compare baseline, label-only, rigid-only, and combined regimes via overlap (DSC, HD95) and plausibility metrics (volume change, HU-histogram JS divergence, negative Jacobians). Label-only achieves the strongest overlap but degrades plausibility; rigid-only significantly improves volume preservation ($p = 0.003$). Combined supervision balances this trade-off, significantly reducing HU deviation ($p = 0.004$) and negative Jacobians ($p < 0.001$) without significant volume change ($p = 0.130$), preventing rib collapse/stretching. The architecture-agnostic rigid loss is extensible to other anatomics for biomechanically plausible longitudinal CT analyses.

References

1. Hering A, Hansen L, Mok TCW, Chung ACS, Siebert H, Hager S et al. Learn2Reg: comprehensive multi-task medical image registration challenge, dataset and evaluation in the era of deep learning. IEEE Trans Med Imaging. 2023;42(3):697–712.
2. Förner L, Wendler T. Anatomy-guided semi-supervised registration with combined rigid and label supervision for improved rib deformation consistency. Proc MLMI. 2026:562–71.
3. Chen J, Frey EC, He Y, Segars WP, Li Y, Du Y. TransMorph: transformer for unsupervised medical image registration. Med Image Anal. 2022;82:102615.
4. Hering A, Murphy K, van Ginneken B. Learn2Reg challenge: CT lung registration – training data. Zenodo, 2020.

© Der/die Autor(en), exklusiv lizenziert an
Springer Fachmedien Wiesbaden GmbH, ein Teil von Springer Nature 2026
H. Handels et al. (Hrsg.), *Bildverarbeitung für die Medizin 2026*,
Informatik aktuell, https://doi.org/10.1007/978-3-658-51100-5_78

Abstract: Time-continuous Sliding Motion Image Registration using Stationary Velocity Fields for Respiratory Motion Interpolation

Ole Gildemeister [1], Johannes Bostelmann [1], Pia Schulz [1], Andra Oltmann [2], Phillip Rostalski [2,3], Jan Modersitzki [1,4], Jan Lellmann [1,4]

[1]Institute of Mathematics and Image Computing, University of Lübeck
[2]Fraunhofer Research Institution for Individualized and Cell-Based Medical Engineering
[3]Institute for Electrical Engineering in Medicine, University of Lübeck
[4]Fraunhofer Institute for Digital Medicine MEVIS, Lübeck
o.gildemeister@uni-luebeck.de

Motivated by the application of respiratory surface electromyography, we propose [1] a motion interpolation framework for computing a time-continuous model of the respiratory cycle based on end-inspiratory and end-expiratory 3D MRI images in the form of a dense deformation map $\phi : \mathbb{R}^3 \times [0, 1] \to \mathbb{R}^3$. The challenge is to incorporate the sliding motion occurring in the pleural cavity, while simultaneously enabling accurate motion interpolation. Such a combination has not been addressed in previous works [2].

To facilitate sliding motion along predefined surfaces, we require an interior local volume Ω_{loc} whose motion is assumed to differ from its surroundings in a sliding fashion. We then obtain ϕ as the composition $\phi := \phi_{\text{loc}} \circ \phi_{\text{glob}}$, where the global diffeomorphism ϕ_{glob} aligns structures outside Ω_{loc}, followed by a local deformation ϕ_{loc} which diffeomorphically aligns the structures inside Ω_{loc}. The result is a dense, piecewise diffeomorphic deformation map with sliding motion along the boundaries of Ω_{loc}.

We model both deformations ϕ_{loc} and ϕ_{glob} via stationary velocity fields, each parameterized by a neural implicit representation. To enforce invariance of Ω_{loc} under the local deformation ϕ_{loc}, we propose a hybrid technique of restricting the velocity field and employing a soft penalty. We validate our approach for registration and motion interpolation experimentally on real-world data.

References

1. Gildemeister O, Bostelmann J, Schulz PF, Oltmann A, Rostalski P, Modersitzki J, Lellmann J. Time-continuous sliding motion image registration using stationary velocity fields for respiratory motion interpolation. Proc SSVM. 2025:404–16.
2. Risser L, Vialard FX, Baluwala HY, Schnabel JA. Piecewise-diffeomorphic image registration: application to the motion estimation between 3D CT lung images with sliding conditions. Med Image Anal. 2013;17(2):182–93.

© Der/die Autor(en), exklusiv lizenziert an
Springer Fachmedien Wiesbaden GmbH, ein Teil von Springer Nature 2026
H. Handels et al. (Hrsg.), *Bildverarbeitung für die Medizin 2026*,
Informatik aktuell, https://doi.org/10.1007/978-3-658-51100-5_79

Resource-efficient Fine-tuning of Stable Diffusion for Synthetic Hand Radiograph Generation

Marten J. Finck [1†], Sina P. Lücke [1†], Niklas C. Koser [2†], Yu Sun [3], Jan-B. Hövener [2], Wojtek Palubicki [4], Sören Pirk [1]

[1]Visual Computing and Artificial Intelligence, Kiel University, Kiel, Germany
[2]i2Lab@Section Biomedical Imaging, Kiel University, University Hospital Schleswig-Holstein, Kiel, Germany
[3]Helmholtz-Zentrum hereon GmbH, Institute of Metallic Biomaterials, Geesthacht, Germany
[4]Mathematics and Computer Science, Adam Mickiewicz University, Poznan, Poland
mafi@informatik.uni-kiel.de

Abstract. The performance of deep learning models in medical image analysis critically depends on the access to large and high-quality datasets. However, ethical, legal, and privacy constraints often limit data availability. Generative models offer a promising solution by producing synthetic training data, yet their resource-efficient fine-tuning remains an open challenge. This study investigates whether stable diffusion (SD) can be adapted using low-rank adaptation (LoRA) with minimal data and computational resources to generate synthetic hand radiographs (X-rays). The aim is not perfect anatomical fidelity but the reproduction of key X-ray characteristics under restrictive conditions. Quantitative and qualitative comparisons of a generic and a medically pre-trained SD 1.4 model show that both can produce visually plausible X-rays despite anatomical imperfections. These findings demonstrate the potential of lightweight fine-tuning methods for medical imaging and underscore the need for systematic research on training efficiency, quality assessment of synthetic data, and integration of synthetic and real datasets in medical AI.

1 Introduction

Deep learning has the potential to revolutionize the field of medical imaging, as it enables analyzing images with unprecedented accuracy and efficiency [1, 2]. However, the success of such models depends on the availability of large, diverse, and high-quality datasets. Besides the common challenges associated with data collection, such as high costs [3] and label inaccuracies introduced by manual annotation [4], curating datasets for medical tasks is further hindered by ethical, legal, and privacy constraints [5]. Consequently, the development of robust and generalizable models is

[†]These authors contributed equally to this work.

© Der/die Autor(en), exklusiv lizenziert an
Springer Fachmedien Wiesbaden GmbH, ein Teil von Springer Nature 2026
H. Handels et al. (Hrsg.), *Bildverarbeitung für die Medizin 2026*,
Informatik aktuell, https://doi.org/10.1007/978-3-658-51100-5_80

often limited by data availability. To address these challenges, synthetic data generation has emerged as a promising solution [6, 7]. Recent progress in diffusion-based models has demonstrated remarkable capabilities in generating high-fidelity and diverse images across various domains [8–10]. In particular, latent diffusion models (LDMs) make the diffusion process computationally more efficient by operating in a compressed latent space while enabling text-conditioned image generation [9]. In the medical domain, diffusion models have shown great potential for data augmentation and improving downstream task performance, such as the classification of pathological structures and the segmentation of anatomical regions [11, 12]. However, the substantial data requirements for training diffusion models often necessitate transferring large pretrained models (originally trained on generic image data) into the medical domain. Several studies have explored this adaptation: Chambon et al. [13] fine-tuned components of stable diffusion (SD) models for chest X-ray synthesis, while Zhang et al. [14] and Kidder et al. [15] used DreamBooth-based fine-tuning to achieve domain-specific generation. More recently, low-rank adaptation (LoRA) has been introduced as a parameter-efficient approach that enables the effective fine-tuning of large diffusion models on small datasets [16–18].

Building upon this line of work, we aim to address three primary research directions: (1) We investigate the efficient fine-tuning of SD models with LoRA for medical imaging using minimal computational resources and a small-scale dataset; (2) We analyze and compare the quality of medical image generation between a generic SD 1.4 model and a RoentGen model pretrained on medical data; and (3) We demonstrate a transferable approach for similar medical applications under comparable resource constraints and derive directions for future research.

2 Materials and methods

In this work, we use the MURA dataset, comprising 40,561 musculoskeletal X-rays of the upper extremities from 14,863 studies on 12,173 patients, acquired between 2001 and 2012 at Stanford Hospital [19]. To evaluate the fine-tuning capabilities of SD models using LoRA, a reduced subset of hand and wrist X-rays (palmodorsal) in the predefined training dataset was used, consisting of 50 training and

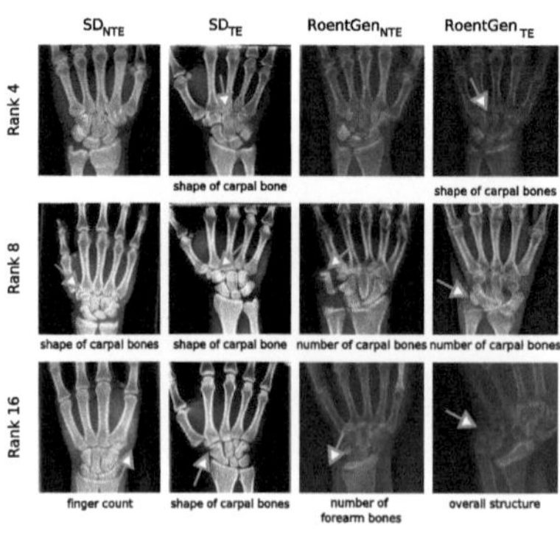

Fig. 1. Example synthetic hand X-rays for the same prompt with different LoRA ranks. The arrows indicate anatomical errors. Prompt: Positive, left hand, fracture at proximal phalanx I and metacarpal I.

Findings	Training (n = 50)	Validation (n = 32)
Negative	13 (26 %)	8 (25 %)
Positive	37 (74 %)	24 (75 %)
Radius fracture	14	8
Arthrosis	13	5
Metacarpus fracture	9	5
Phalanx fracture	8	5
Scaphoid fracture	8	4
Injured joint	5	2
Visible growth plates	4	1
Ulna fracture	3	1
Partial amputation	3	1

Tab. 1. Dataset distribution. Multiple pathologies may coexist in each positively labeled X-ray.

LoRA Rank	Text Encoder	Trainable Parameters
4	No	797,184
4	Yes	1,092,096
8	No	1,594,368
8	Yes	1,889,280
16	No	3,188,736
16	Yes	3,483,648

Tab. 2. Number of trainable parameters (for comparison: The SD 1.4 model has 1,066,235,307 total parameters).

32 validation samples (60/40 split). This is assumed to be a feasible preprocessing workload (resulting from e.g., manual annotations) for individual researchers or small teams. In advance, trivial cases, such as images with amputations or implants, were excluded, and incorrect lateral markings were removed to avoid distortions. The subset was balanced for laterality (left/right) and region (hand/wrist), with positive cases oversampled threefold to reflect clinical prevalence (Tab. 1). For each X-ray, a structured report was created by a medical professional with a radiology license to standardize text input for the diffusion model. Each report comprises: (1) a "Technique" section describing projection plane, imaging technique, affected side, and anatomical region; and (2) an "Impression" section analyzing the X-ray from proximal to distal using standard radiological terminology. Reports were limited to 40 words and prefixed with either "positive" or "negative".

For this study, two models based on the same LDM architecture were evaluated to ensure direct comparability. The first is SD 1.4, consisting of a U-Net, a variational autoencoder (VAE), and a ViT-L/14 text encoder. SD 1.4 was trained on a subset of the LAION-2B(en) dataset using 256 NVIDIA A100 GPUs, where images were encoded into latent representations (f = 8) and text prompts were integrated via cross-attention [9]. As a medically pre-trained counterpart, the RoentGen model [13] was used. RoentGen is an SD 1.4-based model fine-tuned on the MIMIC-CXR dataset, comprising 377,110 chest X-rays and associated reports [20]. Training was performed on 64 NVIDIA A100 GPUs (bf16 precision, 512 × 512 resolution), using only the "Impression" section of the reports. The best-performing checkpoint, fine-tuned on both the U-Net and text encoder, was selected for this study. During inference, 75 denoising steps and a guidance scale of 4 were applied.

Experiments were conducted in Google Colaboratory [21] using a Tesla T4 GPU (16 GB VRAM) with fp16 precision. As the input images varied in size and were not consistently 512 × 512, they were manually cropped to 256 × 256 which further improved efficiency. Fine-tuning was performed on normalized images within a value range of [-1, 1] for 1,250 epochs with a batch size of 16. Pre-trained SD 1.4 weights were obtained from the CompVis repository on Hugging Face, and RoentGen weights were provided by the authors. During inference, the same configuration as in RoentGen fine-tuning was used to ensure comparability [13].

A total of twelve LoRA fine-tuning experiments were conducted, comparing ranks 4, 8, and 16 for each model. Following Chambon et al. [13], two variants were tested: (1) U-Net adaptation only, and (2) joint U-Net and text encoder adaptation, with the text encoder rank fixed at 4. In line with Hu et al. [16], LoRA was applied to the linear projection layers within the attention modules. Experiments were denoted as $\text{Model}_{x\text{NTE}}$ and $\text{Model}_{x\text{TE}}$, where x indicates the U-Net rank. Hyperparameters were optimized iteratively based on t-SNE distributions, loss curves, and Euclidean distances between validation and synthetic image features. The best results were obtained with the AdamW optimizer (weight decay 0.1, $\beta_1 = 0.9$, $\beta_2 = 0.999$, $\epsilon = 1 \times 10^{-8}$), an initial learning rate of 1×10^{-4}, and cosine scheduling to 1×10^{-6}. This configuration yielded images 33% closer to validation features and 17% more self-consistent.

3 Results

To assess the optimal LoRA rank, parameter reduction and training time were recorded to evaluate fine-tuning efficiency. Model performance was evaluated at three checkpoints evenly distributed across training. For each checkpoint, 32 synthetic X-rays were generated using prompts from the validation set. Image quality was quantified using the Fréchet inception distance (FID) [22] and further assessed qualitatively. To examine generalization and potential overfitting, a t-SNE analysis of latent image representations was performed. A radiologist and an orthopedic specialist evaluated the generated images. The assessment comprised: (1) a discrimination task, where experts distinguished real from synthetic X-rays, and (2) a detailed analysis of anatomical correctness on pre-sorted images (good, medium, bad).

LoRA fine-tuning substantially reduced trainable parameters (Tab. 2). The parameter count scaled linearly with rank and increased by approximately 300k when including the text encoder. Training times ranged from 1 h 54 min to 2 h 4 min, indicating that rank had minimal influence on duration.

As shown in Tab. 3, FID values fluctuated non-linearly during training, and no consistent correlation between rank or text encoder adaptation and performance was observed. The best-performing model was $\text{SD}_{4\text{NTE}}$ (FID = 153.85 at checkpoint 834), closely followed by $\text{RoentGen}_{16\text{TE}}$ (FID = 158.43). Visual inspection confirmed $\text{SD}_{4\text{NTE}}$ produced the most realistic hand X-rays, aligning with quantitative results (Fig. 1). Since FID is limited for small datasets and ignores anatomical fidelity, greater emphasis was placed on qualitative evaluation. The t-SNE analysis indicated distinct clustering of generated and real images, with overlapping point clouds but

Experiment	↓ FID CKPT 417	CKPT 834	CKPT 1250
SD_{4NTE}	167.60	**153.85**	**166.68**
SD_{8NTE}	187.14	182.14	184.62
SD_{16NTE}	184.50	173.64	167.60
SD_{4TE}	**165.14**	163.94	168.47
SD_{8TE}	195.33	194.77	197.24
SD_{16TE}	176.42	190.11	179.75
$RoentGen_{4NTE}$	169.84	161.80	**166.05**
$RoentGen_{8NTE}$	180.66	181.89	194.14
$RoentGen_{16NTE}$	202.69	186.32	195.01
$RoentGen_{4TE}$	174.54	178.72	184.46
$RoentGen_{8TE}$	**161.88**	175.18	174.33
$RoentGen_{16TE}$	182.87	**158.43**	168.81

Tab. 3. FID values for all experiments and checkpoints. Lower values indicate better generative performance.

no identical samples, providing no visual evidence of overfitting or data replication. In the expert evaluation, both medical specialists correctly identified the synthetic samples, confirming that even the best models do not yet reach clinical realism. During detailed analysis, the radiologist highlighted several anatomical inaccuracies, particularly in the representation of carpal bones, joint alignments, and fracture morphology. RoentGen images often showed unphysiological vertical whitening lines, while SD occasionally misrepresented epiphyseal joints and arthritic changes. The orthopedic specialist categorized deficiencies into seven main areas: (1) insufficient similarity to real X-rays, (2) soft tissue abnormalities, (3) bone inconsistencies in number, position, or morphology, (4) joint abnormalities, (5) proportion errors, (6) abnormal bone density, and (7) unrealistic pathological patterns. Despite these issues, both experts noted that SD produced more plausible X-rays than RoentGen, especially regarding arthroses, fractures, and soft tissue overlays, and that inexperienced viewers might mistake some SD-generated images for authentic ones.

Finally, the catastrophic forgetting analysis (Figs. 2a, 2b) showed that after fine-tuning, both models lost the ability to generate images from their original domains-

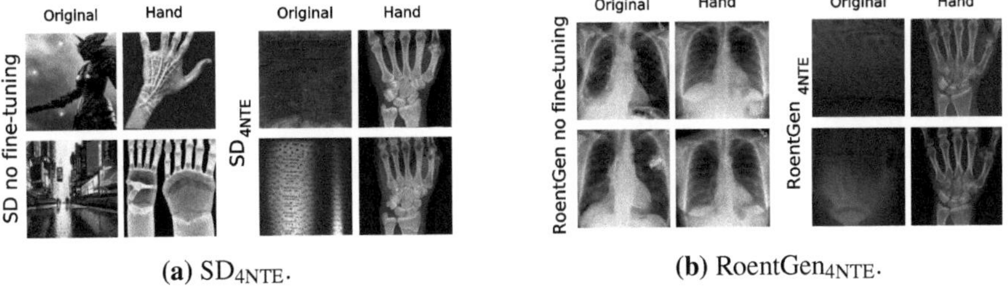

(a) SD_{4NTE}. (b) $RoentGen_{4NTE}$.

Fig. 2. Assessment of catastrophic forgetting using prompts from the original domain and prompts describing hand X-rays before as well as after fine-tuning.

SD no longer produced generic images, while RoentGen continued to output chest X-rays prior to adaptation-indicating significant representational overwrite.

4 Discussion

In this work, we developed a resource-efficient fine-tuning approach to adapt pre-trained LDMs for synthesizing hand X-rays using text prompts. The LoRA implementation reduced the trainable parameters by a factor of around 1000, with a training time of approximately 2 hours regardless of rank. According to the quantitative analysis, SD_{4NTE} and $RoentGen_{16TE}$ achieved the lowest FIDs. The qualitative analysis, however, revealed that $RoentGen_{4NTE}$ is superior to the quantitatively best RoentGen model in terms of visual and anatomical plausibility. The medical experts consulted were able to perform the discrimination task without errors and found in the detailed analysis of the synthetic images that anatomical structures were reproduced correctly in some cases. Nevertheless, difficulties arose in particular with the representation of the carpal bones and contrasts. Both experts considered that the results of SD_{4NTE} (checkpoint 1250) tended to be slightly more favorable, implying no relevant influence of pre-training on medical data. Overfitting is not observed in either SD_{4NTE} or $RoentGen_{4NTE}$. As no mitigation strategies, such as experience replay [23] or elastic weight consolidation [24], were applied, catastrophic forgetting is apparent.

Our study is subject to certain limitations that may influence the generalizability and significance of the results. The training dataset was deliberately small and limited to a single projection, which may restrict the models' ability to learn diverse features. Anatomical correctness was assessed only via perceptual metrics and expert feedback, and downstream task evaluation was not performed. Additionally, automatic generation of radiological reports remains absent, limiting scalability for downstream training.

The models developed here open several avenues for future research. (1) Fine-tuning with larger and more diverse datasets could help optimize the tradeoff between anatomical correctness and computational efficiency. (2) The development of specific metrics, such as bone distances or angles, would enable a more precise and holistic assessment of anatomical fidelity. (3) Expanding expert evaluation and assessing inter- and intra-rater variability would strengthen the reliability of the findings. (4) The clinical relevance of these models could be investigated through downstream tasks (e.g., fracture detection), which would require generating corresponding labels alongside synthetic images to produce fully annotated datasets for training.

Acknowledgement. This work was supported by the IDIR-Project (Digital Implant Research), a cooperation financed by Kiel University, University Hospital Schleswig-Holstein and Helmholtz Zentrum Hereon. We would also like to express our sincere gratitude to Dr. med. Thomas Lange for his medical expertise and insightful guidance, which greatly contributed to the success of this project.

References

1. Kazerouni A, Aghdam EK, Heidari M et al. Diffusion models in medical imaging: a comprehensive survey. Med Image Anal. 2023;88:102846.
2. Shen D, Wu G, Suk HI. Deep learning in medical image analysis. Annu Rev Biomed Eng. 2017;19(1):221–48.
3. Fredriksson T, Mattos DI, Bosch J, Olsson HH. 2D medical image synthesis using transformer-based denoising diffusion probabilistic model. Product-focused Software Process Improvement. Vol. 12562. Cham: Springer International Publishing, 2020:202–16.
4. Lienen J, Hüllermeier E. Mitigating label noise through data ambiguation. Proc AIII CAI. 2024;38(12):13799–807.
5. Price WN, Cohen IG. Privacy in the age of medical big data. Nat Med. 2019;25(1):37–43.
6. De Melo CM, Torralba A, Guibas L et al. Next-generation deep learning based on simulators and synthetic data. Trends Cogn Sci. 2022;26(2):174–87.
7. Nikolenko SI. Synthetic data for deep learning. arXiv: 1909.11512. 2019.
8. Ho J, Jain A, Abbeel P. Denoising diffusion probabilistic models. Proc NeurIPS. 2020;33:6840–51.
9. Rombach R, Blattmann A, Lorenz D et al. High-resolution image synthesis with latent diffusion models. Proc IEEE/CVF CVPR. 2022:10684–95.
10. Song Y, Sohl-Dickstein J, Kingma DP et al. Score-based generative modeling through stochastic differential equations. arXiv preprint: 2011.13456. 2020.
11. Pan S, Wang T, Qiu RLJ et al. 2D medical image synthesis using transformer-based denoising diffusion probabilistic model. Phys Med Biol. 2023;68.
12. Yang Y, Fu H, Aviles-Rivero AI et al. DiffMIC: dual-guidance diffusion network for medical image classification. Proc MICCAI. 2023:95–105.
13. Chambon P, Bluethgen C, Delbrouck JB et al. A vision-language foundation model for the generation of realistic chest X-ray images. Nat Biomed Eng. 2024.
14. Zhang S. Dreambooth-based image generation methods for improving the performance of CNN. Proc IEEE ICETCI. 2023:1181–4.
15. Kidder BL. Advanced image generation for cancer using diffusion models. Biol Meth Prot. 2024,9(1).
16. Hu EJ, Shen Y, Wallis P et al. LoRA: low-rank adaptation of large language models. arXiv: 2106.09685. 2021.
17. Mueller M, Hein M. LoGex: improved tail detection of extremely rare histopathology classes via guided diffusion. arXiv preprint: 2409.01317. 2024.
18. Xu Y, Liang J, Zhuo Y et al. TDASD: generating medically significant fine-grained lung adenocarcinoma nodule ct images based on stable diffusion models with limited sample size. Comput Methods Programs Biomed. 2024;248:108103.
19. Rajpurkar P, Irvin J, Bagul A et al. MURA: large dataset for abnormality detection in musculoskeletal radiographs. arXiv preprint: 1712.06957. 2017.
20. Johnson AE, Pollard TJ, Berkowitz SJ et al. MIMIC-CXR: a de-identified publicly available database of chest radiographs with free-text reports. Sci Data. 2019;6(1):317.
21. Google colaboratory. `colab.research.google.com/`. Accessed: 2025-03-12.
22. Heusel M, Ramsauer H, Unterthiner T et al. GANs trained by a two time-scale update rule converge to a local nash equilibrium. Proc NIPS. 2017;30.
23. Rolnick D, Ahuja A, Schwarz J, Lillicrap T, Wayne G. Experience replay for continual learning. Proc NeurIPS. 2019;32.

24. Kirkpatrick J, Pascanu R, Rabinowitz N, Veness J, Desjardins G, Rusu AA et al. Overcoming catastrophic forgetting in neural networks. Appl Math. 2017;114(13):3521–6.

Kidney Cancer Detection Using 3D-based Latent Diffusion Models

Jen Dusseljee, Sarah de Boer, Alessa Hering

Department of Medical Imaging, Radboudumc, Nijmegen, The Netherlands
sarah.deboer@radboudumc.nl

Abstract. In this work, we present a novel latent diffusion-based pipeline for 3D kidney anomaly detection on contrast-enhanced abdominal CT. The method combines denoising diffusion probabilistic models (DDPMs), denoising diffusion implicit models (DDIMs), and vector-quantized generative adversarial networks (VQ-GANs). Unlike prior slice-wise approaches, our method operates directly on an image volume and leverages weak supervision with only case-level pseudo-labels. We benchmark our approach against state-of-the-art supervised segmentation and detection models. This study demonstrates the feasibility and promise of 3D latent diffusion for weakly supervised anomaly detection. While the current results do not yet match supervised baselines, they reveal key directions for improving reconstruction fidelity and lesion localization. Our findings provide an important step toward annotation-efficient, generative modeling of complex abdominal anatomy.

1 Introduction

Kidney cancer has a yearly incidence rate of approximately 400,000 new cases worldwide. Since patients often remain asymptomatic until advanced stages, automatic detection of kidney tumors on computed tomography (CT) scans could positively affect patient outcomes. Artificial intelligence (AI) provides promising avenues in this field, and has been effectively applied to kidney lesion segmentation [1]. However, most approaches rely on supervised learning requiring large annotated datasets that are time-consuming to create and may generalize poorly to rare abnormalities.

To address these problems, un- or weakly supervised methods can be used. These methods leverage the idea that lesions can be identified as deviations from healthy anatomy. Reconstruction-based methods use generative models to synthesize healthy image reconstructions. Subtracting the reconstruction from the input yields an anomaly map highlighting potential lesions. In particular, diffusion models, have recently demonstrated effectiveness in medical anomaly detection [2, 3].

Despite the prevalence of 3D architectures in medical imaging, most diffusion-based anomaly detection methods still process images slice by slice, potentially overlooking valuable inter-slice dependencies and volumetric structural information inherent in 3D imaging data. To enable efficient 3D processing, latent diffusion [4]

© Der/die Autor(en), exklusiv lizenziert an
Springer Fachmedien Wiesbaden GmbH, ein Teil von Springer Nature 2026
H. Handels et al. (Hrsg.), *Bildverarbeitung für die Medizin 2026*,
Informatik aktuell, https://doi.org/10.1007/978-3-658-51100-5_81

enhances efficiency by operating in the compressed latent space of autoencoders, such as VQ-GANs [5], reducing computation while preserving image quality. Existing work has shown that, using latent diffusion, realistic 3D CT volumes can be generated, enabling the construction of fully volumetric generative pipelines [6]. Additionally, latent diffusion has shown promise for out-of-distribution detection [7], a task closely related to anomaly detection.

This work makes two main contributions: (1) a novel 3D weakly supervised anomaly detection framework combining DDIM, DDPM and VQ-GAN; and (2) a benchmark comparison with supervised methods for kidney abnormality detection, filling a gap in existing diffusion model literature.

2 Materials and methods

2.1 Proposed method

We propose a novel method for kidney anomaly detection in full 3D CT images. Our pipeline combines diffusion-based anomaly detection [2] with an existing latent diffusion architecture [6] for efficient 3D processing. An overview of the pipeline can be seen in Figure 1. The following subsections describe each component in more detail, along with their design decisions.

2.1.1 Pre-processing. Each input CT scan is resampled to 1 mm isotropic resolution. To select the ROI, kidney segmentation masks are obtained using TotalSegmentator [8] (fast preset), and 96×96×128 mm patches are extracted around each kidney. Focusing only on these areas leads to more efficient processing, while reducing false positives outside of the kidneys.

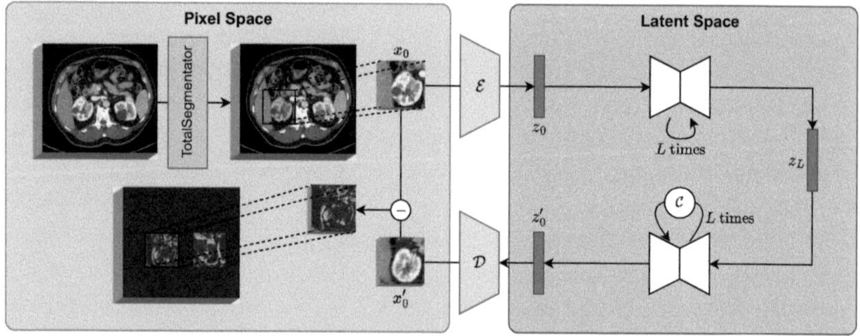

Fig. 1. Overview of the proposed anomaly detection pipeline. Kidney patches, extracted using TotalSegmentator masks, are encoded into a latent space via a VQ-GAN. The latent patch undergoes L forward (noising) diffusion steps, followed by L reverse (denoising) steps with classifier guidance. The denoised latent patch is decoded to produce a healthy reconstruction. Subtracting this from the original yields the anomaly map.

2.1.2 Anomaly detection using latent diffusion models.

Diffusion-based anomaly detection. We adopt denoising diffusion probabilistic models (DDPMs) [9], which generate realistic samples through an iterative denoising process. For anomaly detection, an input image is first corrupted with Gaussian noise via the forward diffusion process and subsequently reconstructed using the reverse denoising process of a model trained exclusively on healthy data. The resulting reconstruction represents a healthy approximation of the input. An anomaly map is then obtained by computing voxel-wise differences between the original image and the healthy reconstruction.

Implicit models for anatomically accurate reconstruction. A key limitation of DDPM-based anomaly detection is the inherent stochasticity of the sampling process, which may introduce anatomical inconsistencies between the original image and its reconstruction. These deviations can lead to false positive detections and reduced anomaly detection performance [2, 3]. To address this limitation, we compare them with denoising diffusion implicit models (DDIMs) [10]. In contrast to DDPMs, the forward and reverse processes of DDIMs can be formulated as exact inverses, allowing for more anatomically accurate reconstructions [2]. However, due to the deterministic nature of DDIM sampling, classifier guidance [11] is required to explicitly steer the reconstruction toward healthy tissue.

Latent diffusion for efficient 3D processing. To enable efficient processing of 3D medical images, we apply latent diffusion [4], where the diffusion process operates in a compressed latent space rather than directly in pixel space. Specifically, we adopt the architecture introduced in [6], which is designed for 3D medical image synthesis and employs a vector-Quantized generative adversarial network (VQ-GAN) [5] as the autoencoder model. Classifier guidance is performed directly within this latent space.

2.1.3 Post-processing. After performing anomaly detection for each kidney patch, we compose the results back into a full-scan anomaly map. This map is then resampled to the original resolution. To reduce noise and false positives in the anomaly map, we apply morphological opening and closing, followed by a hole filling algorithm. Finally, we remove instances smaller than 20 voxels or <3mm in diameter.

2.2 Generating pseudo-labels

The VQ-GAN, DDIM, DDPM, and classifier models are trained on a private dataset from Radboudumc. Contrast-enhanced thorax-abdomen/abdomen CT scans (slice thickness $\leq$ 1 mm) acquired between 2008 and 2021 were included, totaling 8,377 scans from 7,571 studies of 6,800 patients, yielding 5,095 left and 5,099 right kidneys. Pseudo-labels were derived from radiology reports: kidneys with reported lesions, cysts, or tumors were labeled unhealthy; those described as normal or unmentioned were labeled healthy. Kidneys with stones, calcifications, necrosis, atrophy, or prior removal were excluded.

2.3 Training details

We implemented VQ-GAN and DDPM (with DDIM sampling and classifier guidance) based on [6]. The VQ-GAN was trained for 100k iterations on the full dataset using an A100 GPU (batch size 4) in 1 day. The DDPM, with 1000 timesteps, was trained for 250k iterations on healthy kidney images (batch size 40) over 3 days on an A100. A U-Net-based classifier, using the encoder path with a linear head, was trained on a balanced pseudo-labeled dataset (1,162 healthy and 1,162 unhealthy kidneys) for 100 epochs (batch size 32) with early stopping, achieving a validation AUC of 0.70 and a test AUC of 0.56.

2.4 Benchmarks and datasets

We compare our weakly supervised approach to two state-of-the-art supervised baselines. One model is used as-is from prior work, while the other is retrained to serve as a detection-specific benchmark. The first baseline is a pretrained nnU-Net [12] for kidney and lesion segmentation [1], trained with 5-fold cross-validation on the supervised dataset. For detection benchmarking, we train nnDetection [13] with 5-fold cross-validation on the same data, reserving a 20% subset as a holdout test set. The baselines are trained on a combination of the KiTS23 [14] training set and the Radboudumc kidney abnormality dataset [15]. Hyperparameter tuning for the proposed method is done on a validation fold from the nnDetection setup. A test set of 30 CT scans with fully annotated segmentation masks from Radboudumc was used as a test set to compare the proposed method, nnDetection and nnU-Net.

3 Results

3.1 Detection and segmentation performance

We measure segmentation performance using Dice similarity coefficient (DSC) and lesions are reported as detected when an intersection-over-union (IoU) of 0.2 is reached. A hyperparameter sweep for both DDPM and DDIM was conducted. The DDPM achieved the highest DSC on the validation set with a noise level of $L = 500$ and classifier guidance strength $s = 1600$. The DDIM achieved optimal performance at $L = 500$ and $s = 1800$. These optimal hyperparameters were subsequently used to evaluate segmentation performance on the hold out test set of the nnDetection dataset, and the private test set. The results are reported in Table 1. To determine the confidence threshold, we applied the Otsu method [16], as proposed in [2].

3.2 Qualitative analysis

Figure 2 presents a visual comparison between the reconstructions produced by the best-performing DDPM and DDIM models. The figure also shows the resulting difference map and the predictions after post-processing. Case a) shows a lesion present on the border of the kidney that was correctly detected by both models. Case

Tab. 1. Segmentation and detection performance of optimal configurations for all methods on both test sets at an IoU threshold of 0.2.

	DSC ↑	Precision ↑	Recall ↑	F1-score ↑
nnDetection Test				
DDPM	**0.12 (±0.10)**	0.02 (±0.04)	0.16 (±0.30)	0.03 (±0.06)
DDIM	0.07 (±0.09)	0.01 (±0.09)	0.04 (±0.18)	0.02 (±0.10)
nnDetection	N/A	**0.51 (±0.33)**	**0.85 (±0.26)**	**0.63 (±0.26)**
Radboudumc Test				
DDPM	0.08 (±0.10)	0.01 (±0.02)	0.15 (±0.28)	0.02 (±0.03)
DDIM	0.08 (±0.11)	0.02 (±0.10)	0.03 (±0.07)	0.02 (±0.05)
nnDetection	N/A	0.51 (±0.28)	**0.73 (±0.28)**	0.55 (±0.24)
nnU-Net	**0.68 (±0.25)**	**0.78 (±0.30)**	0.67 (±0.29)	**0.69 (±0.26)**

b) shows multiple lesions within the kidney that were, none of which were detected by either model. Case c) shows a small lesion within the kidney that was found by our DDPM-based method, but missed by our DDIM-based method. Case d) shows a lesion that falls well outside the region of interest. Both models evidently struggle with this kind of lesion, with DDPM inpainting a completely new kidney.

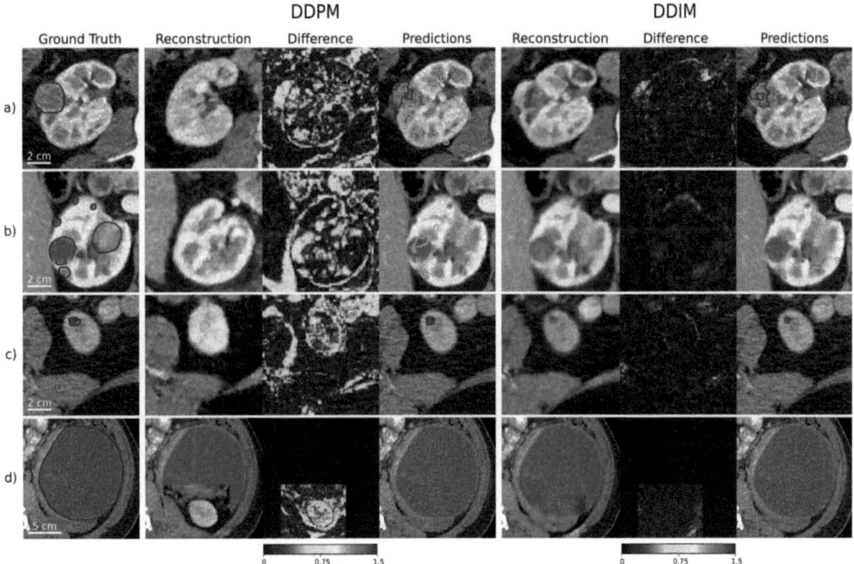

Fig. 2. Visual comparison of diffusion-based reconstructions on four example images.

Tab. 2. Segmentation and detection performance of both unsupervised methods and nnDetection on the nnDetection test set for different lesion sizes at an IoU threshold of 0.2.

Size (cm)	Model	DSC ↑	Precision ↑	Recall ↑	F1-score ↑
	DDPM	**0.03 (±0.05)**	0.01 (±0.02)	0.14 (±0.29)	0.02 (±0.04)
≤ 2 (n = 69)	DDIM	0.02 (±0.05)	0.01 (±0.03)	0.02 (±0.13)	0.01 (±0.05)
	nnDetection	N/A	**0.18 (±0.24)**	**0.77 (±0.35)**	**0.44 (±0.24)**
	DDPM	**0.09 (±0.14)**	0.08 (±0.19)	0.18 (±0.37)	0.10 (±0.22)
2–4 (n = 58)	DDIM	0.03 (±0.11)	0.02 (±0.1)	0.05 (±0.22)	0.03 (±0.14)
	nnDetection	N/A	**0.25 (±0.33)**	**0.94 (±0.22)**	**0.62 (±0.26)**
	DDPM	**0.07 (±0.14)**	0.09 (±0.28)	0.11 (±0.31)	0.09 (±0.28)
4–7 (n = 37)	DDIM	0.00 (±0.02)	0.00 (±0.00)	0.00 (±0.00)	0.00 (±0.0)
	nnDetection	N/A	**0.26 (±0.39)**	**0.84 (±0.37)**	**0.73 (±0.30)**
	DDPM	**0.02 (±0.06)**	0.00 (±0.00)	0.00 (±0.00)	0.00 (±0.00)
> 7 (n = 30)	DDIM	0.00 (±0.02)	0.00 (±0.00)	0.00 (±0.00)	0.00 (±0.00)
	nnDetection	N/A	**0.43 (±0.43)**	**0.72 (±0.44)**	**0.69 (±0.34)**

3.3 Evaluation at different lesion sizes

Table 2 shows the evaluation results at different lesion sizes. Evaluation was done using only the lesions in the reference masks that fall within the given size range. Remaining reference lesions with a matching prediction (IoU ≥ 0.2) were considered true positives, while the reference lesions without a matching prediction were considered as false negatives. Unmatched predictions within the size range were counted as false positives. Cases without reference lesions within the given size range were excluded. The number of remaining cases is reported within parentheses for each size range.

4 Discussion

While our diffusion-based methods did not yet match the performance of the supervised baselines in segmentation accuracy or detection sensitivity, this study provides valuable insights into the challenges and potential of diffusion-based reconstruction in complex anatomical regions. While prior work demonstrated viability in 2D brain MRI [2], abdominal CT's greater variability in anatomy and contrast enhancement patterns may contribute to reduced performance. Both detection and segmentation performance are especially low for the largest lesion sizes, with DDIM failing to detect any lesions ≥ 4 cm in diameter and DDPM failing for any lesion ≥ 7 cm.

Visual inspection revealed that while our DDPM-based pipeline often correctly highlighted lesions, anatomical reconstruction artifacts frequently overshadowed true lesions, creating larger intensity differences than the lesions themselves. The false positives caused by these artifacts lead to low precision, especially when evaluating only lesions with a diameter ≤ 2 cm. Post-processing helped reduce false positives, but risked removing smaller lesions. Future work should investigate the use of false positive reduction networks [17]. Interestingly, DDIM with classifier guidance, which was introduced to mitigate anatomical reconstruction artifacts [2], was outperformed by DDPM without classifier guidance, likely due to the limited performance of the classifier trained on pseudo-labels, which would have a stronger impact on DDIM's deterministic sampling than on DDPM's stochastic sampling. Simplex noise offers a promising alternative to Gaussian noise for reducing reconstruction artifacts in DDPM [3].

Additionally, alternatives to latent diffusion can be explored. Patch-based approaches [18] operate directly in pixel space, eliminating the need for the classifier to operate in latent space, potentially leading to more effective guidance. Alternatively, wavelet diffusion [19] has been shown to be more efficient than latent diffusion, while leading to better results for healthy inpainting in brain MRI [20].

We expect that performance can be significantly improved through a combination of these complementary strategies: false positive reduction, improved guidance mechanisms, and alternative diffusion architectures.

Acknowledgement. This research is funded by the European Union under HORIZON- HLTH-2022: COMFORT (101079894). Views and opinions expressed are however those of the author(s) only and do not necessarily reflect those of the European Union or European Health and Digital Executive Agency (HADEA). Neither the European Union nor the granting authority can be held responsible for them.

References

1. de Boer S, Häntze H, Venkadesh KV et al. Robust kidney abnormality segmentation: a validation study of an AI-based framework. arXiv: 2505.07573. 2025.
2. Wolleb J, Bieder F, Sandkühler R, Cattin PC. Diffusion models for medical anomaly detection. Proc MICCAI. 2022.
3. Wyatt J, Leach A, Schmon SM, Willcocks CG. AnoDDPM: anomaly detection with denoising diffusion probabilistic models using simplex noise. Proc IEEE/CVF CVPR. 2022.
4. Rombach R, Blattmann A, Lorenz D et al. High-resolution image synthesis with latent diffusion models. Proc IEEE/CVF CVPR. 2022.
5. Esser P, Rombach R, Ommer B. Taming transformers for high-resolution image synthesis. Proc IEEE/CVF CVPR. 2021.
6. Khader F, Müller-Franzes G, Tayebi Arasteh S et al. Denoising diffusion probabilistic models for 3D medical image generation. Sci Rep. 2023;13(1).
7. Graham MS, Pinaya WHL, Wright P et al. Unsupervised 3D out-of-distribution detection with latent diffusion models. Proc MICCAI. 2023.
8. Wasserthal J, Breit HC, Meyer MT et al. TotalSegmentator: robust segmentation of 104 anatomic structures in CT images. Radiol Artif Intell. 2023;5.
9. Ho J, Jain A, Abbeel P. Denoising diffusion probabilistic models. Proc NeurIPS. 2020;33.
10. Song J, Meng C, Ermon S. Denoising diffusion implicit models. arXiv: 2010.02502. 2022.
11. Dhariwal P, Nichol A. Diffusion models beat GANs on image synthesis. Proc NeurIPS. 2021;34.
12. Isensee F, Jaeger PF, Kohl SA et al. nnU-net: a self-configuring method for deep learning-based biomedical image segmentation. Nat Methods. 2021;18(2).

13. Baumgartner M, Jäger PF, Isensee F, Maier-Hein KH. nnDetection: a self-configuring method for medical object detection. Proc MICCAI. 2021.
14. Heller N, Isensee F, Trofimova D et al. The KiTS21 challenge: automatic segmentation of kidneys, renal tumors, and renal cysts in corticomedullary-phase CT. arXiv: 2307.01984. 2023.
15. Humpire-Mamani GE, Builtjes L, Jacobs C et al. Dataset for: kidney abnormality segmentation in thorax-abdomen CT scans. Zenodo, 2023.
16. Otsu N. A threshold selection method from gray-level histograms. IEEE Trans Syst Man Cybern. 1979;9(1).
17. Hendrix W, Hendrix N, Scholten ET et al. Deep learning for the detection of benign and malignant pulmonary nodules in non-screening chest CT scans. Commun Med. 2023;3(1).
18. Bieder F, Wolleb J, Durrer A et al. Memory-efficient 3D denoising diffusion models for medical image processing. Proc MIDL. 2024:552–67.
19. Phung H, Dao Q, Tran A. Wavelet diffusion models are fast and scalable image generators. Proc IEEE/CVF CVPR. 2023:10199–208.
20. Durrer A, Wolleb J, Bieder F et al. Denoising diffusion models for 3D healthy brain tissue inpainting. Proc DGM. 2024.

Abstract: Uncertainty-aware ControlNet Bridging Domain Gaps with Synthetic Image Generation

Joshua Niemeijer[1], Jan Ehrhardt[1,2], Heinz Handels[1,2], Hristina Uzunova[3]

[1]German Aerospace Center, Braunschweig, Germany
[2]Institute of Medical Informatics, University of Lübeck, Germany
[3]German Research Center for Artificial Intelligence, Lübeck, Germany
Joshua.Niemeijer@dlr.de

Diffusion Models, in combination with so-called ControlNets, can generate labeled synthetic training data. To establish control over the segmentation label, the ControlNet is trained on the labeled data, which is also used for training the segmentation network. The resulting synthetic data, therefore, is drawn from the same distribution as the segmentation network's training data and does not provide any novel information beyond it. This work aims to guide the generation process towards producing novel, meaningful training samples. We present UnIACorN, an approach that models the uncertainties of a given segmentation model. UnIACorN [1] is based on a Multi-ControlNet architecture that fuses the noise predictions of a semantic ControlNet and an uncertainty ControlNet. The semantic ControlNet is conditioned on the segmentation mask. Additionally, we introduce a novel uncertainty-guided ControlNet that generates images based on epistemic uncertainty. To train the uncertainty ControlNet, we first compute the segmentation network's epistemic uncertainty on images, both from the labeled and unlabeled distributions. The epistemic uncertainty is high if the given image information was not part of the training distribution. We, therefore, obtain the relationship between uncertainty and image information. The uncertainty ControlNet is trained to predict the image given the corresponding epistemic uncertainty. During the diffusion process, the noise predictions of the Semantic ControlNet and the Uncertainty ControlNet are fused. Therefore, the stepwise generation process is guided by both conditions. We sample the uncertainty value from the Gaussian distribution of uncertainties obtained on the unlabeled set. The segmentation label is retained from the original labeled distribution. The segmentation network trained on a combination of synthetic and real data exhibits improved generalization to novel OCT image distributions. UnIACorN enables the segmentation network to learn from its own uncertainty.

References

1. Niemeijer J, Ehrhardt J, Handels H, Uzunova H. Uncertainty-aware ControlNet: bridging domain gaps with synthetic image generation. Proc IEEE/CVF ICCV. 2025:4184–93.

© Der/die Autor(en), exklusiv lizenziert an
Springer Fachmedien Wiesbaden GmbH, ein Teil von Springer Nature 2026
H. Handels et al. (Hrsg.), *Bildverarbeitung für die Medizin 2026*,
Informatik aktuell, https://doi.org/10.1007/978-3-658-51100-5_82

Rethinking Diversity Metrics in Medical Imaging with Wasserstein Distance

Marvin Seyfarth [1,2,3], Salman U. H. Dar [1,2,3], Sandy Engelhardt [1,2,3]

[1]Institute for Artificial Intelligence in Cardiovascular Medicine, Department of Cardiology, Angiology, Pneumology, Heidelberg University Hospital, Heidelberg, Germany
[2]Heidelberg Faculty of Medicine, Heidelberg University, Germany
[3]DZHK (German Centre for Cardiovascular Research), Partner Site Heidelberg/Mannheim, Heidelberg, Germany
Marvin.Seyfarth@med.uni-heidelberg.de

Abstract. Generative models are increasingly used in medical imaging for tasks such as data augmentation and privacy-preserving sharing. Beyond realism, it is crucial that generated images capture clinically relevant diversity, including variations in anatomy and pathology. Dataset diversity is often assessed using the multi-scale structural similarity index (MS-SSIM), which operates in pixel space. However, we show that MS-SSIM is highly sensitive to small perturbations and quickly saturates, failing to capture intrinsic anatomical variability. To address this, we introduce Wasserstein distance diversity *WAD-Div*, a feature-space metric that computes k-nearest neighbor distance distributions and quantifies diversity via Wasserstein distances to a reference. Experiments on chest X-ray and lung CT datasets demonstrate that *WAD-Div* reliably reflects dataset diversity and distributional similarity, whereas MS-SSIM can be misleading under simple augmentations. WAD-Div provides a robust framework for evaluating medical image dataset diversity beyond pixel-level measures.

1 Introduction

Generative models are increasingly used in medical imaging for data augmentation [1] or data sharing [2]. Beyond realism, a key requirement is *diversity*: generated samples should capture clinically relevant variability in pathology and acquisition-related properties. Quantifying diversity ensures models do not collapse to limited representations of the underlying data distribution. A good diversity metric should be robust to irrelevant variations (e.g., small pixel-level or translational / rotational changes), sensitive to intrinsic diversity, interpretable with bounded values, capture task-relevant differences, and be comparable across datasets of varying sizes and modalities. The most common diversity metric in medical imaging [3], mean pairwise MS-SSIM [4], operates in pixel space. While easy to compute, it might therefore be sensitive to noise and simple augmentations, causing datasets with few unique samples to appear artificially diverse, and it scales poorly to large datasets, due

© Der/die Autor(en), exklusiv lizenziert an
Springer Fachmedien Wiesbaden GmbH, ein Teil von Springer Nature 2026
H. Handels et al. (Hrsg.), *Bildverarbeitung für die Medizin 2026*,
Informatik aktuell, https://doi.org/10.1007/978-3-658-51100-5_83

to quadratic dependency of sample size. Feature-space approaches address some of these issues by evaluating diversity in embeddings from pretrained networks. Metrics like recall [5] measure alignment to a reference distribution, assuming meaningful structure is captured. However, they redefine diversity relative to a potentially biased reference, penalize valid out-of-distribution samples, and rely on k-nearest neighbor (kNN) [6] spheres, whose radii are determined by the distance to the k-th nearest neighbor. As a result, sphere sizes vary with local latent distances and across datasets, and different choices of k effectively change the notion of diversity, introducing sensitivity to hyperparameters and outliers. We propose a Wasserstein distance [7] based diversity metric, *WAD-Div*, that moves beyond the conventional "coverage of kNN spheres" used in recall metrics, and instead quantifies diversity by comparing the full distribution of kNN distances in embedding space between a set and a reference. Varying k probes diversity at different scales, providing an interpretable, flexible measure that is robust, sensitive, and comparable across datasets.

We systematically analyze MS-SSIM limitations and introduce WAD-Div, a feature-space metric quantifying diversity via Wasserstein distances between distributions of top-k nearest-neighbor distances. By comparing local kNN distance distributions to a reference, WAD-Div emphasizes intra-dataset variability or alignment with a real reference, rather than global feature coverage. Code will be made publicly available at: `https://github.com/Cardio-AI/wad-div`.

2 Materials and methods

To capture structural diversity beyond pixel space, we evaluate distance distributions in a pretrained feature space. Let $\mathbf{F} = \{\mathbf{f}_1, \ldots, \mathbf{f}_N\}$ be feature embeddings, and $d(\mathbf{f}_i, \mathbf{f}_j)$ their pairwise squared Euclidean distances. For each $\mathbf{f}_i$, the k nearest distances form $\mathcal{D}_i^{(k)}$, and the union over all samples yields the empirical k-NN distance distribution P_{obs}. Diversity is quantified as the first Wasserstein distance between the cumulative distribution functions F_x of P_{obs} and a reference P_{ref}

$$\text{WAD-Div} = \int_{-\infty}^{\infty} |F_{\text{obs}}(x) - F_{\text{ref}}(x)| \, \mathrm{d}x \tag{1}$$

Note that the Wasserstein distance in Eq. 1 is computed on the one-dimensional distribution of scalar kNN distances, not on the multivariate feature embeddings. Larger values indicate greater deviation from the reference and thus higher diversity. Normalization ensures $W_{\text{norm}} \in [0, 1]$

$$W_{\text{norm}} = \frac{W}{W + s} \tag{2}$$

Here, s is chosen by anchoring the scale to a maximally diverse reference: letting $W_{\max}$ denote the Wasserstein distance of this reference, we set $s = W_{\max}(1 - t)/t$ with a target saturation level $t \approx 0.99$, ensuring $W_{\text{norm}} \approx 1$ for maximally diverse data.

Reference distributions define baselines for interpreting WAD-Div. We consider three options:

Tab. 1. Sensitivity of MS-SSIM (↓ = higher diversity) and WAD-Div (↑ = higher diversity) to common minor augmentations in 2D Chest X-rays and 3D Lung CT.

	Noisy	Blurred	Intensity	Rotated
MS-SSIM Chest X-ray	0.49 (0.08)	0.99 (0.00)	0.99 (0.00)	0.76 (0.10)
MS-SSIM Lung CT	0.86 (0.03)	0.99 (0.00)	0.99 (0.01)	0.80 (0.06)
WADiv Chest X-ray	0.90	0.01	0.34	0.14
WADiv Lung CT	0.15	0.03	0.08	0.22

- *Zero:* $P_{\text{ref}} = \delta(x)$, representing identical samples.
- *Exponential:* $P_{\text{ref}}(x) = \lambda e^{-\lambda x}$, allowing limited variability near zero. The rate λ is chosen such that a target percentile x_{ref} of the observed kNN distances satisfies $P(X \leq x_{\text{ref}}) = p_{\text{target}}$. We fix $p_{\text{target}} = 0.95$ and vary x_{ref} across the 25th, 50th, and 75th percentiles.
- *Empirical:* a real dataset with known diversity serving as reference.

Varying the neighborhood size k captures local to global diversity: small k emphasizes fine-scale variation, large k captures overall structural diversity. Unless otherwise indicated, $k = 3$ for all experiments. We evaluated on Chest X-ray images [8] and Lung CT scans [9]. Feature embeddings are extracted using ResNet-50 models pretrained on RadImageNet (2D) [10] and MedicalNet (3D) [11].

3 Results

3.1 Experiment 1: Augmentation Sensitivity

Datasets were constructed from a single source image per modality by applying Gaussian noise (σ=0.05–0.15), contrast/brightness shifts, Gaussian blur (0.5–2.0), and ±5° rotations, yielding 100 images for Lung CT and 200 images for Chest X-ray. Diversity was evaluated using MS-SSIM by computing the mean and standard deviation of pairwise MS-SSIM scores across all image pairs, while WAD-Div was computed using the zero reference distribution. Augmentation sensitivity is summarized in Tab 1. Even when datasets contain only minor augmented versions of a single image (small noise or rotations), MS-SSIM can yield low pairwise similarity scores, falsely suggesting high diversity.

Noise strongly influences both metrics. In 2D Chest X-rays, WAD-Div increases with noise and intensity changes but remains stable under blurring or rotation. In 3D CT, networks are more robust to noise and intensity yet more sensitive to rotations. These trends reflect feature-extractor biases, emphasizing the need for robust, task-specific embeddings when assessing diversity.

3.2 Experiment 2: Intrinsic Diversity

Datasets with increasing numbers of unique images were evaluated using WAD-Div with zero and exponential references. The total number of samples was fixed, with non-unique samples representing slightly rotated versions of the unique ones, as defined in experiment 1. When assessing intrinsic diversity we observe that as the number of unique samples increases, the mean pairwise MS-SSIM initially drops, reflecting added structural variability, but quickly plateaus (Fig. 1), indicating limited sensitivity to further diversity. In contrast, WAD-Div increases consistently with the number of unique samples (Fig. 2). For the zero-peak reference, growth is near-linear at small n_{unique}, steeper in the mid-range, and slower near the maximum, reflecting incremental gains, rapid expansion as diverse samples accumulate, and eventual saturation. With an exponential reference, trends are similar, with smaller absolute distances and tunable slope via λ. Normalized WAD-Div ([0, 1]) retains a clear monotonic trend, confirming reliable capture of global diversity dynamics.

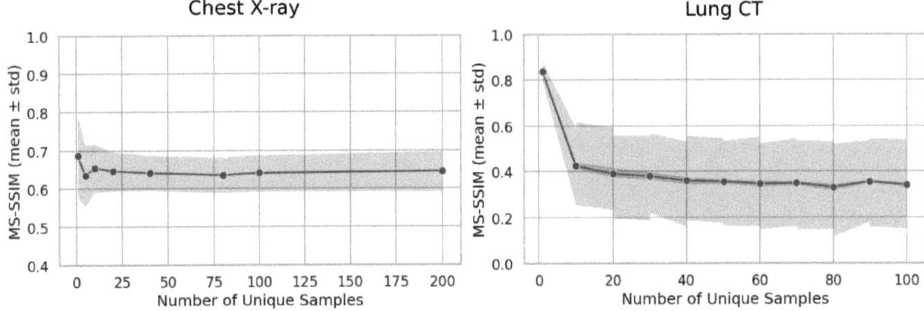

Fig. 1. MS-SSIM as a measure of intrinsic diversity. Left 2D Chest X-ray, right 3D Lung CT.

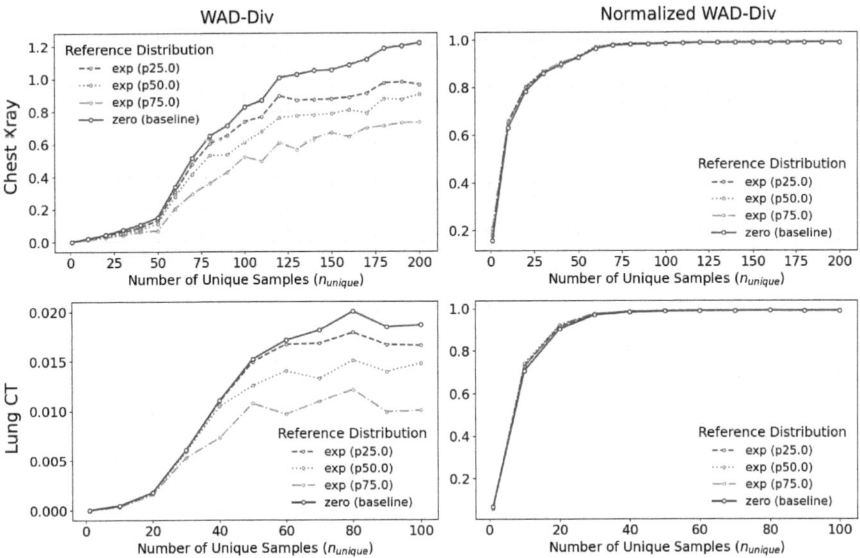

Fig. 2. Intrinsic dataset diversity via WAD-Div. Top: Chest X-ray, Bottom: Lung CT. Left: raw WAD-Div scores, Right: normalized values across reference distributions.

3.3 Distance distribution matching across scales

To assess how WAD-Div reflects similarity between observed and reference datasets, we computed it for varying n_{unique} with the reference distribution set to the fully unique dataset. As shown in Fig. 3, Wasserstein distance to the reference decreases with increasing n_{unique}, indicating convergence toward the variability of the reference distribution. Extending this across multiple k values (Fig. 4) shows consistent behavior across local and global scales.

4 Discussion

MS-SSIM, a common pixel-based metric, is highly sensitive to noise and minor augmentations and quickly saturates as unique samples increase, limiting its ability to quantify intrinsic dataset diversity. In contrast, the proposed WAD-Div metric operates in a learned feature space, using Wasserstein distances of kNN distance distributions to capture intra-dataset variability more reliably and enable meaningful

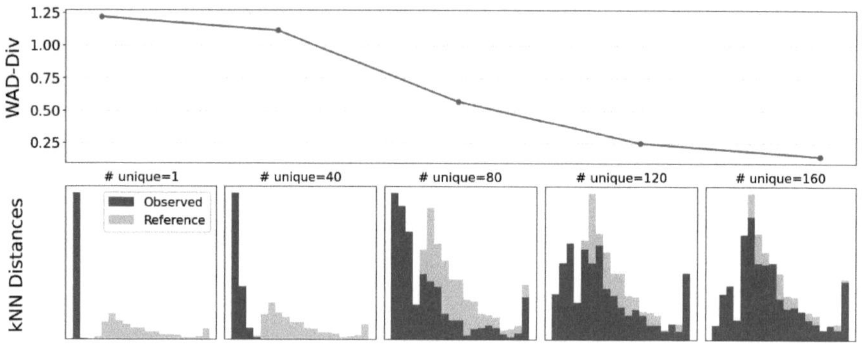

Fig. 3. Chest X-ray embedding similarity. Top: WAD-Div vs. number of unique samples (n_{unique}) for $k = 3$. Bottom: observed (blue) and reference (gray) kNN distance distributions.

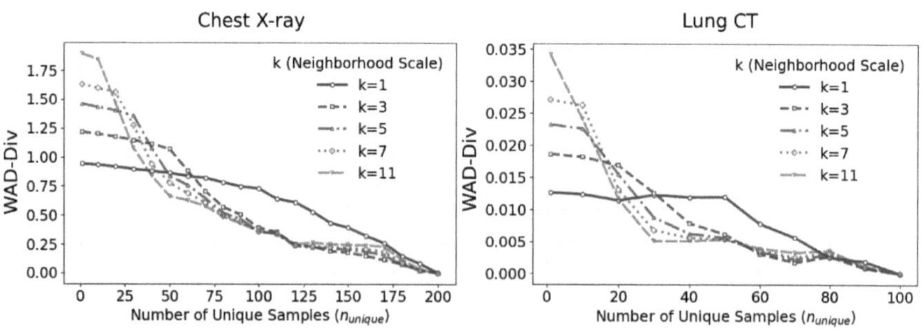

Fig. 4. Multi-scale WAD-Div curves. Distribution matching across datasets with varying numbers of unique samples for 2D Chest X-ray (left) and 3D Lung CT (right).

comparisons across dataset scales. These results have direct implications for evaluating generative model diversity. Small perturbations (e.g., noise or rotations) can inflate diversity estimates for both MS-SSIM and WAD-Div. However, WAD-Div's response depends on the robustness of the pretrained feature extractor. For instance, noise strongly increased normalized WAD-Div in 2D Chest X-rays but had little effect in 3D Lung CTs, likely because the feature network was trained on inherently noisier modalities. This underscores the importance of using embeddings resilient to pixel-level or geometric perturbations. Future work may employ task-specific or self-supervised feature spaces to better capture practitioner-defined notions of diversity [12]. Pixel-based metrics remain less selective, allowing generative models to appear diverse WAD-Div offers a more robust and interpretable framework for assessing diversity in both real and synthetic medical datasets, highlighting the advantages of feature-space over pixel-based approaches.

Acknowledgement. This work was supported by Heidelberg Faculty of Medicine at Heidelberg University, by the Multi-DimensionAI project of the Carl Zeiss Foundation (P2022-08-010) and by the EU-Horizon Project *DVPS* (101213369). The authors acknowledge *1*- the data storage service SDS@hd supported by the Ministry of Science, Research and the Arts Baden-Württemberg (MWK) and the German Research Foundation (DFG) through grant INST 35/1314-1 FUGG and INST 35/1503-1 FUGG, *2*- the state of Baden-Württemberg through bwHPC and the DFG through grant INST 35/1597-1 FUGG.

References

1. Pinaya WHL et al. Brain imaging generation with latent diffusion models. Deep Generative Models. Ed. by Mukhopadhyay A, Oksuz I, Engelhardt S, Zhu D, Yuan Y. (Lecture Notes in Computer Science). Springer, Cham, 2022.
2. DuMont Schütte A, Hetzel J, Gatidis S et al. Overcoming barriers to data sharing with medical image generation: a comprehensive evaluation. NPJ Digit Med. 2021;4:141.
3. Deo Y, Jia Y, Lassila T, Smith WAP, Lawton T, Kang S et al. Metrics that matter: evaluating image quality metrics for medical image generation. arXiv: 2505.07175. 2025.
4. Wang Z, Simoncelli E, Bovik A. Multiscale structural similarity for image quality assessment. Proc ACSSC. 2003.
5. Kynkäänniemi T, Karras T, Laine S, Lehtinen J, Aila T. Improved precision and recall metric for assessing generative models. arXiv: 1904.06991. 2019.
6. Cover T, Hart P. Nearest neighbor pattern classification. IEEE Trans Inf Theory. 1967.
7. Rubner Y, Tomasi C, Guibas LJ. The earth mover's distance as a metric for image retrieval. Int J Comput Vis. 2000.
8. Wang X, Peng Y, Lu L, Lu Z, Bagheri M, Summers RM. ChestX-Ray8: hospital-scale chest X-ray database and benchmarks on weakly-supervised classification and localization of common thorax diseases. Proc IEEE CVPR. 2017.
9. Setio AA, Traverso A, de Bel T, Berens MS, van den Bogaard C, Cerello P et al. Validation, comparison, and combination of algorithms for automatic detection of pulmonary nodules in computed tomography images: the LUNA16 challenge. Med Image Anal. 2017.

10. Mei X, Liu Z, Robson PM, Marinelli B, Huang M, Doshi A et al. RadImageNet: an open radiologic deep learning research dataset for effective transfer learning. Radiol Artif Intell. 2022.
11. Chen S, Ma K, Zheng Y. Med3D: transfer learning for 3D medical image analysis. arXiv preprint: 1904.00625. 2019.
12. Dar SUH, Seyfarth M, Ayx I, Papavassiliu T, Schoenberg SO, Siepmann RM et al. Unconditional latent diffusion models memorize patient imaging data. Nat Biomed Eng. 2025.

Opportunistic Breast Cancer Risk Stratification From Low-dose Chest CT Using Multiple Instance Learning

Yaqiong Ni[1], Adarsh Bhandary Panambur[1], Chang Liu[1], Tri-Thien Nguyen[1,2], Siming Bayer[1,3], Huang Juan[4], Sun Jiayu[4], Lv Su[4], Andreas Maier[1]

[1]Pattern Recognition Lab, Friedrich-Alexander-University Erlangen-Nuremberg, Erlangen, Germany
[2]Radiological Institute, University Clinic Erlangen, Erlangen, Germany
[3]Siemens Healthineers, Erlangen, Germany
[4]West China Hospital, Sichuan University, Chengdu, China
yaqiong.ni@fau.de

Abstract. Breast cancer screening in Asian populations faces significant challenges due to high breast density prevalence, which reduces mammographic sensitivity. Low-dose computed tomography (LDCT) scans acquired for lung cancer screening capture breast tissue and present an opportunity for opportunistic breast cancer risk assessment. This study develops and evaluates deep learning frameworks using multiple instance learning (MIL) for breast cancer risk stratification from LDCT scans combined with clinical features. Two complementary approaches were developed: an individual breast model using attention mechanisms for slice-level interpretability, and a bilateral model employing global pooling to capture asymmetry patterns. Evaluated on 60 patients, the individual model achieved 72.7% accuracy with AUC 0.85, while the bilateral model achieved 75.0% accuracy with AUC 0.87. Both models successfully stratified patients into medium-risk (BI-RADS 3–4) and high-risk (BI-RADS 5–6) categories, providing interpretable outputs through attention maps and asymmetry visualizations. This represents the first comprehensive, proof-of concept study demonstrating the feasibility of automated breast cancer risk assessment from opportunistic LDCT imaging.

1 Introduction

Breast cancer represents the leading malignancy among women globally, with approximately 2.3 million new cases diagnosed annually [1]. Early detection through screening significantly improves survival outcomes, yet current screening approaches face critical limitations, particularly in Asian populations [2]. Mammography, the standard screening modality, shows reduced effectiveness in women with dense breast tissue, which is highly prevalent in Asian populations. Dense breast tissue both increases cancer risk and reduces mammographic sensitivity, creating a population particularly vulnerable to delayed diagnosis [3]. Concurrent with these breast screening challenges, low-dose computed tomography (LDCT) has emerged as the

© Der/die Autor(en), exklusiv lizenziert an
Springer Fachmedien Wiesbaden GmbH, ein Teil von Springer Nature 2026
H. Handels et al. (Hrsg.), *Bildverarbeitung für die Medizin 2026*,
Informatik aktuell, https://doi.org/10.1007/978-3-658-51100-5_84

standard approach for lung cancer screening in high-risk populations. Large-scale trials have demonstrated LDCT's effectiveness in reducing lung cancer mortality, leading to widespread adoption of annual LDCT screening programs [4]. Importantly, these chest CT scans routinely capture the entire breast tissue within their field of view, yet this information typically goes unutilized for breast cancer risk assessment. Given that millions of LDCT scans are performed annually for lung cancer screening and other thoracic indications, systematic analysis of breast tissue in these existing scans could enable opportunistic screening without requiring additional radiation exposure, cost, or patient visits [5]. LDCT offers several advantages for breast tissue evaluation compared to conventional screening approaches. The volumetric three-dimensional imaging eliminates tissue superposition that occurs in projection mammography, potentially improving detection of lesions obscured by overlying tissue. Unlike mammography, CT imaging maintains consistent sensitivity across all breast density categories, addressing a critical limitation of traditional screening in dense-breasted women. The standardized Hounsfield unit measurements enable objective quantitative tissue characterization [6]. Additionally, bilateral breast coverage in a single acquisition facilitates comprehensive asymmetry assessment, an important indicator of malignancy risk routinely evaluated by radiologists [7]. Despite these potential advantages, several critical gaps exist in current research. No comprehensive framework has been developed for systematic breast cancer risk assessment from routine chest LDCT scans. Existing CT-based approaches require detailed slice-level annotations, making large-scale deployment impractical due to annotation burden and cost. Current Multiple Instance Learning (MIL) approaches for medical imaging do not address bilateral organ analysis or automatic asymmetry learning. Furthermore, most deep learning approaches lack the interpretability necessary for clinical acceptance, as radiologists require understandable outputs that can be verified and integrated into diagnostic reasoning.

This study addresses these gaps by developing and evaluating deep learning frameworks specifically designed for opportunistic breast cancer risk stratification from LDCT using MIL with weakly-supervised learning. The key contributions include: (1) development of two complementary MIL architectures optimized for different clinical scenarios, (2) implementation of bilateral analysis capturing asymmetry patterns without explicit feature engineering, (3) integration of imaging features with established clinical risk factors, and (4) generation of interpretable outputs suitable for clinical validation and deployment. To our knowledge, this represents the first systematic pilot investigation of automated breast cancer risk assessment from opportunistic LDCT imaging, with potential implications for expanding screening access in populations where traditional approaches face significant barriers.

2 Material and methods

2.1 Dataset description and preprocessing pipeline

Our dataset comprised LDCT scans from 60 patients collected at a tertiary medical center in China. Patient demographics included ages 35–72 years (mean: 52.3 ± 9.8),

BMI 18.2–31.5 kg/m^2 (mean: 24.1 ± 3.6), and breast density distribution following ACR BI-RADS categories [8]: A (15%), B (38%), C (35%), and D (12%). Family history of breast cancer was present in 5% of patients. LDCT acquisition used standard thoracic screening protocols with 5 mm slice thickness. Board-certified radiologists assigned BI-RADS categories (1–6) to each breast independently. The dataset composition was: BI-RADS 3 (42%), BI-RADS 4 (31%), BI-RADS 5 (19%), and BI-RADS 6 (8%), with BI-RADS 1–2 excluded from analysis to focus on clinically actionable risk stratification rather than normal screening cases. For risk stratification, we grouped BI-RADS 3–4 as *medium risk* and BI-RADS 5–6 as *high risk*. Figure 1 illustrates the preprocessing pipeline designed to enhance breast tissue features from LDCT scans. Raw images underwent four sequential operations: (1) Hounsfield windowing (center = −500 HU, width = 1500 HU) to emphasize breast soft tissue while suppressing bone and air; (2) automated breast tissue segmentation using pre-computed masks, following the approach of Liu et al. [9], to isolate breast parenchyma from the chest wall and surrounding structures; (3) Contrast-Limited Adaptive Histogram Equalization (CLAHE, clipLimit = 2.0, tileSize = 8 × 8) applied only within the segmented breast region to enhance local contrast while limiting noise amplification in LDCT; and (4) channel-wise z-score normalization with values clipped to $[-3, 3]$ to ensure stable network training.

2.2 Proposed MIL architecture

We tested several baselines (2D CNNs, RNNs, 3D CNNs, multi-head attention) and none gave both good accuracy and practicality. 2D/RNN models reached 65–69% but lacked stability or interpretability, and 3D models were worse due to data and memory limits. We therefore chose MIL, which fits the volume-as-bag setup, works with only breast-level labels, and gives attention weights for interpretability.

2.2.1 Individual breast model. Each breast is processed independently. We use MobileNetV2 [10] as a lightweight feature encoder (≈891k parameters in our configuration) to extract a 128-dimensional feature vector per slice. A 64-dimensional

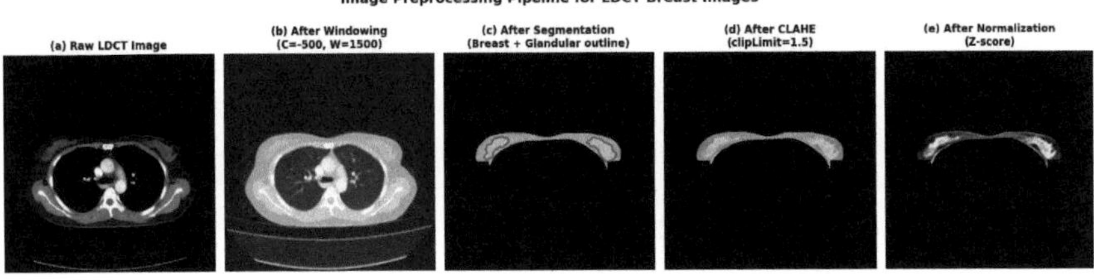

Fig. 1. LDCT preprocessing pipeline: (a) raw image, (b) HU windowing (C= −500, W= 1500), (c) breast segmentation, (d) CLAHE, (e) z-score normalization.

Tab. 1. Performance comparison of model configurations on the test set. The individual model shows stable behavior across class-weightings.

Model	Config	Accuracy	Sens.	Spec.	AUC
Individual	Balanced	**72.7%**	75.0%	71.4%	**0.85**
Individual	High-risk	54.5%	75.0%	42.9%	0.70
Individual	Conservative	63.6%	25.0%	85.7%	0.65
Bilateral	Balanced	37.5%	100%	0.0%	0.50
Bilateral	High-risk	**75.0%**	66.7%	80.0%	**0.87**
Bilateral	Conservative	50.0%	100%	20.0%	0.60

attention module learns instance weights over slices to highlight diagnostically relevant levels. The attention-weighted image feature is then concatenated with eight clinical variables (age, BMI, breast density, family history, and derived features) and passed through fully connected layers to predict a binary label: medium risk (BI-RADS 3–4) vs. high risk (BI-RADS 5–6).

2.2.2 Bilateral model. To exploit side-to-side comparison, we process left and right breasts with an EfficientNet-B0 backbone [11] using shared weights. In the bilateral setting, attention-based aggregation tended to concentrate on one breast or a small subset of slices, limiting effective use of breast laterality information and leading to unstable training. To address this, we apply global average pooling to obtain one feature vector per breast. We then compute four explicit asymmetry descriptors: (i) direct difference, (ii) absolute difference, (iii) normalized difference, and (iv) element-wise maximum between left and right features. These asymmetry features are concatenated with the two unilateral breast features and clinical variables to form the final patient representation. The patient-level risk is defined as the maximum predicted risk across both breasts, reflecting clinical practice.

2.2.3 Training and evaluation. We trained both models with weighted categorical cross-entropy (class weights = inverse class frequency) to address the predominance of medium-risk cases. Optimization used Adam (lr 10^{-3}), ReduceLROnPlateau (factor 0.5, patience 20), and early stopping (patience 50). Three class-weight schemes were evaluated: balanced, high-risk-focused, and conservative. The balanced configuration uses equal class weights to provide baseline performance without bias toward either class. The high-risk focused configuration assigns increased weight to the positive (high-risk) class to prioritize sensitivity, favoring detection of all potential high-risk cases at the cost of increased false positives. The conservative configuration assigns higher weight to the negative class, optimizing for specificity to reduce false alarm rates while maintaining acceptable sensitivity. Data were split in a patient-aware manner into 67% train (40 patients / 67 breasts), 15% validation (9 / 15), and 18% test (11 / 16). Given the limited cohort size, we opted for a fixed patient-level split rather than cross-validation to preserve a strictly held-out test set. Each experiment was run five times with different random seeds, and mean performance is reported across accuracy, balanced accuracy, sensitivity, specificity, F1-score, and AUC; variability across runs was within 3% (absolute). Training was done in TensorFlow 2.x on an NVIDIA RTX 3090.

3 Results

Both MIL frameworks successfully stratified breast cancer risk from LDCT scans. Table 1 summarizes the test-set performance. The individual breast model achieved its best results with the balanced configuration (72.7% accuracy, 75.0% sensitivity, 71.4% specificity, AUC 0.85), while the bilateral model performed best with the high-risk-focused configuration (75.0% accuracy, 66.7% sensitivity, 80.0% specificity, AUC 0.87). The attention module of the individual breast model provides slice-level weights that make its decisions interpretable. Figure 2 shows an example for Patient 092715 (right breast, high-risk case), where attention weights and Grad-CAM activations align. Attention increases from slice 1 (0.112) to slices 3–4 (0.270–0.271), indicating that the model considers mid-breast levels most informative. Grad-CAM maps confirm this behavior: slices with highest attention (2–4) display the strongest, spatially coherent activations over glandular parenchyma and tissue interfaces, while low-attention slices show only minor responses. Across the test set, correctly classified cases typically exhibited distributed attention with peak weights around 0.22–0.27 over multiple slices. Misclassified cases often showed attention collapse (e.g. 84.4% on a single slice), suggesting overreliance on limited information instead of holistic volume reasoning. Although the bilateral model uses global average pooling instead of attention, it still learns clinically meaningful left–right differences. Figure 3 illustrates this with three complementary visualizations. First (Fig. 3a), pixel-level difference maps for six left–right slice pairs (L0–L5 vs. R9–R14; indices reflect acquisition order) show two typical patterns: focal, high-intensity differences (0.3–0.5) indicating local asymmetry, and broader, moderate differences (0.2–0.3) indicating diffuse tissue mismatch. This pairing is for visualization only;

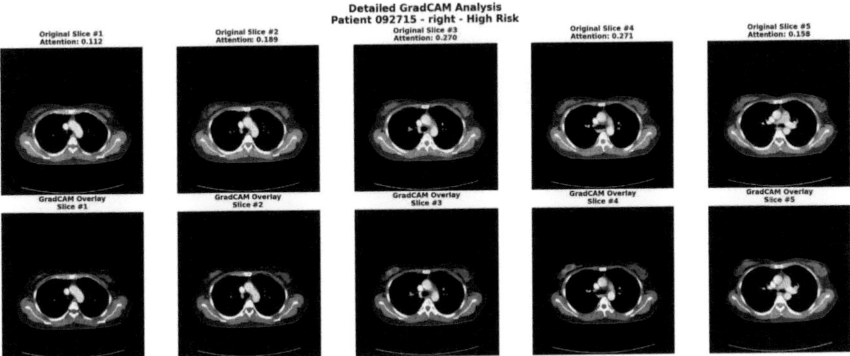

Fig. 2. Attention-Grad-CAM: slices 2–4 get highest attention (0.27) and strongest activations on glandular tissue; low-attention slices show weak responses.

the model itself compares feature vectors, not individual slices. Second (Fig. 3b), the learned 16-D asymmetry representation is sparse: only 6 dimensions show relevant activation, dominated by dimension 3 (value $\approx$ 2.5), followed by dimensions 12, 14, 10, 15, and 6. This indicates that the network compresses bilateral information efficiently, important given the small cohort. Third (Fig. 3c), correlation analysis shows that left and right breast features are moderately correlated ($r = 0.57$), as expected for symmetrical anatomy, but learned asymmetry features have weak negative correlation with unilateral features ($r \approx -0.18$), which means the model extracts complementary information rather than re-encoding the same features. Direct difference features (Diff) correlate with left/right features ($r = 0.57$) but only moderately with learned asymmetry ($r \approx -0.14$), so the asymmetry head captures more than simple subtraction. Quantitatively, high-risk cases showed significantly higher bilateral asymmetry (1.89 ± 0.52) than medium-risk cases (0.74 ± 0.31, $p < 0.001$). Removing asymmetry features dropped accuracy from 75.0% to 66.5%, confirming that bilateral comparison materially improves prediction. Taken together, these results highlight distinct but complementary strengths of individual and bilateral modeling approaches.

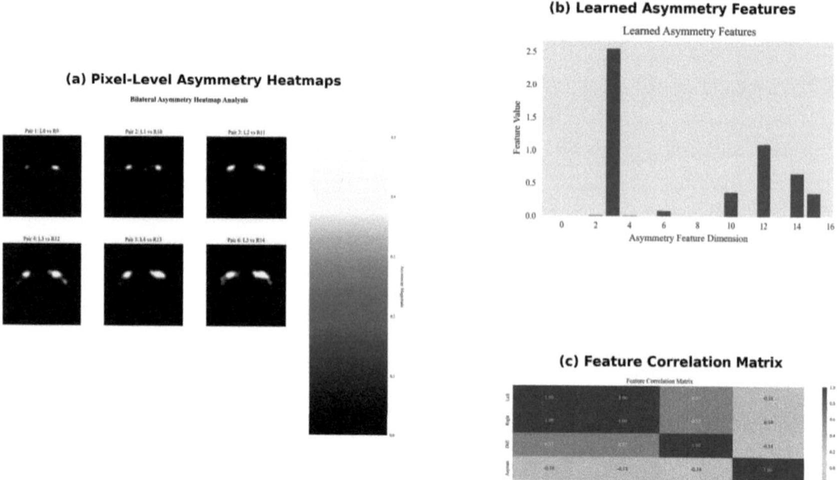

Fig. 3. Bilateral asymmetry analysis: (a) focal vs. diffuse left-right differences; (b) sparse 16-D asymmetry embedding with one dominant dimension; (c) correlations show asymmetry adds complementary information.

4 Discussion

We next interpret the observed performance differences and discuss their clinical implications, limitations, and future directions. The differing impact of class-weighting reflects fundamental differences in how the two models aggregate evidence. While the individual breast model shows better performance across weighting schemes due to its localized slice-level analysis, the bilateral model is highly sensitive to class weighting, as learning meaningful asymmetry patterns benefits from emphasizing high-risk cases during training. Feature-importance analysis showed age was the dominant clinical predictor (0.29), followed by BMI (0.24) and BMI category (0.21); together they explained 74% of the clinical signal, matching breast cancer epidemiology. Breast density contributed modestly (0.09), and family history minimally (0.05) due to low prevalence. This is, to our knowledge, the first automated, weakly supervised breast cancer risk stratification directly from opportunistic LDCT, a modality already acquired in millions of patients and rarely exploited for breast risk. Our bilateral model (AUC 0.87) is close to mammography AI (McKinney 0.889 [12]; Yala 0.76 [13]) despite lower LDCT quality, suggesting 3D context and left-right comparison compensate for 5 mm slices and lack of breast positioning. Even though the comparisons are not direct, we reference mammography-based AI systems only to contextualize feasibility across screening modalities with fundamentally different data scales.The main limitations are the small single-center cohort (n=60), 5 mm slices that can miss small lesions (so this is complementary, not a replacement), and a binary risk setup instead of integration with Gail or Tyrer-Cuzick [14, 15]. The same LDCT could potentially deliver other opportunistic findings (coronary calcium, bone density, steatosis) [16]. While we formulate risk stratification as a binary task due to limited data, future work with larger cohorts will extend the proposed framework to multi-class and ordinal BI-RADS risk stratification. Direct comparison with established state-of-the-art systems was not performed due to fundamental differences in imaging modality, dataset scale, and task definition; however, larger multi-center cohorts will enable more meaningful comparative analyses as well as systematic ablations to quantify the individual contributions of clinical and imaging features. In conclusion, we presented two complementary MIL-based frameworks for breast cancer risk stratification from LDCT. The individual model offers fine-grained interpretability via slice attention, while the bilateral model leverages left-right comparison for higher specificity. Both achieved clinically meaningful performance (AUC up to 0.87) using only weak labels, demonstrating that opportunistic LDCT can be repurposed for breast risk assessment and could help broaden access to early detection in dense-breasted populations.

Disclaimer. This study is intended as a proof-of-concept research investigation and is not designed for clinical deployment.

Acknowledgement. The authors thank West China Hospital, Chengdu, China for providing access to the LDCT data and for their support of this research.

References

1. Kim J, Harper A, McCormack V, Sung H, Houssami N, Morgan E et al. Global patterns and trends in breast cancer incidence and mortality across 185 countries. Nat Med. 2025:1–9.
2. Bae JM et al. Breast density and risk of breast cancer in asian women. J Prev Med Public Health. 2016;49:189–99.
3. Boyd NF, Guo H, Martin LJ et al. Mammographic density and the risk and detection of breast cancer. N Engl J Med. 2007;356(3):227–36.
4. de Koning HJ, van der Aalst CM, de Jong PA, Scholten ET, Nackaerts K, Heuvelmans MA et al. Reduced lung-cancer mortality with volume CT screening in a randomized trial. N Engl J Med. 2020;382(6):503–13.
5. Silvestri GA, Goldman L, Tanner NT, Burleson J, Gould M, Kazerooni EA et al. Outcomes from more than 1 million people screened for lung cancer with low-dose CT imaging. Chest. 2023;164(1):241–51.
6. Chen JH, Chan S, Lu NH, Li Y, Tsai YC, Huang PY et al. Opportunistic breast density assessment in women receiving low-dose chest computed tomography screening. Acad Radiol. 2016;23(9):1154–61.
7. Zheng B, Sumkin JH, Zuley ML, Wang X, Klym AH, Gur D. Bilateral mammographic density asymmetry and breast cancer risk: a preliminary assessment. Eur J Radiol. 2012;81(11):3222–8.
8. Sickles EA, D'Orsi CJ, Bassett LW et al. ACR BI-RADS mammography. ACR BI-RADS Atlas: Breast Imaging Report Data Syst. 2013;5:134–6.
9. Liu S, Salvatore M, Yankelevitz DF, Henschke CI, Reeves AP. Segmentation of the whole breast from low-dose chest CT images. Proc SPIE MI CAD. 2015;9414:94140I.
10. Sandler M, Howard A, Zhu M, Zhmoginov A, Chen LC. MobileNetV2: inverted residuals and linear bottlenecks. Proc IEEE/CVF CVPR. 2018:4510–20.
11. Tan M, Le Q. EfficientNet: rethinking model scaling for convolutional neural networks. Proc ICML. 2019:6105–14.
12. McKinney SM, Sieniek M, Godbole V, Godwin J, Antropova N, Ashrafian H et al. International evaluation of an AI system for breast cancer screening. Nature. 2020;577(7788):89–94.
13. Yala A, Lehman C, Schuster T, Portnoi T, Barzilay R. A deep learning mammography-based model for improved breast cancer risk prediction. Radiology. 2019;292(1):60–6.
14. Gail MH, Brinton LA, Byar DP, Corle DK, Green SB, Schairer C et al. Projecting individualized probabilities of developing breast cancer for white females who are being examined annually. J Natl Cancer Inst. 1989;81(24):1879–86.
15. Tyrer J, Duffy SW, Cuzick J. A breast cancer prediction model incorporating familial and personal risk factors. Stat Med. 2004;23(7):1111–30.
16. Pickhardt PJ, Pooler BD, Lauder T, Rio AM del, Bruce RJ, Binkley N. Opportunistic screening for osteoporosis using abdominal computed tomography scans obtained for other indications. Ann Intern Med. 2013;158(8):588–95.

Abstract: The Missing Piece

A Case for Pre-training in 3D Medical Object Detection

Katharina Eckstein [1,2,3†], Constantin Ulrich [1,2†], Michael Baumgartner [1,4,5,6], Jessica Kächele [1,2,3], Dimitrios Bounias [1,2], Tassilo Wald [1,4,5], Ralf Floca [1,7], Klaus H. Maier-Hein [1,2,3,4,5,8]

[1]German Cancer Research Center (DKFZ), Division of Medical Image Computing, Heidelberg, Germany
[2]Medical Faculty Heidelberg, Heidelberg University, Heidelberg, Germany
[3]German Cancer Consortium (DKTK), German Cancer Research Center (DKFZ), Core Center Heidelberg, Germany
[4]Helmholtz Imaging, DKFZ, Heidelberg, Germany
[5]Faculty of Mathematics and Computer Science, Heidelberg University, Germany
[6]Work done while at DKFZ; now at Siemens Healthineers.
[7]Heidelberg Institute of Radiation Oncology (HIRO), National Center for Radiation Research in Oncology (NCRO), Heidelberg, Germany
[8]Pattern Analysis and Learning Group, Department of Radiation Oncology, Heidelberg University Hospital, Heidelberg, Germany
katharina.eckstein@dkfz-heidelberg.de

Large-scale pre-training holds the promise to advance 3D medical object detection, a crucial component of accurate computer-aided diagnosis. Yet, it remains under-explored compared to segmentation, where pre-training has already demonstrated significant benefits. Existing pre-training approaches for 3D object detection rely on 2D medical data or natural image pre-training, failing to fully leverage 3D volumetric information. In this work, originally published in the Proceedings of MICCAI 2025 [1], we present the first systematic study of how existing pre-training methods can be integrated into state-of-the-art detection architectures, covering both CNNs and Transformers. Our results show that pre-training consistently improves detection performance across various tasks and datasets. Notably, reconstruction-based self-supervised pre-training outperforms supervised pre-training, while contrastive pre-training provides no clear benefit for 3D medical object detection.

References

1. Eckstein K, Ulrich C, Baumgartner M, Kächele J, Bounias D, Wald T et al. The missing piece: a case for pre-training in 3D medical object detection. Proc MICCAI. 2026:615–26.

---

† These authors contributed equally to this work.

© Der/die Autor(en), exklusiv lizenziert an
Springer Fachmedien Wiesbaden GmbH, ein Teil von Springer Nature 2026
H. Handels et al. (Hrsg.), *Bildverarbeitung für die Medizin 2026*,
Informatik aktuell, https://doi.org/10.1007/978-3-658-51100-5_85

Comparison of Modern Transformer Architectures and CNN-based Models for MRI-based Age Estimation of the Knee

Marco Pawłowski[1], Dennis Säring[1], Jochen Herrmann[2], Eilin Jopp-van Well[2], Heinz Handels[3]

[1]Fachhochschule Wedel
[2]Universitätsklinikum Hamburg-Eppendorf
[3]Institut für Medizinische Informatik, Universität zu Lübeck
marco.pawlowski@fh-wedel.de

Abstract. MRI-based age estimation offers a non-invasive approach for assessing biological maturity in forensic medicine. This study compares CNN-, transformer- and hybrid-based architectures for knee MRI age classification and bone segmentation, evaluating vision transformer, Swin transformer, DINOv2, attention U-Net, transformer U-Net, and a baseline CNN U-Net on 1,000 images for classification and 3,000 for segmentation.
Pure transformer models failed to train effectively, while attention U-Net and transformer U-Net achieved good segmentation with a dice coefficient of 0.997 but poor classification with an F1-score of 0.751. These results suggest that CNN locality bias is essential for classification, whereas global attention enhances segmentation. Overall, small datasets and the absence of inductive biases limit transformer performance in knee MRI age estimation.

1 Introduction

Determining chronological age is a crucial aspect of forensic medicine, particularly for assessing individuals without legal documentation, such as asylum seekers. Rapid, safe, and objective methods for age determination are therefore of significant societal importance. Recent research has identified magnetic resonance imaging (MRI) as a promising non-invasive tool for this purpose.

1.1 Age estimation

MRI-based age estimation has been investigated across several anatomical regions, including the hand, brain and knee [1–3]. Among these, the knee joint has emerged as a suitable candidate, as the degree of epiphyseal ossification correlates strongly with chronological age [3].

Several approaches have been proposed for automating the assessment of epiphyseal ossification based on MRI. Convolutional neural networks (CNNs) have

© Der/die Autor(en), exklusiv lizenziert an
Springer Fachmedien Wiesbaden GmbH, ein Teil von Springer Nature 2026
H. Handels et al. (Hrsg.), *Bildverarbeitung für die Medizin 2026*,
Informatik aktuell, https://doi.org/10.1007/978-3-658-51100-5_86

demonstrated viable results for fully automated MRI-based age estimation [3]. Previous studies have further shown that segmenting the bone structure prior to age estimation enhances accuracy, and that CNNs provide an effective method for performing this segmentation step [3].

1.2 Aim of this work

This study aims to evaluate transformer-based architectures for MRI-based age estimation and bone segmentation from knee MRIs and compare them against a CNN-based baseline, given the constraints of a limited dataset size.

In this work, age estimation is formulated as a binary classification task (above vs. below 18 years) and a segmentation task for extracting bone structures from knee MRI scans. The study compares CNN-based, transformer-based, and hybrid architectures, with details provided in later sections. Three hypotheses are proposed:

- Hypothesis 1: Data Limitation: Transformer models require large datasets and tend to underfit or converge unstably when trained on small samples.
- Hypothesis 2: Locality Bias: The lack of locality bias in pure transformers hinders their ability to capture fine-grained anatomical structures, reducing performance compared to CNNs or hybrid models.
- Hypothesis 3: Hybrid Advantage: Combining convolutional features with transformer attention, as in the transformer U-Net or attention U-Net, may leverage both local and global context and improve learning on limited datasets.

2 State of the art

Most prior evaluations of CNN and transformer architectures have focused on natural images [4]. In medical imaging, studies have largely relied on publicly available large datasets. For age estimation, transformers have been applied to hand [1] and brain [2] MRIs, but, to our knowledge, knee joint MRI has not yet been explored, motivating the approach of this study.

An overview of CNN, transformer, and hybrid architectures is provided to outline the current state of the art in MRI-based segmentation and age estimation.

2.1 CNN-based models

CNN-based models such as the U-Net have become the standard for medical image segmentation and classification tasks. One of their advantages is their ability to perform well even on relatively small datasets. However, due to their use of localized convolutional kernels, CNNs have limited capacity to capture global contextual information, which can be a significant drawback in complex anatomical patterns [5].

2.2 Transformer-based models

Transformers, originally developed for text processing, have recently become state of the art across many domains due to their ability to model long-range dependencies and global context. This success inspired their adaptation to computer vision tasks, leading to the introduction of vision transformers (ViT) [6, 7]. However, their integration into medical imaging remains an active research topic. In forensic age estimation, datasets are typically small, image quality varies across acquisition sites, and subtle, localized visual cues challenge the assumptions of transformer architectures.

2.3 Hybrid models

In computer vision, ViT have achieved superior performance in large-scale image classification problems, but they typically require extensive datasets to train effectively. To bridge the gap between CNNs and transformers, attention-based architectures such as the attention U-Net [8] and transformer U-Net [9] have been introduced, aiming to combine the local feature extraction of CNNs with the global attention capabilities of transformers. Fig. 1 shows the structure of the transformer U-Net with the transformer layers and the U-Net structure.

3 Experimental framework

This study consists of two experiments: (1) segmentation of knee bone structures, and (2) binary age classification distinguishing individuals above and below 18 years. Both tasks were performed using a consistent dataset and shared preprocessing pipeline.

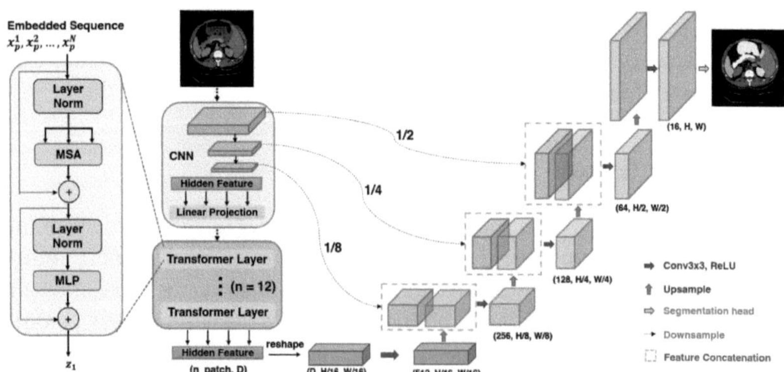

Fig. 1. Overview of the TransUNet, on the left schematic of the transformer layer; on the right architecture of the TransUNet [9].

3.1 Dataset and preprocessing

182 MRI scans were collected from University Medical Center Hamburg-Eppendorf and included 41 subjects for up to three time points. All scans were T1-weighted coronal images. Images were cropped to 450x450 voxel around the knee plate. Ground-truth segmentation masks were created by medical experts. For the segmentation all 3444 slices were individually used. For the classification seven slices with the intercondyloid eminence in the center were selected. This created a dataset of 1295 individual slices.

3.2 Model configurations

Six model architectures were implemented for comparison:

1. U-Net (baseline CNN model) [5],
2. Attention U-Net (CNN with attention gates) [8],
3. Transformer U-Net (hybrid convolutional-transformer) [9],
4. Vision transformer (ViT) [7],
5. Swin transformer [10], and
6. DINOv2 transformer with linear classifier [11].

3.3 Training protocol

All models were trained using AdamW optimizer. Hyperparameter like batchsize, learning rate, weight decay and drop-out factor, were individually searched via grid- and random search. Data augmentation strategies included translation, rotation and scaling. DINOv2, Swin und ViT were tested without and with pretraining on ImageNet.

3.4 Evaluation

Segmentation was evaluated with Dice similarity coefficient (DSC) and intersection-over-union (IoU) based on expert-generated ground truth, while classification used accuracy, recall, and F1-score. The dataset was divided into 80% training and 20% validation.

4 Results

This section presents the quantitative and qualitative results for both the segmentation and age classification tasks. All models were evaluated under identical training conditions described in the previous section. The goal is to assess the performance differences between CNN-based, transformer-based, and hybrid architectures and to evaluate the hypotheses formulated earlier.

Model	DSC (↑)	IoU (↑)
U-Net (baseline)	0.758	0.962
Attention U-Net	0.775	**0.970**
Transformer U-Net	**0.776**	0.968
Vision Transformer (ViT)	-	-
Swin Transformer	0.469	0.634
DINOv2 Transformer	-	-

Tab. 1. Quantitative results for MRI knee bone segmentation. ViT and DINOv2 were not able to create a segmentation mask. transformer U-Net and attention U-Net achieved the best results.

4.1 Segmentation results

4.1.1 Quantitative evaluation. The segmentation task was evaluated using DSC and IoU. Tab. 1 summarizes the results for all models.

4.1.2 Qualitative evaluation. Representative segmentation outputs are shown in Fig. 2, illustrating differences in structural consistency and edge precision across models.

4.2 Age classification results

4.2.1 Quantitative evaluation. Classification performance was measured in terms of accuracy, recall and F1-score. Tab. 2 presents the results for all architectures.

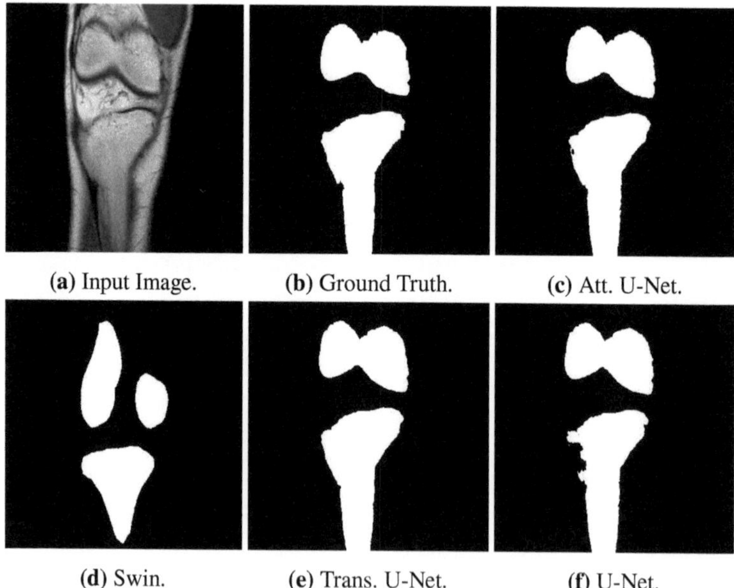

(a) Input Image. **(b)** Ground Truth. **(c)** Att. U-Net.

(d) Swin. **(e)** Trans. U-Net. **(f)** U-Net.

Fig. 2. Comparison of the bone segmentation results. Input MRI slice (a), ground truth segmentation created by an expert (b), attention U-Net (c), Swin transformer (d), transformer U-Net (e), U-Net (f).

Tab. 2. Classification (above vs. over 18 years) results based on knee MRI in terms of accuracy, recall and F1-score.

Model	Accuracy (↑)	Recall (↑)	F1-score (↑)
U-Net (CNN-based baseline)	**0.924**	**0.925**	**0.941**
Attention U-Net	0.645	0.675	0.751
Transformer U-Net	0.771	0.920	0.794
Vision Transformer (ViT)	0.749	0.721	0.831
Swin Transformer	0.545	0.852	0.490
DINOv2 Transformer	0.630	0.630	0.773

4.3 Summary of key findings

Based on the findings of this study and insights from prior research, the following core findings can be summarized.

- The transformer and attention U-Net achieved the best segmentation results.
- The attention U-Net outperformed the standard U-Net in segmentation but not in classification.
- Pure transformer-based models (ViT, Swin, DINOv2) either failed to converge or produced unstable results, likely due to the small dataset size.

Overall, the observed differences between CNN, hybrid, and pure transformer models point to fundamental limitations related to data availability and architectural design, which are further examined in the following discussion of the three hypotheses.

5 Discussion

In knee MRI age estimation, CNNs outperformed pure transformers, which struggled to converge. Hybrid models performed well in segmentation but poorly in classification. Future research should test medical-domain pretraining of transformer and include multi-modal inputs like patient weight and height, which transformers handle more effectively than CNNs.

5.1 Hypotheses evaluation

- Hypothesis 1: Data Limitation: Transformers struggled with limited data, even when pretrained on ImageNet, while U-Net integration improved segmentation, showing hybrids can partially mitigate data constraints.
- Hypothesis 2: Locality Bias: CNN locality bias remains essential for classification, as transformers could not capture subtle epiphyseal features.
- Hypothesis 3: Hybrid Advantage: Hybrid models improved segmentation via global attention but did not enhance classification, indicating global context cannot fully replace locality bias.

6 Conclusion

In summary, transformers alone were unable to learn effectively from the small dataset, while hybrid models captured structural detail but not discriminative cues for age classification. These findings support the hypotheses that data scarcity and locality bias are central to model performance. Global attention aids segmentation, yet CNN-based locality remains essential for classification.

References

1. Zhang J, Chen W, Joshi T, Zhang X, Loh PL, Jog V et al. BAE-ViT: an efficient multimodal vision transformer for bone age estimation. Tomography. 2024;10(12):2058–72.
2. He S, Grant PE, Ou Y. Global-local transformer for brain age estimation. IEEE Trans Med Imaging. 2022;41(1):213–24.
3. auf der Mauer M et al. Towards automated age estimation of young individuals. Düren: Shaker, 2020.
4. Tay Y, Dehghani M, Gupta J, Bahri D, Aribandi V, Qin Z et al. Are pre-trained convolutions better than pre-trained transformers? arXiv: 2105.03322. 2022.
5. Ronneberger O, Fischer P, Brox T. U-net: convolutional networks for biomedical image segmentation. arXiv: 1505.04597. 2015.
6. Vaswani A, Shazeer N, Parmar N, Uszkoreit J, Jones L, Gomez AN et al. Attention is all you need. arXiv: 1706.03762. 2023.
7. Dosovitskiy A, Beyer L, Kolesnikov A, Weissenborn D, Zhai X, Unterthiner T et al. An image is worth 16x16 words: transformers for image recognition at scale. arXiv: 2010.11929. 2021.
8. Oktay O, Schlemper J, Folgoc LL, Lee M, Heinrich M, Misawa K et al. Attention U-net: learning where to look for the pancreas. arXiv: 1804.03999. 2018.
9. Petit O, Thome N, Rambour C, Soler L. U-net transformer: self and cross attention for medical image segmentation. arXiv: 2103.06104. 2021.
10. Liu Z, Lin Y, Cao Y, Hu H, Wei Y, Zhang Z et al. Swin transformer: hierarchical vision transformer using shifted windows. arXiv: 2103.14030. 2021.
11. Oquab M, Darcet T, Moutakanni T, Vo H, Szafraniec M, Khalidov V et al. DINOv2: learning robust visual features without supervision. arXiv: 2304.07193. 2024.

Comparison of Post-hoc Calibration Methods for Neural Network Likelihood Scores

Ole H. Martensen[1], Tobias Strauß [1], Majid Ramedani [2], Martin Dyrba [2]

[1]Department of Mathematics, University of Rostock, Germany
[2]German Center for Neurodegenerative Diseases (DZNE), Rostock, Germany
martin.dyrba@dzne.de

Abstract. This study investigates how to improve the reliability of probability estimates produced by deep learning models for the detection of Alzheimer's disease using MRI data. Although convolutional neural networks (CNNs) can accurately classify neurodegenerative diseases, their softmax outputs often misrepresent true classification probabilities. We evaluated four calibration methods, two parametric (logistic and probit regression) and two non-parametric (isotonic regression and Bayesian binning into quantiles), on data from 474 participants. All models improved the CNN's calibration noticeably without reducing accuracy. Non-parametric methods achieved the best calibration results (expected calibration error ≈ 0.014 and maximum calibration error ≈ 0.025). These findings suggest that non-parametric calibration provides more reliable and clinically useful probability estimates.

1 Introduction

Neurodegenerative diseases are a leading cause of disability worldwide and are strongly associated with aging. With the rapid growth of the elderly population, there is an increasing need for efficient and rapid diagnostic approaches. Magnetic resonance imaging (MRI), particularly T1-weighted scans, is widely used in clinical neuroimaging to study brain structure and detect disease-related changes. In recent years, machine learning and deep learning techniques have demonstrated promising accuracy in analyzing and classifying brain MRI data. Among these, convolutional neural networks (CNNs) have shown remarkable effectiveness in automated disease classification and hold great potential for improving health monitoring systems. In a classification task, a softmax layer at the end of a CNN model converts the output scores into a probability distribution across all possible classes. However, the disease likelihood scores produced by the softmax layer represent the model's relative confidence rather than true statistical probabilities. They also do not provide confidence intervals, both of which are important for clinical decision-making. A pretrained model's output probabilities from the softmax layer do not always reflect true likelihoods. Probability calibration addresses this limitation by adjusting the predicted scores so that they better reflect the observed frequencies in an independent calibra-

© Der/die Autor(en), exklusiv lizenziert an
Springer Fachmedien Wiesbaden GmbH, ein Teil von Springer Nature 2026
H. Handels et al. (Hrsg.), *Bildverarbeitung für die Medizin 2026*,
Informatik aktuell, https://doi.org/10.1007/978-3-658-51100-5_87

tion dataset. Several methods, such as logistic regression, probit regression, isotonic regression, histogram binning, Dirichlet calibration, and temperature scaling, have so far been proposed to perform probability calibration [1]. In this study, we investigated which calibration method provides the most practical utility for empirical clinical data. Specifically, we used a pretrained CNN for Alzheimer's disease detection provided by Dyrba et al. [2] and compared the methods in terms of both calibration effectiveness and the width of the resulting confidence intervals.

2 Materials and methods

2.1 Overview

To overcome the limitations discussed in the Introduction, we applied several established calibration methods to transform the CNN's output scores into more reliable probability estimates. For simplicity, we consider an arbitrary computational model performing binary classification. Let X denote the model's output likelihood score (i.e., the predicted probability or activation corresponding to the Alzheimer-positive neuron of our CNN). Let T represent the true target variable, with $t = 0$ for healthy participants and $t = 1$ for individuals diagnosed with Alzheimer's disease. Let $\mathcal{D} = \{x_1, x_2, \dots x_n\}$ be the set of model outputs for a given dataset. These likelihood scores serve as the basis for the calibration analyses. The source code of all calibration methods is available at `https://github.com/CITlabRostock/probcal`.

2.2 Bootstrapping

To ensure robust evaluation and to quantify variability in the probability estimates, we applied percentile bootstrapping with 500 resamples of the dataset drawn with replacement. For each bootstrap iteration, we retrained all calibration models, allowing us to construct 95% confidence intervals defined by the 2.5th and 97.5th percentiles of the resulting distributions of estimates [3]. For each observation, we computed the mean predicted probability across all resamples for every model, on which the calibration metrics were subsequently evaluated. Additionally, model averaging yields more robust and smoother probability estimates.

2.3 Logistic regression

Logistic regression, also known as Platt scaling, is a simple parametric method used to calibrate model outputs. Conceptually, it transforms the raw output score X into a well-calibrated probability estimate of the true label T. By applying Bayes' theorem to the class-conditional distributions, we can express the posterior probability as $\Pr(T = 1 \mid X = x) = \sigma(a)$ where σ denotes the logistic function, and a is a transformation that depends on the class-conditional probabilities $\Pr(X = x \mid T = t)$ where $t \in \{0, 1\}$. Assuming that the class-conditional distributions are Gaussian with equal covariance matrices, $\Pr(X = x \mid T = t) \sim \mathcal{N}(\mu_t, \Sigma)$, it can be shown that the transformation reduces to a affine function of the input score x: $a = wx + b$.

Thus, by leveraging Bayes' theorem under these assumptions, logistic regression provides a simple yet effective way to map uncalibrated model outputs to well-calibrated probabilities. While the logistic regression takes the logit as link function, in contrast, *probit regression* uses the inverse normal link function, i.e., the cumulated density function $\Phi^{-1}(a)$.

2.4 Bayesian binning into quantiles

The Bayesian binning into quantiles (BBQ) method divides X into B bins to estimate well-calibrated probabilities in a data-driven manner. To prevent empty or sparsely populated bins, the interval is divided based on empirical quantiles rather than fixed-width segments. To do this, the smallest $\frac{|\mathcal{D}|}{B}$ scores form the first bin, the next $\frac{|\mathcal{D}|}{B}$ scores form the second, and so on. Within each bin, probabilities are modeled using a Bayesian estimate based on the Beta distribution [4]. Models with varying numbers of bins B are then averaged to obtain the final calibration function. We varied the number of bins between

$$B_{min} := \max\left\{2, \left\lfloor \frac{n^{\frac{1}{3}}}{C} \right\rfloor\right\} \text{ and } B_{max} := \min\left\{\left\lfloor \frac{n}{20}, \right\rfloor, \left\lfloor n^{\frac{1}{3}} \right\rfloor \cdot C + 1\right\}$$

where the constant C was chosen as 10. It is important to note that BBQ is entirely data-driven and may produce non-monotonic calibration functions as a result.

2.5 Isotonic regression

Isotonic regression is a non-parametric calibration method that fits a non-decreasing step function minimizing the mean squared error (MSE) between predicted probabilities and true target values. The resulting piecewise-constant mapping provides a monotonic transformation from raw scores to calibrated probabilities. Using the pool-adjacent-violators algorithm (PAVA), it achieves an optimal $O(n)$ solution on the calibration set with respect to MSE. Although the estimate is piecewise-constant, it appears smoother after model averaging.

2.6 Experimental setup

To evaluate the effectiveness of the calibration methods, we employed a pretrained CNN originally developed by Dyrba et al. [2] for the detection of Alzheimer's disease from MRI scans. This network had been trained on $N = 663$ structural MRI scans obtained from the Alzheimer's Disease Neuroimaging Initiative (ADNI) and achieved a balanced accuracy of $\approx$ 85–90% as well as AUC ≥ 0.95 across three independent datasets. For testing and calibration, we used MRI data from the german center for neurodegenerative diseases (DZNE) multicenter observational study on longitudinal cognitive impairment and dementia (DELCODE) [5]. The dataset consisted of $N = 474$ participants, including healthy controls, individuals with amnestic mild cognitive impairment (MCI), and patients with Alzheimer's

Tab. 1. Comparison of the calibration scores for the DELCODE dataset.

Model	Accuracy	F1	Log-Loss	Brier	ECE	MCE
Logit	0.7158	0.6966	0.5191	0.1714	0.0679	0.1033
Probit	0.7053	0.6818	0.5185	0.1714	0.0669	0.1008
Isotonic	0.7158	0.6966	0.4965	0.1731	**0.0134**	**0.0227**
BBQ	0.7158	0.6897	**0.4807**	**0.1671**	0.0140	0.0306
CNN	0.7158	0.6966	0.5239	0.1748	0.0803	0.2340

disease (AD) dementia. For the purposes of this study, the MCI and AD groups were labeled as disease-positive ($t = 1$), while healthy participants were labeled as disease-negative ($t = 0$). Model outputs for all participants were obtained from the pretrained CNN, providing predicted likelihood scores for subsequent calibration analysis. We assessed calibration performance using several complementary metrics. All experiments were conducted using an 80/20 train-test split. Accuracy and F1-score provide standard measures of predictive performance, whereas the Brier score (MSE) and the Log-Loss capture both misclassification and calibration error. To isolate calibration quality from overall accuracy, we additionally calculated the expected calibration error (ECE) and maximum calibration error (MCE) [1]. These metrics quantify, respectively, the mean and maximum absolute deviation between the confidence of the prediction and observed accuracy over m quantile bins of the predicted probabilities where m is based on the number of test samples. Collectively, these measures allow a comprehensive evaluation of the effectiveness of each calibration method.

3 Results

Tab. 1 summarizes the quantitative performance of the four calibration methods, along with the uncalibrated CNN outputs for comparison. Across all methods, overall predictive performance remained largely unchanged, with accuracy and F1-score showing minimal variation. This indicates that the calibration procedures primarily affect the alignment of predicted probabilities with observed outcomes rather than the classifier's discriminative ability. The calibration-specific metrics, ECE and MCE, reveal substantial differences between the methods. The raw CNN outputs exhibited the largest calibration errors (ECE = 0.0803, MCE = 0.2340), confirming that although the network is accurate, its probability estimates are poorly aligned with observed outcome frequencies. Both isotonic regression and the BBQ approach substantially reduced calibration errors, achieving the lowest ECE and MCE values (ECE $\approx$ 0.013–0.014, MCE $\approx$ 0.023–0.031). This is consistent with the calibration plots shown in Fig. 1, which demonstrate near-perfect alignment of predicted probabilities with observed outcome frequencies for these two non-parametric methods. In contrast, the parametric methods logistic and probit regression achieved moderate reductions in ECE and MCE (ECE $\approx$ 0.067–0.068, MCE $\approx$ 0.101–0.103). Their calibration functions (Fig. 2) are smoother and narrower due to the parametric constraints but fail to fully capture non-linear deviations in the raw CNN output. Consequently, their estimated confidence intervals are smaller than those of the non-parametric methods.

4 Discussion

The calibration methods logit, probit, and isotonic regression are monotone estimators, while BBQ is a non-monotone approach. Monotone estimators have the advantage of preserving the accuracy of the uncalibrated neural network on the calibration set when the Youden index is used as the decision boundary. On the test set, this property results in only minimal changes in accuracy. In contrast, the non-monotonicity of BBQ can lead to non-monotone confidence intervals (CIs). Logit and probit regression are global parametric models that estimate a single functional relationship across the entire dataset, limiting their ability to capture larger local variations. However, this global nature reduces their susceptibility to local overfitting caused by dataset irregularities. Consequently, global estimators typically produce smoother calibration curves and narrower confidence intervals, whereas local estimators, such as isotonic regression, tend to yield wider intervals.

When evaluating calibration performance, accuracy-based metrics like accuracy or F1 should not be overinterpreted. Since monotone models ensure that accuracy

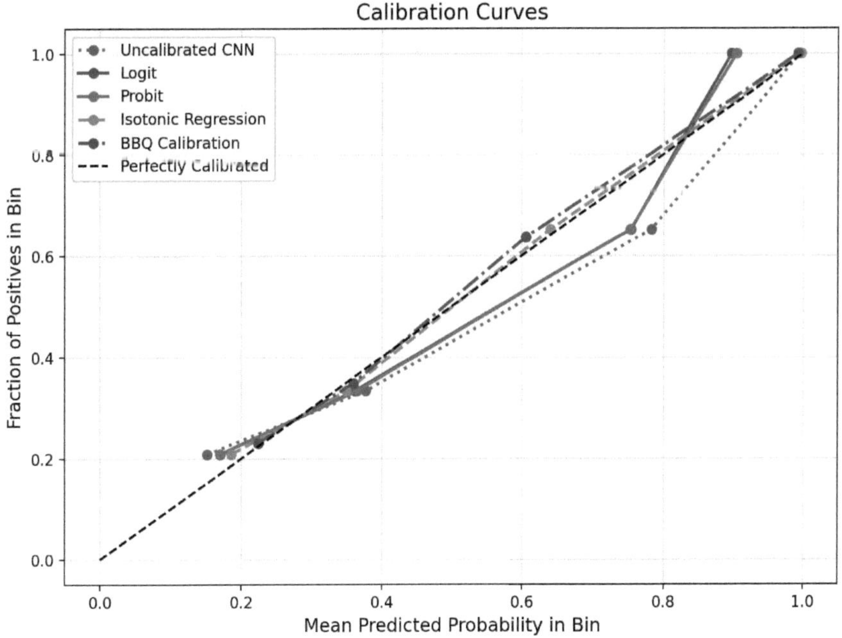

Fig. 1. Calibration plot indicating the reliability of the various calibration methods.

remains nearly unchanged after calibration, the main goal is to remain as close as possible to the discriminative performance of the uncalibrated CNN while improving calibration. The ECE provides a good overall indication of average calibration quality, while the MCE captures the worst-case deviations. However, neither of these metrics reflects the width or quality of the confidence intervals. To assess these aspects, visual inspection and interpretation of calibration plots are necessary. In a medical context, where overestimating confidence intervals is generally preferable to underestimation, isotonic regression and BBQ are the most suitable methods.

Future work will include evaluating additional datasets and calibration techniques. Furthermore, using more advanced bootstrapping methods than simple percentile bootstrapping could provide more reliable uncertainty estimates.

In conclusion, both isotonic regression and BBQ can yield well-calibrated probability estimates, but they differ in terms of computational cost and flexibility. Isotonic regression offers computational efficiency and simplicity. However, it produces reliable and sufficiently smooth results only when combined with model averaging. In settings where model averaging is not employed, BBQ is preferable, provided that its hyperparameters are carefully tuned, as its Bayesian binning framework offers greater flexibility at the cost of increased computational complexity.

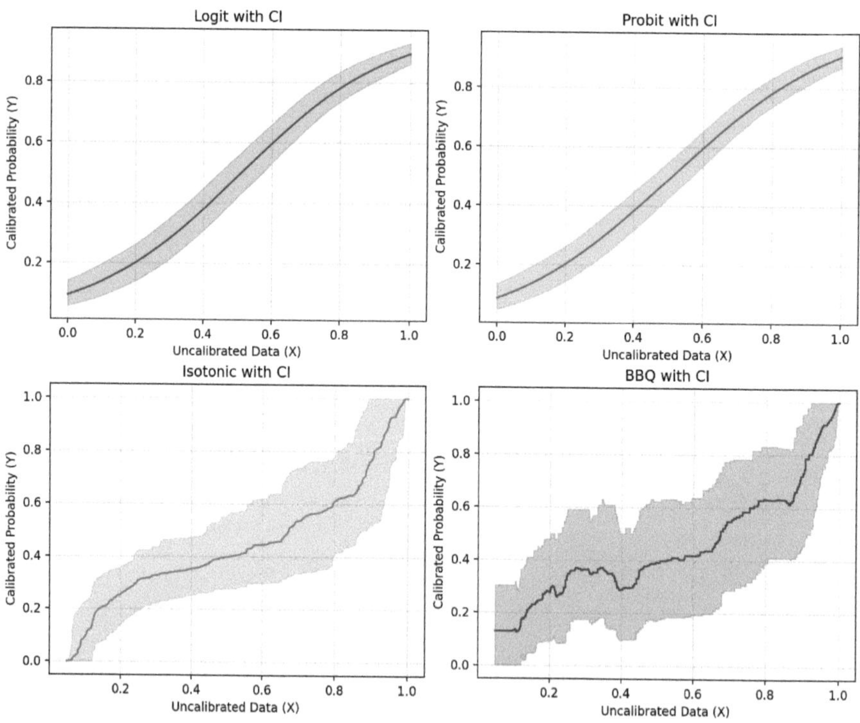

Fig. 2. Comparison of the calibrated probability estimates and confidence intervals derived from four different methods for the DELCODE dataset.

Acknowledgement. We would like to thank A. Spottke, O. Peters, J. Hellmann-Regen, J. Priller, A. Schneider, J. Wiltfang, E. Düzel, K. Buerger, R. Perneczky, S. Teipel, C. Laske and F. Jessen on behalf of the DELCODE study group.

References

1. Silva Filho T, Song H, Perello-Nieto M, Santos-Rodriguez R, Kull M, Flach P. Classifier calibration: a survey on how to assess and improve predicted class probabilities. Mach Learn. 2023;112(9):3211–60.
2. Dyrba M, Hanzig M, Altenstein S, Bader S, Ballarini T, Brosseron F et al. Improving 3D CNN comprehensibility via interactive visualization of relevance maps: evaluation in alzheimer's disease. Alzheimers Res Ther. 2021;13(1):191.
3. Efron B. Better bootstrap confidence intervals. J Am Stat Assoc. 1987;82(397):171–85.
4. Naeini MP, Cooper GF, Hauskrecht M. Obtaining well calibrated probabilities using bayesian binning. Proc AAAI CAI. 2015:2901–7.
5. Jessen F, Spottke A, Boecker H, Brosseron F, Buerger K, Catak C et al. Design and first baseline data of the DZNE multicenter observational study on predementia alzheimer's disease (DELCODE). Alzheimers Res Ther. 2018;10(1):15.

Abstract: Audio-vision Contrastive Learning for Phonological Class Recognition

Daiqi Liu[1], Tomás Arias-Vergara[1,2], Jana Hutter[3], Andreas Maier[1], Paula A. Pérez-Toro[1,2]

[1]Pattern Recognition Lab, Friedrich-Alexander-Universität Erlangen-Nürnberg, Germany
[2]GITA Lab. Facultad de Ingeniería. Universidad de Antioquia UdeA, Medellín, Colombia
[3]Smart Imaging Lab, Friedrich-Alexander-Universität Erlangen-Nürnberg, Germany
daiqi.deutschfau.liu@fau.de

Real-time magnetic resonance imaging (rtMRI) enables detailed visualization of articulatory structures during speech production, making it invaluable for analyzing articulatory-phonological features and advancing clinical speech technologies. While MRI captures the anatomical dynamics of articulation, concurrent audio signals provide complementary acoustic information that enhances temporal resolution in speech processing. Nevertheless, deriving meaningful phonological representations from rtMRI data remains difficult when audio signals are unavailable – situations that commonly arise during MRI scanning due to acoustic noise interference or in cases involving speech disorders such as those seen in glossectomy patients. To address this limitation, we propose a contrastive learning framework for automatically classifying three fundamental articulatory dimensions from MRI data: manner of articulation, place of articulation, and voicing. During training, paired MRI frames and speech segments are encoded separately using vision transformer (ViT) and Wav2Vec2 architectures, respectively, with contrastive learning employed to maximize cross-modal alignment between visual and acoustic representations. Critically, only MRI data is required during inference, enabling phonological classification without audio input. We evaluated four experimental configurations on the USC-TIMIT dataset: unimodal rtMRI, unimodal audio, multimodal middle fusion, and our contrastive learning-based approach. Results show that contrastive learning achieves state-of-the-art performance with an average F1-score of 0.81 across 15 phonological classes, representing absolute improvements of 0.23 over the unimodal baseline and 0.09 over multimodal fusion, thereby confirming the efficacy of cross-modal contrastive representation learning for MRI-based articulatory analysis when audio signals are unavailable [1].

References

1. Liu D, Arias-Vergara T, Hutter J, Maier A, Pérez-Toro PA. Audio-vision contrastive learning for phonological class recognition. Proc TSD. 2025:60–71.

© Der/die Autor(en), exklusiv lizenziert an
Springer Fachmedien Wiesbaden GmbH, ein Teil von Springer Nature 2026
H. Handels et al. (Hrsg.), *Bildverarbeitung für die Medizin 2026*,
Informatik aktuell, https://doi.org/10.1007/978-3-658-51100-5_88

Fracture Morphology Classification
Local Multiclass Modeling for Multilabel Complexity

Cassandra Krause, Mattias P. Heinrich, Ron Keuth

Institut für Medizinische Informatik, Universität zu Lübeck
cassandra.krause@student.uni-luebeck.de

Abstract. Between 15 % and 45 % of children experience a fracture during their growth years, making accurate diagnosis essential. Fracture morphology, alongside location and fragment angle, is a key diagnostic feature. In this work, we propose a method to extract fracture morphology by assigning automatically global AO codes to corresponding fracture bounding boxes. This approach enables the use of public datasets and reformulates the global multilabel task into a local multiclass one, improving the average F1-score by 7.89 %. However, performance declines when using imperfect fracture detectors, highlighting challenges for real-world deployment. Our code is available on GitHub.

1 Introduction

15 % to 45 % of all children suffer a fracture by the end of their growing years [1], with the distal forearm being the most common location. Consequently, proper treatment of wrist bones fractures is particularly important in the paediatric field to avoid permanent deformities or growth disorders. Fracture morphology, alongside location and fragment angle, is a key characteristic for describing fractures [2]. Hence, a reliable morphology classification is crucial for therapy planning. The AO/OTA system (Arbeitsgemeinschaft für Osteosynthesefragen/Orthopaedic Trauma Association) offers a standardized framework for classifying fractures by location and morphology [3]. Based on this system, several deep learning-based approaches for binary fracture classification have emerged lately, ranging from supervised [4] to self-supervised methods [5]. For a finer classification, other approaches include the location of fractures covering radius/ulna and their metaphyse/epiphyses [6] or identify extra-, partial-, and intra-articular fractures [7–9]. Recent work extends the input modality to segmentation and radiology reports to classify the seven most common AO classes [10].Facing challenges, they conclude that a hierarchical stage could be better suited for AO/OTA systems, as it was done by [7, 8]. Both first detecting ROIs and then classifying fractures within two separated models. To our best knowledge, we provide the first study explicitly focusing on fracture morphology with automatic assignment from fracture class to bounding box by separating fracture detection from its classification.

© Der/die Autor(en), exklusiv lizenziert an
Springer Fachmedien Wiesbaden GmbH, ein Teil von Springer Nature 2026
H. Handels et al. (Hrsg.), *Bildverarbeitung für die Medizin 2026*,
Informatik aktuell, https://doi.org/10.1007/978-3-658-51100-5_89

2 Materials and methods

2.1 Dataset

We use the public available GRAZPEDWRI-DX [11] dataset. It holds 20 327 paediatric trauma wrist X-ray images of AP and lateral view combined with bounding boxes and AO codes for 18 090 fractures. For preprocessing, we follow [11] and relative split the dataset into 8:1:1 train/validation/test images, preserving the label distribution.

2.2 Extraction of fracture morphology from AO codes

Since the dataset itself does not provide any fracture morphology labels natively, we have to extract them from the provided AO-codes and fractures' bounding boxes. We rely on the classification of Kaiser and Weinberg for femoral shaft fractures and Salter classification (I-IV) regarding epiphyseal fractures. With this, we create a mapping from the provided global AO codes to their corresponding fracture morphology in collaboration with radiologists. While mapping a single fracture to its AO code is straightforward (1:1), associating multiple fractures with their respective codes is ambiguous, as AO codes are assigned globally to each image. To resolve this, we use the segmentation masks from [10] for the radius, ulna, and their epiphyses, assigning each fracture to the bone with the greatest segmentation overlap within its bounding box (Fig. 1) and thus extract its bone label. Simultaneously, AO codes are assigned to the respective bone labels using a further mapping from AO codes to bone classes. If an AO code refers to fractures occurring in both the radius and the ulna (e.g. 22-D/4.1), it is replaced by their two variants (22r-D/4.1 and 22u-D/4.1 respectively), since two bounding boxes are given in these cases. With this, we can

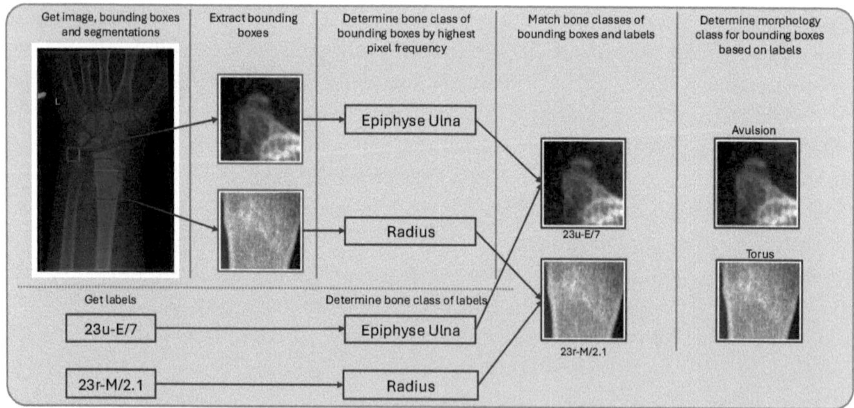

Fig. 1. Proposed pipeline to extract fracture morphology by assigning global AO codes to the corresponding fracture bounding boxes. Therefore, a matching of the bounding boxes and labels is performed based on their corresponding bone class.

map each fracture (bounding box) to an AO-code and vice versa and assign its fracture morphology label (Fig. 1). We find that six of eleven fracture morphology have too few samples to train our models, even after applying loss weighting and oversampling. Consequently, we exclude those from our experiments. Fig. 3 shows the five fracture morphologies extracted from the 18 different AO-codes.

2.3 Experiments

As a lower baseline, we train a CNN on the whole image utilizing morphology classes provided by the global AO-codes. With this, no mapping from morphology class to the fractures exits and hence we only detect their global presence, formulating this task as a multilabel classification (multi-label on full-image). For our multiclass approach, we extract the fracture's bounding boxes as patches and assign their morphology label utilizing our pipeline (Sec. 2.2). On those patches, we train a CNN converting the fracture morphology classification from a multi-label full-image into a multi-class patch-based task. However, extracting those patched requires access to the fractures' bounding boxes and while we use the provided ground truth (GT) bounding boxes as an upper baseline (multi-class on GT BBox) they are not available in a real-world application with unknown images. To overcome this limitation, we also consider the impact of a non-perfect fracture detection. We train a YOLO detector on the same dataset with the GT fracture bounding boxes. Here, we experiment with different confidence thresholds $t \in \{0.01, 0.05, 0.1, 0.5, 0.8, 0.85\}$ for YOLO's fracture detection to further boost its recall, since for a real-world application, an overlooked fracture would be a crucial error. Since a low t results in a higher recall but lower precision, we implement a false-positive reduction (FP-reduction). For this, we extend our classifier with a new "Healthy" class holding all patches proposed by YOLO covering non-fracture image content. We determine such a false-positive by comparing YOLO's predicted bounding box with the GT. If no GT box exist having an IoU of at least 0.5 (threshold of the Pascal VOC challenge), we consider this prediction as false-positive and assign the label "Healthy".

2.4 Training setup

As CNN for classification, we chose an ImageNet-pretrained ResNet18 (`torchvision` implementation). We employ a drop out layer ($p = 0.1$) before the classifier head to lessen overfitting. For the patch-based approach, we remove the stride of the first conv layer with kernel size 7 and its following max pooling to adapt the model's downsample scale to the lower patch resolution. As preprocessing for the full-image baseline, we bilinear resize the images to 384×224 preserving the average aspect ratio of the dataset and providing enough details to detect fine fracture lines. The patches were extracted from the original high-resolution image and bilinear resized to their average size (96×96). We counter class imbalance by employing loss weighting and oversampling via a weighted random sample using the class inverse frequencies as weights. For on-the-fly data augmentation, we use random affine transformations: rotation of $\mathcal{U}(-25°, 25°)$, scaling of $\mathcal{U}(80\,\%, 120\,\%)$,

Tab. 1. Quantitative results across different methods. Multi-label on full-image and multi-class on GT BBox have been trained on GT fracture locations and AO codes. YOLO BBox describes the patched-based multiclass approach using YOLO for fracture detection with given confidence (Conf) and optional FP-reduction.

Model	FP-reduction	Accuracy	F1-score	Precision	Recall
Multi-label on full-image	×	**0.8790**	0.6771	0.6941	0.6631
Multi-class on GT BBox	×	0.7334	**0.7630**	**0.8085**	**0.7334**
YOLO BBox, Conf 0.01	×	0.6603	0.2786	0.7655	0.1761
	✓	0.6593	0.2460	0.7351	0.1545
YOLO BBox, Conf 0.05	×	0.6463	0.2421	0.6872	0.1516
	✓	0.6415	0.2343	0.6893	0.1451
YOLO BBox, Conf 0.5	×	0.6171	0.2126	0.7497	0.1287
	✓	0.6171	0.2126	0.7497	0.1287
YOLO BBox, Conf 0.85	×	0.4775	0.1100	0.8673	0.0607
	✓	0.4751	0.1099	0.7763	0.0603

and translation of $\mathcal{U}(-10\,\%, 10\,\%)$ in width and height. The Adam optimizer minimizes the loss (cross entropy for multiclass and binary cross entropy for mutlilabel) for 200 epochs. We adapt its initial learning rate $1e^{-4}$ using a cosine annealing scheduler with a single cycle and a linear warm-up during the first 20 epochs. For fracture detection, we employ a YOLOv10x (`ultralytics` framework) and train it with a three folded cross validation. For our morphology classification, we then use the model that included the current image in its validation split. We evaluate our experiments with the macro-averaged accuracy, F1-score, precision, and recall. Fractures missed by YOLO (false negatives) are considered errors and are included in the evaluation metrics. Our code is available on GitHub[1].

3 Results

The quantitative results in Tab. 1 show both baselines outperforming the fracture morphology classification employing a YOLO-based fracture detection (with mAP of 0.92). The multi-label approach, taking the whole image as input, yields the highest accuracy. When the GT fracture bounding boxes are used in our patch-based, multi-class approach, we achieve the highest recall, precision and thus F1-score. However, when we use the YOLO to predict the fracture bounding boxes, all metrics, especially recall and thus F1-score decrease. This decrease cannot be recovered by the FP-reduction. Moreover, when comparing their results with its corresponding counterpart without, the FP-reduction hurts the performance across all metrics.

Fig. 2 reveals that reducing the confidence level for the YOLO prediction indeed increases the recall (orange, x-dotted line) and F1-score (blue, circle-dotted line), indicating a boost in the overall performance. As already observed in Tab. 1, the FP-reduction does not increase the performance. When considering the results for

[1] `https://github.com/multimodallearning/FractureMorphologyClassification`

the non-pretrained model (red, cross-dotted line), we find that utilizing ImageNet weights play no crucial role in our setting.

Fig. 3 plots the F1-scores for our five fracture morphologies across all models. Except for “Transverse”, the patch-based approach utilizing the GT fracture bounding boxes yields the highest F1-score (7.89 % on average) with the largest margin (0.7831) on the “Avulsion” class. Again, it can be seen that the F1-scores of the YOLO boxes on lower confidence levels are mostly higher in comparison to higher confidence levels and the FP-reduction does not boost the performances.

4 Discussion

Our proposed method to extract fracture morphology by assigning global AO codes to the corresponding fracture bounding boxes (Fig. 1 allow the reformulation of a global multi-label task to a local multi-class one. Our study reveals, that this reformulation improves the overall performance (7.89 % F1 on average), since it permits only one morphology to be present. However, the real-world usability of the patch-based approach is currently limited by the unreliable YOLO fracture detection (−65.3 % F1 at 0.85 confidence level). To overcome this, we investigated into multiple confidence thresholds for the fracture detection combined with a FP-reduction (extending the classifier with “Healthy” class) to handle the expected increase in false detection.

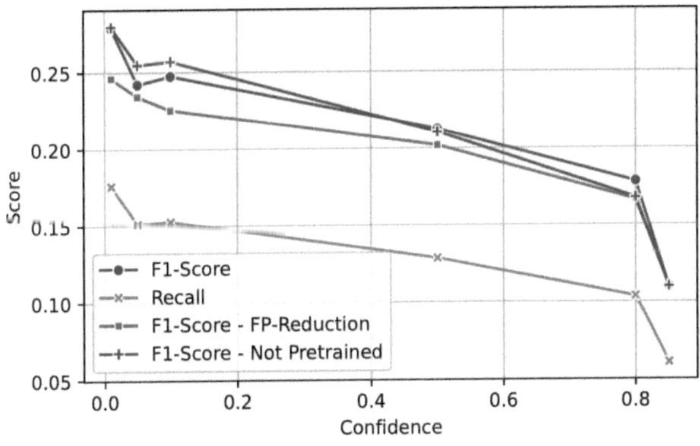

Fig. 2. The impact of FP-reduction and pretraining on F1-scores was analyzed across different YOLO fracture detection confidence levels. The recall curve shows that lowering the confidence threshold increases recall.

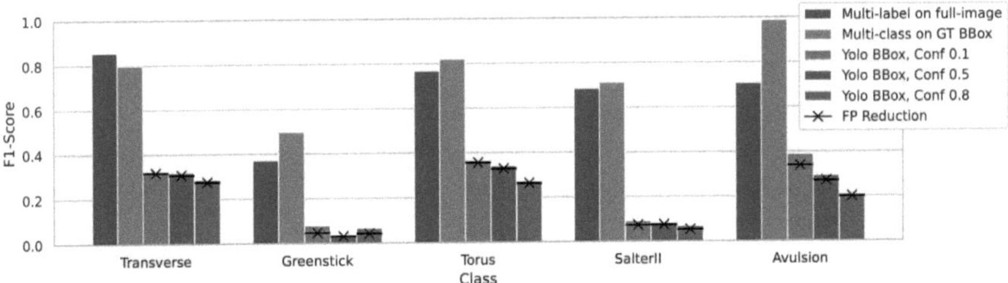

Fig. 3. F1-scores for different fracture morphologies. See the caption of Tab. 1 for brief method descriptions.

While we found a correlation in lowering the confidence level and the performance (−48.44 % F1 at 0.01), the FP-reduction does not yield any improvement. We perform a sanity check by training a binary classifier ("Fracture" and "Healthy") on the YOLO proposed patches with confidence 0.01. This yields a F1-score of 0.5 (not shown in the results) indicating that a (preprocessing) step within our setup might limit the FP-reduction. Hence, extending the fracture morphology classification task with the FP-reduction adds additional difficulty to the already complicated task. The YOLO model frequently misses several bounding boxes (e.g. 2 953 at confidence level of 0.01) that are present within the GT bounding boxes. The addition of these false-negative examples in the evaluation metrics has led to a decrease in metric values, particularly in the recall. While the performance with the GT bounding boxes proofs the potential of our multi-class reformulation, the focus of future work must be on the improvement of fracture detection algorithms to create a real-world application. Furthermore, analysing a more diverse dataset, including more AO codes, would lead to a more generalized solution including more fracture morphologies.

Acknowledgement. This research has been funded by Schleswig-Holstein, Grant Number 22023005. We thank Ludger Tüshaus and Franziska Halm from the University Hospital Schleswig-Holstein for their valuable expertise in extracting fracture morphology from AO codes.

References

1. Kraus R, Schneidmüller D, Röder C. Häufigkeit von Frakturen der langen Röhrenknochen im Wachstumsalter. Dtsch Arztebl Int. 2005;102(12):A–838.
2. Khan H, Monsell F, Duffy S, Trompeter A, Bridgens A, Gelfer Y. Paediatric distal radius fractures: an instructional review for the FRCS examination. Eur J Orthop Surg Traumatol. 2023;33(5):2169–72.
3. Slongo T, Audigé L, Schlickewei W, Clavert JM, Hunter J. Development and validation of the AO pediatric comprehensive classification of long bone fractures. J Pediatr Orthop. 2006;26(1):43–9.
4. Shojib MH, Khan RR, Faiaz A, Ashrafee M, Alfaz N. Classification of wrist fracture from X-ray images using DenseNet-121. Proc ICCIT. 2024:1428–33.
5. Thorat SR, Jha DG, Sharma AK, Katkar DV. Wrist fracture detection using self-supervised learning methodology. Musculoskelet Surg. 2024;8(2):133–41.
6. Binh LN, Nhu NT, Vy VPT, Son DLH, Hung TNK, Bach N et al. Multi-class deep learning model for detecting pediatric distal forearm fractures based on the AO/OTA classification. J Imaging Inform Med. 2024;37(2):725–33.
7. Min H, Rabi Y, Wadhawan A, Bourgeat P, Dowling J, White J et al. Automatic classification of distal radius fracture using a two-stage ensemble deep learning framework. Phys Eng Sci Med. 2023;46(2):877–86.
8. Gan K, Liu Y, Zhang T, Xu D, Lian L, Luo Z et al. Deep learning model for automatic identification and classification of distal radius fracture. J Imaging Inform Med. 2024.
9. Yang F, Cong R, Xing M, Ding B. Study on AO classification of distal radius fractures based on multi-feature fusion. Proc APSDP. 2021;1800(1):012006.

10. Keuth R, Balks M, Tschauner S, Tüshaus L, Heinrich M. Systematic analysis of input modalities for fracture classification. Proc BVM. 2025:203–8.
11. Nagy E, Janisch M, Hržić F, Sorantin E, Tschauner S. A pediatric wrist trauma X-ray dataset for machine learning. Sci Data. 2022;9(1):222.

Deep Learning Framework for Brain Age Prediction Integrating Gray Matter Structure and White Matter Microstructure

MN-FNet

Xinghao Wang[1,2], Marco Maass[3], Yuanheng Zhang[2], Chen Li[4], Xinyu Huang[5], Hongzan Sun[1], Marcin Grzegorzek[2,3]

[1]Department of Radiology, Shengjing Hospital of China Medical University, Shenyang, China
[2]Institut für Medizinische Informatik, Universität zu Lübeck
[3]Deutsches Forschungszentrum für Künstliche Intelligenz GmbH (DFKI)
[4]Northeastern University, Shenyang, China
[5]expandAI GmbH, Lübeck
marcin.grzegorzek@uni-luebeck.de

Abstract. Brain aging is an inevitable process in adulthood, yet there remains a critical need for objective and accurate biomarkers to assess its progression. In this study, we develop a deep learning-based framework for brain age estimation using multiparameter MRI. Structural (T1 and T2 weighted) and diffusion-weighted images were acquired, from which we extracted cortical features, including gray matter volume, surface area, and thickness along with white matter integrity metrics such as fractional anisotropy, mean diffusivity, axial diffusivity, and radial diffusivity. To integrate these multimodal neuroimaging features, we propose MN-FNet (multimodal neurofeature fusion network), a dedicated regression architecture that effectively combines gray matter structure and white matter microstructure. Our model achieves accurate brain age prediction with low estimation error and identifies key neuroanatomical regions associated with aging, additionally providing evidence of hemispheric lateralization as a factor in brain aging. This approach offers a reliable and interpretable tool for brain age estimation, with potential applications in early detection of neurodegenerative conditions.

1 Introduction

Brain aging and its associated neurodegenerative conditions present growing challenges to global health. However, the absence of reliable and objective biomarkers for organ-specific or systemic biological aging has greatly hindered precise assessment of functional decline and degenerative processes. Over the past four decades, researchers have sought biomarkers that can objectively reflect the pace of biological

© Der/die Autor(en), exklusiv lizenziert an
Springer Fachmedien Wiesbaden GmbH, ein Teil von Springer Nature 2026
H. Handels et al. (Hrsg.), *Bildverarbeitung für die Medizin 2026*,
Informatik aktuell, https://doi.org/10.1007/978-3-658-51100-5_90

aging. Advances in multi-omics technologies now allow accurate age prediction using various biological data types [1]. In the study of central nervous system aging, the concept of "brain age" [2] has emerged a neuroimaging based metric derived from magnetic resonance imaging (MRI) that offers a noninvasive approach to evaluate structural and functional brain aging. By modeling the healthy brain as a reference, this method identifies deviations associated with accelerated or delayed aging.

To build such a model, neuroimaging parameters extracted from brain scans of healthy individuals are used to train regression models labeled with chronological age. These models condense complex, multidimensional aging patterns into a single interpretable value "brain age" for each individual. Early detection of age-related brain changes is essential for preventing or delaying neurodegenerative diseases. Research on brain age has expanded rapidly in recent years. Model performance is typically assessed using the mean absolute error (MAE), which quantifies the average absolute difference between predicted brain age and actual age. The discrepancy between these two values is known as the brain age gap (BAG), which has been shown to correlate strongly with other age-related traits, such as cognitive decline and physical fitness, supporting its validity as a biomarker of brain aging. Furthermore, integrating multiple MRI modalities is increasingly common to enhance prediction accuracy and achieve a more comprehensive representation of brain health [3].

In this study, we develop a brain age prediction model based on multimodal MRI data. Our goal is to characterize healthy brain aging and provide an accurate assessment framework for population-level studies. Based on our experimental objectives, we designed a data screening and processing pipeline (Fig. 1).

2 Materials and methods

2.1 Dataset

Neuroimaging data were acquired using 3.0 Tesla MRI scanner with the same model (General Electric 750 W, Milwaukee, WI, USA) in this multicenter study. Data from the study were acquired from 2020 to 2022. All included participants are healthy participants without neurological or psychiatric diagnoses.

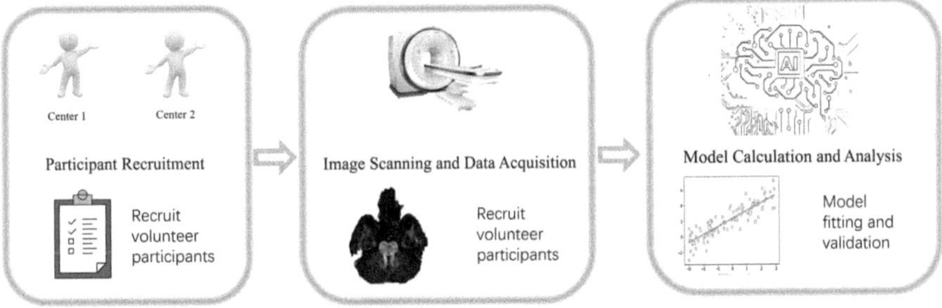

Fig. 1. A full framework for brain age modeling: from image data processing to application validation.

2.2 Image Processing

This study mainly used structure and dispersion sequences from healthy individuals. Regardless of the database type, we implemented a standardized image data processing procedure to minimize variations between sites. For image processing, we mainly used tools such as FSL and FreeSurfer. We cropped and registered structure images to the Montreal Neurological Institute 152 (MNI152) "non-linear 6th generation" standard space structure Template. The regions of interest were defined in the MNI152 space, combining parcellations from the Harvard-Oxford cortical and subcortical atlases. For DTI images, we used the eddy tool. Eddy current and head motion artifacts were removed, and abnormal slices were corrected. We extracted two parameters, fractional anisotropy (FA) and mean diffusivity (MD), to represent the white matter fiber situation.

2.3 Model Establishment

To effectively integrate multimodal neuroimaging features for brain age prediction, we proposed a dedicated deep learning architecture termed the multimodal neurofeature fusion network (MN-FNet). The overall objective of MN-FNet is to learn a non-linear mapping function from high-dimensional, multimodal brain features to a continuous biological age value.

The model processing pipeline consists of three main stages: modality-specific encoding, feature fusion, and regression output (Alg. 2).

Alg. 2 Multimodal Neurofeature Fusion Network (MN-FNet).

Require: Multimodal feature matrices $\mathbf{X}^{(1)} \in \mathbb{R}^{N \times d_1}, \mathbf{X}^{(2)} \in \mathbb{R}^{N \times d_2}$
Ensure: Predicted brain ages $\hat{\mathbf{y}} \in \mathbb{R}^N$

for each sample $i = 1$ to N **do**
  for each modality $m \in \{1, 2\}$ **do**
    $\mathbf{h}_{i,1}^{(m)} \leftarrow \text{ReLU}(\text{BN}(\mathbf{W}_1^{(m)} \mathbf{x}_i^{(m)} + \mathbf{b}_1^{(m)}))$ ▷ Modality-specific encoding
    $\mathbf{h}_{i,2}^{(m)} \leftarrow \text{ReLU}(\text{BN}(\mathbf{W}_2^{(m)} \mathbf{h}_{i,1}^{(m)} + \mathbf{b}_2^{(m)}))$
  end for
  $\mathbf{h}_{\text{fusion},i} \leftarrow [\mathbf{h}_{i,2}^{(1)}; \mathbf{h}_{i,2}^{(2)}]$ ▷ Feature concatenation
  $\mathbf{h}_{\text{fused},i} \leftarrow \text{ReLU}(\mathbf{W}_f \mathbf{h}_{\text{fusion},i} + \mathbf{b}_f)$ ▷ Cross-modal fusion
  $\hat{y}_i \leftarrow \mathbf{w}_o^\top \mathbf{h}_{\text{fused},i} + b_o$ ▷ Age regression output
end for
return $\hat{\mathbf{y}}$

Each modality (e.g., cortical thickness and diffusion metrics) is first encoded through independent fully connected layers with batch normalization and ReLU activation. The resulting features are concatenated and processed through a fusion layer before final age regression. The model is trained to minimize the mean absolute error (MAE) between predicted and chronological ages

$$\mathcal{L} = \frac{1}{N}\sum_{i=1}^{N} |y_i - \hat{y}_i|$$

We use Adam optimizer with dropout regularization to prevent overfitting. The implementation is based on PyTorch framework.

3 Results

The predictive performance of the proposed multimodal neurofeature fusion network (MN-FNet) was quantitatively evaluated and compared against two baseline models: a convolutional neural network (CNN) and a linear regression model. The models were assessed using the MAE between the predicted brain age and the chronological age on both the training and an independent test set (Fig. 2).

As demonstrated, our proposed MN-FNet achieved the lowest prediction error, with an MAE of 2.72 years on the training set and 2.87 years on the test set. This result signifies a superior performance compared to the CNN model, which yielded higher MAEs of 3.52 and 3.67 years on the training and test sets, respectively. The conventional linear regression model, as expected, exhibited the largest prediction error, with an MAE of nearly 7 years. The minimal discrepancy between the training and test errors for MN-FNet further indicates its strong generalization capability without substantial overfitting. In summary, these results confirm that the MN-FNet framework provides a more accurate and robust estimate of brain age from multimodal neuroimaging features than the established baseline approaches.

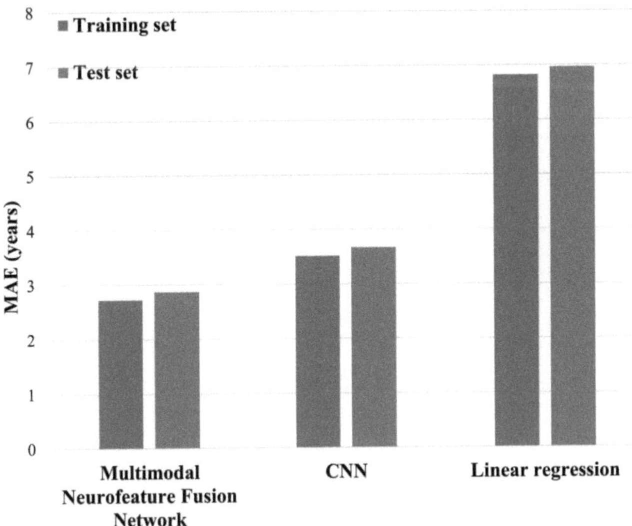

Fig. 2. Comparison of brain age prediction performance (MAE, years) across different models.

4 Discussion

In this study, we developed and validated the MN-FNet, a deep learning framework for brain age estimation that effectively integrates cortical structural and white matter microstructural features. Our model achieved a MAE of 2.87 years on the test set, demonstrating superior performance compared to conventional CNN and linear regression baselines. This result underscores the advantage of explicitly modeling multimodal neuroimaging characteristics for capturing the complex biological processes of brain aging.

The performance of MN-FNet aligns with and advances the current state of brain age prediction. While previous studies have reported MAEs ranging from 5 to 8 years using voxel based morphometry [4], recent deep learning approaches have progressively lowered this error. For instance, the SFCN architecture has shown promise due to its efficiency with 3D data [5]. A notable study by Beheshti et al. [6] achieved an MAE of almost 3 years in healthy controls by incorporating a bias correction technique. Our model's performance, attained through a dedicated multimodal fusion design on a specific population cohort, contributes to this trend of increasing accuracy. Furthermore, our focus on T1 weighted and DTI modalities is supported by literature indicating that these provide the most substantial contributions to brain age prediction, while functional connectivity features show weaker correlations [7].

Neuroanatomically, the features leveraged by our model are grounded in well established hallmarks of brain aging. The observed contributions from cortical thinning, particularly in the left hemisphere, are consistent with findings that language-dominant regions may be more vulnerable to age-related degeneration [8]. Similarly, the importance of white matter integrity, especially in regions like the cingulate gyrus and corpus callosum, echoes prior research linking these tracts to cognitive aging [9]. These structural and microstructural changes are believed to reflect underlying neurobiological mechanisms, including neuronal loss, synaptic reduction, myelin degradation, and neuroinflammation. By quantifying these alterations, the brain age gap derived from our model can serve as a composite biomarker for such processes.

A significant aspect of our work is its focus on an Asian population. It is recognized that brain aging patterns can vary across ethnic groups due to a confluence of genetic, environmental, and socioeconomic factors [10]. Most existing brain age models are derived from European or North American cohorts, potentially limiting their generalizability. Our study helps to address this gap, providing a tool tailored to and validated on a demographic that is underrepresented in neuroaging research.

While this study presents a robust multimodal framework for brain age prediction, several limitations should be acknowledged, which also outline directions for future research:

- The neuroimaging features were extracted using a standardized brain atlas not specifically optimized for the neuroanatomy of the cohort under study, which may introduce a subtle but systematic bias.
- A deliberate trade-off was made between model interpretability and predictive performance. The chosen feature-based, deep learning framework prioritizes

transparency and control over overfitting, potentially at the cost of a marginally higher MAE compared to more complex "black-box" architectures.

- The model was developed and validated on a specific demographic cohort. Its generalizability and performance across diverse ethnic populations remain to be comprehensively evaluated in future multi-center studies.
- The model currently integrates only the two most contributory modalities (T1 and DTI). Incorporating additional imaging sequences, while potentially beneficial, was constrained by data availability and the objective of maintaining a streamlined and clinically applicable pipeline.

Acknowledgement. Thank you to the database personnel for their hard work in data collection, processing, and ethical approval.

References

1. Jylhävä J, Pedersen NL, Hägg S. Biological age predictors. EBioMedicine. 2017;21:29–36.
2. Mishra S, Beheshti I, Khanna P. A review of neuroimaging-driven brain age estimation for identification of brain disorders and health conditions. IEEE Rev Biomed Eng. 2023;16:371–85.
3. Rokicki J, Wolfers T, Nordhøy W, Tesli N, Quintana DS, Alnaes D et al. Multimodal imaging improves brain age prediction and reveals distinct abnormalities in patients with psychiatric and neurological disorders. Hum Brain Mapp. 2021;42(6):1714–26.
4. Baecker L, Garcia-Dias R, Vieira S, Scarpazza C, Mechelli A. Machine learning for brain age prediction: introduction to methods and clinical applications. EBioMedicine. 2021;72:103600.
5. Fu Y, Huang Y, Dong S, Wang Y, Yu T, Niu M et al. SFCNEXT: A simple fully convolutional network for effective brain age estimation with small sample size. Proc IEEE ISBI. 2023:1–5.
6. Beheshti I, Nugent S, Potvin O, Duchesne S. Bias-adjustment in neuroimaging-based brain age frameworks: a robust scheme. Neuroimage Clin. 2019;24:102063.
7. G. A, Anatürk M, Suri S, Kaufmann T, Cole JH, Griffanti L et al. Multimodal brain-age prediction and cardiovascular risk: the Whitehall II MRI sub-study. Neuroimage. 2020;222:117292.
8. Michaelis K, Erickson LC, Fama ME, Skipper-Kallal LM, Xing S, Lacey EH et al. Effects of age and left hemisphere lesions on audiovisual integration of speech. Brain Lang. 2020;206:104812.
9. Archer DB, Schilling K, Shashikumar N, Jasodanand V, Moore EE, Pechman KR et al. Leveraging longitudinal diffusion MRI data to quantify differences in white matter microstructural decline in normal and abnormal aging. Alzheimers Dement (Amst). 2023;15(4):e12468.
10. Moonen JEF, Nasrallah IM, Detre JA, Dolui S, Erus G, Davatzikos C et al. Race, sex, and mid-life changes in brain health: cardia MRI substudy. Alzheimers Dement. 2022;18(12):2428–37.

Abstract: Automated Detection of Focal Bone Marrow Lesions from MRI

A Multi-center Feasibility Study in Patients with Monoclonal Plasma Cell Disorders

Jessica Kächele[1,2,3†], Markus Wennmann[4,5†], Arvin von Salomon[2,4], Peter Neher[1,3,6], Heinz-Peter Schlemmer[4], Klaus Maier-Hein[1,2,6,7], and others

[1]Division of Medical Image Computing, German Cancer Research Center, Germany
[2]Medical Faculty, Heidelberg University, Germany
[3]German Cancer Consortium (DKTK), Partner Site Heidelberg, Germany
[4]Division of Radiology, German Cancer Research Center (DKFZ), Germany
[5]Diagnostic and Interventional Radiology, Heidelberg University Hospital, Germany
[6]Pattern Analysis and Learning Group, Department of Radiation Oncology, Heidelberg University Hospital, Germany
[7]Faculty of Mathematics and Computer Science, Heidelberg University, Heidelberg, Germany

jessica.kaechele@dkfz-heidelberg.de

This retrospective feasibility study aimed to train and test an AI-based algorithm for automated detection of focal bone marrow lesions (FL) on MRI. 444 patients with monoclonal plasma cell disorders were included, focusing on FLs in the left pelvis. Using the nnDetection framework, the algorithm was trained on 334 patients with 494 FLs from center 1 and evaluated on an internal test set (36 patients, 89 FLs) and a multicentric external test set (74 patients, 262 FLs, centers 2–11). On the internal/external test sets, the algorithm achieved a mAP of 0.44/0.34, F1-score 0.54/0.44, sensitivity 0.49/0.34, and a PPV of 0.61/0.61. In two high-quality external subsets, performance approached that of the internal test set (mAP 0.45/0.41, F1-score 0.50/0.53, sensitivity 0.44/0.43, PPV 0.60/0.71). Automated and reference FL counts correlated significantly (internal $r = 0.51$, $p = 0.001$; external $r = 0.59$, $p < 0.001$). These results demonstrate the feasibility and multicentric robustness of automated FL detection and quantification from MRI. [1]

References

1. Wennmann M, Kächele J, von Salomon A, Nonnenmacher T, Bujotzek M, Xiao S et al. Automated detection of focal bone marrow lesions from MRI: a multi-center feasibility study in patients with monoclonal plasma cell disorders. Acad Radiol. 2025;32(10):6012–26.

[†]These authors contributed equally to this work.

© Der/die Autor(en), exklusiv lizenziert an Springer Fachmedien Wiesbaden GmbH, ein Teil von Springer Nature 2026
H. Handels et al. (Hrsg.), *Bildverarbeitung für die Medizin 2026*, Informatik aktuell, https://doi.org/10.1007/978-3-658-51100-5_91

Abstract: Annotation-efficient 3D Body Composition Segmentation

Lena Philipp [1], Maarten de Rooij [1], John Hermans [1], Matthieu Rutten [1], Horst Hahn [2], Bram van Ginneken [1,2], Alessa Hering [1]

[1] Department of Imaging, Radboudumc, Nijmegen, The Netherlands
[2] Fraunhofer MEVIS, Bremen, Germany
lena.philipp@radboudumc.nl

Quantifying body composition from computed tomography (CT) provides valuable insights into metabolic health, disease prognosis, and treatment outcomes. However, the development of 3D segmentation models for body composition analysis has been limited by the extensive manual annotation effort required. We present an annotation-efficient strategy for 3D segmentation of abdominal and pelvic body composition [1], designed to drastically reduce annotation needs while maintaining high accuracy. Our approach combines sparse manual annotations with an iterative self-learning framework that transitions from 2D to 3D segmentation. Only 1% of all training slices were manually annotated. The model was trained on 116 CT scans and evaluated on an internal test set of 20 scans and a reader study of 100 cases. Quantitative performance was assessed using the Dice similarity coefficient. To further assess generalizability and clinical reliability, a multi-reader evaluation was conducted by three experienced radiologists using a standardized scoring protocol to rate the correction effort per segmentation class. The final 3D model achieved Dice coefficients of 0.97 ± 0.01 for skeletal muscle (SM), 0.85 ± 0.04 for inter-/intramuscular adipose tissue (IMAT), 0.94 ± 0.04 for visceral adipose tissue (VAT), and 0.98 ± 0.01 for subcutaneous adipose tissue (SAT). Reader study results confirmed negligible to minimal correction effort for SM, VAT, and SAT, with higher variability for IMAT. These results indicate strong robustness and demonstrate the feasibility of developing accurate 3D body composition models with minimal annotation effort.

References

1. Philipp L, de Rooij M, Hermans J, Rutten M, van Ginneken B, Hering A. Annotation-efficient strategy for segmentation of 3D body composition. Proc MIDL. 2024.

© Der/die Autor(en), exklusiv lizenziert an
Springer Fachmedien Wiesbaden GmbH, ein Teil von Springer Nature 2026
H. Handels et al. (Hrsg.), *Bildverarbeitung für die Medizin 2026*,
Informatik aktuell, https://doi.org/10.1007/978-3-658-51100-5_92

Abstract: Enhancing Deep Learning Methods for Brain Metastasis Detection Through Cross-technique Annotations on SPACE MRI

Tassilo Wald [1,2†], Benjamin Hamm [1,3†], Julius Holzschuh[1], Rami El Shafie [4,5], Andreas Kudak [4,6,7], Balint Kovacs [1,3], Irada Pflüger[8], Bastian von Nettelbladt[4,6,9], Constantin Ulrich [1,3,9], Michael A. Baumgartner [1,2], Philipp Vollmuth [8,10], Jürgen Debus [4,6,7,9], Klaus H. Maier-Hein [1,2,9,11], Thomas Welzel [4,6,9]

[1]German Cancer Research Center (DKFZ), Division of Medical Image Computing
[2]Helmholtz Imaging, DKFZ and Faculty of Mathematics and CS, Heidelberg University
[3]Medical Faculty, Heidelberg University
[4]Radiation Oncology Department, UK Heidelberg
[5]Radiation Oncology Department, UK Göttingen
[6]Heidelberg Institute of Radiation Oncology
[7]Clinical Cooperation Unit Radiation Oncology, DKFZ
[8]Neuroradiology Dep. and Div. for Computational Neuroimaging, UK Heidelberg
[9]NCT Heidelberg, DKTK and HIT, UK Heidelberg
[10]Div. for Comp. Radiology Clinical AI, UK Bonn and Medical Faculty, Bonn University
[11]Pattern Analysis and Learning Group, UK Heidelberg and TLRC
benjamin.hamm@dkfz-heidelberg.de

High-quality annotation plays a crucial role in improving deep learning-based detection of brain metastases (BMs). In this work, originally published in European Radiology Experimental [1], we investigate how annotations derived from SPACE sequences, which offer superior lesion conspicuity compared to MPRAGE, affect detection performance. We compare models trained with normal annotation quality on MPRAGE against those trained with high-quality annotation (HAQ) derived from co-registered SPACE images. Our results show that HAQ significantly enhances detection and delineation performance across multiple datasets, even when applied to MPRAGE inputs. These findings demonstrate that improved annotation quality alone can substantially boost deep learning detection of small BMs, enabling faster and more accurate fully automated diagnosis.

References

1. Wald T, Hamm B, Holzschuh JC, El Shafie R, Kudak A, Kovacs B et al. Enhancing deep learning methods for brain metastasis detection through cross-technique annotations on SPACE MRI. Eur Radiol Exp. 2025;9(1):15.

†These authors contributed equally to this work.

© Der/die Autor(en), exklusiv lizenziert an Springer Fachmedien Wiesbaden GmbH, ein Teil von Springer Nature 2026
H. Handels et al. (Hrsg.), *Bildverarbeitung für die Medizin 2026*, Informatik aktuell, https://doi.org/10.1007/978-3-658-51100-5_93

Abstract: BinaryFormer

Differentiable 1-bit Self-attention for Long-range Transformers in Medical Segmentation and 3D Diffusion Models

Mattias P. Heinrich

Institut für Medizinische Informatik, Universität zu Lübeck
mattias.heinrich@uni-luebeck.de

Vision transformers are essential for medical image analysis thanks to their ability to capture long-range dependencies. However, their quadratic computational cost with sequence length challenges high-resolution 3D tasks such as diffusion models or inpainting. FlashAttention eases memory bottlenecks via local access patterns, yet the computational load remains high. Quantising or binarising weights and activations shows promise in CNNs but often degrades accuracy and requires high-precision training. In transformers, work has focused on quantised linear layers or sparse attention, while binary attention remains largely unexplored.

Originally presented as oral at MIDL 2025 [1], our work introduces a novel differentiable binary attention mechanism that enables 1-bit precision computation of self-attention during both training and inference. Our method combines bitwise hamming distances with learnable scalar weighting of queries and keys to provide gradients. In theory it achieves 16–32× improvements in computational and memory efficiency over floating-point attention. We evaluate BinaryFormer on challenging tasks with sequence lengths of N>1000: image classification without patch embedding, semantic 2D MRI segmentation, and 3D high-resolution diffusion modelling for inpainting and synthesis. Across all tasks, our binary attention achieves competitive performance while greatly reducing resource demands. For faster inference, binarisation-aware training with a straight-through estimator is sufficient, whereas our hamming Attention is essential for fully binary precision training.

Future work will explore integrating binarisation into other transformer components, e.g. linear weight matrices, and investigating alternative backpropagation schemes using trainable attention biases. These directions may further enhance the efficiency of low-precision transformers for medical imaging and beyond. Code is available at `https://github.com/mattiaspaul/binaryformer`.

References

1. Heinrich MP. BinaryFormer: 1-bit self-attention for long-range transformers in medical image segmentation and 3D diffusion models. Proc MIDL. 2025.

© Der/die Autor(en), exklusiv lizenziert an
Springer Fachmedien Wiesbaden GmbH, ein Teil von Springer Nature 2026
H. Handels et al. (Hrsg.), *Bildverarbeitung für die Medizin 2026*,
Informatik aktuell, https://doi.org/10.1007/978-3-658-51100-5_94

Neural Instance Optimization for Lesion Segmentation in Follow-up CT

Sina Walluscheck [†], Vanja S. Cangalovic[†], Tanja Lossau, Stefan Heldmann, Jan H. Moltz

Fraunhofer Institute for Digital Medicine MEVIS
sina.walluscheck@mevis.fraunhofer.de

Abstract. The increasing volume of CT imaging data and the limited availability of radiologists pose challenges for timely and accurate cancer assessment. While lesion diameters are routinely measured in clinical workflows, volumetric analysis remains uncommon due to the time-intensive nature of manual segmentation. Automated segmentation methods enable precise, reproducible, and efficient quantification of tumor burden over time. By leveraging information from prior examinations, longitudinal analysis can further enhance the accuracy and consistency of follow-up segmentations.
We propose an approach for longitudinal lesion segmentation through neural instance optimization (NIO). A pre-trained segmentation network is fine-tuned on a patient's prior scan to capture individual lesion-specific characteristics, which are subsequently leveraged during inference on the follow-up examination. The proposed method is applied on two public datasets. While promising results are achieved on synthetic longitudinal data (median Dice of 0.74/0.83 without/with NIO), no quantitative improvement was achieved on the second real-world longitudinal dataset. Our experiments reveal the potential of the proposed method but also its limited ability to deal with domain shifts between prior and follow-up present in real-world scenarios.

1 Introduction

The growing number of CT examinations, combined with limited radiologist capacity, places substantial pressure on cancer diagnosis and longitudinal monitoring. In current clinical practice, lesion diameters are manually measured and tracked over time, whereas volumetric quantification, although more accurate, is rarely performed due to the burden of manual segmentation. Automated and robust segmentation methods are therefore essential to enable consistent and efficient quantification of tumor burden across time points. To be practical in a clinical setting, such methods must minimize the need for manual correction, thereby reducing radiologists' workload.

Longitudinal lesion segmentation offers the opportunity to incorporate information from previous time points in order to refine the follow-up segmentation.

[†]These authors contributed equally to this work.

© Der/die Autor(en), exklusiv lizenziert an
Springer Fachmedien Wiesbaden GmbH, ein Teil von Springer Nature 2026
H. Handels et al. (Hrsg.), *Bildverarbeitung für die Medizin 2026*,
Informatik aktuell, https://doi.org/10.1007/978-3-658-51100-5_95

A multitude of prior work deals with lesion segmentation in the context of longitudinal brain imaging, a domain characterized by limited anatomical variability across time points. Rokuss et al. [1] integrate prior information by weighting feature differences between latent representations of prior and follow-up images. Patel et al. [2] propose a joint registration-segmentation framework that enhances lesion detection sensitivity. Conversely, our work targets improvements in segmentation quality rather than detection. In the more challenging setting of whole-body lesion segmentation, Rokuss et al. [3] present *LesionLocator*, which combines registration and segmentation in a densely promptable U-Net, injecting propagated prior masks as an additional input channel, while Yassine et al. [4] fuse temporal cues via self-attention over channel-concatenated features from separately encoded time points.

We propose the use of neural instance optimization (NIO) as lightweight, lesion-specific adaptation strategy. NIO has already been introduced in the field of medical image processing and successfully used in deformable image registration to overcome performance losses due to distribution shifts during inference [5]. We apply NIO to fine-tune a pre-trained segmentation network on the prior and apply the adapted model to the follow-up. Image-specific fine-tuning techniques have shown promise in related medical imaging settings, such as interactive refinement [6]. In contrast to this work, we target longitudinal consistency by adapting on the prior and evaluating at follow-up without architectural changes. We deliberately do not compare our method with related approaches, as we are presenting a proof of concept and investigating limitations in the evaluation. The contributions in this work are as follows:

1. We implement NIO for longitudinal lesion segmentation on a pre-trained nnU-Net described in Sec. 2.2 and detail a practical setup (decoder-only updates and augmentations) in Sec. 2.3 that preserves global features while adapting to lesion-specific characteristics.
2. We conduct an evaluation of the proposed method on two public datasets including synthetic and real-world longitudinal data (Sec. 2.4 and Sec. 2.5).
3. Experimental results are critically discussed in Sec. 3 and Sec. 4 to highlight potential and current limitations of the proposed method.

2 Materials and methods

2.1 Proposed workflow

Our workflow aims to improve lesion segmentation on follow-up scans by fine-tuning a pre-trained model on a corresponding prior scan and its segmentation mask. Assuming that lesions retain similar appearance characteristics between time points, this adaptation enables lesion-specific model refinement while data augmentation and partial weight freezing mitigate overfitting.

For each lesion, a patch is extracted around the region of interest in the prior scan. The prior and follow-up images are registered to determine the corresponding patch location in the follow-up scan.

NIO is applicable in any context in which a high-quality segmentation of the lesion in the prior image is provided, regardless of whether the segmentation was obtained through fully automatic, semi-automatic, or manual approaches. Fig. 1 illustrates a semi-automatic workflow scenario, in which an initial AI-based segmentation may require manual refinement. The model is then fine-tuned over a small number of iterations and subsequently applied to the registered follow-up patch, producing a refined and temporally consistent segmentation.

2.2 Pre-trained segmentation model

We employ a state-of-the-art nnU-Net [7] trained on a diverse collection of public and proprietary datasets comprising a total of 10,922 lesions throughout the body. Training patches are uniformly resampled to a voxel size of 1.0 in z dimension, each patch is centered on the center of mass of a single lesion, and the network learns to segment only this central lesion. The extracted patches have a size of $128x128x112$.

2.3 Lesion-specific fine-tuning

Let x_t denote the prior image, x_{t+1} the follow-up image, and θ the parameters of the pre-trained model. The segmentation of the prior image before fine-tuning is $f(\theta, x_t)$, with y_t representing the (optionally corrected) annotation mask. The fine-tuning objective combines binary cross-entropy and Dice loss

$$\mathcal{L}(\theta) = \mathcal{L}_{\text{BCE}}(f(\theta, x_t), y_t) + \mathcal{L}_{\text{Dice}}(f(\theta, x_t), y_t) \tag{1}$$

Fine-tuning is performed with the Adam optimizer and an initial learning rate of 1×10^{-4}. Only decoder layers are updated to preserve global features while adapting

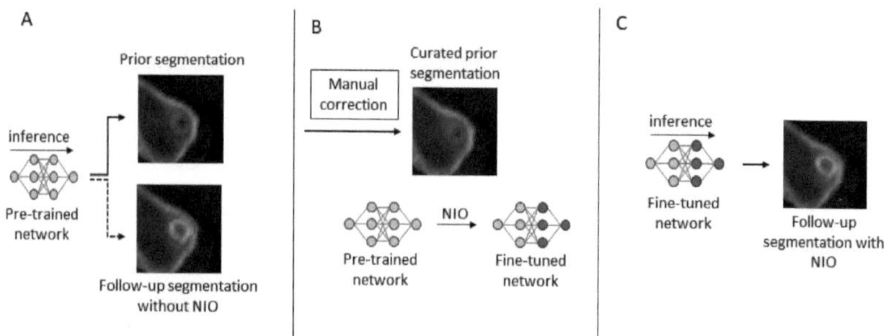

Fig. 1. Potential integration of the proposed neural instance optimization (NIO) in a semi-automatic workflow. (A) A pre-trained network produces an initial segmentation for the prior image. (B) The baseline segmentation might be manually refined or accepted by a radiologist. The resulting lesion mask is subsequently used as training sample for NIO. (C) The fine-tuned model generates a refined follow-up segmentation which is more consistent to the refined prior segmentation compared to a follow-up segmentation without NIO (dashed arrow in A).

to instance-specific characteristics. A batch size of three and data augmentation (comprising local morphological transformations via elastic deformations, rotation and scaling, and image-level alterations in the form of noise, blur, brightness and contrast transforms) are used to prevent overfitting. The adapted model parameters θ^* are subsequently used to segment x_{t+1}.

2.4 Synthetic LesionLocator dataset

The LesionLocator test dataset [3] contains lesion images compiled from various publicly available sources, along with artificially generated follow-up images derived from prior lesions using probabilistic augmentation. Although not based on real longitudinal acquisitions, the synthetic generation process ensures consistent lesion masks, enabling controlled evaluation of temporal adaptation. We follow the data split proposed by Grauw et al. [8], using 1,816 lesions for evaluation.

2.5 AutoPET/CT IV dataset

For real-world longitudinal evaluation, we use the autoPET/CT IV challenge dataset, comprising paired scans of 300 melanoma patients acquired at two distinct time points. We adhere to the official validation and test split. After excluding lesions with topological changes between time points, such as splits, merges, new appearances, or disappearances, the resulting evaluation set includes 60 patients with 477 lesions.

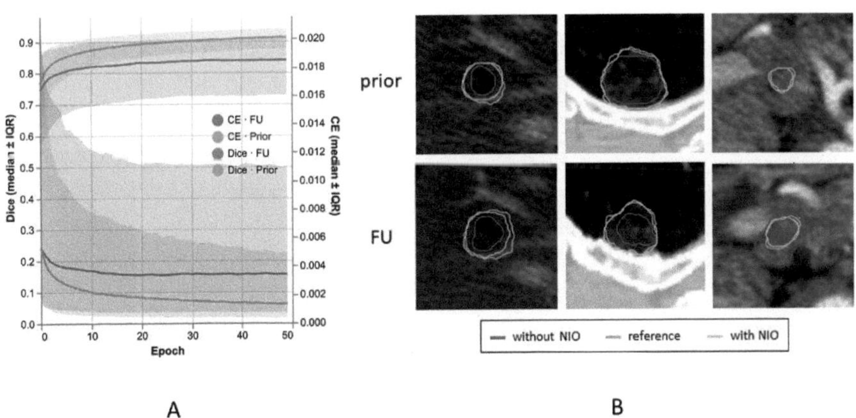

Fig. 2. Results on the synthetic dataset. (A) Learning curves for Dice scores and cross-entropy loss on prior and follow-up images. (B) Qualitative examples illustrating segmentation refinement after fine-tuning.

3 Results

3.1 Synthetic LesionLocator dataset

To evaluate our method, we compute the Dice score on the follow-up images after every fine-tuning epoch. Fig. 2A presents the learning curves of Dice and cross-entropy loss during fine-tuning on synthetic test cases over 50 epochs, aggregated across all lesions. The value for epoch zero corresponds to the performance of the baseline segmentation model without NIO. The plots for prior and follow-up images demonstrate that performance steadily improves without signs of overfitting. Fine-tuning increases the median Dice score on follow-up images from 0.74 (baseline) to 0.83 (fine-tuned), while qualitative results in Fig. 2B show visibly refined segmentations on follow-up images.

3.2 autoPET/CT IV dataset

We conduct the same evaluation on the real-world longitudinal autoPET/CT IV dataset. The results (Fig. 3A) reveal that while fine-tuning effectively adapts to prior images, the aggregated follow-up Dice scores slightly decline. Nevertheless, qualitative inspection identifies several improved follow-up segmentations, some examples of which are shown in Fig. 3B. This discrepancy between synthetic and real-world performance underscores the sensitivity of NIO to annotation consistency and imaging conditions.

4 Discussion

Our findings suggest that NIO can enhance longitudinal lesion segmentation when prior and follow-up images exhibit comparable appearance and consistent anno-

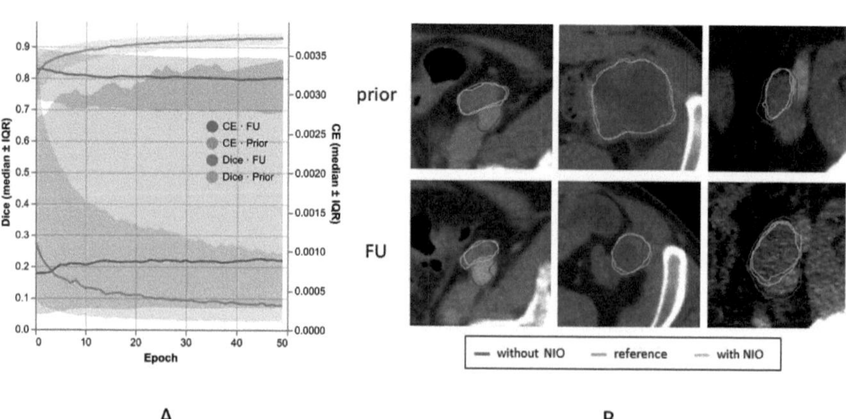

Fig. 3. Results on the autoPET/CT IV dataset. (A) Learning curves for Dice scores and cross-entropy loss on prior and follow-up images. (B) Qualitative examples illustrating segmentation refinement after fine-tuning.

tations. On synthetic data, the method yielded clear quantitative and qualitative improvements. However, on real-world data, inconsistencies in annotation quality, image resolution, and acquisition protocols as well as substantial anatomical changes limited transferability. In particular, the autoPET/CT IV dataset introduces several challenges, most notably annotation inconsistencies between prior and follow-up images, which undermine the initial assumption that prior lesions provide relevant shape and appearance cues for fine-tuning.

These discrepancies highlight the need for carefully curated longitudinal datasets to meaningfully evaluate temporal adaptation methods. A promising direction for future research is to filter test cases using a metric other than the Dice score, similar to the approach of Zhou et al. [9], in order to retain only well-predicted cases for evaluation and thereby mitigate the impact of annotation inconsistencies. Furthermore, domain shifts between prior and follow-up acquisitions pose challenges related to those encountered in Test-Time Adaptation, where optimization under domain shift can lead to performance degradation [10]. Future work should therefore focus on developing mechanisms to effectively counteract these effects.

Two simplifying assumptions in our experimental setup currently constrain generalization. First, the model was trained to segment only the central lesion which is perfectly centered within the input patch, allowing the model to rely on absolute position information, while real-world applications must remain robust to registration inaccuracies. Second, our evaluation currently excludes lesions undergoing topological changes, limiting analysis to stable lesion configurations (i.e. no splitting, merging or disappearing is taken into account). In future work, we plan to conduct a reader study in which radiology experts assess whether the follow-up segmentations refined by our method are more consistent, accurate, and require fewer manual corrections than those of a static baseline model.

Acknowledgement. This work was supported by the German Federal Ministry of Research, Technology, and Space (BMFTR) under grant number 01QE2404B as part of the ALTRIS (Automated Lung Tracking Image Software) consortium project.

References

1. Rokuss M, Kirchhoff Y, Roy S, Kovacs B, Ulrich C, Wald T et al. Longitudinal segmentation of MS lesions via temporal difference weighting. arXiv: 2409.13416. 2024.
2. Patel J, Ahmed SR, Chang K, Singh P, Gidwani M, Hoebel K et al. A deep learning based framework for joint image registration and segmentation of brain metastases on magnetic resonance imaging. Proc MLHC. 2023:565–87.
3. Rokuss M, Kirchhoff Y, Akbal S, Kovacs B, Roy S, Ulrich C et al. LesionLocator: zero-shot universal tumor segmentation and tracking in 3D whole-body imaging. arXiv: 2502.20985. 2025.
4. Yassine W, Charachon M, Hudelot C, Ardon R. LiFE-net: longitudinal information fusion for enhanced lesion detection in unsupervised learning contexts. Proc MIML. 2025.
5. Mok T, Li Z, Xia Y, Yao J, Zhang L, Zhou J et al. Deformable medical image registration under distribution shifts with neural instance optimization. Proc MIML. 2023:126–36.

6. Wang G, Li W, Zuluaga MA, Pratt R, Patel PA, Aertsen M et al. Interactive medical image segmentation using deep learning with image-specific fine tuning. IEEE Trans Med Imaging. 2018;37(7):1562–73.
7. Isensee F, Petersen J, Klein A, Zimmerer D, Jaeger PF, Kohl S et al. nnU-Net: self-adapting framework for U-net-based medical image segmentation. arXiv: 1809.10486. 2018.
8. de Grauw MJJ, Scholten ET, Smit EJ, Rutten MJCM, Prokop M, van Ginneken B et al. The ULS23 challenge: a baseline model and benchmark dataset for 3D universal lesion segmentation in computed tomography. Med Image Anal. 2025;102:103525.
9. Zhou Y, Wu J, Liao W, Zhang S, Zhang S, Wang G. TEGDA: test-time evaluation-guided dynamic adaptation for medical image segmentation. Proc NYSDS. 2025.
10. Chen Z, Ye Y, Pan Y, Xia Y. Gradient alignment improves test-time adaptation for medical image segmentation. arXiv: 2408.07343. 2024.

Automated Segmentation and Biomarker Analysis in OCT Images using a Transformer-based Framework

Lukas Mechs[1,2], Stefan B. Ploner[1,2], Yunchan Hwang[2], Muhammad U. Jamil[3], Nadia K. Waheed[3], James G. Fujimoto[2], Andreas Maier[1]

[1]Pattern Recognition Lab, Friedrich-Alexander-Universität Erlangen-Nürnberg, Germany
[2]Research Laboratory of Electronics, Massachusetts Institute of Technology, USA
[3]Department of Ophthalmology, New England Eye Center, USA
lukas.mechs@fau.de

Abstract. Accurate segmentation of retinal layers in optical coherence tomography (OCT) is crucial in the diagnosis of various retinal diseases, including the early detection of age-related macular degeneration (AMD). The ellipsoid zone (EZ), a hyperreflective layer associated with photoreceptor integrity, plays a critical role in disease assessment but poses challenges for automated analysis, as degeneration in pathologic eyes leads to variable visibility and structural alterations. This study introduces a fully automated method for segmenting the anterior EZ boundary using a Transformer-based architecture derived from UNETR. The proposed network produces two outputs (1) a sub-pixel depth position, indicating the location of the anterior EZ boundary and (2) a presence prediction, representing the probability that the EZ is present at that position. The model is trained only on the prediction of the depth position, while the presence prediction is derived from the 3D output feature map. Trained on 68 high-resolution volumetric OCT scans with an axial resolution of 2.7 µm, the proposed method achieved a mean Median Absolute Error of 1.11 µm and a 12% failure rate at a 4 µm threshold for sub-pixel EZ boundary localization. For EZ presence prediction, it reached 0.96 accuracy and an ROC AUC of 0.86. Qualitative evaluation confirmed anatomically consistent predictions across healthy and diseased retinas. Furthermore, a derived EZ-based biomarker showed a gradual increase with disease severity in AMD, highlighting its potential for both early detection and disease staging. These findings demonstrate the robustness and clinical relevance of the proposed framework.

1 Introduction

Vision is essential to navigating daily life, yet vision impairment remains a significant global health issue. In 2020, an estimated 596 million people had impaired vision worldwide, 43 million of whom were blind. Among the leading causes of these conditions was age-related macular degeneration (AMD) [1]. Optical coherence tomography (OCT) enables non-invasive visualization of retinal layers and plays a

© Der/die Autor(en), exklusiv lizenziert an
Springer Fachmedien Wiesbaden GmbH, ein Teil von Springer Nature 2026
H. Handels et al. (Hrsg.), *Bildverarbeitung für die Medizin 2026*,
Informatik aktuell, https://doi.org/10.1007/978-3-658-51100-5_96

central role in the early detection of retinal diseases [2]. Among these layers, the ellipsoid zone (EZ), shown in Fig. 1, is of particular interest for its potential as an early biomarker. In OCT images, it appears as a bright, hyperreflective band whose continuity indicates photoreceptor integrity, but it becomes disrupted in AMD [3].

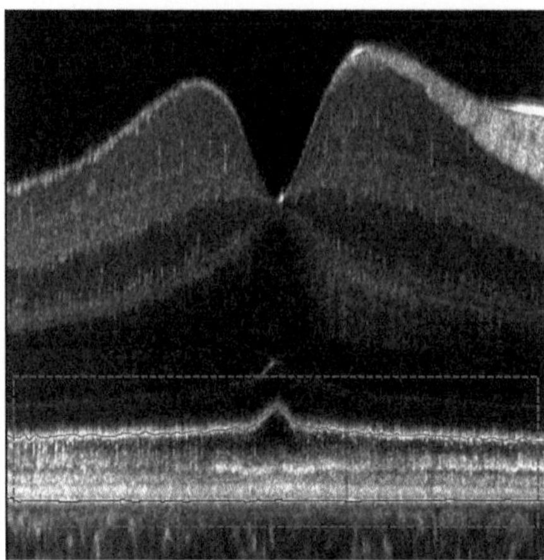

Fig. 1. Clinical OCT B-scan. The red dashed box highlights the region of interest, the outer retina, which is used as the input to the network. The EZ is marked by the red line. The Bruch's Membrane (BrM) is marked by the blue line.

Recent advances in high-resolution OCT imaging [4] enable near-histological visualization, offering new opportunities to detect early retinal biomarkers. Achieving this requires precise 3D analysis of retinal layers, particularly the EZ, whose degeneration often causes variable visibility and structural alterations. To address these challenges, automated methods for accurately segmenting retinal layers have been an active area of research. He et al. proposed a structured layer surface segmentation framework for retinal OCT that integrates surface topology into an end-to-end model. Using a residual U-Net with dual outputs for pixel-wise layer segmentation and soft-argmax surface regression, their fully convolutional design yields smooth, continuous and topologically consistent surface estimates [5]. Karbole et al. extended these concepts to 3D boundary segmentation. Leveraging high-resolution OCT with motion correction and volumetric merging, their approach introduced the depth map regression network, a 3D U-Net variant employing a soft-argmax layer for sub-pixel boundary localization [6]. While the framework demonstrated accurate 3D boundary estimation for the posterior end of the retinal pigment epithelium (RPE), generalization to the EZ is limited. The EZ can be absent in certain disease stages and often shows strong local elevations as well as intensity variations.

To address these challenges, this study presents a fully automated approach for segmenting the anterior EZ boundary using a Transformer-based architecture. In addition to estimating the depth position of the anterior EZ boundary, the method also predicts its presence, explicitly accounting for cases where the EZ is weak or absent. Combined with volumetrically merged high-resolution OCT, these features demonstrate the potential to measure subtle pathological variations in early AMD.

2 Materials and methods

The dataset consists of 68 volumetric OCT images from 52 different subjects. The mean age is 70.91 ± 14.58 years, ranging from 27 to 94. The dataset contains images from different disease stages: healthy (14), early amd (12), intermediate amd (20), advanced amd (3) and other diseases (19). The OCT images were captured using a high-resolution OCT device, which was previously described in [4]. Each subject underwent acquisition of six sequential OCT volumes, covering a 6 × 6 mm retinal area centered on the fovea. A lateral spacing of 12 × 12 µm was used, resulting in a sampling grid of 500 A-scans and 500 B-scans. The axial voxel spacing was 0.89 µm. The initial OCT volumes had a resolution of 1600 × 500 × 500 voxels (depth × width × height). To further improve image quality, the sequential scans were motion corrected and volumetrically fused [7, 8]. Ground truth labels for the EZ were generated using a semi-automatic two-step approach. First, the EZ boundary was automatically estimated by detecting the first strong dark-to-bright transition along each A-scan using gradient information. In the second step, the preliminary surface was manually refined B-scan by B-scan to produce the final ground truth map. The dataset was split into 52 training, 8 validation and 8 test volumes. For the validation and test sets we randomly selected three healthy subjects and five pathologic subjects to ensure a balanced distribution of disease conditions across the subsets.

The input resolution of the OCT volumes is 256 x 496 × 496 voxels (depth × width × height), corresponding to the axial and two transversal directions. Each volume was cropped to include the region above Bruch's Membrane (BrM) and 10 pixels below it. The data dimensions were rearranged to meet the input requirements of the network. For memory efficiency, the input volumes were divided into overlapping windows of size 256 x 128 × 128 voxels (depth × width × height) with an overlap of 0.5 between adjacent windows.

For the automated prediction of the anterior boundary of the EZ, we propose an architecture that is based on the UNETR by Hatamizadeh et al. [9]. The architecture integrates a transformer-based encoder with a convolutional decoder in a U-Net-like structure. The transformer encoder captures global context, while the CNN decoder with skip connections fuses it with local details to reconstruct high-resolution outputs. The network outputs a 3D heatmap in which each voxel represents the confidence that the EZ boundary lies at the corresponding spatial position. To obtain the continuous distance prediction suitable for our task, a soft-argmax function is applied along the vertical axis, converting the heatmap into a predicted Y-coordinate. During training, supervision is applied only to the predicted coordinates using a Smooth L1 loss, which provides robustness to noisy or uncertain annotations. The presence prediction is derived directly from the predicted heatmap, by computing two quantities for each vertical axis of the 3D heatmap: the total activation energy obtained by a log-sum-exp (LSE) operation, which provides a smooth and numerically stable measure of overall activation strength and the maximum activation (max) along the depth axis. These values are then combined into a contrast-based confidence measure

$$p_{\text{presence}} = \sigma(\text{LSE}) \cdot \sigma(\max - \text{LSE}) \tag{1}$$

Tab. 1. Metrics of the test set.

Case	Disease Stage	Median Absolute Error	Failure rate	Accuracy	ROC AUC
Case 1	Healthy	0.52 µm	0.021	0.967	0.752
Case 2	Healthy	0.46 µm	0.020	0.986	0.767
Case 3	Healthy	0.63 µm	0.011	0.959	0.940
Case 4	early AMD	1.13 µm	0.148	0.992	0.917
Case 5	intermediate AMD	2.66 µm	0.368	0.930	0.797
Case 6	intermediate AMD	0.82 µm	0.146	0.982	0.905
Case 7	AMD	1.09 µm	0.133	0.883	0.860
Case 8	other disease	1.58 µm	0.087	0.952	0.925
Mean		1.11 µm	0.117	0.956	0.858

where $\sigma(\cdot)$ denotes the sigmoid function. The first term, $\sigma(\mathrm{LSE})$, reflects the overall activation strength and indicates the likelihood that an EZ-related signal is present, while the second term, $\sigma(\max - \mathrm{LSE})$, measures how sharply this response is localized. When the EZ layer is clearly present, the heatmap exhibits a strong, narrow peak. In contrast, if the EZ is absent or ambiguous, the response becomes weak and broad. Because this computation is derived solely from the heatmap output, no additional parameters are trained for presence estimation.

The model was trained for 220 epochs using the Adam optimizer with a learning rate of 8e-5 and a weight decay of 1e-5. The best model was reached after 101 epochs.

After inference, the predicted depth maps were processed through a dedicated post-processing script to quantify the biomarker of interest. Only predictions exceeding the presence prediction threshold of 0.595 were considered. The threshold was computed using the F1-optimized method. Along each A-scan, the distance between the predicted position of the anterior EZ boundary and the next local maximum in posterior direction was computed and subsequently averaged per case.

3 Results

We performed a quantitative evaluation on the eight held-out test cases. The performance of the distance prediction was evaluated using the median absolute error (MAE) per case and a failure rate, defined as the proportion of A-scans with an absolute error exceeding 4 µm. The accuracy (threshold = 0.595) and the receiver operating characteristic (ROC) AUC were used to evaluate the performance of the presence prediction. The results for all test cases are summarized in Tab. 1.

The notably lower performance in Case 5 can be attributed to the darker overall image intensity and the weak or highly elevated appearance of the EZ, which makes depth position estimation particularly challenging.

To illustrate the network performance, Fig. 2 presents qualitative results for two representative cases: Case 3 (healthy) and Case 5 (intermediate AMD). In the healthy case, the predicted anterior EZ boundary aligns closely with the reference annotation and follows the true layer smoothly, even in regions with moderate intensity variation or elevated boundary. This demonstrates stable performance under normal retinal conditions. In the diseased case, the prediction remains largely accurate but shows local deviations where the EZ signal is weak or the EZ itself is highly elevated. These shifts reflect the structural irregularities typical of pathological tissue. Nonetheless, the predicted boundaries remain anatomically plausible, indicating that the model is robust to signal loss and morphological changes.

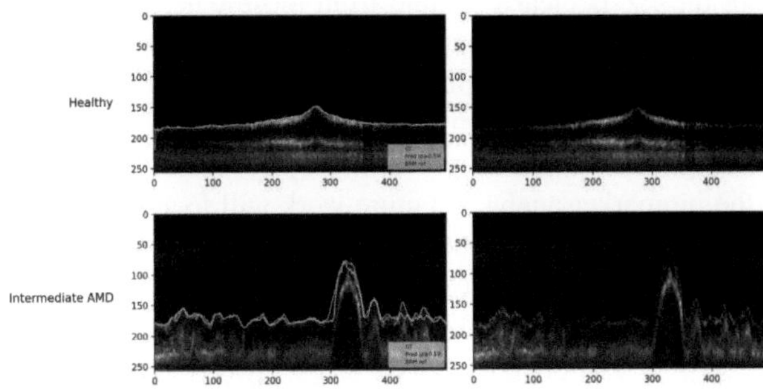

Fig. 2. Top: Slice 249 of Case 3 with and without labels (67 years, healthy). Bottom: Slice 239 of the challenging Case 5 with and without labels (70 years, intermediate AMD).

In addition, we analyzed the computed biomarker across all 68 OCT volumes, defined as the distance between the predicted position of the anterior EZ boundary and the next local maximum along the axial direction for each disease stage (Fig. 3).

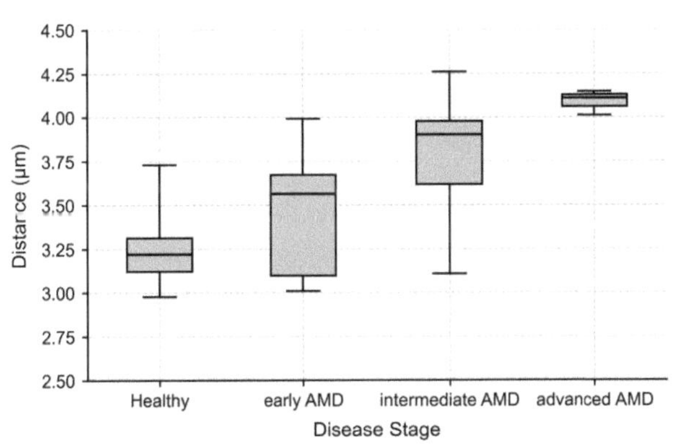

Fig. 3. Box plots of the distance per disease stage between the predicted anterior EZ boundary position and the next local maximum.

A consistent trend was observed, with the mean distance gradually increasing across disease stages, suggesting that the network captures fine-grained structural variations that may reflect early changes associated with disease severity.

4 Discussion

The results demonstrate that the proposed network accurately predicts the anterior EZ boundary across different retinal conditions. Quantitative metrics confirm precise localization, while qualitative analysis shows consistent performance on healthy scans and anatomically consistent predictions in diseased cases. The gradual increase of the computed distance measured across disease stages further indicates that the model captures subtle structural variations in the retinal layers, which commercial OCT's 5–7 µm axial resolution would be too coarse to capture. The findings also confirm that deriving the presence prediction directly from the heatmap is a valid and effective approach. Although not explicitly trained, the presence measure reliably distinguishes regions where the EZ is clearly visible from those where it is weak or absent. This suggests that the heatmap representation inherently encodes both boundary position and layer confidence, enabling presence estimation to emerge naturally from the learned spatial response while keeping the model simple and robust. Despite these promising results, the study is limited by the small dataset and the exploratory nature of the biomarker analysis. Future work will focus on larger-scale validation and a more detailed investigation of the derived biomarker, which shows potential as an early and progressive indicator of AMD.

Acknowledgement. DFG project 508075009, NIH projects R01EY011289 and R01EY034080.

References

1. Burton MJ, Ramke J, Marques AP, Bourne RRA, Congdon N, Jones I et al. The lancet global health commission on global eye health: vision beyond 2020. Lancet Glob Health. 2021;9(4):e489–551.
2. Huang D, Swanson EA, Lin CP, Schuman JS, Stinson WG, Chang W et al. Optical coherence tomography. Science. 1991;254(5035):1178–81.
3. Chen S, Abu-Qamar O, Kar D, Messinger JD, Hwang Y, Moult EM et al. Ultrahigh resolution OCT markers of normal aging and early age-related macular degeneration. Ophthalmol Sci. 2023;3(3):100277.
4. Lee B, Chen S, Moult EM, al. et. High-speed, ultrahigh-resolution spectral-domain OCT with extended imaging range using reference arm length matching. Transl Vis Sci Technol. 2020;9(7):12.
5. He Y, Carass A, Liu Y, Jedynak BM, Solomon SD, Saidha S et al. Structured layer surface segmentation for retina OCT using fully convolutional regression networks. Med Image Anal. 2021;68:101856.
6. Karbole W, Ploner SB, Won J, Marmalidou A, Takahashi H, Waheed NK et al. 3D deep learning-based boundary regression of an age-related retinal biomarker in high resolution OCT. Proc BVM. 2024:350–5.
7. Ploner S, Chen S, Won J, Husvogt L, Breininger K, Schottenhamml J et al. A spatiotemporal model for precise and efficient fully-automatic 3D motion correction in OCT. Proc MICCAI. 2022:517–27.
8. Ploner S, Won J, Schottenhamml J, Girgis J, Lam K, Waheed N et al. A spatiotemporal illumination model for 3D image fusion in optical coherence tomography. Proc IEEE ISBI. 2023:1–5.

9. Hatamizadeh A, Tang Y, Nath V, Yang D, Myronenko A, Landman BA et al. UNETR: transformers for 3D medical image segmentation. Proc IEEE/CVF WACV. 2022:1748–58.

Data-driven Model Adaptation Enhances Lesion Segmentation

ULS+

Rianne Weber †, Niels Rocholl †, Max de Grauw, Mathias Prokop, Ewoud Smit, Alessa Hering

Department of Medical Imaging, Radboud University Medical Center, Nijmegen, The Netherlands
Rianne.Weber@radboudumc.nl

Abstract. In this study, we present ULS+, an enhanced version of the universal lesion segmentation (ULS) model. The original ULS model segments lesions across the whole body in CT scans given volumes of interest (VOIs) centered around a click-point. Since its release, several new public datasets have become available that can further improve model performance. ULS+ incorporates these additional datasets and uses smaller input image sizes, resulting in higher accuracy and faster inference.
We compared ULS and ULS+ using the Dice score and robustness to click-point location on the ULS23 Challenge test data and a subset of the Longitudinal-CT dataset. In all comparisons, ULS+ significantly outperformed ULS. Additionally, ULS+ ranks first on the ULS23 Challenge test-phase leaderboard. By maintaining a cycle of data-driven updates and clinical validation, ULS+ establishes a foundation for robust and clinically relevant lesion segmentation models.[2]

1 Introduction

Cancer remains one of the leading causes of mortality worldwide, and its burden is projected to continue rising. By 2050, the global cancer incidence is predicted to increase by 77%, reaching 35.3 million cases [1]. Correspondingly, radiologists are experiencing a steady growth in workload [2]. A substantial part of this workload arises from the longitudinal assessment of disease burden in oncologic imaging, where radiologists must identify, measure, and track target lesions over time according to the response evaluation criteria in solid tumors (RECIST) guidelines. This process requires consistent lesion localization and quantification across time points, which is both time-consuming and prone to variability.

Artificial intelligence (AI) offers opportunities to support radiologists in this workflow by automating parts of the lesion assessment process. AI-based methods

† These authors contributed equally to this work.

[2] Code and weights available at https://github.com/DIAGNijmegen/oncology-uls-plus

© Der/die Autor(en), exklusiv lizenziert an Springer Fachmedien Wiesbaden GmbH, ein Teil von Springer Nature 2026
H. Handels et al. (Hrsg.), *Bildverarbeitung für die Medizin 2026*, Informatik aktuell, https://doi.org/10.1007/978-3-658-51100-5_97

have shown promise for lesion detection, segmentation, and classification, and can serve as building blocks for automated lesion tracking and response evaluation. Recent studies have demonstrated the feasibility of combining registration-based lesion matching with volumetric segmentation to support longitudinal tumor response assessment in CT imaging [3]. These approaches aim to improve the consistency of lesion measurements and reduce observer variability in follow-up evaluations.

To further advance automatic lesion quantification, the universal lesion segmentation (ULS) baseline model [4] was introduced in 2023 as part of the ULS23 challenge. ULS adopts a click-centered, interactive segmentation paradigm. Unlike methods designed for full-volume, exhaustive lesion segmentation, ULS allows a radiologist to select a specific lesion with a single click point. The model then rapidly returns a complete 3D mask from a localized volume of interest (VOI), thereby aligning with the focused, click-guided use case prevalent in interactive follow-up workflows.

Given the limited interaction required, as well as the lesion-specific training data used to develop this model, the ULS baseline has significant potential for use in clinical practice. However, since the release of the ULS model, new and valuable public datasets have been released that may enrich the training data of this model and thus improve its performance. In addition, the model shows limited robustness to click point location; when indicating different voxels in a lesion as the center voxel, the resulting lesion segmentations may differ.

In this study, we present ULS+, an improved version of the ULS model. Our contributions to the ULS model are twofold: (1) we extend the training data by incorporating additional publicly available whole-body CT lesion datasets, focusing specifically on lesions for which the original ULS model performed sub-optimally; and (2), we enhance robustness to click-point variation through train-time augmentation by sampling random lesion voxels as VOI center. We evaluate ULS+ against the ULS baseline in terms of both segmentation performance and click-point robustness, demonstrating its potential as a more reliable foundation for automated lesion analysis and longitudinal tracking.

2 Materials and methods

The ULS+ model builds upon the original ULS baseline by modifying the training data, input configuration, and augmentation strategy to improve generalization and robustness to click-point variation. The main differences between the two models are visualized in Fig. 1 and described in more detail below.

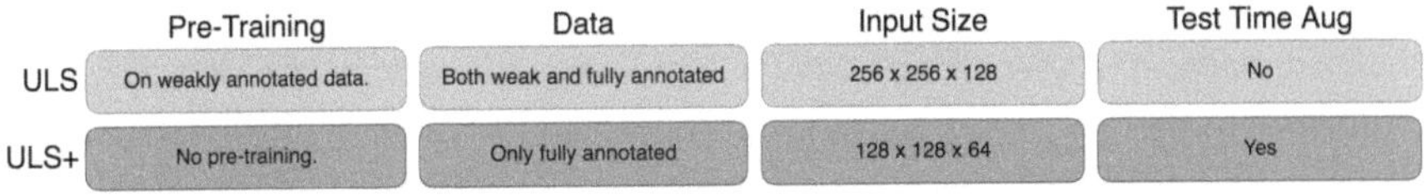

Fig. 1. Differences between the ULS model and the ULS+ model.

Tab. 1. Overview of training data used for ULS+. *Only the fully annotated data of ULS was used. **Longitudinal-CT refers to task 2 of the AUTOPET challenge. ***Images from the liver, pancreas, colon and lung tasks were used.

Dataset	Location	Number of lesions	Reference
ULS*	Whole body	5737	[4]
Longitudinal-CT**	Whole body	4973	[5]
MSD***	Whole body	1314	[6]
WORC GIST	Gastrointestinal	248	[7]
WORC CRLM	Liver (metas.)	96	[7]
CLM	Liver (metas.)	479	[8]
WAW-TACE	Liver (prim.)	360	[9]
CECT	Liver (prim.)	1274	[10]
MSWAL	Abdominal	2638	[11]

2.1 Datasets

The original ULS model was trained on both a fully annotated and a weakly annotated dataset. To increase overall annotation quality and reduce training time, only the fully annotated part of this data was used for ULS+. In addition, ULS+ was trained on six more datasets. These datasets include both liver-specific sets and sets with multiple lesion types. Details on the added data can be found in Tab. 1.

For each dataset, the center voxel of each lesion mask was determined, around which a VOI of $128 \times 128 \times 64$ voxels was cropped. If the cropped image included lesion masks unrelated to the central lesion, these masks were excluded. This resulted in one lesion mask per cropped image.

2.2 Lesion shifting

To increase robustness to click-point variability, we introduced a train-time augmentation strategy that simulates different user click points. For each lesion, we sampled two additional random click points within the lesion mask. We then cropped VOIs from the original CT scans centered around these new points, applying zero-padding if the crop extended beyond the original image boundaries. This yielded three spatially shifted variations of the same lesion for training.

2.3 Training

Training was performed on an NVIDIA L40S GPU using the nnUNet v2 framework [12] with a residual encoder (size L). We trained the model for 1000 epochs using standard settings, but with resampling disabled and the patch size set to equal the input image. Notably, we reduced the ULS+ input dimensions to $128 \times 128 \times 64$, compared to the $256 \times 256 \times 128$ used in the baseline. This reduction was prioritized to minimize inference latency for interactive clinical workflows on standard hardware, and because the larger volume proved redundant for click-centered tasks where only the central lesion is targeted.

Unlike the baseline, we omitted weakly supervised pretraining to simplify the pipeline, as prior experiments showed it yielded negligible improvements. Integrating other pretraining techniques was outside the scope of this study and remains a direction for future work.

2.4 Evaluation

To accurately compare the original ULS model to ULS+, we used the same test data as used in the ULS23 challenge. Additionally, we tested the models on a held-back part of the Longitudinal-CT dataset (20%, split on patient level). While we recognize that part of the Longitudinal-CT set was used to train ULS+ and not to train the original ULS model, this dataset is still valuable because it contains more lesion types than the ULS23 challenge test set. This allows for more extensive organ-level evaluation.

The original ULS model does not make use of test-time augmentation because this increases inference time. However, given its smaller input size, ULS+ allows for the use of test-time augmentation without rendering the model unusably slow in clinics. Therefore, this was turned on for the evaluation of ULS+.

To evaluate the robustness of the models to variations in user input, we simulated the variability of user-provided click-points using the mechanism (Sec. 2.2). For each lesion, we generated three segmentations by cropping the input VOI around different points: one centered on the lesion's centroid (P_{normal}), and two centered on random points sampled within the lesion mask (P_{aug1} and P_{aug2}) to simulate "off-center" clicks. This process results in slightly shifted input volumes for the model. The robustness score was defined as the mean pairwise Dice similarity between the resulting three segmentations

$$\text{Robustness} = \frac{1}{3}\left[\text{Dice}(P_{\text{normal}}, P_{\text{aug1}}) + \text{Dice}(P_{\text{normal}}, P_{\text{aug2}}) + \text{Dice}(P_{\text{aug1}}, P_{\text{aug2}})\right] \quad (1)$$

This metric ranges from 0 to 1, where higher scores indicate greater robustness to click-point placement and more consistent predictions despite shifts in the cropped input volume.

3 Results

Tab. 2 summarizes performance on the ULS23 and Longitudinal-CT test sets. Overall, ULS+ consistently outperforms the original ULS model in terms of both Dice score and robustness across both datasets, with all improvements being statistically significant. The gains are more pronounced on the Longitudinal-CT dataset.

Per-lesion plots in (Fig. 2 (Dice) and Fig. 3 (robustness)) show that ULS+ generally shifts scores toward higher dice and robustness values, but it is not uniformly better for every lesion type (e.g., adrenal and bone lesions). These exceptions occur in lesion categories with very small sample counts. Qualitative examples of both successful and challenging cases are shown in Fig. 4.

Tab. 2. Comparison of the original ULS model and ULS+ on both the ULS23 and Longitudinal-CT datasets. *Indicates statistical significance ($p < 0.0001$ using a paired two-tailed t-test with Bonferroni correction for multiple testing).

	ULS23		Longitudinal-CT	
	Dice	Robustness	Dice	Robustness
ULS baseline	0.74 ± 0.20	0.81 ± 0.24	0.68 ± 0.23	0.85 ± 0.19
ULS+	0.78 ± 0.15*	0.86 ± 0.20*	0.79 ± 0.14*	0.90 ± 0.16*

ULS+ was submitted to the test phase of the ULS23 challenge and achieved first place on the leaderboard with a challenge score of 0.749. For further details on the challenge, we refer the reader to the original ULS paper [4].

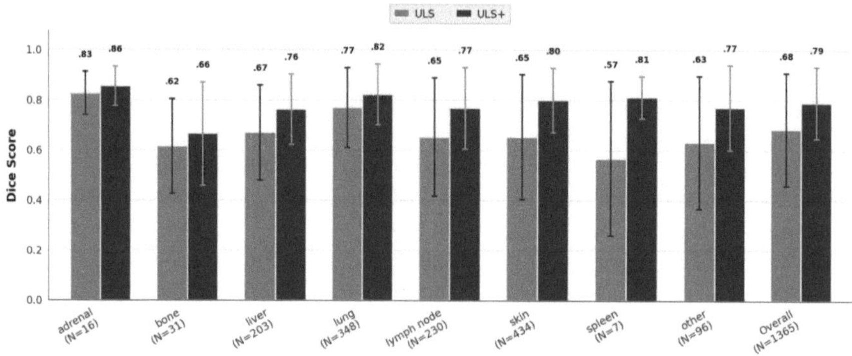

(a) Longitudinal-CT test set.

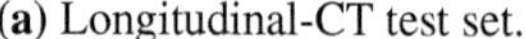

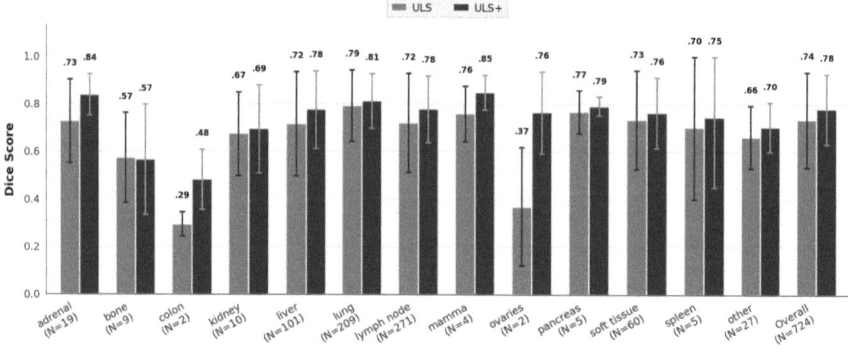

(b) ULS23 Challenge test set.

Fig. 2. Dice scores of the original ULS model and ULS+ on two different test sets, stratified by lesion location.

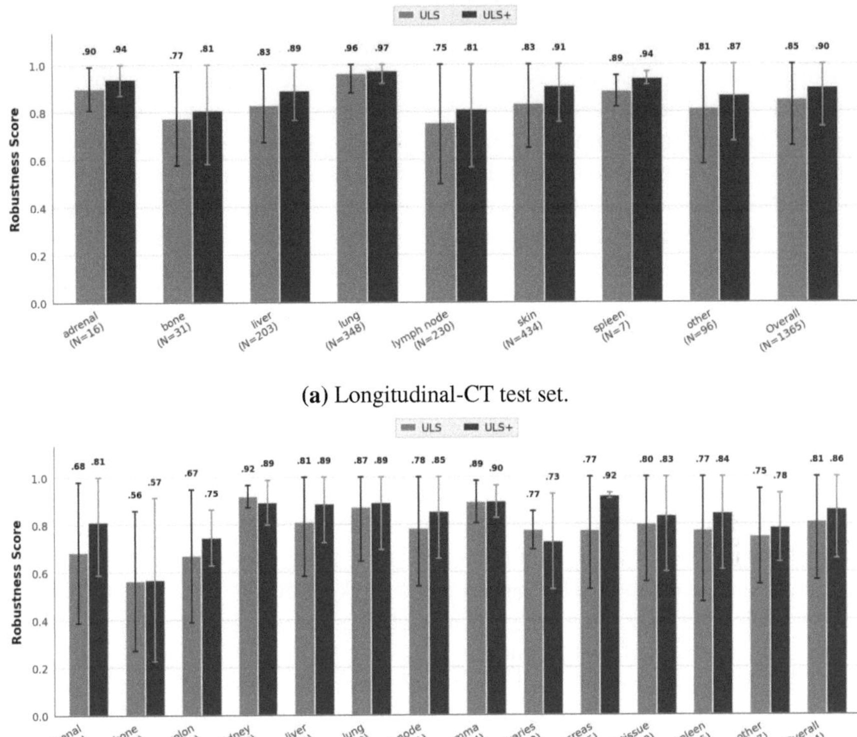

(**a**) Longitudinal-CT test set.

(**b**) ULS23 Challenge test set.

Fig. 3. Robustness scores (Eq. 1) of the original ULS model and ULS+ on two different test sets, stratified by lesion location.

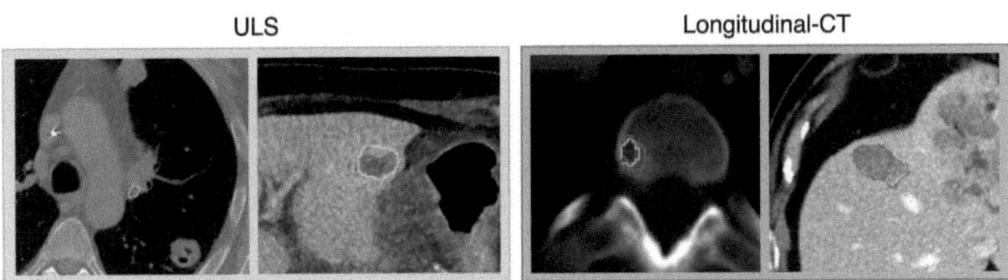

Fig. 4. Example segmentations of the ULS and ULS+ model on both datasets on lesions from different locations. Blue: ground truth, red: ULS, yellow: ULS+. Note that for visibility of this figure, some lesions are zoomed in on while preserving surrounding context. Therefore, in this visualization, some lesions may not appear centered.

4 Discussion

This study introduces ULS+, an improved version of the universal lesion segmentation (ULS) model, designed to enhance segmentation accuracy and robustness to click-point variation. Despite using a smaller input size and no pretraining, ULS+ achieved higher Dice scores and improved robustness to click point location on two separate datasets. Improvements were relatively homogeneous across lesion location, which may be attributed to the fact that the newly added training data contains cases of lesions across the whole body, providing enrichment for all these lesion types.

The ULS+ framework incorporates four primary updates: the inclusion of expanded, fully annotated multi-organ data, the implementation of click-point augmentation, the transition to a $128 \times 128 \times 64$ input size and test-time augmentation. While these changes collectively coincide with the observed performance gains, the specific contribution of each factor has not yet been isolated. Consequently, a systematic ablation study and a dedicated same-dimension comparison are planned as future work to quantify the individual impact of these components.

Although several of the newly added datasets were specific to liver lesions, the observed performance gains were not limited to this organ. The similar improvement in Dice score across all lesion types suggests that the benefits of the new data extend beyond organ-specific information, strengthening the model's capacity for whole-body lesion segmentation. The slightly lower click-point robustness in skeletal and undefined lesions may reflect the intrinsic challenges of these structures, such as small size and unclear lesion boundaries.

It should be noted that in addition to better performance, the ULS+ model is faster than the original. ULS takes input images of $256 \times 256 \times 128$, whereas ULS+ uses an input image size of $128 \times 128 \times 64$. Inference with ULS+ takes around 0.5 seconds on an NVIDIA A100 SXM4 GPU when applying test-time augmentation. This combination of increased performance and high speed makes it more realistically applicable in clinical settings, where time efficiency is highly valued. The smaller input size introduces the inherent limitation that lesions extending beyond the input field of view cannot be fully segmented in a single forward pass. A sliding-window inference strategy would address this, but was outside the scope of this study.

Our study shows the value of iterative retraining and updating AI models with new, relevant data. As more and more valuable, well-annotated medical imaging data becomes publicly available, preexisting models may benefit from this added information without requiring significant adaptations to architecture. This paradigm supports the sustainability and continual improvement of clinical AI tools, ensuring that deployed systems evolve alongside advances in data availability and imaging practice. By maintaining a cycle of data-driven updates and clinical validation, ULS+ can serve as a foundation for robust, transparent, and clinically relevant lesion segmentation models.

To facilitate reproducibility the code, data and trained model weights are available at `https://github.com/DIAGNijmegen/oncology-uls-plus`.

References

1. Bizuayehu HM, Dadi AF, Belachew T, Alene KA, Ross H et al. Global disparities of cancer and its projected burden in 2050. JAMA Netw Open. 2024;7(11):e2443198.
2. Bruls RJM, Kwee RM. Workload for radiologists during on-call hours: dramatic increase in the past 15-years. Insights Imaging. 2020;11(1):121.
3. Hering A, Westphal M, Gerken A, Almansour H, Maurer M, Geisler B et al. Improving assessment of lesions in longitudinal CT scans: a bi-institutional reader study on an AI-assisted registration and volumetric segmentation workflow. Int J Comput Assist Radiol Surg. 2024;19(9):1689–97.
4. de Grauw M, Scholten E, Smit E, Rutten M, Prokop M, van Ginneken B et al. The ULS23 challenge: a baseline model and benchmark dataset for 3D universal lesion segmentation in computed tomography. Med Image Anal. 2025;102:103525.
5. Gatidis S, Hepp T, Frh M, La Fougre C, Nikolaou K, Pfannenberg C et al. A whole-body FDG-PET/CT dataset with manually annotated tumor lesions. Sci Data. 2022;9(1):601.
6. Antonelli M, Reinke A, Bakas S, Farahani K, Kopp-Schneider A, Landman BA et al. The medical segmentation decathlon. Nat Commun. 2022;13(1):4128.
7. Starmans MPA, Timbergen MJM, Vos M, Padmos GA, Grünhagen DJ, Verhoef C et al. The WORC database: MRI and CT scans, segmentations, and clinical labels for 930 patients from six radiomics studies. bioRxiv. 2021.
8. Simpson AL, Peoples J, Creasy JM, Fichtinger G, Gangai N, Keshavamurthy KN et al. Preoperative CT and survival data for patients undergoing resection of colorectal liver metastases. Sci Data. 2024;11(1):172.
9. Bartnik K, Bartczak T, Krzyziski M, Korzeniowski K, Lamparski K, Wgrzyn P et al. WAW-TACE: a hepatocellular carcinoma multiphase CT dataset with segmentations, radiomics features, and clinical data. Radiol Artif Intell. 2024;6(6):e240296.
10. Luo J, Wan X, Du J, Liu L, Zhao L, Peng X et al. Comprehensive multi-phase 3D contrast-enhanced CT imaging for primary liver cancer. Sci Data. 2025;12(1):768.
11. Wu Z, Zhao Q, Hu M, Li Y, Xue H, Jiang Z et al. MSWAL: 3D multi-class segmentation of whole abdominal lesions dataset. Proc MICCAI. 2026:378–88.
12. Isensee F, Jaeger PF, Kohl SAA, Petersen J, Maier-Hein KH. nnU-net: a self-configuring method for deep learning-based biomedical image segmentation. Nat Methods. 2021;18(2):203–11.

Autorenverzeichnis

Adams LC, 298
Adomeit S, **139**
Akbal S, 83
Al-Haj Hemidi Z, **33**
Alhalabi O, 118
Alikarrar M, **55**
Allgaier A, **177**
Allmendinger F, 118
Amft O, 218
Ammeling J, **18**, 193, 203
Andresen J, 1, **93**, 245
Arias-Vergara T, 450
Aubreville M, 18, 193, 203, 375, **393**
Auer C, 100, 218
Aulich J, 146
Aung T, 354
Aust O, 400
Azouzi Z, **162**

Banerjee S, **203**, 375
Barkhausen J, 1, 335, 345
Barth E, 345
Bäßler J, 139
Batvinskas A, 146
Bäuerle A, 90
Bauer J, 195
Bauer JW, 299
Baumgartner M, 194, 435
Baumgartner MA, 466
Baumgärtner T, 226
Baumgart S, **70**
Bayer S, 10, 34, 328, 387, 427
Beer M, 90, 132
Bergler C, 354
Bertram CA, 193, 203, 393
Bhandary Panambur A, **10**, 427
Bischof A, 345
Bi Y, **108**
Böhringer J, 139
Bolenz C, 368
Bolten J, 118
Bornmann J, 177
Bosma J, 48, 92
Bostelmann J, **106**, 402
Bounias D, 269, 435
Bracci J, **285**
Braren R, 194
Braun M, 226
Breininger K, 18, 110, 203, 321
Bressem KK, 298
Brinker TJ, 315
Brucher R, 177
Brügge NS, 63
Buess L, 84
Builtjes L, **92**, **381**
Bundschuh RA, 139
Buser M, 298
Buzug TM, 156

Cangalovic VS, 468
Cepeda S, 124
Chmelik J, 292
Clarenbach R, 108
Clunie D, 194
Conrad J, 239
Conrad T, 203

Dar SH, 420
Datchev A, 146
de Boer S, 48, 411
de Grauw M, 482
de Rooij M, 465
Debus J, 118, 466
Deng M, 118
Deubner N, 70
Dias Almeida S, 194
Diekmann S, 277
Diem A, 299
Djoumsi ST, **354**
Donovan TA, 203, 393
Dörfer C, 239
Drees D, 132
Drömann D, 1
Dusseljee J, **411**

© Der/die Herausgeber bzw. der/die Autor(en), exklusiv lizenziert an Springer Fachmedien Wiesbaden GmbH, ein Teil von Springer Nature 2026
H. Handels et al. (Hrsg.), *Bildverarbeitung für die Medizin 2026*, Informatik aktuell, https://doi.org/10.1007/978-3-658-51100-5

Dyrba M, 443

Ebert F, 269
Eckstein K, **435**
Ehrhardt J, 1, 63, 76, 419
Ehses V, 219
Eichhorn H, 146
Eichkorn T, 118
Eixelberger T, **368**
El Shafie R, 466
Elser Y, 1
Engelhardt S, 420
Engelson S, **1**
Engster JC, 156
Erceg I, 400
Ergler T, 337
Erick FX, 170

Fagni F, 321
Fan F, 400
Felsner L, **146**, 267
Ferrero V, 154
Finck MJ, **403**
Fiorina E, 154
Fischer M, 118, **194**, 315
Fischer SM, **267**
Floca R, 269, 435
Förner L, 139, 307, **401**
Franz AM, 177, 226
Friedrich T, 335
Fujimoto JG, 475
Furtner A, **185**

Gallée L, **132**
Ganz J, 18
Gastreich de Llanes E, 139
Gehrmann T, 239
Geissler K, 26, **277**
Gemeier C, 299
Gerdes H, 345
Ghotbi R, 108
Gildemeister O, **402**
Giske K, 269
Glüer C, 239
Goncalves M, 375
Gorges T, 111
Gosch T, 203
Götz M, 90, 132, 194
Graetz C, 239
Grimm R, 277
Grzegorzek M, 458
Gutbrod M, 131, **362**
Guttmann-Gruber C, 195
Gu M, 34, 400

Haas J, 345
Hahn H, 465
Hamm B, 466
Handels H, 1, 63, 76, 93, 245, 419, 436
Hansen CJ, **239**
Hanstein M, 118
Häntze H, **298**
Härteis S, 354
Heinrich MP, 33, 451, **467**
Heldmann S, 26, 468
Hellwege L, **156**
Hering A, 48, 92, 298, 381, 411, 465, 482
Hermans J, 465
Herrmann J, 436
Hester S, 203
Hillenhagen H, 90
Hille G, 219
Hirsch D, **76**
Hoegen-Saßmannshausen P, 118
Holzapfel K, 218
Holzschuh J, 466
Hövener J, 239, 403
Hrubovcak J, 292
Huang L, 108
Huang X, 458
Huang Y, 270, 400
Huber T, 219
Huettl F, 219
Hümmer C, 55
Hutter J, 450
Hwang Y, 475

Ikuma T, 252
Ivanovska T, 354

Jäkel O, 269
Jamil MU, 475

Jiang Z, 108, 169
Jiayu S, 427
Jopp-van Well E, 436
Juan H, 427
Jungk C, 118

Kächele J, 435, **464**
Kafali SG, 146
Kahrs B, 63, 93
Kainz B, 170
Kaltenecker C, 203
Kappler S, 55
Karlas A, 108
Kasprzak J, 154
Käster T, 345
Kats E, 33
Katzmann A, 285
Kauba C, 299
Keck T, 1
Kepp T, 63, 93, 245
Keuth R, 451
Khajarian S, **218**
Khamseh S, **337**
Kiechle J, 267
Kirchhoff Y, 83, 292
Kist A, 40, 259
Kist AM, 70, 252
Klausmann L, **131**
Kleesiek J, 194
Klemm F, 146
Klinger R, 146
Kloeckner R, 335
Kloehn P, 239
Klopfleisch R, 203
Knybel L, 292
Kohlbrandt T, **26**
Köhler G, 109
Kollster A, 239
Kolokolnikov G, **233**
Komposch J, 226
König L, 118
Kopp M, 40
Koser NC, 403
Kovacs B, 83, **269**, 466
Kramer F, 124

Krause C, **451**
Kreher B, 210, 217
Krejci K, 292
Kudak A, 118, 466
Kunduk M, 252

Laimer M, 299
Lang DM, 267
Lang H, 219
Lapa C, 139
Larsen D, 252
Laufer M, **345**
Leal dos Reis F, 345
Leepagorn P, 146
Leijten L, 48
Leiniger A, 177
Lellmann J, 106, 402
Lemberger-Viehmann L, 354
Leth AJ, 146
Liemberger B, 195
Liermann J, 269
Lisson CG, 132
Lisson CS, 132
Liu C, 427
Liu D, **450**
Li C, 458
Li X, **169**
Lossau T, 468
Lücke SP, 403
Lurz D, **40**, **259**

Maass M, 458
Maerkl R, 131
Maier-Hein K, 83, 109, 118, 194, 315, 464
Maier-Hein KH, 269, 435, 466
Maier A, 10, 19, 34, 55, 84, 111, 162, 210, 217, 270, 285, 328, 334, 337, 387, 400, 427, 450, 475
Mairhöfer D, 345
Maisch P, 368
Malzacher T, 226
Marco N, 315
Martensen OH, **443**
Martinek L, 292
Martinetz T, 345

Mechs L, **475**
Meine H, 277
Mei S, 34, 328, 334, **400**
Miah M, **84**
Mirzaei Z, 400
Modersitzki J, 402
Moltz JH, 468
Morales C, 226
Mouton C, 239
Muckenhuber A, 194
Müller-Diesing F, 375
Müller D, 124
Müller JP, 170

Navab N, 108, 169
Neag G, 400
Neher P, 118, 194, 464
Neubig L, 40, **252**, 259
Nguyen T, 10, 427
Niemeijer J, **419**
Niklas M, 269
Ni Y, **427**
Nohel M, 109, **292**
Nolden M, 194

Obreja B, 48
Ochmann J, **170**
Oltmann A, 402
Osuala R, 267

Palm C, 131, 362
Palubicki W, 403
Pawłowski M, **436**
Peeken JC, 267
Peeters D, 48
Pennazio F, 154
Peretzke R, 109, **118**, 194
Pérez-Toro PA, 328, 450
Petersen E, 133
Peter N, 315
Pflüger I, 466
Philipp L, 48, **465**
Pirk S, 403
Ploner SB, 475
Porsche N, 203, **375**
Prodinger C, 299
Prokop M, 92, 482
Puttinger C, 299
Putz F, 270

Rafecas M, 154
Raghunath A, 19, 111
Rakshit J, 219
Ramedani M, 443
Rauber D, 131, 362
Regnery S, 118
Reguli S, 292
Reinke Z, 185
Remmele S, 100, 218
Riener A, 193
Rijhwani NP, **315**
Ristow I, 233
Rist L, 285
Ritschl L, 55
Rizoudis A, **124**
Robra L, 177
Rocholl N, 482
Rohleder M, 217
Roider J, 245
Rokuss M, **83**, 292
Ropinski T, 90
Rosbach E, **193**
Roser J, 154
Rose G, 219
Roßkopf J, 226
Rostalski P, 402
Rothert J, **219**
Rotkopf LT, 83
Roy S, 83
Rueckert D, 146
Rueckert T, 131
Rutten M, 465

Saalfeld S, 219
Salz JL, 219
Santarossa M, 245
Säring D, 436
Schaar M, 156
Scheuplein J, 55, **210**, **217**, 337
Scheurer E, 139
Schierholz S, 1

Schillinger M, 110, 321
Schlager P, 299
Schlemmer H, 83, 464
Schlereth M, **110**, **321**
Schmalhofer M, 233
Schmidt J, 218
Schmitz B, 226
Schmutzenhofer N, **307**
Schnabel JA, 146, 267
Schneider L, 34, 328, 334
Schneider R, 162
Schröter P, 118
Schüffler P, 194
Schulz P, 402
Schwimmbeck M, **100**, 218
Seibel MS, **63**, 245
Seyfarth M, **420**
Sieren M, 345
Sieren MM, 1, 335
Smit E, 48, 482
Stanic G, 269
Stille M, 156
Strauß T, 443
Stroblberger C, 203
Sühling M, 285
Sun H, 458
Sun Y, **34**, 328, 334, 387, 400, 403
Suprijadi J, 109
Sutariya D, **133**
Su L, 427
Syben C, 55

Tababi M, **226**
Tagscherer J, **48**
Taskin B, 90
Tawk B, 269
Tehlan K, 139, 307, **353**
Thies M, 334, 400

Ude-Schoder K, 299
Uhl A, 195, 299
Ulrich C, 83, **109**, 194, 292, 435, 466
Uzunova H, 419

v. Dresky C, **245**
van der Graaf F, 48
van Ginneken B, 92, 465
Vik T, 277
Vogele D, 132
Volk K, 177
Vollmuth P, 466
von Busch H, 277
von der Burchard C, 245
von Nettelbladt B, 466
von Salomon A, 464
Vorberg L, 162, 285

Wagner F, 34, 162, 400
Waheed NK, 475
Wald T, 83, 109, 435, **466**
Walluscheck S, **468**
Wally V, 195
Wang A, **270**
Wang J, **387**
Wang X, **458**
Weber F, 19, **111**
Weber R, **482**
Wegner F, 335
Weig F, 132
Weiler F, 335
Weiss V, 203
Well L, 233
Welponer T, 299
Welzel T, 466
Wendler T, 139, 185, 307, 353, 401
Wendrich S, 307
Wennmann M, 464
Wenzel M, 277
Werner J, **154**
Werner R, 233
Wessel L, 118
Weykamp F, 269
Wichelmann S, **335**
Wies C, 315
Wilm F, 18
Wimmer G, **299**
Wittenberg T, 100, 368
Wolf D, **90**
Wolz F, 337

Xiao S, 194

Xin D, **195**

Yadav B, **19**
Ye C, 34, **328**, **334**
Yildiran SR, 131

Zauner R, 299
Zhang Y, 458
Ziegler S, 109, 194
Zillner A, 177

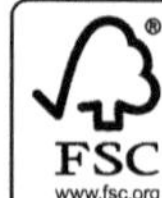

MIX
Papier aus verantwortungsvollen Quellen
Paper from responsible sources
FSC® C105338

If you have any concerns about our products,
you can contact us on
ProductSafety@springernature.com

In case Publisher is established outside the EU,
the EU authorized representative is:
Springer Nature Customer Service Center GmbH
Europaplatz 3, 69115 Heidelberg, Germany

Printed by Libri Plureos GmbH
in Hamburg, Germany